CLINICAL PEDIATRIC ENDOCRINOLOGY

Solomon A. Kaplan, M.D.

Professor of Pediatrics
UCLA School of Medicine
Los Angeles, California

W. B. SAUNDERS COMPANY
Harcourt Brace Jovanovich, Inc.
Philadelphia/London/Toronto/Montreal/Sydney/Tokyo

W. B. SAUNDERS COMPANY
Harcourt Brace Jovanovich, Inc.

The Curtis Center
Independence Square West
Philadelphia, PA 19106

Library of Congress Cataloging-in-Publication Data

Clinical pediatric endocrinology

Rev. ed. of: Clinical pediatric and adolescent
endocrinology. 1982.
Includes bibliographical references.
1. Pediatric endocrinology. I. Kaplan, Solomon A.
II. Clinical pediatric and adolescent endocrinology.
[DNLM: 1. Endocrine Diseases—in adolescence. 2. Endo-
crine Diseases—in infancy & childhood. WS 330 C641]
RJ418.C57 1990   618.92'4   89-10780
ISBN 0-7216-5283-2

CLINICAL PEDIATRIC ENDOCRINOLOGY   ISBN 0-7216-5283-2

Printed in the United States of America.

Last digit is the print number: 9   8   7   6   5   4   3

This book is dedicated to our students, houseofficers and
fellows for their constant vigilance, to our physician colleagues with whom we participate in a mutual responsibility
to our patients and to our families without whose tolerance
and patience this book would have been an even more
arduous task.

CONTRIBUTORS

HANS HENNING BODE, M.D.
Associate Professor of Pediatrics, Harvard Medical School, Boston, Massachusetts; Massachusetts General Hospital, Shriners Burns Institute, Boston, Massachusetts
Disorders of the Posterior Pituitary

CHRISTOPHER CRAWFORD
Research Assistant, Cornell University Medical College, New York, New York
The Adrenal Cortex

PATRIZIA DEL BALZO
Assistant Professor of Pediatrics, Bambino Gesu' Hospital, Rome, Italy
The Adrenal Cortex

DELBERT A. FISHER, M.D.
Professor of Pediatrics and Medicine, UCLA School of Medicine, Los Angeles, California; Harbor-UCLA Medical Center, Torrance, California
The Thyroid

MITCHELL E. GEFFNER, M.D.
Associate Professor of Pediatrics, Division of Endocrinology and Metabolism, UCLA School of Medicine, Los Angeles, California
Hypoglycemia

SOLOMON A. KAPLAN, M.D.
Professor of Pediatrics, UCLA School of Medicine, Los Angeles, California; Attending Pediatrician, UCLA Medical Center, Los Angeles, California
Growth and Growth Hormone: Disorders of the Anterior Pituitary

BARBARA M. LIPPE, M.D.
Professor of Pediatrics, UCLA School of Medicine, Los Angeles, California; Chief, Division of Pediatric Endocrinology and Metabolism, UCLA Center for Health Sciences, Los Angeles, California
Primary Ovarian Failure

FRANCIS MIMOUNI, M.D.
Associate Professor of Pediatrics, Assistant Professor of Obstetrics and Gynecology, University of Cincinnati, Cincinnati, Ohio; Attending Neonatologist, Children's Hospital Medical Center, Cincinnati, Ohio
Parathyroid and Vitamin D-Related Disorders

MARIA I. NEW, M.D.
Professor and Chairman, Department of Pediatrics, Harold and Percy Uris Professor of Pediatric Endocrinology and Metabolism, Cornell University Medical College, New York, New York; Pediatrician-in-Chief, Department of Pediatrics, The New York Hospital, New York, New York
The Adrenal Cortex

ROBERT L. ROSENFIELD, M.D.
Professor of Pediatrics and Medicine, University of Chicago Pritzker School of Medicine; Head, Section of Pediatric Endocrinology, Wyler Children's Hospital, Chicago, Illinois
The Ovary and Female Sexual Maturation

PHYLLIS W. SPEISER, M.D.
Assistant Professor of Pediatrics, Cornell University Medical College, New York, New York; Assistant Attending Pediatrician, The New York Hospital, New York, New York
The Adrenal Cortex

MARK A. SPERLING, M.D.
Vira I. Heinz Professor and Chairman, Department of Pediatrics, University of Pittsburgh, Pittsburgh, Pennsylvania; Pediatrician in Chief, Children's Hospital of Pittsburgh, Pittsburgh, Pennsylvania
Diabetes Mellitus

DENNIS M. STYNE, M.D.
Professor of Pediatrics, University of California, Davis, California; Chair of Pediatrics, University of California Medical Center, Sacramento, California
The Testes: Disorders of Sexual Differentiation and Puberty

REGINALD C. TSANG, M.B.B.S.
Professor of Pediatrics, Obstetrics and Gynecology, University of Cincinnati, Cincinnati, Ohio; Director, Neonatal Division, Children's Hospital Medical Center, Cincinnati, Ohio
Parathyroid and Vitamin D-Related Disorders

MARY L. VOORHESS, M.D.
Professor of Pediatrics, School of Medicine, State University of New York at Buffalo; Attending Pediatrician, Co-Director, Division of Endocrinology, Children's Hospital of Buffalo, Buffalo, New York
Disorders of the Adrenal Medulla and Multiple Endocrine Adenomatosis Syndromes

PREFACE

Bringing out the second edition of this textbook, predictably, has been a challenging experience. Quantum information leaps in Pediatric Endocrinology over the past seven years have necessitated the rewriting of nearly half the chapters and extensive revision of all the others. Many advances have been the result of careful clinical observation and this method of furthering the acquisition of knowledge continues to be the mainstay of learning in all clinical sciences. In the recent past, however, explosive advances in the basic sciences such as molecular biology, have provided us with new information on the pathogenesis of disease, new tools for diagnosis and new methods for the manufacture of therapeutic agents. As always, Endocrinology has been in the vanguard of the advance and it is no accident that two of the first agents for human use synthesized by molecular biological technology have been hormones, human insulin and human growth hormone.

The authors of the chapters of this book, whatever their expert knowledge of these new fields of endeavor, have never lost sight of the goals and title of this book, that this is a book by clinicians for clinicians. Our objective has been to provide guidance for the physician caring for pediatric patients with endocrine problems. We have not shied away from covering the necessary background for the clinical information contained in its pages but we have done our best to avoid lengthy forays into the areas of biochemistry, molecular biology and neuroanatomy. For those interested, an extensive bibliography lists sources where this information may be obtained in greater detail.

Comprehensive reorganization of this second edition has resulted in the reordering of the list of contributors to the first edition with the inevitable substitution for respected authorities, but with the assembly of what the editor believes is the best roster of experts available to him. We express our sorrow at the passing of one of our most illustrious contributors to the first edition, Alfred Bongiovanni, whose death is mourned by his many friends and colleagues throughout the world. His pioneering contributions to the field of Pediatric Endocrinology will assure a respected place for him in the history of our specialty and of medical science in general.

I wish to express my thanks to the contributors to this book who met their deadlines and enabled us to expedite its publication. Also I wish to thank my colleague Dr. S. Douglas Frasier who kindly edited my contribution. Finally, I wish to thank the many readers of the first edition who generously offered comments and suggestions that were invaluable in the planning and writing of the second edition.

Solomon A. Kaplan

CONTENTS

1

GROWTH AND GROWTH HORMONE: Disorders of the Anterior Pituitary

Solomon A. Kaplan

NORMAL GROWTH[1,2]

The term *growth* is used to describe change in size with maturation. Normal growth can occur only if the individual is healthy. Thus, measurement of height and weight is an essential part of the physical examination to determine if the individual's health is normal. Acute illnesses do not impair growth significantly, but long-standing illness of the bowel, kidney, heart, lung, and so on may lead to marked change in growth rate. Physicians who take care of children should have measuring devices available that permit an accurate determination of *length*. Children who can stand erect steadily should have their height measured by a device that is fixed to a wall or some other sturdy support. The standing height is best measured by having the subject stand with heels, buttocks, thoracic spine, and head touching the device. It is advisable to have the subject stand as tall or erect as possible to counter the slouching that tends to become more marked as the day progresses. A sliding device that projects from the measuring device and is made to rest firmly on the subject's head is useful in providing reproducible measurements.

"Stadiometers" have also been used to measure height. These somewhat more expensive instruments have self-balancing devices that do not require the head-measuring block to be held in the hand. In that case the measurer is free to use the hands to raise the subject to full height by upward pressure on the mandibular rami. For infants a useful device is a boxlike structure that accommodates the head on one side and has a movable slab to press against the soles of the feet on the other. Length measurements of infants are particularly difficult to make, and erroneous results are obtained unless great care is exercised. *Sitting height* is a most important measurement for any child with a growth disturbance and is measured by seating the subject on a box with the back resting against the measuring device. In general, measurements of sitting height are more accurate in determining the relative lengths of the legs and trunk than measurements of the distances between the pubic tubercles and the top of the head and bottoms of the feet.

Standards of growth have been compiled by the National Center for Health Statistics of the United States Government. These standards are based on accurate measurements made on large, nationally representative samples of children. Seven centiles (5, 10, 25, 50, 75, 90, and 95) have been calculated for both height and weight. The growth measurements are listed in Tables 1–1, 1–2, 1–3, 1–4, and 1–5. Growth charts based on these data are available and are most useful in diagnosis and treatment of growth problems (Figs. 1–1, 1–2, 1–3, and 1–4). The charts are applicable to virtually all racial groups in the United States provided the growth patterns of the parents are taken into account.

To determine if a child is abnormally short when his or her parents are short one can use the following maneuver. Obtain the derived midparental height by averaging the parents' heights after first adding 13 cm to the mother's height if the subject is a boy or subtracting 13 cm from the father's height if the subject is a girl. Determine the growth

1

TABLE 1–1.   SMOOTHED CENTILES OF RECUMBENT LENGTH IN CENTIMETERS, FOR MALES AND FEMALES, BIRTH TO 36 MONTHS*

	Centile						
Sex and Age	5th	10th	25th	50th	75th	90th	95th
Male							
Birth	46.4†	47.5	49.0	50.5	51.8	53.5	54.4
1 month	50.4	51.3	53.0	54.6	56.2	57.7	58.6
3 months	56.7	57.7	59.4	61.1	63.0	64.5	65.4
6 months	63.4	64.4	66.1	67.8	69.7	71.3	72.3
9 months	68.0	69.1	70.6	72.3	74.0	75.9	77.1
12 months	71.7	72.8	74.3	76.1	77.7	79.8	81.2
18 months	77.5	78.7	80.5	82.4	84.3	86.6	88.1
24 months	82.3	83.5	85.6	87.6	89.9	92.2	93.8
30 months	87.0	88.2	90.1	92.3	94.6	97.0	98.7
36 months	91.2	92.4	94.2	96.5	98.9	101.4	103.1
Female							
Birth	45.4	46.5	48.2	49.9	51.0	52.0	52.9
1 month	49.2	50.2	51.9	53.5	54.9	56.1	56.9
3 months	55.4	56.2	57.8	59.5	61.2	62.7	63.4
6 months	61.8	62.6	64.2	65.9	67.8	69.4	70.2
9 months	66.1	67.0	68.7	70.4	72.4	74.0	75.0
12 months	68.8	70.8	72.4	74.3	76.3	78.0	79.1
18 months	76.0	77.2	78.8	80.9	83.0	85.0	86.1
24 months	81.3	82.5	84.2	86.5	88.7	90.8	92.0
30 months	86.0	87.0	88.9	91.3	93.7	95.6	96.9
36 months	90.0	91.0	93.1	95.6	98.1	100.0	101.5

* Statistics from National Center for Health Statistics. See reference 1 for method of smoothing by cubic-spline approximation.
† Recumbent length given in centimeters.

TABLE 1–2.   SMOOTHED CENTILES OF WEIGHT IN KILOGRAMS, FOR MALES AND FEMALES, BIRTH TO 36 MONTHS*

	Centile						
Sex and Age	5th	10th	25th	50th	75th	90th	95th
Male							
Birth	2.54†	2.78	3.00	3.27	3.64	3.82	4.15
1 month	3.16	3.43	3.82	4.29	4.75	5.14	5.38
3 months	4.43	4.78	5.32	5.98	6.56	7.14	7.37
6 months	6.20	6.61	7.20	7.85	8.49	9.10	9.46
9 months	7.52	7.95	8.56	9.18	9.88	10.49	10.93
12 months	8.43	9.84	9.49	10.15	10.91	11.54	11.99
18 months	9.59	9.92	10.67	11.47	12.31	13.05	13.44
24 months	10.54	10.85	11.65	12.59	13.44	14.29	14.70
30 months	11.44	11.80	12.63	13.67	14.51	15.47	15.97
36 months	12.26	12.69	13.58	14.69	15.59	16.66	17.28
Male							
Birth	2.36	2.58	2.93	3.23	3.52	3.64	3.81
1 month	2.97	3.22	3.59	3.98	4.36	4.65	4.92
3 months	4.18	4.47	4.88	5.40	5.90	6.39	6.74
6 months	5.79	6.12	6.60	7.21	7.83	8.38	8.73
9 months	7.00	7.34	7.89	8.56	9.24	9.83	10.17
12 months	7.84	8.19	8.81	9.53	10.23	10.87	11.24
18 months	8.92	9.30	10.04	10.82	11.55	12.30	12.76
24 months	9.87	10.26	11.10	11.90	12.74	13.57	14.08
30 months	10.78	11.21	12.11	12.93	13.93	14.81	15.35
36 months	11.60	12.07	12.99	13.93	15.03	15.97	16.54

* Statistics from National Center for Health Statistics. (see legend for Table 1–1).
† Weight given in kilograms.

TABLE 1–3. SMOOTHED CENTILES OF STATURE IN CENTIMETERS, FOR MALES AND FEMALES, 2 TO 18 YEARS*

	Centile						
Sex and Age	5th	10th	25th	50th	75th	90th	95th
Male							
2.0 years	82.5†	83.5	85.3	86.8	89.2	92.0	94.4
3.0 years	89.0	90.3	92.6	94.9	97.5	100.1	102.0
4.0 years	95.8	97.3	100.0	102.9	105.7	108.2	109.9
5.0 years	102.0	103.7	106.5	109.9	112.8	115.4	117.0
6.0 years	107.7	109.6	112.5	116.1	119.2	121.9	123.5
7.0 years	113.0	115.0	118.0	121.7	125.0	127.9	129.7
8.0 years	118.1	120.2	123.2	127.0	130.5	133.6	135.7
9.0 years	122.9	125.2	128.2	132.2	136.0	139.4	141.8
10.0 years	127.7	130.1	133.4	137.5	141.6	145.5	148.1
11.0 years	132.6	135.1	138.7	143.3	147.8	152.1	154.9
12.0 years	137.6	140.3	144.4	149.7	154.6	159.4	162.3
13.0 years	142.9	145.8	150.5	156.5	161.8	167.0	169.8
14.0 years	148.8	151.8	156.9	163.1	168.5	173.8	176.7
15.0 years	155.2	158.2	163.3	169.0	174.1	178.9	181.9
16.0 years	161.1	163.9	168.7	173.5	178.1	182.4	185.4
17.0 years	164.9	167.7	171.9	176.2	180.5	184.4	187.3
18.0 years	165.7	168.7	172.3	176.8	181.2	185.3	187.6
Female							
2.0 years	81.6	82.1	84.0	86.8	89.3	92.0	93.6
3.0 years	88.3	89.3	91.4	94.1	96.6	99.0	100.6
4.0 years	95.0	96.4	98.8	101.6	104.3	106.6	108.3
5.0 years	101.1	102.7	105.4	108.4	111.4	113.8	115.6
6.0 years	106.6	108.4	111.3	114.6	118.1	120.8	122.7
7.0 years	111.8	113.6	116.8	120.6	124.4	127.6	129.5
8.0 years	116.9	118.7	122.2	126.4	130.6	134.2	136.2
9.0 years	122.1	123.9	127.7	132.2	136.7	140.7	142.9
10.0 years	127.5	129.5	133.6	138.3	142.9	147.2	149.5
11.0 years	133.5	135.6	140.0	144.8	149.3	153.7	156.2
12.0 years	139.8	142.3	147.0	151.5	155.8	160.0	162.7
13.0 years	145.2	148.0	152.8	157.1	161.3	165.3	168.1
14.0 years	148.7	151.5	155.9	160.4	164.6	168.7	171.3
15.0 years	150.5	153.2	157.2	161.8	166.3	170.5	172.8
16.0 years	151.6	154.1	157.8	162.4	166.9	171.1	173.3
17.0 years	152.7	155.1	158.7	163.1	167.3	171.2	173.5
18.0 years	153.6	156.0	159.6	163.7	167.6	171.0	173.6

* Statistics from National Center for Health Statistics (see legend for Table 1–1).
† Stature given in centimeters.

centile on which the midparental height falls. Extrapolation of the child's anticipated growth along his or her channel, taking the skeletal age into account, should yield an adult height within plus or minus 5 cm of the derived mean adult height. If the growth extrapolation is different from the midparental height by 5 cm or more, then the growth of the child should not be ascribed simply to parental short stature.

Growth increments are most important criteria on which to base a diagnosis of the cause of short stature. Irrespective of where the child's height or weight is found to plot on the growth curve, if the increment in growth over the recent 6 or 12 months is normal, it is most unlikely that an active dis-order impairing growth exists in the individual. Children recovering from an illness or undergoing treatment for one or children with idiopathic growth delay, after an initial period of growth delay, will show normal or greater than normal growth increments. For example, if the height measurement of a child plots below the 5th centile on the growth chart, and if the height increment over a period of 6 months or 1 year is normal, it is improbable that the child is suffering from an active disorder leading to growth failure. Growth increments normally vary considerably throughout the life of the child. The normal growth increment in the first 6 months of life is 16 to 17 cm and in the second 6 months about 8 cm. In the sec-

TABLE 1–4. SMOOTHED CENTILES OF WEIGHT IN KILOGRAMS, FOR MALES AND FEMALES, 2 TO 18 YEARS*

	Centile						
Sex and Age	5th	10th	25th	50th	75th	90th	95th
Male							
2.0 years	10.49†	10.96	11.55	12.34	13.36	14.38	15.50
3.0 years	12.05	12.58	13.52	14.62	15.78	16.95	17.77
4.0 years	13.64	14.24	15.39	16.69	17.99	19.32	20.27
5.0 years	15.27	15.96	17.22	18.67	20.14	21.70	23.09
6.0 years	16.93	17.72	19.07	20.69	22.40	24.31	26.34
7.0 years	18.64	19.53	21.00	22.85	24.94	27.36	30.12
8.0 years	20.40	21.39	23.09	25.30	27.91	31.06	34.51
9.0 years	22.25	23.33	25.40	28.13	31.46	35.57	39.58
10.0 years	24.33	25.52	28.07	31.44	35.61	40.80	45.27
11.0 years	26.80	28.17	31.25	35.30	40.38	46.57	51.47
12.0 years	29.85	31.46	35.09	39.78	45.77	52.73	58.09
13.0 years	33.64	35.60	39.74	44.95	51.79	59.12	65.02
14.0 years	38.22	40.64	45.21	50.77	58.31	65.57	72.13
15.0 years	43.11	46.06	50.92	56.71	64.72	71.97	79.12
16.0 years	47.74	51.16	56.16	62.10	70.26	77.97	85.62
17.0 years	51.50	55.28	60.22	66.31	74.17	83.58	91.31
18.0 years	53.97	57.89	62.61	68.88	76.04	88.41	95.76
Female							
2.0 years	9.95	10.32	10.96	11.80	12.73	13.58	14.15
3.0 years	11.61	12.26	13.11	14.10	15.50	16.54	17.22
4.0 years	13.11	13.84	14.80	15.96	17.56	18.93	19.91
5.0 years	14.55	15.26	16.29	17.66	19.39	21.23	22.62
6.0 years	16.05	16.72	17.86	19.52	21.44	23.89	25.75
7.0 years	17.71	18.39	19.78	21.84	24.16	27.39	29.68
8.0 years	19.62	20.45	22.26	24.84	27.88	32.04	34.71
9.0 years	21.82	22.92	25.27	28.46	32.44	37.60	40.64
10.0 years	24.36	25.76	28.71	32.55	37.53	43.70	47.17
11.0 years	27.24	28.97	32.49	36.95	42.84	49.96	54.00
12.0 years	30.52	32.53	36.52	41.53	48.07	55.99	60.81
13.0 years	34.14	36.35	40.65	46.10	52.91	61.45	67.30
14.0 years	37.76	40.11	44.54	50.28	57.09	66.04	73.08
15.0 years	40.99	43.38	47.82	53.68	60.32	69.54	77.78
16.0 years	43.41	45.78	50.09	55.89	62.29	71.68	80.99
17.0 years	44.74	47.04	51.14	56.69	62.91	72.38	82.46
18.0 years	45.26	47.47	51.39	56.62	62.78	72.25	82.47

* Statistics from National Center for Health Statistics (see legend for Table 1–1).
† Weight given in kilograms.

ond year growth normally exceeds 10 cm, in the third year it exceeds 8 cm, and in the fourth year 7 cm. Between the fourth and 10th years the growth rate is 5 to 6 cm per year. In general, if the growth increment of the subject is within the normal range, it is unlikely that active or progressive disease is present. Assessment of the normal growth velocity for a particular age span can be made by measuring the growth increment along the 50th centile of the growth chart for that age span. Charts depicting normal growth velocities for height have been developed by Tanner and Davies,[3] and are available commercially.

Growth of the Osseous System[4,5]

The major factor contributing to growth is the lengthening of the skeleton. Longitudinal growth of the bones occurs by endochondral ossification, in which growth of the bone occurs by transformation of cartilage into osseous tissue. This process of endochondral ossification occurs largely in the tubular bones of the extremities but is also characteristic of the vertebral bodies. Increase in width of bones occurs from development of skeletal tissue directly from fibrous membrane. This is the mechanism by which thickening of the bones of the calvarium, the flat parts of the pelvis and sca-

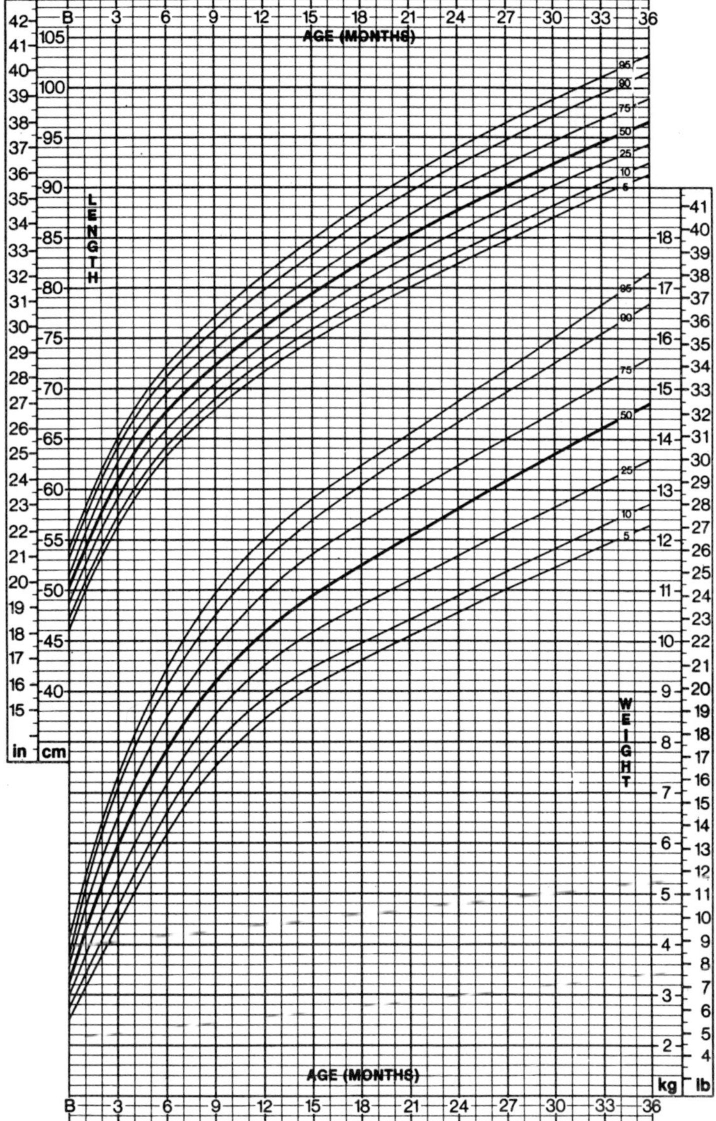

FIGURE 1-1. NCHS centiles for length and weight for age, boys, birth to 36 months. (From Moore WM: Children are different. *In* Johnson TR, Moore WM (eds): Physical Growth. Columbus, OH, Ross Laboratories, 1978, p 16.)

pulae, and the body of the mandible occurs. The diaphysis of tubular bones of the extremities also thickens by the laying down of bone directly from the fibrous periosteum. In general, length of bones is increased by the process of growth in cartilage, or endochondral ossification, while increase in the girth of bones occurs through membranous ossification.

The first signs of endochondral ossification begin in the fetus during the seventh week, and growth begins to spread from the center of the bone, which is referred to as the primary center. Subsequently, secondary centers of ossification develop in many bones, usually at a much later date and at other sites, mostly at the extremities of the bone. Initially cartilage undergoes ossification in fetal life, but this process is short lived, as osteoclasts invade the cartilage with proliferation of the blood vessels. Accompanying the proliferation of blood vessels are the bone-forming cells, osteoblasts, which form layers of bone on those remnants of the calcified cartilage that have not been destroyed by the osteoclasts. The development of cavities in spongy bone is the result of osteoclastic activity. In a bone such as the femur, none of the bony tissue present in the adult was present at birth because the size of the marrow cavity in the adult is greater than the size of the femur at birth.

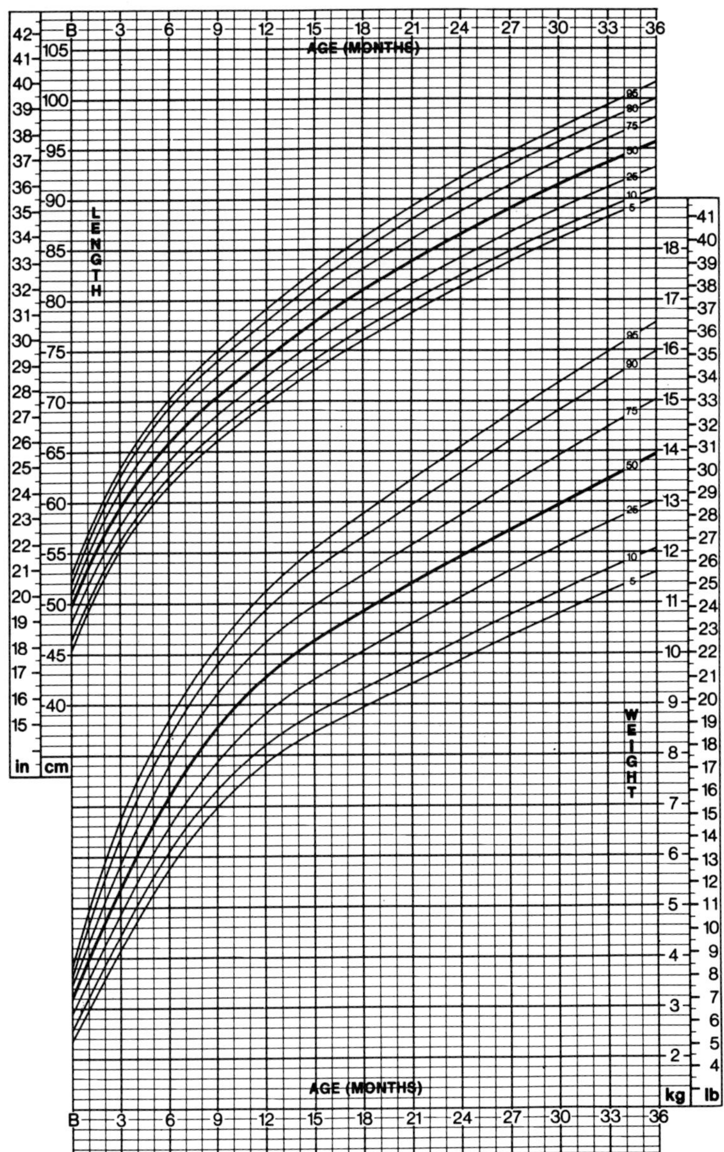

FIGURE 1–2. NCHS centiles for length and weight for age, girls, birth to 36 months. (From Moore WM: Children are different. *In* Johnson TR, Moore WM (eds): Physical Growth. Columbus, OH, Ross Laboratories, 1978, p 18.)

This example illustrates the marked turnover of structures that occurs from the inception of development of a bone until its growth ceases. Even after growth ceases, turnover of calcium and other chemical components of the bone continues actively.

While many short or flat bones ossify entirely from the primary center, all the long bones and some of the flat bones develop secondary centers that appear in the cartilage of the extremities of the bone. With few exceptions these secondary centers appear after birth. Ossification in these centers proceeds in a manner identical to that in the primary centers, with ossification of cartilage and invasion of osteoclasts and osteoblasts. The part of the bone ossified from the primary center is the diaphysis, while the part developed from the secondary center is referred to as the epiphysis. As the secondary center is progressively ossified, the cartilage is replaced by bone until only a thin plate of cartilage, the epiphyseal plate, separates the diaphyseal bone from the epiphysis. The part of the diaphysis that abuts on the epiphysis is referred to as the metaphysis and represents the growing end of the bone. As long as the epiphyseal cartilage plate persists, both the diaphysis and epiphysis continue to grow, the growth being much greater in the diaphysis. Eventually the osteoblasts cease to multiply, and the

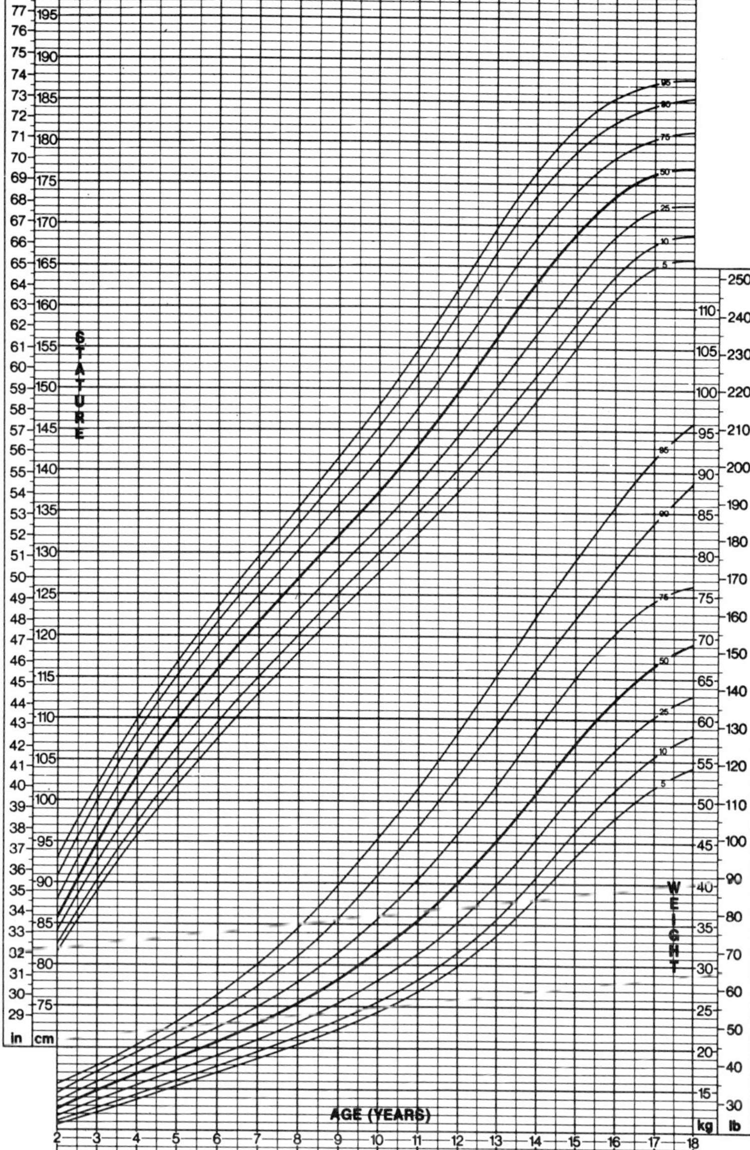

FIGURE 1–3. NCHS centiles for stature and weight for age, boys, 2 to 18 years. (From Moore WM: Children are different. *In* Johnson TR, Moore WM (eds): Physical Growth. Columbus, OH, Ross Laboratories, 1978, p 20.)

epiphyseal plate is ossified. The osseous structures of the diaphysis and epiphysis are fused and growth ceases. If the bone forms part of a joint, however, articular cartilage persists. This articular cartilage does not participate in further growth of the bone.

Skeletal Age

The length of an individual is determined by the length of the skeleton, growth of which is determined largely by lengthening of the diaphysis. In bones with normal structure (e.g., those that are not affected by skeletal dysplasia) the growth potential of the diaphysis depends on the progression of ossification within the epiphysis. It is possible to assess the growth potential of the bone by the degree of ossification of the epiphysis. It was first recognized that epiphyseal ossification was severely delayed in hypothyroidism, but it has been established that many other factors influence the progression of epiphyseal ossification. Measurement of epiphyseal center development or skeletal age has become a valuable tool in the classification of growth retardation and in the prediction of ultimate height.

The first standards for skeletal age were established by Todd in 1937 and subse-

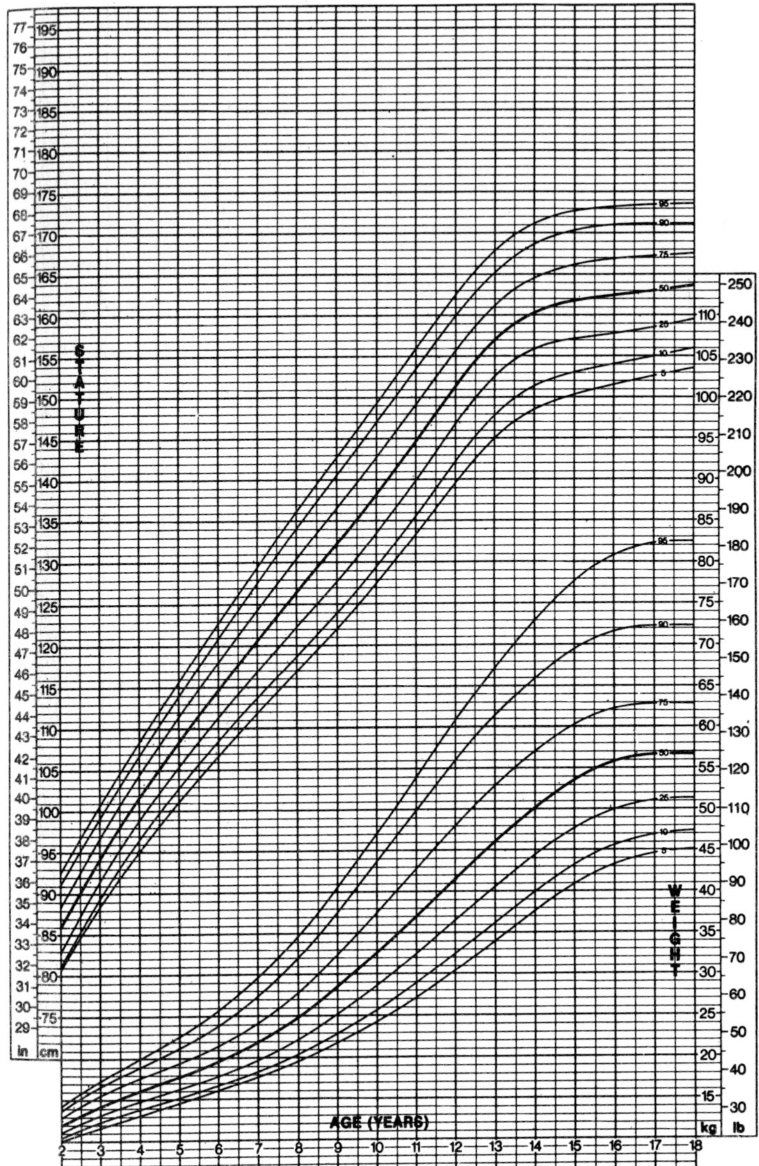

FIGURE 1–4. NCHS centiles for stature and weight for age, girls, 2 to 18 years. (From Moore WM: Children are different. *In* Johnson TR, Moore WM (eds): Physical Growth. Columbus, OH, Ross Laboratories, 1978, p 21.)

quently further developed by Greulich and Pyle.[5] Radiographs of the bones of an individual are compared with the normal standards, and the individual is assigned a skeletal age. Thus a convenient means is available for expressing the potential for growth of the individual.

Several methods for the assessment of skeletal age have been developed, and there is no unanimous agreement on which method is best. Examination of radiographs of all bones of the body of a growing child would be tedious and expensive, and the radiation exposure would be undesirable. Considerable effort has been made, there-

fore, to determine if a portion of the skeleton could be used as an index of development of the rest of the skeleton. Although the hand and wrist do not contribute to the height of the individual, radiographs of this part of the body have proven valuable in assessment of skeletal age. Discrepancies between the two sides are generally insignificant, and standards have been developed that use only the left hand and wrist. Using the radiographs of 100 normal children, Greulich and Pyle compiled the *Radiographic Atlas of Skeletal Development of the Hand and Wrist*, the second edition of which was published in 1959 and is cur-

TABLE 1–5. MEAN SITTING HEIGHT TO LOWER SEGMENT RATIOS*

Age (Years)	Boys	Girls
0.5–1.4	1.81	1.86
1.5–2.4	1.61	1.80
2.5–3.4	1.47	1.44
3.5–4.4	1.36	1.36
4.5–5.4	1.30	1.29
5.5–6.4	1.25	1.24
6.5–7.4	1.20	1.21
7.5–8.4	1.16	1.16
8.5–9.4	1.13	1.14
9.5–10.4	1.12	1.11
10.5–11.4	1.10	1.08
11.5–12.4	1.07	1.07
12.5–13.4	1.06	1.07
13.5–14.4	1.04	1.09
14.5–15.4	1.05	1.10
15.5–16.4	1.07	1.12
16.5–17.4	1.08	1.12
17.5–18.4	1.09	1.12

*Calculated from data taken from Bayer LM, Bayley N: Growth Diagnosis. Chicago, University of Chicago Press, 1959.

rently used extensively.[5] The standards of males differ from those of females, especially in the adolescent years, but significant differences may be found at other ages. The films chosen for the *Atlas* were radiographs of children no more than 2 per cent older or younger than the age represented, and those chosen for inclusion in the *Atlas* represented the best approximation to the anatomic mode. In many instances films covering several examinations from the same individual were used. For the first 18 months of age, the standards are 3 months apart but, subsequently, longer intervals of time separate the standards.

In interpreting the films, account is taken of distal parts of the radius and ulna, the carpals, the metacarpals, and all the phalanges. A careful and detailed comparison of each bone of the subject with the standard is necessary, and it is preferable to proceed in a predetermined order to examine each bone. The *Atlas* provides descriptions of the features of the bones that should be assessed as well as line drawings of these features.

It is well to recognize that sources of error exist in the interpretation of skeletal age films and that such interpretation must be made with great caution. A problem frequently encountered is one of discrepancy between different centers and, often, the development of the carpal bones does not correlate well with the development of the distal centers. It has long been known that different centers have different degrees of predictive value in terms of potential growth. The relative value of different centers has been assessed by Garn and associates by longitudinal evaluation of radiographic information on the skeletal development of a large number of boys and girls and its correlation with the age of appearance of other centers.[6] The predictive ranking varies between boys and girls. In boys, the predictive ranking for epiphyseal centers in the hand was highest for the distal segment of the fifth, fourth, and third fingers, followed by the epiphysis of the third metacarpal. The lowest predictive ranking was found for the carpal capitate, lunate, and hamate centers. For girls, the epiphyses of the third, fifth, and fourth metacarpals gave the highest orders of ranking in the hand and wrist; the lowest rankings were given by the carpal capitate, lunate, and hamate. None of the carpal bones of the hand was listed in the top 20 for either sex.

More recently, Tanner and Whitehouse have attempted to refine the method of assessment of skeletal age by establishing a series of standard appearances or stages through which each bone passes.[7] Each bone of the radiograph of the subject's hand is matched with the standard and is assigned a numerical score. The scores are summed to give a skeletal maturity score for the whole hand and wrist. A centile status in skeletal maturity is then assigned to the subject just as it is for height and weight. Originally the Tanner-Whitehouse system did not discriminate between the sexes, but in the revised system, the Tanner-Whitehouse 2 system, girls and boys are assigned somewhat different scores for each stage of bone development. At any age the total score is higher for girls than for boys. Separate standards are given for bone age based only on the radius, ulna, metacarpals, and phalanges (RUS) or only on the carpal bones.

Delay in osseous maturation is paralleled by delay in dental maturation to a large degree. Tooth formation and status of eruption as seen in radiographs may be used to develop an assessment of *dental age*.[6] Perhaps because it involves additional radiation exposure, this assessment is not usually a part of the clinical investigation of children with short stature. However, clinical examination of the teeth to determine their eruption pattern and questions regarding the time of appearance of both deciduous and permanent teeth are most useful in predicting whether skeletal age may be delayed.

Determination of skeletal age is perhaps the most important laboratory test used in determining the etiology of growth disorders and the prognosis for children with them. It is important to realize, however, that errors in interpretation frequently occur. These can be minimized if the films are interpreted by an individual with experience in reading them and if comparisons are made with films taken previously. At any age the standard deviation for interpretation is about 10 per cent of the chronologic age. By and large, when there is a discrepancy between the carpal bones and the distal centers, it is better to assign greater weight to the distal centers because they tend to correlate better with growth potential.

Although the standards of the *Atlas* are based largely on Caucasian children, they may be used for other racial groups living in the United States. The osseous maturation of American-born Japanese children was found to be much closer to that of Caucasian-American children than to that of Japanese living in Japan in the first few years after World War II. Genetic factors also contribute to the pattern of osseous maturation. Significant parent-child similarities in hand-wrist ossification have been found to occur, and (as will be discussed later in greater detail) ossification patterns found in individuals with inherited skeletal dysplasias may be detectable in their parents and siblings.

Knowledge of skeletal age is of great importance in the diagnosis and treatment of infants and children with growth disorders for two reasons. First, growth retardation is classified into two broad categories depending on whether (1) there is an intrinsic disease of the bone that has led to shortening of the diaphysis without significant delay of epiphyseal maturation or (2) there are factors outside the skeletal system that impair growth and epiphyseal maturation, such as hypothyroidism or malnutrition. Thus, evaluation of the skeletal age greatly assists in the diagnosis of the cause or category of growth retardation. Second, the growth potential of the individual can be estimated from the individual's height at the time of examination and the skeletal age. It is necessary to realize, however, that any such prediction is only a rough estimate and attempts at accurate prediction are unwise. Several reasons for this exist. It has been

pointed out that accurate skeletal age interpretation may be quite difficult and that significant errors are made even by experienced observers. In addition, progression of skeletal age does not necessarily parallel height increments, particularly in children with skeletal dysplasia. A similar discrepancy often occurs in children treated over several years for severe hypothyroidism. Discordance between skeletal development and growth is particularly likely to occur in children with sexual precocity, in whom estrogens and androgens produced in excess generally accelerate skeletal age to a greater degree than height age.

Tables for prediction of ultimate height based on the individual's height, skeletal age, sex, age, and growth rate have been published.[5,8] Using skeletal age for prediction of ultimate height it is also possible to make a rough calculation as follows. Measure the individual's height, plot it on a standard growth curve, and extrapolate the value horizontally to the age on the chart that is equal to the bone age. If the point of extrapolation falls between the 5th and 95th centiles, then a guarded prediction of normal adult stature can be given. The closer the extrapolated value is to the 50th centile, the more good reason there is for optimism.

Growth deficiency may be classified into two broad categories:

Primary growth deficiency: In this category there is an intrinsic defect in the skeletal system as a result of either a genetic defect of or prenatal damage to the skeletal system. In this form of growth disorder the potential normal bone growth (and, therefore, body growth) is impaired. Skeletal age is not delayed or is delayed much less than is height age.

Secondary growth deficiency: Growth is retarded because factors, generally outside the skeletal system, delay osseous maturation. These factors may be endocrine, nutritional, metabolic, or unknown, as in the syndrome of idiopathic (constitutional) growth delay. In this form of growth retardation the skeletal age and the height age may be delayed to nearly the same degree. (Height age of an individual is defined as the age at which the individual's height is at the 50th centile.) In secondary growth deficiency, the potential often exists for reaching normal adult height.

A distinction between these two categories of growth impairment is necessary because their causes, prognoses, and diagnostic approaches are different. Difficulties with this classification may arise in some instances in which the skeletal age is delayed to a lesser degree than the height age. In general, however, a distinction between primary and secondary categories of growth failure can be made from the clinical findings and from a knowledge of the skeletal age.

Early attempts at classification divided growth impairment into the broad categories of nanosomia primordialis (short stature from birth) and nanosomia infantilis (short stature recognized after birth in later infancy). In general, primordial short stature was associated with no delay of bone age (when this measurement was introduced later), whereas infantile nanosomia was generally associated with delay of epiphyseal maturation. This distinction based on time of onset of growth delay holds up reasonably well in the light of newer information on causes of growth impairment, but examples of discrepancies are numerous. For example, in hypochondroplasia, a form of chondrodystrophy, the syndrome is usually not recognized until at least 1 or 2 years after birth. In this disorder bone age is generally not significantly delayed. On the other hand, important causes of growth retardation with significant delay in skeletal maturation may date from birth. This is usually the case in congenital hypothyroidism, for example.

PRIMARY DISTURBANCES OF GROWTH

1. Skeletal dysplasias

2. Chromosomal abnormalities

3. Congenital errors of metabolism

4. Intrauterine growth retardation
   a. Fetal infections
   b. Exposure of the fetus to toxins (ethanol, nicotine, drugs, etc.)
   c. Impaired fetal nutrition
   d. Severe maternal illness
   e. Unknown causes

5. Miscellaneous syndromes of primary growth failure (progeria, Russell-Silver syndrome, Seckel syndrome, Noonan syndrome, and so on)

6. Genetic short stature

In most instances of this category, growth deficiency begins before birth. Impairment of diaphyseal growth occurs without an equivalent degree of delay in skeletal age. In most instances, the antenatal disturbance is permanent, and the outlook for normal adult height is poor. In a few instances, however, infants who are small for their gestational age at birth can recover some growth potential and grow to a normal height.

Skeletal Dysplasias

Over 100 disorders have been described that fall into the category of skeletal dysplasias. Very little is known about the vast majority of these disorders except for clinical descriptions. An international group of experts met in 1977 to recommend a classification that modified previously used terminologies.[9] Because the list of disorders is so complex, only a modified version of the classification will be presented here, followed by a description of some of the more important types.

I. Osteochondrodysplasias: this category includes abnormalities of cartilage or bone development or both
   A. Defects of growth of tubular bones or spine
      1. Identifiable at birth
         a. Achondroplasia
         b. Spondyloepiphyseal dysplasia congenita
         c. Achondrogenesis types I and II
         d. Thanatophoric dysplasia
         e. Campomelic dysplasia
         f. Chondroectodermal dysplasia (Ellis-van Creveld syndrome)
         g. Kniest dysplasia
         h. Miscellaneous
      2. Identifiable in later life
         a. Hypochondroplasia
         b. Dyschondrosteosis (Leri-Weill)
         c. Metaphyseal chondrodysplasias
         d. Spondylometaphyseal dysplasias
         e. Multiple epiphyseal dysplasia
         f. Miscellaneous
   B. Disorganized development of cartilage and fibrous components of skeleton
      1. Fibrous dysplasias
      2. Enchondromatoses
      3. Cherubism
      4. Miscellaneous
   C. Abnormalities of cortical diaphyseal structure or metaphyseal structure

     1. Osteogenesis imperfecta (congenita and tarda)
     2. Osteopetrosis
     3. Diaphyseal dysplasia
     4. Miscellaneous

II. Dysostoses: this category comprises malformations of individual bones singly or in combination
  A. Cranial and facial involvement
     1. Cranial and craniofacial dysostoses
     2. Acrocephalosyndactyly
     3. Miscellaneous
  B. Axial involvement
     1. Vertebral segmentation defects (including Klippel-Feil syndrome)
     2. Miscellaneous
  C. Extremity involvement
     1. Camptodactyly
     2. Cardiomelic syndromes (Holt-Oram, etc.)

A full listing of the skeletal dysplasias is provided in the *International Nomenclature of Constitutional Diseases of Bone.*[9] A detailed discussion of all the different disorders is beyond the scope of this book. The following is a discussion of the more important forms of skeletal dysplasia leading to short stature.

Achondroplasia (Fig. 1–5)

Achondroplasia is the commonest form of chondrodystrophy. The disorder is recognizable at birth. It is inherited as an autosomal dominant trait, but as many as 80 per cent of all cases have no family history and are considered as new mutations. Increased paternal age appears to be a contributing factor. When achondroplastic dwarfs marry, 75 per cent of their offspring are affected and 25 per cent are expected to be homozygous for the achondroplastic genes. Such infants appear to inherit a very severe form of the disease, and many die early in life because movement of the thoracic cage is severely compromised.

The typical heterozygotic form of achondroplasia is characterized by disproportionate shortening of the limbs, especially in their proximal segments. The hands are short and broad and appear large compared to the abbreviated limbs. Wideness of the proximal phalanges leads to difficulty in opposing the fingers, and a space between the third and fourth digits gives the hand a

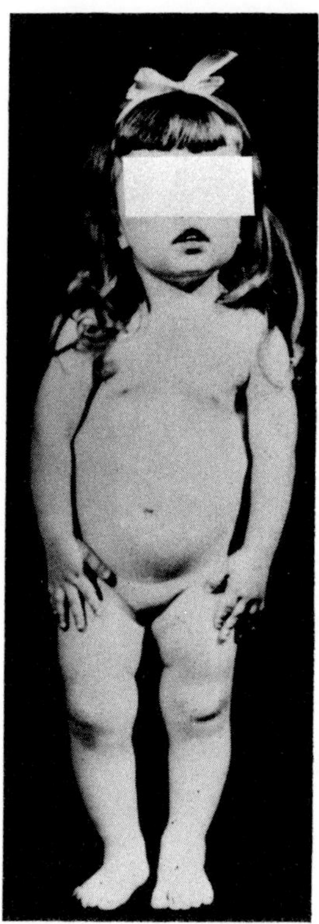

FIGURE 1–5. Typical achondroplasia in a child.

three-pronged or trident appearance. The trunk is less involved, but because of accentuated lumbar lordosis and pelvic tilt, the buttocks are prominent. The head is large and the forehead protrudes. The nasal bridge is depressed and the mandible is prognathic. The foramen magnum is small and internal hydrocephalus may develop. Intelligence is usually normal unless brain function is impaired as a consequence of hydrocephalus. Mean adult height for achondroplastic men is about 132 cm and for women about 123 cm. Standard growth charts have been published for achondroplasia[10] as well as for diastrophic dysplasia, spondyloepiphyseal dysplasia congenita, and hypochondroplasia.[11]

The radiologic features of achondroplasia include shortening of the skull base, small foramen magnum, and large skull vault. The long tubular bones are short, especially the proximal ends of the femur and humerus. The pelvis is short and broad. The acetabular roofs are narrow, and the sacrosciatic notches are deep. The distances between the vertebral pedicles narrow between L1 and L5 instead of increasing in width, as is the case normally.

Very little is known about the nature of the disturbance in achondroplasia. Although previous studies have suggested that the organization of the ossifying cells is irregular, recent studies have failed to substantiate this. The chondrocytes and matrix are apparently normal.

At present no treatment is available for short stature due to achondroplasia.

Hypochondroplasia (Fig. 1–6)

Although hypochondroplasia resembles a milder form of achondroplasia, the two disorders are clearly different and do not occur in the same family. There is considerable variation in clinical forms of this disorder, although most individuals with hypochondroplasia are taller than those with achondroplasia.[11] The individuals are short and stocky, and as in achondroplasia, they show abnormal ratios of upper to lower segments characteristic of short-limbed dwarfism. In addition, the arm span is less than the height. The hands are short but do not have a trident appearance. As in achondroplasia, the trunk is nearly normal in size.

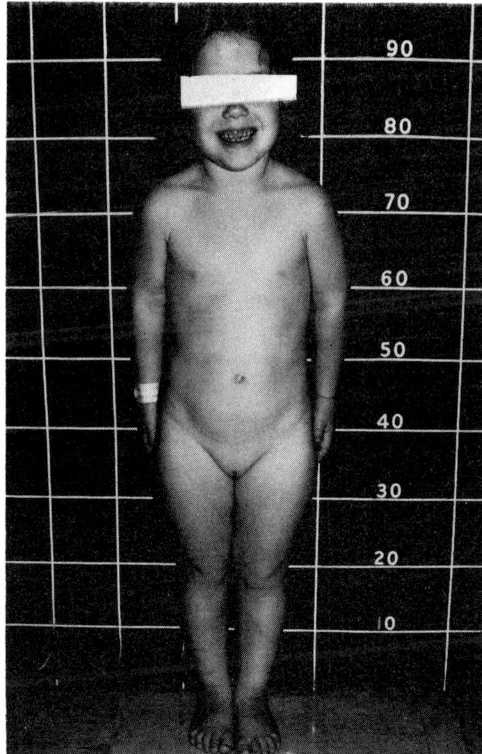

FIGURE 1–6. Hypochondroplasia in a child. The general appearance is normal except for shortness, which is particularly marked in the upper and lower extremities.

The parallelism between achondroplasia and hypochondroplasia extends to the radiologic findings. The long bones may show some flaring of the epiphyses. There is also some flaring of the pelvis, and the sacrosciatic notch is narrowed. The distances between the vertebral pedicles diminishes from L1 to L5, and the pedicles appear short. A mild concavity of the posterior surface of the vertebral bodies may be seen.

Hypochondroplasia is also inherited as a dominant trait, and the condition is more frequently familial. Subjects with this disorder often seek advice from the endocrinologist because the nature of the skeletal disorder is less evident than in achondroplasia.

The rare disorder *thanatophoric dwarfism* can be confused with achondroplasia at birth, but the thorax is very narrow and usually is unable to sustain respiration for long. *Grebe disease* is a nonlethal form of short-limbed dwarfism in which the trunk and cranium are normal. The disease is inherited as an autosomal recessive trait. *Diastrophic dwarfism* is characterized by short limbs, club feet, scoliosis, hip dysplasia, and hand malformations. The term "diastrophic" implies twisting. The condition is clearly evident at birth.

Epiphyseal Dysplasias

Epiphyseal dysplasias are a group of disorders characterized by short stature associated with poor development of epiphyseal ossification centers. Eventually the epiphyses appear but they are small, irregular, and fragmented. Occasionally this disorder is confused with Legg-Calvé-Perthes disease. *Spondyloepiphyseal dysplasia* is characterized by shortening of the trunk with eventual development of kyphosis and scoliosis. Although the limbs appear long in relation to the trunk, they are really abnormally short. In the congenital form, abnormal ossification of the epiphyseal centers may be seen at birth; when the epiphyses develop, they are short, irregular, fragmented, and flattened. The congenital form is transmitted as an autosomal dominant trait, and there is marked clinical and genetic variability. The tarda form is transmitted as an X-linked trait, and the shortness is generally not noticed until ages 5 to 10. The dwarfism is much milder, but severe osteoarthritis may develop early in adult life. Radiographs show a mild flattening of the vertebral bodies and the disk spaces appear narrow.

Chromosomal Abnormalities

Most chromosomal abnormalities lead to disturbances of growth. An exception is Klinefelter syndrome. Other anomalies of chromosomal number, morphology, and organization generally lead to growth impairment. These are associated with mental retardation and clearly evident somatic anomalies. Both intrauterine and postnatal growth are impaired in the syndromes of trisomy of chromosomes 18 and 15, deletion of chromosome 5, and most other chromosomal anomalies. In these subjects, growth retardation is rarely a major cause of concern, and the search for its cause does not pose a serious diagnostic dilemma.

Down Syndrome

The commonest chromosomal disorder is trisomy of chromosome 21, leading to Down syndrome, which occurs in approximately 1 in 600 live births. Short stature is characteristic of but not always present in this syndrome. At birth, the average weight of Down syndrome infants is 400 to 600 gm less than normal full-term infants and their mean length is 2 to 3 cm less than normal. The small size at birth is partly due to the fact that Down syndrome infants have shorter periods of gestation, which average about 1 week less than normal, a slight but statistically significant difference. The difference in size at birth cannot be accounted for entirely by the shorter gestational period, however. The short stature is due to involvement of the skeleton in the widespread disease in which every cell in the body (or many cells in some mosaics) has abnormal quantities of genetic material. Shortness of stature continues throughout life. The ranges of adult heights in Down syndrome in one series were 135 to 170 cm for males and 127 to 158 cm for females. Other factors, such as congenital heart disease or hypothyroidism, may contribute to impairment of growth in this disorder.

Few subjects with Down syndrome are referred to growth or endocrine clinics for diagnosis of the cause of short stature because the diagnosis of the disorder is relatively easy. The growth of the subject is sometimes considered an important issue, and attempts have been made by some to accelerate it.

Skeletal age is often normal and sometimes even advanced at birth, but subsequently children with Down syndrome experience relative retardation of skeletal development. The delay in skeletal maturation is not as marked as the delay in growth, however. Treatment of Down syndrome with anabolic steroids may improve growth rate temporarily. The disadvantages and potential adverse effects of such treatment are discussed in the general section "Principles of Treatment of Growth Retardation" on page 52.

Turner Syndrome

Gonadal dysgenesis (Turner syndrome) is an important cause of growth retardation and must always be considered in the search for a cause for growth retardation in the female. The syndrome is described in considerable detail in Chapter 9, and only some of the aspects of the syndrome that are important in assessment of growth retardation are considered here. Any girl with growth retardation must be examined carefully for signs of gonadal dysgenesis. A large number of subjects with Turner syndrome do not have signs clearly indicative of the presence of the syndrome. It may be necessary, therefore, to proceed with laboratory testing for the disorder in short girls with none of the typical signs of the disorder. Girls with gonadal dysgenesis frequently have abnormally short limbs. If the cause of short stature is not evident, and if the subject is a female with short-limbed dwarfism characterized by an abnormally high upper-to-lower segment ratio, presence of gonadal dysgenesis must be suspected.

Skeletal Anomalies with Known Disorders of Metabolism[9,12]

The *mucopolysaccharidoses* are a group of disorders characterized by a variety of skeletal anomalies, storage of mucopolysaccharides in the tissues, and excretion of mucopolysaccharides in the urine. Only those generally associated with growth retardation will be considered here. These disorders are characterized by diffuse involvement of the skeletal system, including the epiphyses, metaphyses, and diaphyses. The skeletal anomalies often include poorly modeled tubular bones. The metacarpal bones are bottle shaped, and the basal phalanges are cylindrical. The ribs are flat and spatulate. The vertebral bodies are short in the sagittal plane, and because their anterior and posterior surfaces are concave, they are said to have a "beaked" appearance. The lower ribs are club shaped. The bones of the arm and forearm are short, and their epiphyseal ends are irregular. In Morquio syndrome the shafts of the long bones are normal in length and shape, but the outlines of their epiphyseal ends are irregular. The vertebrae are flat and irregular with wide disk spaces. In Morquio syndrome severe spinal and chest deformities lead to marked kyphosis and scoliosis. The arms are relatively long and extend to the knees. The joints are enlarged and the muscles and ligaments are flaccid.

Depending on the clinical, biochemical, and genetic findings, at least 12 different types of mucopolysaccharidoses have been described, including the syndromes of Hurler, Scheie, Hunter, Sanfilippo, Morquio, and Maroteaux-Lamy. In addition to skeletal dysplasia, physical anomalies may include clouding of the cornea, cardiovascular anomalies, and mental retardation. Most disorders are transmitted as autosomal-recessive traits, although the Hunter syndromes are transmitted through an X-linked gene. There is excessive urinary excretion of mucopolysaccharide substances, including dermatan sulfate, heparan sulfate, keratin sulfate, and chondroitin sulfates A and C. The syndromes are caused by deficiencies of lysosomal enzymes, including α-L-iduronidase, sulfoiduronate sulfatase, sulfamidase, N-acetyl-D-glucosaminidase, hexosamine-6-sulfate sulfatase, and β-glucuronidase. No treatment for these disorders is currently available.

Intrauterine Growth Retardation[13,14]

Growth of the fetus may be inhibited by any one factor or a combination of several factors. In many instances such growth impairment augurs poorly for normal postnatal growth and attainment of normal adult height. Exceptions to this rule are occasionally seen. Healthy infants of multiple births are examples of low birth weight subjects in whom postnatal growth is characterized by "catch-up" growth and normal adult height. Generally, normal infants born prematurely will have caught up with full-term infants by the second year of life, depending on the degree of prematurity and the absence of congenital malformations and serious perinatal complications.

Infections of the fetus may lead to serious congenital anomalies and growth retardation. Among the best recognized are rubella, toxoplasmosis, cytomegalovirus, and herpes simplex. Intrauterine growth retardation may occur in infants whose mothers have contracted other infections during pregnancy, although the association between the infection and growth impairment of the fetus is often difficult to establish. Transplacental transmission of *toxic substances*, such as results from alcohol ingestion by the mother or smoking, also impairs fetal growth. The peculiar facies and other phenotypic features of the fetal alcohol syndrome[15] and the fetal hydantoin syndrome are well described.[16] Maternal illness such as *toxemia, hypertension,* or *malnutrition* or ingestion of *drugs* for therapeutic or other purposes may impair fetal growth. A rare but interesting cause of fetal growth impairment is *congenital diabetes mellitus,* in which absence of insulin in the fetus impairs fetal growth in length and weight. After birth, growth accelerates with insulin treatment until the infant reaches normal dimensions. The role of *placental insufficiency* in producing intrauterine growth retardation is often difficult to determine. The placenta normally undergoes involution in the last few weeks of pregnancy, and it may be difficult to distinguish normal involution from placental insufficiency by anatomic and microscopic examination of the placenta.

The classification of intrauterine growth retardation has been assigned to all infants born after normal gestational length with a birth weight of less than 2000 gm[13] or to prematurely born infants whose size is small for gestational age. Unlike prematurely born infants, those with intrauterine growth retardation do not experience respiratory distress at birth because their lungs are generally sufficiently mature to produce adequate quantities of surfactant. Congenital anomalies may be present, however, leading to other cardiopulmonary symptoms and signs. Newborn infants abnormally small for gestational age experience hypoglycemia much more frequently than do normal-sized infants. The underlying mechanisms for this disturbance of carbohydrate metabolism are not known.

Intrauterine growth retardation with persistent postnatal growth impairment is usually classified under the category of primary disturbances of skeletal growth even though there may be no demonstrable anatomic lesions of the skeleton. In this disorder, as in all other disorders of primary skeletal growth disturbances, it is not possible to account for growth impairment by abnormalities of the endocrine system, or of nutrition, or by generalized metabolic or toxic disturbances. Skeletal age is normal, or if delayed, the retardation is significantly less than the retardation in somatic growth. Children subsequently diagnosed as having growth hormone (GH) deficiency are usually normal in size at birth. This may be because the vast majority of cases of GH deficiency are acquired after birth and not necessarily because GH is not required for fetal growth. Infants with gene deletions, on the other hand are apparently small at birth. The subject of GH deficiency due to GH gene defects is discussed on pages 33–34.

Miscellaneous Syndromes of Primary Growth Failure

Grouped together under this heading are several syndromes of unknown etiology identifiable because of typical patient phenotype. In these syndromes there is no evidence of systemic disease, and the skeletal age is generally not delayed. If it is delayed, the retardation in height age is much greater than the delay in skeletal age. No specific treatment is available, and the children generally do not reach normal height as adults. A complete description of all syndromes in which growth is impaired is beyond the scope of this book. The reader is referred to other sources for more extensive descriptions of these many syndromes. Only a few of those syndromes in which the initial or major concern is growth retardation will be discussed here. In many instances growth failure has a prenatal onset, and the syndromes could well be included in the list of intrauterine growth retardation syndromes. Their grouping into a separate category is arbitrary.

Russell-Silver Syndrome[17,18]

In 1954, Russell reported the cases of five children with prenatal onset of growth retardation, craniofacial dysostosis, and disproportionately short limbs.[17] The facies had a triangular shape, and the frontal bones a bossed appearance. Two of the five children also had asymmetry. In 1964, Silver reported on two unrelated children with

asymmetry and short stature.[18] The consensus is that the two reports described the same disorder, and it is now referred to as the Russell-Silver syndrome.

The asymmetry of the body is usually of the extremities. An incurving or shortening of the fifth finger is also often seen. In about one third of the patients, pubertal development, characterized by enhanced gonadotropin secretion, occurs early. Other features of the syndrome are mental retardation, dislocation of the hips, dislocation of the radius and ulna at the elbow, hypoglycemia, renal anomalies, and hypospadias. Nearly all cases have been sporadic, but in rare instances a parent may show some of the features of the disorder.

Noonan Syndrome[19,20]

In this disorder certain phenotypic resemblances to Turner syndrome are present, but the two are separate disorders. The syndrome is found in males but can also affect females. The subjects with this syndrome have short stature, low-set or abnormal ears, low posterior hair lines, neck webbing, pectus excavatum, cubitus valgus, vertebral column anomalies (spina bifida occulta, hemivertebrae), small penis, and cryptorchidism. Mental retardation occurs in about one half of subjects. Less frequent manifestations are ptosis, hypertelorism, nerve deafness, high arched palate, and simian creases of the hands. Edema of the dorsum of the hand and foot may be found. There are several important differences from Turner syndrome. The congenital heart lesions are on the right side of the heart (pulmonic stenosis, etc.) in Noonan syndrome, whereas in Turner syndrome the left side is involved (see Chapter 9). The chromosome constitution in Noonan syndrome is appropriate (e.g., 46XY). Although often sporadic, the syndrome has occurred in several families in which a vertical mode of dominant inheritance has been found.

Progeria (Hutchinson-Gilford Syndrome)[21]

This disorder generally manifests itself within the first 2 years of life, although the birth weight on average is low. Over 60 cases have been described in the world literature. The course is one of inexorable progression of loss of subcutaneous fat, growth failure, alopecia, joint stiffness, and thinning of the skin. Diffuse involvement of the cardiovascular system occurs in the first decade of life. There is generalized atherosclerosis, and angina, hypertension, congestive heart failure, myocardial infarction, and cerebral vascular accidents occur. Generalized hyperlipidemia occurs, but it is not certain whether the degenerative changes in the vascular system are related to hyperlipidemia or to a progressive generalized disorder of connective tissue. Although the disorder resembles premature senility, it is by no means certain that it represents a telescoping of the normal three- to fourscore life span into two decades. The affected subjects are short, and skeletal age is either appropriate for chronologic age or slightly delayed. Intelligence is generally normal.

Bloom Syndrome

Bloom syndrome[22] is characterized by prenatal onset of growth delay. The syndrome is distinguished by facial telangiectatic erythema involving the cheeks and nose. The erythema is accentuated by exposure to sunlight. Other features include dolichocephaly and malar hypoplasia. Intelligence is normal. There appears to be a propensity for development of malignancy of the lymphoreticular system. When cells from these patients are cultured in vitro, chromosome breakage and rearrangement frequently occurs.

Seckel Syndrome

In Seckel syndrome[23] growth retardation occurs prior to birth. Mental retardation is typical and is associated with microcephaly and premature synostosis (Fig. 1–7). Facial hypoplasia with prominence of the nose has led to use of the term "bird-headed" dwarfism. The ears are low set and often malformed. Anomalies of the peripheral skeleton include clinodactyly of the fifth finger, absence of phalangeal epiphyses, and hypoplasia of the proximal radius. The disorder appears to be transmitted as an autosomal-recessive trait.

Rubenstein-Taybi Syndrome

The combination of broad thumbs and toes, facial anomalies, mental retardation, and short stature is found in the Rubenstein-Taybi syndrome.[24] The abnormal facies are characterized by slanting palpebral fissures,

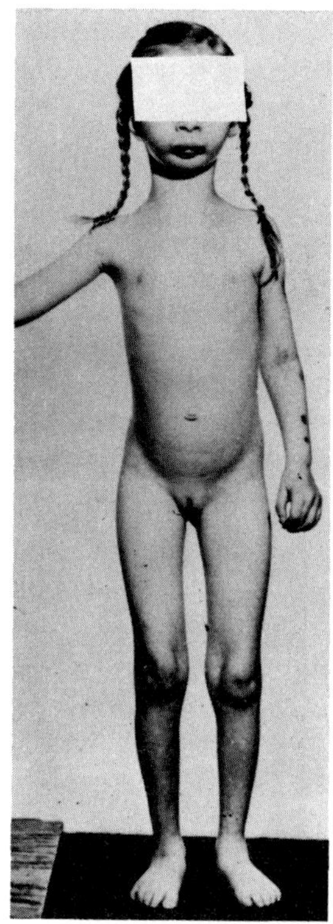

FIGURE 1–7. Child with Seckel type of dwarfism.

a beaked nose and prominent nasal septum, strabismus, and low-set or malformed ears. The forehead is prominent. Anomalies of the eyes, heart, kidneys, and spine have been reported. Skeletal age may be somewhat delayed. Cryptorchidism is present in virtually every subject.

Prader-Willi Syndrome[25]

The Prader-Willi syndrome is characterized by short stature, which is usually present at birth. The children are mentally retarded. Typical of the syndrome are micromelia, infantile hypotonia, small penis, cryptorchidism, obesity, and a tendency to abnormal carbohydrate tolerance. In rare instances children with many features of this syndrome have been found to have hypopituitarism. It is not clear if these cases are variants of the syndrome. Hypogonadism often becomes evident when the subjects reach adult life. A deletion involving chromosome 15 is found in many but not all patients with this syndrome.

Genetic Short Stature

The inheritance of growth is multifactorial. Tall parents tend to have tall children, and short parents tend to have short children. Because so many genetic factors enter into the picture of growth, however, frequent discrepancies occur between expected and achieved height when the midparental height is taken into account. A method for estimating if the growth pattern of a child falls within the expected genetic limits has been described previously in this chapter (p. 1). Perhaps the most striking type of genetic short stature is that seen among the African pygmies, in whom evolutionary selection of short stature genes has led to virtual elimination of genes for normal stature.[26] The multifactorial nature of the inheritance is underscored by the fact that unions between pygmies and Bantu individuals of normal height tend to produce offspring intermediate in height between the two parents (allowing for sexual differences). In other parts of the world, the union of two individuals—one genetically tall and the other genetically short—often leads to a similar result. So many genetic factors are involved in growth, however, that the predictions based on the heights of the parents are often inaccurate.

SECONDARY DISTURBANCES OF GROWTH

1. Undernutrition
    a. Protein-calorie malnutrition
    b. Kwashiorkor
    c. Specific vitamin deficiencies (e.g., vitamin D)
    d. Specific mineral deficiencies (e.g., zinc and iron)
2. Disorders of the bowel
    a. Regional enterocolitis (Crohn disease)
    b. Ulcerative colitis
    c. Malabsorption syndromes
    d. Celiac syndrome
    e. "Short bowel" syndrome following surgery
    f. Chronic gastroenteritis
    g. Cystic fibrosis of the pancreas
3. Disorders of the kidney
    a. Congenital anomalies (e.g., polycystic kidney disease)
    b. Chronic glomerulonephritis
    c. Pyelonephritis and obstructive uropathy
    d. Nephrotic syndromes
    e. Renal tubular acidosis
    f. Bartter and Liddle syndromes
    g. Syndromes of Fanconi and Lowe
    h. Nephrogenic diabetes insipidus
4. Disorders of the heart and circulation
    a. Patent ductus arteriosus
    b. Ventricular septal defect
    c. Tetralogy of Fallot
    d. Atrioventricular canal
    e. Aortic stenosis
    f. Pulmonic stenosis
    g. Transposition of great vessels
    h. Coarctation of the aorta
5. Deprivation (psychosocial) dwarfism
6. Metabolic disorders of carbohydrate, lipid, and protein metabolism
7. Chronic infections
8. Drugs
9. Disorders of the hematopoietic system
10. Disorders of the lungs
11. Miscellaneous chronic disorders (dysautonomia, etc.)
12. Endocrine disorders
    a. Growth hormone deficiency
    b. Hypothyroidism
    c. Gonadal dysgenesis
    d. Glucocorticoid excess
    e. Pseudohypoparathyroidism
    f. Premature epiphyseal fusion
        i. Androgen excess
        ii. Estrogen excess
13. Idiopathic (constitutional) growth delay

Malnutrition and Growth Impairment

Malnutrition is by far the commonest cause of growth retardation throughout the world. Disturbance of nutrition can take the form of gross undernutrition, in which there is a deficiency of total calorie and protein intake, or a form of malnutrition in which total intake of calories is not substantially below normal standards but in which there are substantial reductions in intake of essential food constituents such as essential amino acids or vitamins. Following periods of food deprivation, normal growth and intellectual development may resume if the deficiency is corrected.[27,28] With protein undernutrition such as occurs in kwashiorkor, normal growth cannot be reestablished without a supply of essential amino acids irrespective of the total caloric intake. In children with marasmus, circulating levels of GH may be high but the hormone is unable to stimulate protein anabolism because of lack of necessary substrates.[29] In the diencephalic syndrome of emaciation GH concentrations in the plasma are often increased.[30] This condition occurs in young infants and children who are emaciated despite apparently adequate food intake. A tumor is present, usually in the anterior hypothalamus or floor of the third ventricle, and neurologic abnormalites may be present. Whether the GH concentrations are high because of the emaciation or because of a disturbance of the neurohypophysial regulation of GH secretion is not known. In cases of generalized undernutrition, specific vitamin deficiencies may not be detectable. Circumstances may arise in which caloric intake is adequate, but specific vitamin deficiencies may occur. This can occur in American infants, for example, who live in inner cities where there is not much sunlight and who are receiving breast milk without vitamin supplementation.[31] Vegetarian diets that have adequate amounts of calories, vitamins, (including D and B_{12}), high-quality protein, and calcium should be adequate for normal growth in infancy or later in life.[32] Children receiving such diets should be monitored and dietary advice given if signs of growth retardation or vitamin deficiency develop, however.

Specific deficiencies of minerals such as *zinc* and *iron* may lead to growth retardation. Male subjects living in Iran and Egypt have been described as having syndromes of dwarfism and hypogonadism associated with hepatosplenomegaly.[33] Some of the subjects had schistosomiasis and hookworm infestations, but these were not considered to account for the dwarfism in all subjects. Evidence has been presented that zinc deficiency may have played a role in the growth retardation. The diet of the subjects consisted largely of bread that may have contained sufficient phosphate and phytate to form complexes with heavy metals, impairing absorption of zinc and iron. In animals, induced zinc deficiency leads to growth retardation and testicular atrophy. Whether zinc deficiency can occur in individuals in developed countries who are ingesting average diets has not been determined. It seems unlikely to be a factor in growth or pubertal delay, however, unless an individual's diet has an abnormal content of factors leading to malabsorption of zinc. Zinc deficiency in the United States seems confined to individuals with disturbances such as chronic malabsorption and acrodermatitis enteropathica and to those dependent on parenteral nutrition when the sustaining solutions do not contain adequate zinc. Zinc deficiency is a very unlikely cause of growth impairment in an individual who is otherwise in good health.

Bowel Disorders as Causes of Growth Disturbances

Growth impairment is typical of chronic disease of the gastrointestinal tract. Diseases that are characterized by chronic vomiting or diarrhea, whether due to infections, chronic inflammations, intolerance of constituents of the diet, or tumors of the bowel, often cause growth impairment because of insufficient absorption of nutriments. Intolerance of protein, such as gluten enteropathy (celiac disease), incomplete hydrolysis or absorption of mono- and disaccharides, and malabsorption of fat, such as occurs in liver or pancreatic insufficiency, can all lead to marked growth impairment. The diagnosis is usually easily made from the history and physical examination. Retardation of skeletal maturation is characteristic in growth retardation due to disease of the gastrointestinal tract.

A number of diseases of the bowel, however, may cause growth retardation without obvious evidence of bowel involvement. Chief among these in the United States is regional enteritis (Crohn disease). Children with this disorder may suffer marked growth delay for several months or years before typical symptoms of the bowel disease develop.[34] In the United Kingdom celiac disease often has been reported to lead to growth retardation before symptoms such as diarrhea occur.[35] This disorder is less prevalent in the United States but, presumably, the disease can also masquerade as idiopathic growth retardation west of the Atlantic Ocean.

Another important bowel disorder that can impair growth before significant disease of the bowel or lungs is manifest is cystic fibrosis of the pancreas. The author has also encountered a case of mild Hirschsprung disease in which denial of symptoms of constipation for many years confused the diagnosis and in which normal growth resumed following corrective surgery. All these disorders, whether they manifest symptoms of bowel disease or not, are characterized by delay of skeletal age.

When faced with the problem of growth retardation for which no obvious cause is discernible, the physician must consider disease of the bowel. In parts of the world where there is a high prevalence of celiac disease, measurement of the serum titer of antigliadin antibodies or biopsy of the bowel have been recommended as diagnostic maneuvers in any child with persistent growth failure. Chronic anemia and increased sedimentation rate may be clues to the presence of regional enteritis. Persistent failure to grow at a normal rate may require radiographic or biopsy study of the bowel. Measurement of sweat electrolyte concentration to exclude cystic fibrosis of the pancreas should be considered in any case of persistent growth failure.

Disorders of the Kidney and Growth Disturbances[36–38]

Renal failure can impair growth through any one of several mechanisms. The severe biochemical disturbances that are associated with uremia create a milieu in which normal growth cannot be achieved. Among the consequences of renal failure are acidosis, disturbances of body fluid tonicity, hyperphosphatemia, hypocalcemia, hyperparathyroidism with renal osteodystrophy, impaired synthesis of dihydroxyvitamin D, anemia, and hypertension. With so many factors, it may be impossible to evaluate the contribution of each one to the disturbance of growth. The result is very clearly one of tissue resistance to growth factors. For example, occurrence of insulin resistance in uremia has been known for a long time. An additional factor in production of short stature is treatment of the disease. Glucocorticoids, large doses of which may be necessary to control the renal disease, have long been known to impair growth.

Among the best studied factors in renal disease is acidosis.[36] This is present in a majority of children with renal disease who have growth retardation but is rare in children with renal disease who are growing normally. Treatment of acidosis can lead to substantial acceleration of growth, but such treatment alone is rarely effective if acidosis is part of a broader picture of renal failure. Administration of alkali may produce dramatic increases in growth in children with idiopathic renal tubular acidosis.[38] By itself,

increased retention of nitrogen in the serum does not appear to impair growth.

The role of undernutrition as a factor in growth retardation with renal disease may be of considerable importance. Children with chronic renal failure tend to have poor appetites. Their need to drink large volumes of fluid if they have concentrating deficiencies and their reluctance to take solid food may aggravate the state of poor nutrition. Renal osteodystrophy is a complex constellation of events, including impaired synthesis of dihydroxycholecalciferol, absorption of calcium from the intestine, and impaired excretion of phosphate and acidosis.

Recent dramatic improvement in the treatment of end-stage renal disease has led not only to the prolongation of the lives of the children but also to some improvement in their growth rates.[39] This improvement in growth has not been uniform, however, and in the recent past attempts to accelerate growth have been made by treatment with GH.[40] Some of the initial responses have been encouraging but at the time of writing of this chapter the treatment is still considered experimental.

Disorders of the Heart and Circulation and Growth[41–44]

Several surveys of children with congenital heart disease have shown that growth retardation occurs frequently in this disorder. A study of 890 patients in 1962 showed that 27 per cent were below the 3rd centile for height and weight. Growth retardation was more prevalent in the cyanotic group, in which 40 per cent were below the 3rd centile for height and weight. In the cyanotic group, growth retardation was particularly marked in tetralogy of Fallot with pulmonic atresia or in anomalies in which both major vessels arose from the right side of the heart. In acyanotic malformations, growth retardation was much less severe, occurring in 8 per cent of patients with coarctation of the aorta, in 13 per cent with atrial septal defect, in 15 per cent with pulmonic stenosis, in 15 per cent with aortic stenosis, in 22 per cent with patent ductus arteriosus, and in 23 per cent with ventricular septal defect.[41] These percentages are not always closely duplicated in other studies. There is a general trend for growth retardation to be more severe if congestive heart failure supervenes early. In these subjects, growth retardation persists, perhaps because congestive heart failure, occurring early, has a permanent detrimental effect on growth. Birth weight may be significantly low in some children with congenital heart disease, but in over 95 per cent of such patients birth weights are appropriate for gestational age. Premature delivery is more frequent than in infants without congenital heart disease, occurring in up to 10 per cent of infants.

Following corrective surgery, a large increase in weight tends to occur, especially in patients with uncomplicated ventricular septal defect, aortic stenosis, atrioventricular canal, or pulmonic stenosis. Following repair of transposition of the great vessels, there is some increase in weight, but this tends to be maintained between 1 and 2 standard deviations below the mean. Surgical correction of congenital heart lesions improves linear growth rate, especially in children with ventricular septal defect and heart failure in infancy, patent ductus arteriosus, tetralogy of Fallot, atrioventricular canal, and aortic stenosis. Shunting procedures in patients with tetralogy of Fallot lead to increases in growth less frequently than does corrective surgery. In general, patients with normal growth prior to surgery do not experience an acceleration in growth following surgery. Children with growth retardation who do not experience an increase in growth after surgery may do so partly because the heart anomaly has not been completely corrected and a residual defect remains.

Aside from the abnormal cardiovascular dynamics in these patients, other factors play a role in their growth retardation. This is evidenced by the fact that even when the congenital anomaly is completely corrected, growth failure may persist. Some do not grow because the heart lesion is one expression of generalized damage to the developing fetus. The damage may be exogenous, such as occurs in rubella, or endogenous, such as occurs with chromosomal anomalies in Down and Turner syndromes. In these children the growth disorder is only partly ascribable to insufficiency of the circulation. As mentioned previously, severe congestive heart failure in infancy is associated in many instances with permanent growth retardation even if the cardiovascular abnormality undergoes total correction. The role of inadequate nutrient intake in the growth retardation of children with congenital heart disease is not clearly established.

Deprivation (Psychosocial) Dwarfism[45–48]

Normal interaction between infants and children and the environment is necessary for normal growth and development. The syndrome of growth failure with anorexia and weight loss (among other signs and symptoms) has long been recognized in infants separated from their mothers. It has been referred to as "anaclitic depression" and was first considered to involve only institutionalized infants. Subsequently, however, it became evident that the same disturbance could happen in infants and children who were not thriving in their homes with their natural mothers. These infants often improved following removal from their parents to another environment. Among the factors responsible for this pattern of behavior are social isolation, cruelty and neglect, institutional upbringing, adverse child-rearing practices less severe than "cruelty and neglect," separation experiences, and socioeconomic deprivation. These influences are particularly likely to affect infants, but older children are vulnerable as well.

Growth failure may be the direct result of failure, deliberate or otherwise, of the parent or guardian to provide adequate protein or other essential nutrients. In addition, it is possible that the adverse environment may lead the child to develop anorexia. Another possible mechanism is that the adverse environment may produce abnormal physiologic responses such as disturbance of bowel function or of endocrine or metabolic function.

The prevalence of psychosocial dwarfism varies considerably among age groups. Several reports have confirmed that deprivation is an important cause of dwarfism in infants. In infants in whom a careful history, physical examination, and simple laboratory testing for anemia, renal disease, and hypothyroidism do not reveal a cause for growth retardation, psychosocial factors are found to be responsible for the growth retardation in more than half of the cases. In older children, deprivation dwarfism also occurs but is responsible for a smaller percentage of all cases of short stature.

The history obtained in cases of psychosocial dwarfism may not always reveal the true nature of the disorder. The parent or guardian may be unwilling to disclose the true nature of the relationship between the child and its environment. In some instances the responsible adult is unaware of his or her failure to carry out adequate parenting. The parents may themselves be socioeconomically deprived and unable to fulfill their obligations to the child despite their best efforts. The syndrome also occurs among the affluent, some of whom may leave much of their parenting responsibilities to others. In any case, the possibility of deprivation dwarfism must always be borne in mind if no other cause for growth retardation can be found, and careful inquiries should be made to gain information on the relation of the child to the environment. The behavior of the child may be quite characteristic. If the child is old enough, bizarre polydipsia may occur, with the child often drinking water from toilet bowls, gutters, or fish tanks. The appetite may be voracious. The child may rummage for food among garbage cans and beg or steal food from friends, neighbors, and stores. These unusual patterns may continue throughout the day and night.

Physical examination will often show that the child is afraid of adults and recoils from offered love and affection until he or she realizes that not all other individuals are abusive. Physical examination generally does not uncover any abnormalities. In some instances, however, evidence of child abuse, such as fractures, bruising, and periosteal and subdural hemorrhages, may be found.

Laboratory tests, if they are to be done, are best carried out before admission to the hospital is contemplated. Hospitalization should be carried out only if it is considered necessary to observe the child in circumstances in which a change in the influence of parenting is necessary. Admission of the child to the hospital for tests that are painful and require periods of starvation may not be helpful in uncovering the cause of the growth failure.

Studies of older children with deprivation dwarfism have shown evidence of hypopituitarism in some cases. Deficiency of growth hormone may occur; less frequently there may be adrenocorticotropic hormone (ACTH) deficiency; and even less frequently thyroid-stimulating hormone (TSH) deficiency is found. In some instances hypercortisolemia has been reported, possibly as a result of the chronic stress. Irrespective of whether endocrine abnormalities are found, delay in skeletal maturation occurs. Administration of GH to these individuals, however, may not be helpful in restoring normal growth. The proper treatment, and the most successful, is restoration of a normal environment. In those instances of child abuse in which trauma to the brain leads to hypopituitarism, hormonal treatment is also necessary.

Metabolic Disorders and Growth Retardation

Disturbances of metabolism of carbohydrate, protein, and lipids are often associated with growth impairment. Growth retardation and pubertal delay are characteristic of several types of *glycogen storage disease*, especially type I in which the defect is in activity of glucose-6-phosphatase.[49] Marked growth retardation and also delay of pubertal development occur in this disorder. The disease is characterized also by hepatomegaly, ketonuria, hypoglycemia, and increased concentrations of pyruvate, urate, and free fatty acids in the plasma. Successful treatment of this disorder to control hypoglycemia is often attended with improved growth velocity. The disorders of carbohydrate metabolism are discussed in detail in Chapter 5. Several defects of *amino acid* and *protein metabolism* may lead to growth retardation. In these, mental retardation and metabolic disturbances such as of hydrogen ion concentration frequently dominate the clinical course, and advice is rarely sought for separate treatment of growth retardation. Some disorders of glycoprotein metabolism are associated with severe skeletal dysplasia. These have been discussed previously in this chapter (pp. 14–15). Abnormalities of *mucolipid metabolism* may also be associated with dysostosis multiplex[12] and growth retardation. Several disturbances of lipid storage may impair growth, among other physiologic functions. A full discussion of these abnormalities is beyond the scope of this book.

Infections as Causes of Growth Retardation

Chronic infections are important causes of growth failure worldwide. In many developing countries malnutrition and chronic infections are both responsible for growth retardation and the effects of each are difficult to separate. It is evident, however, that chronic infections with intestinal and systemic parasites, for example, schistosomiasis, hookworm, and roundworm, do act as serious deterrrents to normal growth.[50] Acquired immune deficiency syndrome is rapidly becoming an important cause of growth impairment in children throughout the world. Other disturbances of the immune system, such as chronic granulomatous disease of childhood, may also lead to growth failure.[51]

Drugs as Causes of Growth Retardation

A number of drugs and other pharmaceutical agents may cause growth impairment, especially if they are ingested in large doses over long periods of time. Some of these (e.g., glucorticoids, anabolic agents) are discussed in other parts of this chapter. One widely used pharmacologic agent that has been associated with growth retardation is methylphenidate, used for the treatment of hyperkinetic chidren. A review of several published reports suggests that use of this agent is associated with a temporary retardation in growth velocity but has no effect on adult height.[52] Following use of dextroamphetamine for treatment of the hyperkinetic state, transient weight loss may occur, but tolerance soon develops and there seems to be no effect on adult height or weight. Short stature may occur in other situations in which children undergo long-term treatment with drugs, such chemotherapy for malignancy.[53]

Hematopoietic Disorders and Growth

Children with sickle cell disease experience significantly progressive retardation in height and weight velocity beginning before the age of 2 years.[54] By the age of 9 years the average height of children with the homozygous form of the disease is about 1 standard deviation below the mean for normal controls. Delay in weight gain and skeletal maturation parallels the retardation in height increment. Puberty is delayed, but while permanent hypogonadism does occur it is unusual. The factors leading to growth impairment are not understood but do not appear to involve the endocrine system in the prepubertal child. Children with the SC form of the disease do not appear to have growth retardation.

Longitudinal measurements of height, weight, and skeletal maturation in children with thalassemia show that prepubertal growth is generally normal.[55] Endocrine disorders do occur in these children, probably as a result of frequent transfusions and damage from hemosiderosis. These disorders include hypogonadotropic hypogonadism, hypoparathyroidism, and reduced adrenocortical reserve.[56]

Pulmonary Disease and Growth Impairment

Children with mild or moderately severe asthma generally do not experience significant delay in growth. If glucocorticoids in large doses are used for treatment, as is sometimes necessary, growth retardation may occur.[57] Growth retardation may also occur in children with severe asthma who are not treated with glucocorticoids. The growth retardation is accompanied by a deceleration of skeletal maturation. If the severity of the asthma diminishes and the dose of glucocorticoids is reduced, normal growth is resumed and adult height is often normal. It appears that doses in excess of 45 mg cortisone/sq m/day (or other glucocorticoid equivalent dose) must be administered over a prolonged time to produce growth retardation.[58]

Short stature and pubertal delay are characteristic findings in children with cystic fibrosis of the pancreas, in which disease the lungs are severely affected.[59] The growth impairment in this disorder is probably due to several factors, pancreatic and pulmonary insufficiency as well as chronic infections.

Endocrine Causes of Growth Retardation: Growth Hormone

With the exception of growth hormone deficiency, all endocrine causes of short stature are discussed in other chapters.

Synthesis and Secretion of Growth Hormone

Human growth hormone (hGH) is a single-chain polypeptide consisting of 191 amino acids with a molecular weight of approximately 21,500. Intramolecular disulfide bonds link positions 53 and 165, and 182 and 189.[60] There is considerable homology between hGH and prolactin. Significant species differences occur, and only GH isolated from pituitaries of anthropoid apes and humans is effective in the human.[61] Recently hGH has been synthesized by bacteria in which recombinant DNA techniques have been used.[62]

The pituitary gland is formed in fetal life from two separate sources.[4] The anterior portion is derived from a tubular diverticulum that grows up from the primitive oral cavity, Rathke's pouch. The pituitary stalk (infundibulum) and posterior lobe have their origins in a hollow diverticulum that grows downward from that part of the brain that will later form the third ventricle. The anterior and posterior portions undergo fusion, and the anterior portion develops lateral buds that grow upward to cover the stalk with a thin layer of cells known as the *pars tuberalis.* The connection of the posterior lobe with the brain persists, but the lumen of Rathke's pouch is obliterated. Embryonic remnants of the pouch, known as the pharyngeal pituitary, may persist and may function after embryonic life.

The anterior part of the pituitary constitutes about 75 per cent of the weight of the pituitary and is referred to as the *adenohypophysis.* The part derived from the inferior surface of the developing brain is referred to as the *pars distalis* or *neurohypophysis.* Between the adenohypophysis and neurohypophysis, colloidal cyst remnants may be found, and this area is referred to as the *pars intermedia.* The medium eminence represents a thickening of the floor of the third ventricle from which the hypophyseal stalk extends to the neurohypophysis. It contains fiber tracts from the tuber cinereum and supraoptic and paraventricular nuclei to the neurohypophysis. There are no significant neural connections, however, between the hypothalamus and anterior pituitary. GH releasing hormone (GHRH) has been localized by immunohistochemical techniques to neurons of the arcuate (infundibular) nucleus (Fig. 1–8). In this nucleus, the neurons containing dopamine tend to concentrate in the dorsomedial portions, whereas GHRH occupies a more lateral and inferior location. A large number of hormones and transmitters has been located in the arcuate nucleus, including dopamine, galanin, γ-aminobutyric acid (GABA), GHRH, neuropeptide Y, neurotensin, pancreatic polypeptide, proenkephalin A, prolactin, pro-opiomelanocortin, somatostatin, and substance P. Somatostatin has also been detected in the parvocellular division of the paraventricular nucleus.[63,64]

The blood supply to the pituitary consists of a systemic arterial supply, a portal blood system, and venous drainage.[65] The arterial supply is derived from the superior hypophysial artery, a branch of the internal carotid artery. The venous portal system originates from specialized straight terminal arterioles in the median eminence, from which blood is collected in a series of parallel veins coursing down the anterior sur-

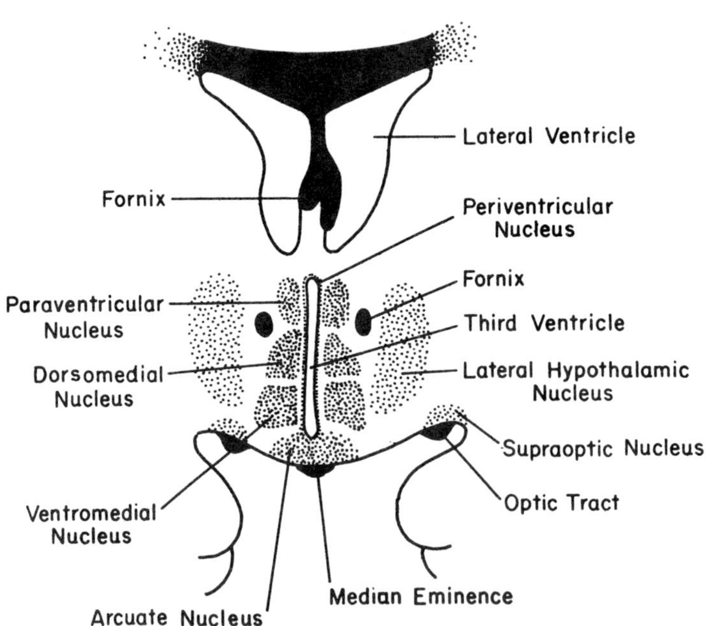

FIGURE 1–8. Cross-section through the hypothalamus showing the relationship of the arcuate nucleus to surrounding structures. (From Lechan RM: Neurology of pituitary hormone regulation. In Molich ME (ed): Pituitary Tumors: Diagnosis and Management. Endocrinology and Metabolism Clinics of North America, Vol 16. Philadelphia, WB Saunders Company, 1987, p 503.)

face of the pituitary, and terminates in the sinusoidal capillaries of the adenohypophysis. This portal system has come to be recognized as the pathway by which hypothalamic releasing and inhibiting substances are transmitted to the anterior pituitary (Fig. 1–9). These substances play a major role in regulating secretion of the hormones of the anterior pituitary. The blood supply of the posterior lobe is entirely separate from that of the anterior lobe, arising as it does from the inferior hypophysial arteries. Hypothalamic regulation of the posterior lobe is exerted entirely through neural connections. The only significant nerves found in the anterior pituitary are vasomotor nerves accompanying the arterioles. Blood from both lobes drains into the cavernous sinus.

The concept of regulation of anterior pituitary function by factors produced in the hypothalamus and carried to the anterior pituitary by portal blood vessels is now established.[66] Growth hormone circulates in the plasma in multiple forms, a 22,000 molecular weight form (native GH), a 20,000 molecular weight form, and a "big" form composed of several monomers (not linked by covalent bonds) with a molecular weight of in excess of 100,000.[67] The clinical signifi-

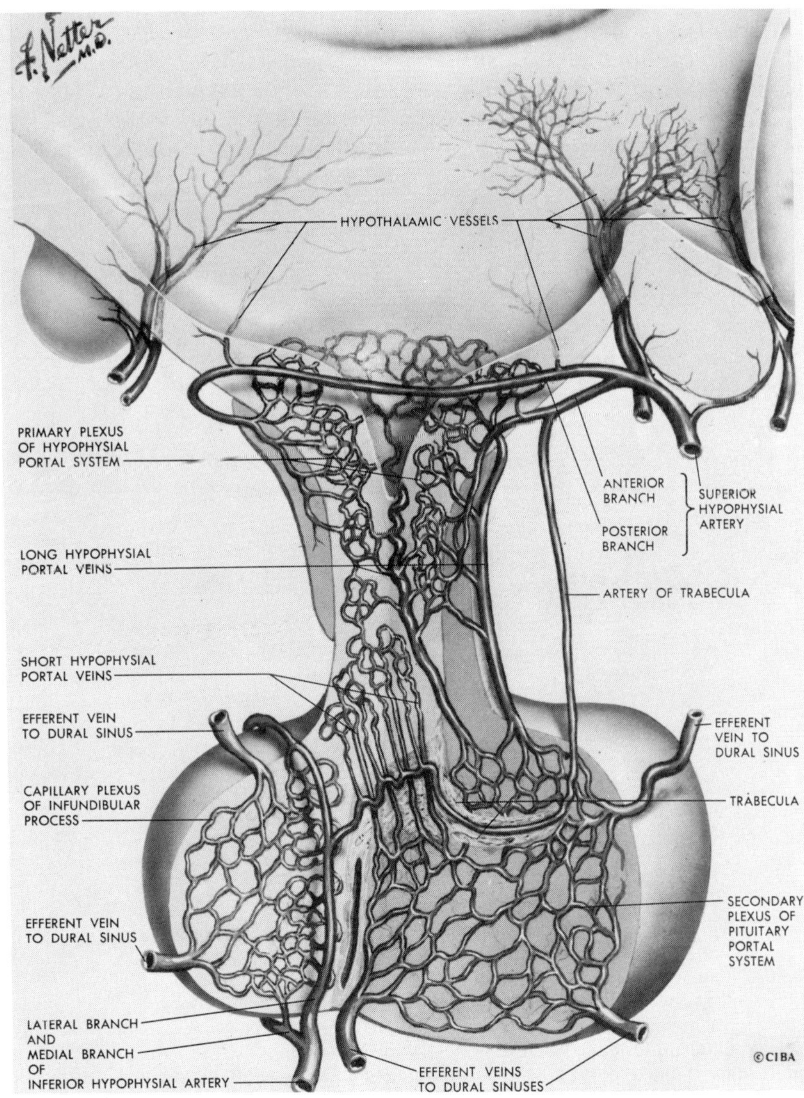

FIGURE 1–9. The main components of the hypothalamic-pituitary portal system. (From Netter FH: The Ciba Collection of Medical Illustrations. Vol. 4, Endocrine System and Selected Metabolic Diseases. 1965.)

cance of these forms of circulating GH is un-clear. Growth hormone also circulates in the plasma bound to a specific high-affinity car-rier protein.[68] The carrier protein may be related to the GH receptor, because it does not appear to circulate in subjects with the Laron type of growth deficiency.[69]

Secretion of GH occurs in a series of ir-regular bursts throughout the day and night.[70] For much of the time, concentra-tions in the blood plasma are below the lim-its of detection. Surges of secretion may occur, leading to concentrations in the plasma as high as 60 ng/ml in normal indi-viduals. The most consistent surge comes after sleep begins and correlates well tem-porally with development of phases 3 and 4, or slow-wave electroencephalographic rhythms. With advancing age from puberty to adolescence, the number of GH surges increases sharply. While factors such as sleep, postprandial decline of blood glucose concentration, and stress account for some

of the secretory surges, many of the surges appear to be spontaneous (Fig. 1–10).

Increased secretion of GH occurs in re-sponse to *hypoglycemia* and increased con-centrations of *amino acids* in the blood, but only when the degree of variation in glucose or amino acid concentration is greater than normally occurs.[70] Abnormally high concen-trations of free fatty acids inhibit GH secre-tion. The nocturnal surge cannot be sup-pressed by induced hyperglycemia unless it is extreme (greater than 400 mg/dl). It ap-pears, therefore, that the surges of growth hormone secretion are not related to fluc-tuation in plasma glucose, amino acids, or free fatty acids but to intrinsic neural mech-anisms. Secretion of GH also appears un-related to secretion of prolactin, TSH, or ad-renal glucocorticoids.

Sleep-associated GH release occurs irres-pective of what time of day the subject goes to sleep. If sleep is delayed GH secretion is delayed, and if the sleep pattern is reversed

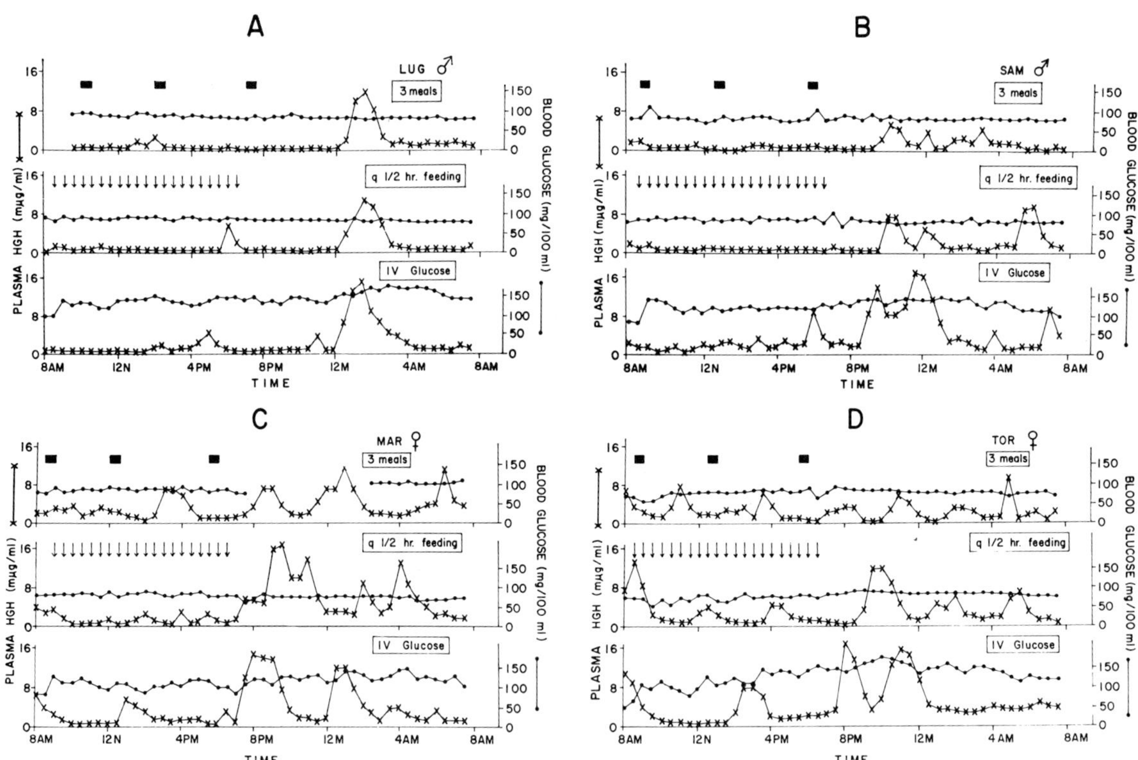

FIGURE 1–10.   Variation in plasma GH levels over 3-day periods in four normal subjects. Ingestion of meals was followed by periods in which growth hormone levels were generally low. Subsequently there were bursts of secretion that were apparently unrelated to food intake or change in blood glucose concentration. Ingestion of small meals frequently was also generally associated with persistently low concentrations of GH in the plasma, although, again, bursts of secretion were still observed. The secretory pattern is not significantly different from that observed during oral feeding, even though the blood glucose concentration is significantly higher. (From Goldsmith SJ, Glick SM: Rhythmicity of human growth hormone secretion. Mt Sinai J Med 37:501, 1970.)

and the subject goes to sleep during the day, GH secretion will occur with phases 3 and 4 of the daytime sleep.[71] The close temporal correlation between the GH surge and the development of slow-wave rhythm sleep, even in blind people, has led to the conclusion that the two are closely associated. The association is close only for the slow-wave rhythm that develops after the subject falls asleep. Other bursts of slow-wave activity during the day or night, however, are not associated with GH secretion.

The presence of GH-releasing activity in the hypothalamus was long suspected, but it is present in such small amounts that its existence was masked by the more abundant somatostatin, which has the opposite effect. Three human pancreatic peptides with GH-releasing activity have been sequenced. They contain 37, 40, and 44 amino acids, respectively.[72] These peptides are apparently identical to those found in the pituitary. It is likely that the smaller peptides are proteolytic degradation products of hpGRF-44, the 44-amino-acid peptide. All three molecular species are biologically active, although the smaller one is less active than the others. The NH_2-terminal group is essential for activity. GHRH appears to be species specific, and rat GHRH, for example, has a different structure from the human variety.

Bolus injection of GHRH (50 μg in adults) is followed by a sharp increase in GH levels in the serum. Following subsequent injections, however, the response is smaller and gradually diminishes. Continuous infusion of GHRH also does not lead to sustained increases in GH secretion.[73]

In an effort to determine the usefulness of GHRH as a diagnostic agent it was administered to 574 European children with apparently normal GH secretion, partial GH deficiency, or severe GH deficiency.[74] The mean concentrations of GH achieved in the serum were 45.8, 29.2, and 16.8 μU/ml, respectively, for the three groups. Chihara et al. administered repeated doses by infusion and injection to children with various forms of GH deficiency. In some of the subjects repeated injections were necessary to elicit GH responses.[75] A priori one would expect patients with pituitary lesions to fail to respond to GHRH while those with hypothalamic deficiency should respond. Schriock et al. administered repeated doses of GHRH to 13 patients with GH deficiency in different schedules to determine the usefulness of the agent in the diagnosis of hypothalamic

deficiency.[76] They administered GHRH every 2 hours for 12 doses, the first and last 5 μg/kg and all the others 1 μg/kg. Some subjects responded to a single injection but others required multiple injections. They concluded that hypothalamic deficiency cannot be excluded on the basis of impaired response to one injection and that the number of injections required to establish a diagnosis of hypothalamic dysfunction is quite variable. Studies have been carried out to determine if GHRH can be used for the treatment of children with GH deficiency.[77,78] Over a treatment period of 6 months or longer, it was found that a dose of at least 1 μg/kg given every 3 hours (8 μg/ kg/day) administered by a pump was necessary to promote growth. Antibodies to GHRH were found in 11 of the 24 children who participated in the study, but they did not appear to blunt the response to GHRH. Whether a sustained-release GHRH preparation may be effective in the long-term promotion of growth acceleration in children with GH deficiency is not known.

The presence in hypothalamic extracts of material inhibiting GH release led to identification of the inhibiting material as a tetradecapeptide, subsequently named somatostatin.[79] This material was particularly concentrated in the median eminence of the hypothalamus. Somatostatin inhibits GH secretion induced by several stimuli, including electrical stimulation of the hypothalamus, sleep, and administration of L-dopa, pentobarbital, morphine, chlorpromazine, insulin, and arginine. Somatostatin also blocks thyrotropin-releasing hormone (TRH)-induced TSH release but does not affect TRH-induced prolactin release. It does not block basal secretion of follicle-stimulating hormone (FSH), luteinizing hormone (LH), TSH, or the induction of LH or FSH secretion by luteinizing hormone–releasing hormone (LRH). It reduces growth hormone secretion in acromegaly and ACTH secretion in Nelson syndrome. The effect of somatostatin injected into the bloodstream is quite transient, lasting less than 5 min. Following this, rebound secretion of GH occurs. Somatostatin analogs, however, persist for much longer times in the body. Their use in the treatment of GH-secreting tumors is discussed later in this chapter (p. 56).

Animal experiments have shown that stimulation of other parts of the brain, such as the basolateral amygdala, results in GH secretion. Stimulation of other areas, such as the preoptic area and corticomedial amygdala, inhibits secretion of GH. Thus it appears that surges of GH secretion can follow activity of parts of the brain well removed from the hypothalamus. Coincidentally, high concentrations of somatostatin have been found in the preoptic area and the amygdala as well as in other parts of the brain, including the cerebral cortex, thalamus, cerebellum, brainstem, spinal cord, and pineal gland. At present, the role of these extrahypothalamic areas in regulation of GH secretion is not fully understood. It would appear that the effects of sleep and stress on its secretion originate beyond the hypothalamus. It is possible, that impulses or secretory processes ranging as far away from the hypothalamus as the cerebral cortex may influence the secretion of GH.

Aside from the effects of somatostatin on the secretion of GH, the action of this peptide is widespread throughout the body. It inhibits insulin and glucagon secretion by the pancreatic islets, gastrin secretion by the pancreatic cells, calcitonin secretion by the thyroid, ACTH secretion by the pituitary cells, and the effects of vasoactive intestinal polypeptide on fluid transport in the colon. Its inhibitory effect on TSH secretion by the pituitary has been alluded to previously (p. 27). It also appears to counter the effects of prostaglandins in certain systems.

Neurotransmitters in the central nervous system play important roles in control of secretion of GH.[80] The catecholamines epinephrine and norepinephrine, given alone, have no effect on GH secretion, but if administered with a β-blocking agent such as propranolol, they do elicit a GH response. This increased secretion is inhibited, however, if an α-blocking agent such as phentolamine is administered. In addition, α-adrenergic blockers such as phentolamine block GH secretion induced by insulin hypoglycemia, glucagon, amphetamines, aminophylline, L-dopa, and possibly arginine. The GH secretory response to insulin-induced hypoglycemia is also blocked by reserpine and chlorpromazine. Clonidine, an α_2-adrenergic receptor agonist, is a potent stimulant of GH secretion and is widely used as a testing agent for GH deficiency.[81]

L-dopa has also been shown to stimulate GH release. This effect is not due to conversion of L-dopa to norepinephrine. The GH secretory spike, however, is blocked if catecholamine reuptake is inhibited by imipramine and by methscopolamine. The sleep spike of GH secretion is inhibited by high concentrations of nonesterified fatty acids as well as by very high concentrations of glucose in the blood. *Serotonin* also appears to be involved in the regulation of GH secretion. Administration of 5-hydroxytryptophan, a serotonin precursor, increases GH release, and this effect can be blocked by administration of cyproheptadine, a serotonin receptor blocker. Release of GH is also enhanced by *GABA* and *enkephalin*. Methscopolamine, an anticholinergic agent, inhibits the sleep-associated secretion of GH. Conversely, piperidine, a cholinergic receptor stimulant, enhances sleep-induced and insulin-stimulated GH secretion.[82]

Exercise is characteristically associated with an increase in GH secretion.[83] The GH response occurs while free fatty acid concentrations increase, but if the exercise is prolonged, free fatty acid concentrations continue to increase while GH secretion diminishes. Growth hormone secretion during exercise is enhanced by protein ingestion but may be obliterated by glucose ingestion. The stimulus for increased GH secretion during exercise is not known, but it may be related to the degree of *stress* induced in the individual, because it is more prolonged in physically unfit than in physically fit individuals. In addition to physical stress, *psychic stress* may enhance GH secretion, as may occur during repeated venipunctures.[84] *Surgery*, including mastectomy and cholecystectomy, induces GH secretion, as does hemorrhage involving 13 to 20 per cent of the blood volume.[84]

Intravenous administration of *vasopressin* has been reported to increase GH secretion, but intramuscular vasopressin does not produce such an increase consistently. The effects of vasopressin administration appear to be quite variable.[84]

Administration of *glucocorticoids* in doses considerably in excess of normal production rates leads to a blunting of the GH response to hypoglycemia.[85] High doses of glucocorticoids, may produce considerable attenuation of the GH response, whereas lower doses for longer periods of time may be without effect. Administration of 4 to 8 mg of dexamethasone in a single dose may inhibit GH secretion in an adult, but a dose of 1 mg does not. *Estrogens*[84] enhance the GH secretory response following administration of insulin, arginine, or vasopressin and exercise. Women ingesting oral contraceptives experience enhancement of GH release following insulin hypoglycemia or infusion of arginine intravenously. The effect is due to the estrogen component of the contraceptive. *Progestational agents* such as medroxyprogesterone appear to suppress GH release. The mechanisms by which estrogens enhance GH secretion are not understood but may be related to enhanced sensitivity of the GH-releasing mechanism to other stimuli.[84] *Androgens*, too, appear to enhance secretion of GH following induction of hypoglycemia by insulin. Administration of 400 mg of testosterone for 1 or 2 days is followed by increased secretion of GH.[86] Generally, GH responses to insulin hypoglycemia are greater in magnitude after puberty in both males and females.

The *thyroid* plays an important part in modulating GH secretion.[87] Secretion of GH is decreased in hypothyroid individuals and is restored to normal with appropriate thyroid medication. Restoration of the GH response to normal occurs within 3 to 4 weeks of beginning thyroid medication in hypothyroid individuals.

Actions of Growth Hormone[14,88]

Growth hormone is a potent anabolic agent, promoting increase in size of virtually all tissues of the body. Balance studies show considerable retention of nitrogen, phosphorus, potassium, and calcium when GH is administered to hypopituitary subjects. Among the most striking effects are those exerted on bone and cartilage. Following administration of GH in vivo, linear growth of cartilage is accelerated, but increased growth of the epiphysis and premature epiphyseal fusion do not occur. The result is a lengthening of the osseous structures leading to increased tallness. Human subjects with GH deficiency show a diminution of bone mineral content and bone width and also delayed skeletal maturation. The effects in the bone and epiphysis are due to increased protein synthesis. Growth hormone promotes accretion of calcium in the deficient subject, partly by enhancing calcium absorption from the intestine. It has been suggested that GH enhances production of parathormone and, therefore, the synthesis of 1,25-dihydroxyvitamin D, but the evidence is conflicting. The primary effect of GH may be to enhance synthesis of protein in calcium-containing tissues. Increased calcium absorption from the intestine would then occur as a secondary

phenomenon. Type 1 procollagen concentrations in the blood are low in children with GH deficiency and increase into the normal range with GH treatment.[89] Increased protein synthesis also occurs in many other tissues, such as skeletal muscle, liver, kidneys, heart, and the erythropoietic system.[90] Although changes in components of the immune system, such as numbers of B cells and T helper-to-suppressor ratios, have been reported following GH therapy, there is no good evidence that this leads to increased susceptibility to infection.[91]

In those tissues in which its effects have been studied, GH appears to enhance DNA-directed RNA and protein synthesis. This is accompanied by increased transport of amino acids into the cells from extracellular sources. After GH administration, urea production is decreased, suggesting that amino groups normally converted to urea are transaminated to enhanced synthesis of nonessential amino acids. In the human, administration of GH leads to a diminution in urea and amino acid concentrations in the serum. There also occurs a diminution in concentration of inorganic phosphate in the serum.

The effects of GH on carbohydrate metabolism are complex.[92] Intravenous injection of GH is followed by a fall in blood glucose concentration within 20 min. Animal experiments suggest that this fall is caused by enhanced transport of glucose into intracellular compartments of adipose and skeletal muscle cells. These hypoglycemic effects, however, were generally thought to occur only after injection of large doses of GH, but use of more modest doses has also been followed by transient hypoglycemia.

In the child with GH deficiency oral glucose tolerance tests may show impaired ability to dispose of the carbohydrate load, although the blood sugar concentrations achieved are generally lower than in the diabetic state. This impairment of carbohydrate tolerance is associated with significantly diminished insulin production. If insulin is administered to GH-deficient children, lower blood glucose levels are reached and this suggests enhanced insulin sensitivity in the GH-deficient subject. Following administration of GH in therapeutic doses, 0.1 IU/kg three times weekly for several weeks or months, carbohydrate tolerance deteriorates further in spite of increased insulin secretion. In states of GH excess, such as acromegaly, marked impairment of carbohydrate tolerance develops in association with enhanced insulin secretion. There appears to be little evidence for an "insulin-like" action of GH. In the GH-deficient state, impaired secretion of insulin occurs because of pancreatic islet hypoplasia. When GH is administered to deficient individuals, the pancreatic islets are stimulated to produce more insulin. In spite of this, carbohydrate tolerance is not improved because GH antagonizes the effect of insulin on its target organs. Thus, in states of both GH deficiency and excess, altered carbohydrate tolerance is the result of the opposing effects of GH on insulin secretion and insulin action. How GH stimulates insulin secretion is not known. The peripheral antagonism of GH on insulin action does not appear to be due to effects of GH on the insulin receptor (Figs. 1–11, 1–12, and 1–13).

Growth hormone also exerts important actions on lipid metabolism. Growth hormone deficiency is generally accompanied by increased deposition of fat in subcutaneous stores. Injection of GH into such individuals leads to depletion of these stores and their transport to the liver. Within a few hours of administration of GH a rise in plasma nonesterified fatty acids occurs, following an earlier reduction in plasma free fatty acid concentration. This reduction is not related to enhanced secretion of insulin and its

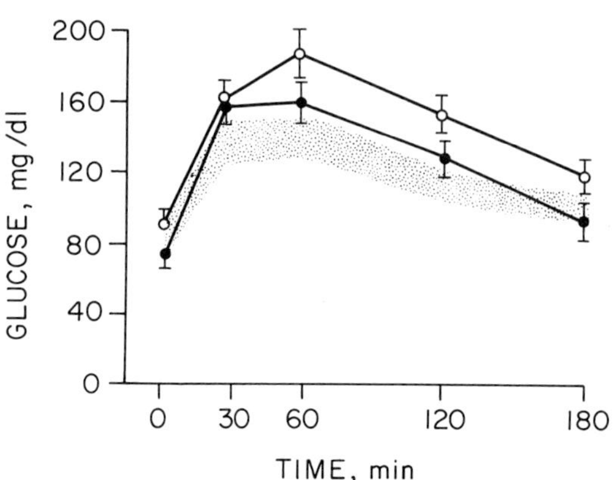

ORAL GLUCOSE TOLERANCE TEST

FIGURE 1–12. Glucose concentrations in the blood of children with growth hormone deficiency before (closed circles) and after (open circles) treatment with growth hormone. The shaded area is the range for normal children. (From Lippe BM, Kaplan SA, Golden MP, et al: Carbohydrate tolerance and insulin receptor binding in children with hypopituitarism: Responses following acute and chronic growth hormone administration. J Clin Endocrinol Metab 53:507, 1981.)

mechanism is not understood. In acromegalic subjects, levels of free fatty acids in the serum are not higher than in GH-deficient subjects.

Somatomedins[93–95]

The concept of somatomedins as mediators of the effects of GH arose from the inability of investigators to demonstrate effects of GH on cartilage in vitro. When GH is administered to deficient animals in vivo, it enhances incorporation of precursors such as sulfate and thymidine into cartilage. Growth hormone does not produce these effects in vitro and neither does serum from hypophysectomized animals. Serum from hypophysectomized animals or GH-deficient humans who have received GH several hours previously, however, does stimulate sulfate incorporation into cartilage. The hypothesis was advanced, therefore, that GH does not act on its target organs directly but generates another factor that mediates its effects. This factor is referred to as somatomedin. Originally, the term *sulfation factor* was used because of the observed effects on sulfate incorporation into cartilage proteoglycans. Subsequently a term of more generalized applicability, *somatomedins*, came into general use following the observation that plasma extracts with sulfation factor activity stimulate other biochemical

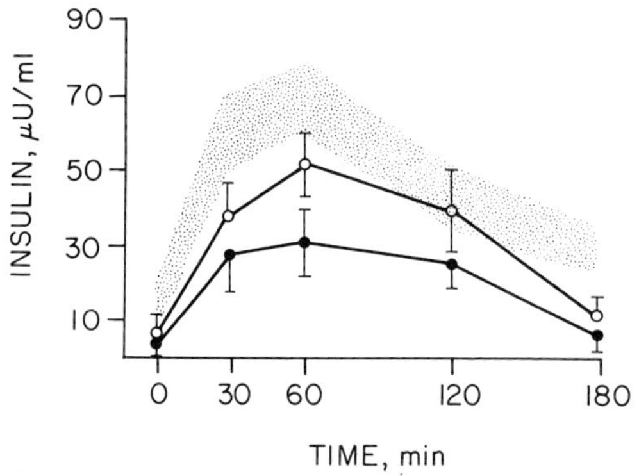

ORAL GLUCOSE TOLERANCE TEST

FIGURE 1–11. Insulin concentrations in the serum of children with growth hormone deficiency before (closed circles) and after (open circles) treatment with growth hormone. The shaded area is the range for normal children. (From Lippe BM, Kaplan SA, Golden MP, et al: Carbohydrate tolerance and insulin receptor binding in children with hypopituitarism: Responses following acute and chronic growth hormone administration. J Clin Endocrinol Metab 53:507, 1981.)

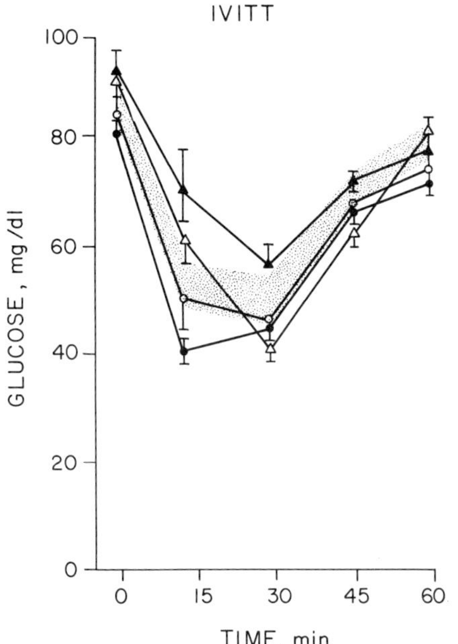

FIGURE 1–13. Glucose concentrations in the blood of children with GH deficiency after injection of insulin, 0.07 U/kg intravenously. Closed circles, before treatment; open circles, after several months of treatment with GH; closed triangles, after short-term treatment with GH in large doses in children undergoing conventional treatment with GH; open triangles, long-term treatment with GH followed by intensive short-term treatment with GH. The shaded area covers the range in normal controls. (From Lippe BM, Kaplan SA, Golden MP, et al: Carbohydrate tolerance and insulin receptor binding in children with hypopituitarism: Responses following acute and chronic growth hormone administration. J Clin Endocrinol Metab 53:507, 1981.)

functions of cartilage, muscle, adipose tissue, and tumor cells in tissue culture.

Somatomedins are peptides with molecular weights of about 7000 to 8000 that circulate in the plasma bound to carrier proteins. These bound complexes have molecular weights of about 50,000 and 150,000 and the concentration in the serum of the largest is GH dependent.[96] The factor that is thought to mediate the effects of GH is now referred to as somatomedin C. It appears that the substances characterized as somatomedins A and B are not related to action of GH. It has also been established that somatomedin C is identical to insulin-like growth factor I (IGF-I).[96] It is a single-chain polypeptide with a molecular weight of about 6000, A, B, and C domains homologous to the A and B chains and connecting peptide of proinsulin, and a D domain extending from the COOH-terminal of the A chain.[97] The structure of IGF-II has considerable homology with IGF-I. Its relationship to GH is not established.

Somatomedin C binds to receptor sites in hepatocytes, chondrocytes, adipocytes, placental circulating monocytes and lymphocytes, and several lines of cultured human cells. Among its effects are stimulation of amino acid transport and synthesis of DNA, RNA, and proteins including proteoglycans and collagen. Insulin-like activities include stimulation of intracellular transport of glucose and incorporation of glucose into glycogen in skeletal muscle. It stimulates glucose uptake and lactate production in heart muscle and glucose transport, glucose oxidation to carbon dioxide, and glucose residue incorporation into lipids. Somatomedins have mitogenic properties in tissue culture systems. In addition to these numerous actions in vitro, some in vivo actions have also been observed. These include enhanced incorporation of glucose into glycogen and lipid, a decrease in serum nonesterified fatty acids, and enhanced glycine incorporation into protein. Another effect observed is a prolonged reduction in blood glucose concentrations. Infusion of somatomedin C into hypophysectomized rats has been followed by an increase in growth rate.[96]

Accurate quantitation of somatomedin C in the plasma has been attended by considerable difficulties. Until highly purified or synthetic somatomedin C became available relatively insensitive bioassays, radioreceptor assays, and competitive binding assays were used. With the advent of radioimmunoassays other problems such as the presence of carrier proteins had to be solved because these interfere with the assay. Failure to solve these problems has led to lack of agreement in the field and conflicting results. Recent studies suggest that a desirable method to remove these interfering proteins is by acid chromatography prior to performance of the reaction with antibody.[98] With the availability of purified or synthetic somatomedin C it appears that 200 ng of somatomedin C is approximately equivalent to 1 unit, the amount of somatomedin C determined by older bioassay methods to be present in 1 ml pooled adult plasma.[99]

The concentrations of somatomedin C in the serum vary considerably with the age of the subject. Bala et al.[100] found mean levels in the newborn to be about 0.4 unit/ml. The mean values fall to less than 0.1 unit/ml in the first few weeks of postnatal life and then gradually increase to about 0.4 unit/ml in the first 3 to 5 years. There is a sharp increase in early puberty to mean levels of about 2.4 and 2.0 units/ml in girls and boys, respectively, these highest values being reached at about ages 13 to 14. The concentrations fall in the late teens to means of about 1 to 1.2 unit/ml. In order to interpret results of radioimmunoassays, therefore, it is essential that the laboratory's normal values for the subject's age are known.

Dependence of Somatomedins on Growth Hormone and Other Factors.   In general, somatomedin C activity tends to parallel that of GH secretion. Variation in levels may reflect the degree of GH deficiency. In states of GH excess, the concentration of somatomedins tends to be high, and levels as high as five times those of normal may be found.

Normal concentrations of somatomedin C are maintained in pregnant animals even after hypophysectomy. It has been inferred that chorionic somatomammotropin sustains the level of somatomedin activity in such experimental models. Somatomedin C activity is blunted by glucocorticoids. Increases of somatomedin C levels at puberty are thought to be mediated by estrogens and androgens. In hypothyroidism somatomedin C levels are diminished. After removal of craniopharyngiomas, children may grow normally even though normal GH release cannot be demonstrated. These children may have normal levels of somatomedin C. Another condition in which somatomedin C levels do not correlate well with GH levels is kwashiorkor, in which high levels of GH are not associated with correspondingly high levels of somatomedins, possibly because of impaired hepatic responses to GH. In poorly controlled diabetics, adequate insulin therapy may lead to improved somatomedin C levels. Starvation may be associated with low levels of somatomedin C which may be increased to normal on refeeding. Chronic liver disease and chronic renal disease may also be characterized by low levels of somatomedin as measured by bioassay.

Somatomedin levels have been measured in individuals with short stature not caused by hypopituitarism. In general, levels have been found to be normal in patients with Turner syndrome or achondroplasia and also in African pygmies. It has also been suggested that somatomedin levels are increased in individuals who are tall for their age and that levels are correlated to some extent with growth velocity. There is no evidence, however, that growth velocity or stature in normal individuals is correlated with GH secretion.

The premise that the actions of GH are mediated by somatomedin C circulating in the plasma after being generated in the liver by action of GH is by no means firmly established. In the first place, it is clear that numerous factors other than GH secretion modulate somatomedin levels. Second, somatomedins have insulin-like actions. It is remarkable that the mediator of actions of a hormone could have effects typical of an antagonist. Third, evidence is beginning to accumulate that GH in physiologic concentrations has direct effects on certain peripheral tissues. Erythrocyte precursors of subjects with Laron-type dwarfism with in vivo GH resistance demonstrate resistance to stimulation by GH in vitro.[101] It is evident that while somatomedins are growth factors whose presence often correlates well with growth and normal nutrition, the evidence that somatomedins are the mediators of effects of GH is by no means conclusive. It is possible that GH stimulates production of somatomedin C in its target cells and somatomedin C exerts its effects as a second messenger in these cells. Leakage of somatomedin C into the blood may be responsible for the correlation observed between GH secretion and somatomedin C levels in the plasma. Evidence favoring the concept that GH influences growth by acting directly on its target tissues is presented by Isaksson et al.[102]

Causes of Growth Hormone Deficiency

1. Congenital
   a. Septo-optic dysplasia
   b. Midline facial or skull defects
   c. Congenital absence of the pituitary
   d. Miscellaneous syndromes

2. Trauma
   a. Accidental, including birth injuries
   b. Surgical damage, including stalk section
   c. Child abuse (battered child) syndrome

3. Infections and other inflammatory diseases
   a. Viral encephalitides

b. Bacterial infections

c. Fungal infections

d. Nonspecific hypophysitis (? autoimmune)

4. Vascular
    a. Aneurysmal malformations of the pituitary vessels
    b. Pituitary infarction

5. Irradiation

6. Toxic sequelae of chemotherapy for malignancies

7. Tumors of the hypothalamus and pituitary—craniopharyngioma, glioma, pinealoma, and so on

8. Histiocytosis

9. Sarcoidosis

10. Idiopathic
    a. Sporadic
    b. Hereditary (including GH gene deletions)

11. Unresponsiveness to growth hormone (Laron type)

Deficiency of growth hormone may result from disease of the hypothalamus or pituitary. The use of GHRH to determine whether the deficiency is in the pituitary or hypothalamus has been discussed previously (p. 27). If an associated deficiency of thyrotropin or gonadotropins exists, use of TRH or gonadotropin-releasing hormone (GRH) may help in elucidating the site of the defect. Thus, in a subject with combined GH and thyrotropin deficiency due to hypothalamic disease, injection of TRH will produce normal or exaggerated secretion of thyrotropin. Classification of causes of GH deficiency according to whether the defect is in the hypothalamus or pituitary is often impractical.

Idiopathic Hypopituitarism. The commonest form of GH deficiency is the *idiopathic type,* that is, one in which no organic lesion can be found during life.[84] The nature of the disorder remains enigmatic. It has been suggested that an autoimmune defect may be responsible as in other autoimmune diseases of the endocrine system, such as chronic lymphocytic thyroiditis, but there is no proof that this mechanism is generally responsible for the development of idiopathic hypopituitarism. Most cases are spontaneous, but some are inherited. It has been estimated as occurring in about 1 of every 60,000 live births in the United Kingdom.[103]

Retrospective studies of the histories of children with idiopathic growth hormone deficiency[104,105] show a high incidence of perinatal problems such as breech births, forceps deliveries, and early vaginal bleeding. Prolonged, or unusually short, labors frequently occur in hypopituitary subjects, as do signs of intrapartum fetal distress or asphyxia. It has been suggested that these perinatal insults may lead to hypopituitarism. On the other hand, if the fetal endocrine system has a participatory role in the induction of labor, it is conceivable that the pituitary or hypothalamic disorder in the fetus itself contributes to abnormal labor and neonatal morbidity.

The GH gene is located on the long arm of chromosome 17.[106,107] The gene has five coding sequences or exons and four introns. Adjacent to the GH gene (GH-N) are four analogs with more than 90 per cent homology with the GH gene. They have been designated the CS-L (silent nonexpressed gene), the chorionic somatomammotropin analog (CS-A) gene, the GH-V gene, an analog of the GH-N gene, and the CS-B gene, an analog of the CS-A gene. Other than the GH-N gene, none of the genes codes for GH in humans. Some are not expressed and others code for proteins the functions of which are not known.

Deletion of the GH-N gene leads to a syndrome referred to as GH deficiency type IA, originally described by Illig et al.[108] The subjects typically have impairment of growth beginning before birth. The length of the infants is only slightly below average but is significantly reduced when their weight and the size of their siblings are taken into account. They have a normal response to GH therapy when this is first begun but develop resistance to GH subsequently because of the appearance of neutralizing GH antibodies. As a consequence, the subjects are extremely short in adult life. The appearance of antibodies is consistent with the concept that the individual's immune system recognizes the GH administered as a foreign protein because the genome has never had the capacity to code for it. The deficiency is transmitted by an autosomal-recessive mode of inheritance. Growth hormone deficiency type IB is similar except that small quantities of GH are present in the serum of the subjects. The disorder is also transmitted by an autosomal-recessive mode of inheritance. No abnormalities in the GH gene have been detected, and children with this disorder do not develop antibodies in sufficient quantities to impair response to GH treatment.

A form of GH deficiency classified as type II is similar to type IB but is inherited in an autosomal-dominant pattern. One other form of inherited GH deficiency has been described in which there is no abnormality in the GH gene and there is no increased propensity for development of neutralizing antibodies. This disorder is transmitted by an X-linked form of inheritance and is classified as type III GH deficiency.[109] In all these forms of genetically transmitted GH deficiency the hormone deficiency is restricted to GH. Case reports have been published in which one of two apparently monozygous twins had isolated GH deficiency, but linkage markers to the GH gene have not been studied in such cases.[110]

Autopsy studies of subjects with idiopathic GH deficiency have been done only on rare occasions. An autopsy examination was performed on a 78-year-old man with proven isolated growth hormone deficiency inherited as a recessive trait.[111] The pituitary gland appeared normal in size and shape on gross examination. Histologic examination showed normal distribution of cell types, and on electron microscopy secretory granules were seen in all the pituitary parenchymal cells. Release of these granules by emiocytosis was not observed in the somatotropes but appeared normal in the basophils, thyrotropes, and gonadotropes. No abnormality of the hypothalamus was seen. This form of GH deficiency appears to be one of secretion rather than impaired synthesis. Little information is available on the autopsy findings of sporadic cases of idiopathic hypopituitarism. From in vivo studies of patients with combined deficiency of GH and TSH, it appears that the hypothalamus is more frequently affected than is the pituitary. In one study of 13 such subjects, administration of TRH led to normal or increased TSH secretion in 10.[112]

In addition to variation in the site of primary organ deficiency, considerable variation also exists in the number of hormones whose secretion is defective. Testing for gonadotropin deficiency of the hypothalamus is not possible in children. It has been suggested, however, that when GH-deficient subjects are tested in their adolescent and adult years, a high proportion will show gonadotropin deficiency.[113] In one study of 35 children with idiopathic GH deficiency, 16 were found to have isolated GH deficiency, 7 had GH deficiency and TSH deficiency, 4 had GH and ACTH deficiency, and 8 had deficiency of GH, TSH, and ACTH. Of those with isolated GH deficiency, 3 of 5 developed puberty by the age of 14. In those with multiple hormone deficiencies who had reached the age of 14, only 1 had developed signs of puberty.[114]

The *clinical features* of GH deficiency are as follows. Usually birth weight and length are normal, except in infants with absence of GH secretion as a result of deletion or abnormality of the GH gene. In infants with idiopathic GH deficiency growth retardation is not apparent until some time after birth, but signs such as hypoglycemia may be manifested in the neonatal period. When GH deficiency develops in the first year, the subjects tend to be thin rather than obese, as is usually the case when GH deficiency develops later on.[115] Characteristic of GH deficiency in early infancy is the development of *hypoglycemia*, occurrence of which in a short child should alert the physician to the possibility that growth hormone deficiency exists. Males with this disorder often have a micropenis.[115] In some instances the hypoglycemia is related to concomitant deficiency of ACTH, but GH deficiency itself can lead to hypoglycemia. This can be proved by the fact that glucocorticoid treatment does not ameliorate the hypoglycemia in many cases, whereas GH treatment does. The hypoglycemia at this age is generally of the fasting type and may be associated with the presence of ketone bodies in the blood and urine. The tendency to spontaneous hypoglycemia tends to disappear between the second and fifth years of life. Recurrent episodes of hypoglycemia may cause permanent cerebral damage and convulsive disorders. Hypoglycemia may occur in the newborn and may be associated with prolonged hyperbilirubinemia.

Growth hormone deficiency leads to abnormal rates of development of the facial bones, leading to protrusion of the frontal bones and poor development of the bridge of the nose. Dental eruption is delayed, and the development and setting of the permanent teeth are irregular. Closure of the anterior fontanel may be delayed for several years. Delay of skeletal maturation is universal, and epiphyseal development is usually delayed to a degree equivalent to the delay in somatic growth. The hair is thin and nail growth is poor. The voice is high pitched. The penis is often quite small, and the apparent abnormality of this organ is accentuated by truncal obesity (Figs. 1–14, 1–15, and 1–16). Delay of puberty is frequent and may be due to deficiency of GH itself. However, if gonadotropin function is intact, puberty will develop sooner or later, much sooner if the subject is treated with GH injections.

If GH deficiency is accompanied by TSH deficiency, symptoms of hypothyroidism may be present in addition. In general, these symptoms are not as marked as in states of primary hypothyroidism. The patient may experience no more than some dryness of the skin, while other symptoms of hypothyroidism such as constipation and cold intolerance may be absent. Thyroid-stimulating hormone deficiency may develop simultaneously with GH deficiency, or it may develop insidiously subsequently. In some instances, TSH deficiency may be induced by therapy with GH (this will be discussed in the section "Treatment of Growth Hormone Deficiency.") Symptoms and signs of concomitant ACTH deficiency are quite subtle and unless the pituitary-adrenal axis is tested by administration of in-

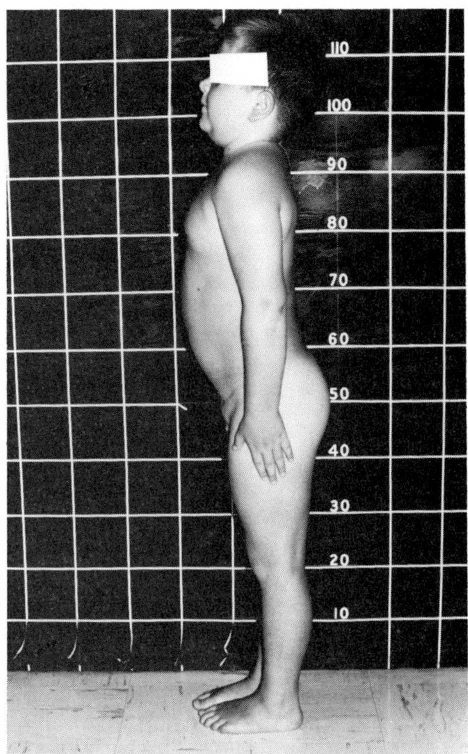

FIGURE 1–15. Boy with GH deficiency, lateral view.

sulin or metyrapone, the deficiency may remain uncovered. An important indication of ACTH deficiency is the development of hypoglycemia. Because hypoglycemia may be due to GH deficiency itself, it is often only possible to determine which hormone deficiency is responsible by treating the subject with GH or glucocorticoids. Mineralocorticoid deficiency is rare in children with hypopituitarism, since aldosterone secretion is largely independent of pituitary ACTH stimulation.

The radiologic signs of GH deficiency include delay in maturation of the epiphyses. The delay is often extreme and its magnitude is related to how long GH deficiency has been present. In a series of 44 subjects (nearly all children), the volume of the sella turcica was found to be abnormally small in about one half.[116]

Tumors of the Brain.[117]   After the idiopathic form, tumors of the brain represent the most frequent cause of GH deficiency. Although tumors in several locations in the brain may have indirect effects on the hypothalamus through anatomic distortion of the brain, the most frequent tumors to impair hypothalamic-pituitary function are midline brain tumors. This group of pathologically diverse tumors includes cranio-

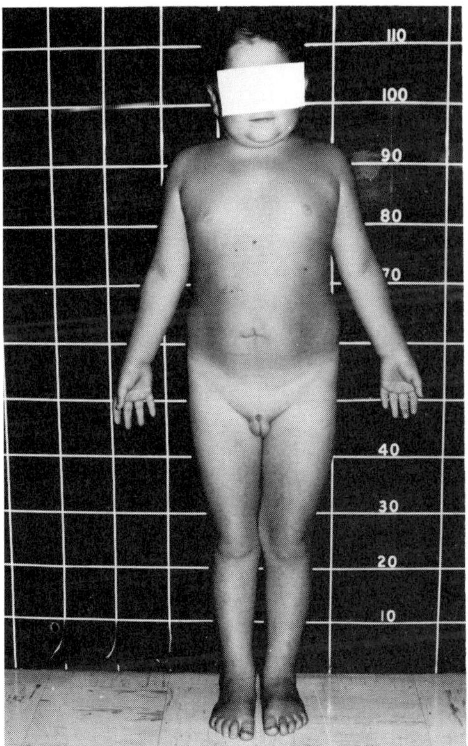

FIGURE 1–14. Boy with typical phenotypic manifestations of GH deficiency. The features of shortness, obesity, and small phallus are illustrated.

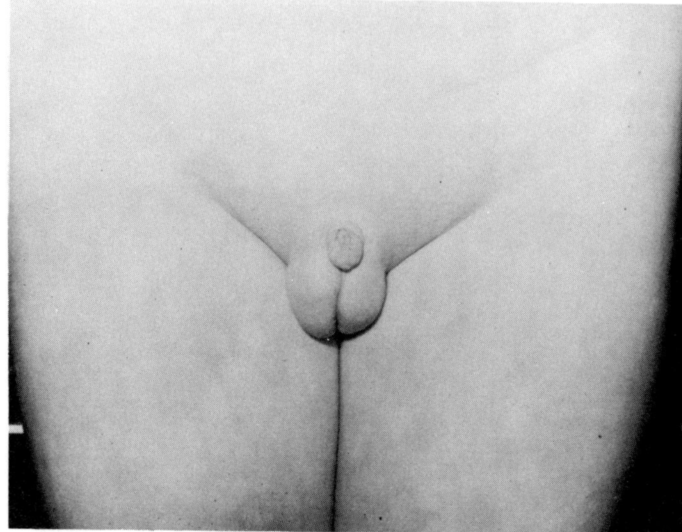

FIGURE 1–16.   Genitalia of boy with GH deficiency. The penis is typically very small.

pharyngioma and glioma of the optic nerve. Rarer tumors causing disturbances of endocrine function are ectopic pinealomas (recently reclassified as germinomas) and various intraventricular neoplasms such as colloid cysts of the third ventricle, papillomas of the choroid plexus, and ependymomas of the third ventricle. Tumors arising from the pituitary are rare causes of endocrine deficiency in children. These include chromophobe adenomas and prolactin-secreting tumors.

Craniopharyngioma. This tumor is believed to arise from remnants of Rathke's pouch, the diverticulum from the roof of the primitive oral cavity that leads to formation of the adenohypophysis. The tumor itself arises from rests of squamous cells at the junction of the adenohypophysis and the neurohypophysis. Although present at birth, the tumor grows very slowly and may not give rise to symptoms or signs for years or even decades. In about 45 per cent of cases the tumor is confined to the suprasellar region. In the rest it involves both suprasellar and infrasellar structures. As it grows it may develop cystic areas. The tumor mass grows forward to compress the optic chiasm, downward to compress the pituitary gland, and upward to impinge on the third ventricle. The tumor is highly variable in histologic structure. It may contain solid masses of epithelial cells, which may become squamous as they line cystic areas. Degeneration of areas of the tumor with calcification and even bone formation may be found. Connective tissue resembling tooth pulp may be

seen. Malignant degeneration is virtually unknown.

The most important feature of craniopharyngioma is its propensity to grow to large sizes without producing typical signs of increased intracranial pressure, such as headache, vomiting, and oculomotor abnormalities. In younger children such symptoms are more likely to occur, but in older children growth impairment may be the only symptom. Visual symptoms, when they occur, vary in nature and intensity. Abnormalities include papilledema with secondary optic atrophy and bitemporal hemianopsia because of compression of the medial tracts of the optic chiasm and nerves. Visual field defects are variable, however, and homonymous hemianopsia may also occur because of compression of the optic nerves. In a series of 34 children with this tumor, 22 had increased intracranial pressure, 21 impaired vision, 14 endocrine abnormalities, 14 papilledema, 3 ataxia, 27 calcification, 17 erosion of the sella, and 8 psychological symptoms.[118] Other symptoms include periods of visual and olfactory hallucinations, abnormalities of the sleep cycle, and dementia. These may be due to involvement of the hypothalamus. Seizures may occur because of involvement of the medial aspect of the temporal lobe. Rarely, ataxia is seen because of involvement of the red nucleus and its connections with the cerebellum.

The most frequent symptom of involvement of the endocrine system is growth failure. In a series of 20 subjects with craniopharyngioma, impairment of GH secretion was found in all but one.[119] The patient with craniopharyngioma may complain only of growth failure and may not have headaches or visual impairment. These subjects are frequently obese, as are many children with GH deficiency. Any child with unexplained growth retardation, obesity, and delayed skeletal maturation should be screened for the presence of a craniopharyngioma by having radiographs taken of the skull and more precise imaging performed if necessary.

Pituitary function is impaired frequently in patients with craniopharyngioma because the tumor is in a location that makes it likely that expansion will damage the hypothalamus or the pituitary itself.[119] Deficiency of ACTH secretion occurs less often than GH deficiency. Thyroid deficiency, however, occurs frequently. In many instances this is caused by direct involvement of the pituitary. In others, administration of TRH produces a normal or exaggerated TSH response, indicating that the hypothyroidism is due to hypothalamic deficiency. Prolactin secretion, surprisingly, tends to be only moderately increased, if at all, in subjects with craniopharyngioma even though the hypothalamus is frequently compressed by the tumor. Gonadotropin deficiency is found in nearly all patients with craniopharyngioma. Low levels of FSH and LH are common, as is a poor response to LRH. Diabetes insipidus is found in 25 to 50 per cent of patients prior to surgery.

Radiographic examination of subjects with craniopharyngioma reveals curvilinear areas of suprasellar calcification in 80 to 90 per cent and distortion of the sella turcica in most of the others (Figs. 1–17 and 1–18). Computed tomography will usually readily identify the tumor by the presence of cystic changes or thickening of the capsule. If cystic changes are absent, however, the tumor may be difficult to detect. Magnetic resonance imaging may be preferable in some cases, but computed tomography is more sensitive for the detection of minute amounts of calcification. Craniopharyngiomas give rise to slightly hypo- or hyperintense images with T_1-weighted magnetic resonance imaging but are markedly hypointense in T_2-weighted images.[120] Most subjects have increased concentrations of protein in spinal or ventricular fluid.

Other tumors in the area that may produce effects similar to craniopharyngioma include optic glioma, chromophobe adenoma, suprasellar meningioma, astrocytoma, and germinoma. The differential diagnosis between these tumors may not be easy prior to surgery.

Primary treatment of the tumor is by surgery. Prognosis depends on whether the tumor can be completely removed. If not, there is a great likelihood that it will recur and eventually cause death. Occasionally, evacuation of a cyst will temporarily relieve symptoms of pressure. Without surgery, life expectancy is 3 to 4 years from the onset of symptoms. About 40 per cent of all patients appear to survive for 8 years or more.

Results of surgical treatment of 42 patients

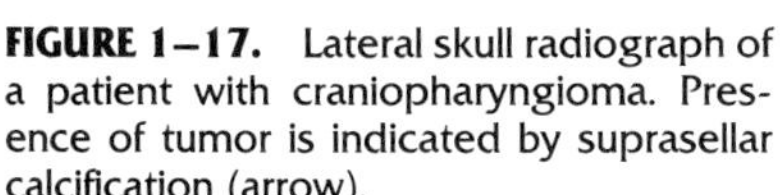

FIGURE 1–17. Lateral skull radiograph of a patient with craniopharyngioma. Presence of tumor is indicated by suprasellar calcification (arrow).

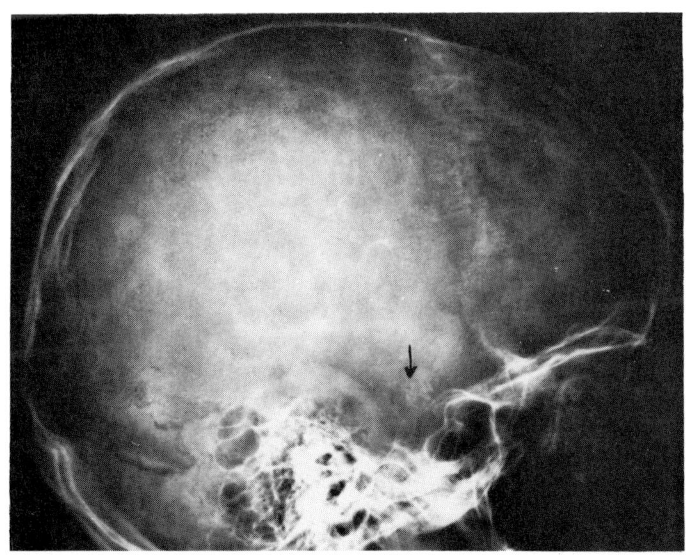

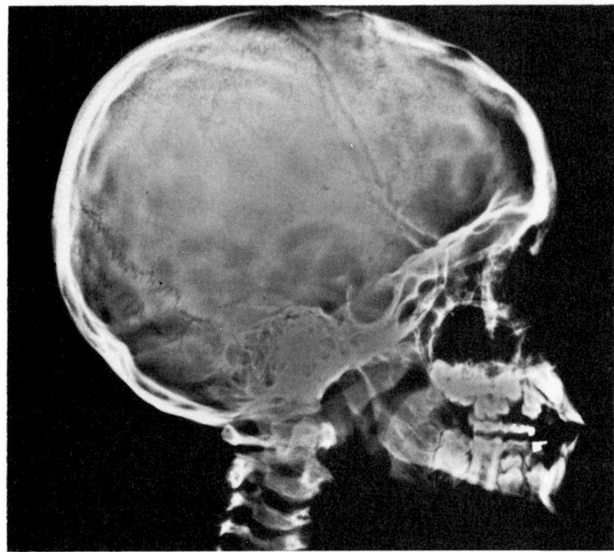

FIGURE 1–18. Lateral skull radiograph of a patient with craniopharyngioma. The tumor caused enlargement of the pituitary fossa.

with craniopharyngioma have been presented.[121] Following surgery, endocrine function always deteriorated and never improved. One of the most distressing sequelae of surgery for craniopharyngioma is rapid and extreme weight gain. The reason for this is not clear and several hypotheses have been advanced to explain it. Involvement of the appetite control center in the hypothalamus may be responsible. Another unexplained sequel of surgery for craniopharyngioma is normal or excessive growth, even though the usual stimulatory tests fail to evoke normal secretion of growth hormone into the blood. Considerable controversy has surrounded the question of optimal treatment of craniopharyngioma for many years. Radical excision in the hands of some has led to long-term survival, but even in these cases there are recurrences as long as 20 years after surgery. On the other hand, partial excision when the tumor cannot be removed in toto and subsequent irradiation may be followed by fewer deaths and fewer recurrences. Radiation itself, however, carries some hazards, as will be discussed later in this chapter. Nevertheless, the approach of limited excision and irradiation is considered by some to be highly satisfactory if the tumor cannot be removed without seriously endangering vital structures in the area of the tumor.

Other Tumors.   Other tumors that are associated with hypopituitarism include chromophobe adenomas, which are rare in children. Germinomas, meningiomas, gliomas, colloid cysts of the third ventricle, ependymomas, and metastatic carcinomas may impair function of the pituitary and hypothalamus. In adults, metastases from breast carcinoma are among the most frequently associated with hypofunction of the pituitary. Ependymomas and germinomas arising at some distance from the hypothalamus may spread to the floor of the third ventricle by seeding and give the appearance of multiple tumors. Sarcomas of the pituitary have also been reported to cause hypopituitarism. Tumors outside the cranium but extending into the pituitary-hypothalamic area, such as craniopharyngeal carcinoma and Hodgkin disease of the nasopharynx, may also cause hypopituitarism.

Congenital Malformations of the Brain

Septo-optic Dysplasia.[122–124]   The combination of optic nerve anomalies and agenesis of the septum pellucidum has been known for about 40 years. Only recently, however, has it been recognized that this combination of abnormalities also extends to impaired function of the hypothalamus and pituitary. The syndrome of hypopituitarism associated with septo-optic dysplasia is now considered a common cause of GH deficiency, ranking behind the idiopathic and brain tumor categories as perhaps the third most frequent cause of hypopituitarism in children.

The factors responsible for development of this congenital anomaly are not known. There is no evidence that the condition is inherited, although it does occasionally occur in siblings. A remarkable observation made by several writers is the unusually young age of many of the mothers. Both sexes appear affected, and there is an increase in frequency among first born. The dysplasia is considered a form of holoprosencephaly because it is a result of abnormal induction of tissue from the forebrain. Hypopituitarism may be a consequence of extension of the anterior midline abnormalities into the hypothalamus. About 70 per cent of those studied by pneumoencephalograph show absence of the septum pellucidum, but optic nerve hypoplasia and hypopituitarism occur without demonstrable abnormality of the septum pellucidum.

The endocrine deficiencies involve several hormones of both anterior and posterior pituitary lobes. Growth hormone deficiency is the most frequent abnormality, but TSH and ACTH deficiencies also occur. The primary defect is in the hypothalamus. Vasopressin deficiency may also occur. The lesions of the optic nerve are not always easily discernible. They consist of hypoplasia of the optic nerve heads, an abnormality that is more quantitative than qualitative and may only be appreciated if photographic measurements of the diameters of the optic nerve heads are made. The optic nerve lesion may be unilateral. The disk may have an inner hypoplastic margin and a halo. In any case, amblyopia is quite marked, and searching nystagmus is characteristic of the syndrome.

Other features of the syndrome are hypoglycemia in the newborn period, prolonged jaundice, apnea, and hypotonia. Also described is the occurrence of hepatomegaly, psychomotor retardation, and receding mandible. In some instances growth failure may not be evident in the first few years of life. Hypoglycemia (and possibly jaundice) is due to growth hormone or ACTH deficiency in the newborn. Few patients have reached the age of sexual maturity and thus far there is no evidence that gonadotropin deficiency is a part of this disorder. In rare instances subjects with septo-optic dysplasia have even developed sexual precocity.

Other Forms of Holoprosencephaly. The association of hypopituitarism with other forms of holoprosencephaly has also been noted.[125,126] During the third week of fetal life, the prechordal mesoderm migrates forward to an area anterior to the notochord, and this process is necessary for induction and morphogenesis of the forebrain. Various external malformations occur, which, when severe, may lead to cyclopia. Less severe malformations may result in hypertelorism, absence of the philtrum or nasal septum, herniation of the brain through the base of the skull, and cleft lip and palate. Involvement of the brain may be associated with hypopituitarism. In some cases the pituitary is absent, and death may occur shortly after birth as a result of glucocorticoid deficiency. The disorder may be genetically transmitted, and there may be a variation in expression of the disorder in different members of the family. Growth hormone deficiency may not be present.

The issue of whether GH deficiency also occurs more frequently in patients with cleft lip and palate has been raised.[127] It would appear that the defect may involve the pituitary in some instances. On the other hand, we have studied several short children with cleft lip and palate and have not found deficiency of GH secretion in any of them. The issue is not yet resolved. It is of interest that many subjects with the syndrome of holoprosencephaly do not have defects of olfaction as occurs in Kallmann syndrome. Another rare congenital malformation is the association of GH deficiency with the development of a single central upper incisor and abnormalities in development of the nose.

Histiocytosis.[128,129] Histiocytosis X consists of three types of disorders: disseminated acute, disseminated chronic, and the solitary form. Initially the solitary form may affect one bone only. Subsequently, additional lesions may develop in other bones or parenchymatous organs. The etiology of the disorder is not known. The disorders were once referred to as Hand-Schüller-Christian disease, eosinophilic granuloma, and Letterer-Siwe disease but are now grouped together under the title of histiocytosis X. The histologic appearances of the different disorders are not clearly distinguishable, and one form of the disorder may progress to another. Lesions of bone are commonly found in association with anemia, skin eruptions, seborrhea of the scalp and external ear canals, stomatitis, hepatomegaly, and pulmonary infiltrates. Infiltration of the skull may produce lucent areas of bone loss and, if the orbits are involved, proptosis.

Growth retardation occurs in about half of the cases of chronic disseminated histiocytosis. It may also occur in association with solitary lesions. A large proportion of cases have inadequate responses to GH stimulation tests. Loss of normal GH secretory capacity can occur at any time during progression of the disease. Other manifestations of GH deficiency in patients with histiocytosis are abnormal glucose tolerance tests, increased sensitivity to administration of insulin, and pubertal delay. Other hormones of the anterior pituitary may be involved but less frequently than GH. Assessment of FSH, LH, and TSH functions has often shown these to be normal. Involvement of the posterior pituitary with diabetes insipidus, however, is quite common.

Treatment of the disorder depends on the nature of involvement of the organ systems of the body. Combinations of prednisone, vinblastine, 6-mercaptopurine, methotrexate, and vincristine have been used with considerable success. The disease process can often be arrested, but if diabetes insipidus develops, it is generally permanent. Short stature is sometimes a consequence of therapy. Glucocorticoid therapy may impair growth. Chemotherapy and irradiation of the skull can also lead to hypopituitarism.

Irradiation of the Brain.   Treatment of tumors of the brain, face, head, or neck frequently requires the use of irradiation. Such irradiation, whether directed at the hypothalamic-pituitary area or other portions of the head, may lead to impairment of pituitary function.[130,131] The hormone most frequently affected is GH. In fact, it is rare for other hormones to be involved. Deceleration of growth is often the first sign of damage and may occur within a few months of the course of radiation. On the other hand, reports have appeared that it may take as long as 10 years or more for evidence of pituitary dysfunction to appear. The hypothalamus is primarily affected, and pituitary dysfunction is presumably due to impaired release of GHRH.[132] Damage to the hypothalamus may occur following treatment of tumors with such diverse origins as retinoblastoma, sarcoma of the middle ear, nasopharyngeal carcinoma, and tumors of the cervical lymph nodes. The higher the dose of radiation to the brain the greater is the likelihood of hypothalamic dysfunction. Doses such as those used for the treatment of leukemia may possibly be followed by GH deficiency,[133] but courses in excess of 5000 rads are more likely to do so.[131] Use of GH for the treatment of children with irradiation-induced GH deficiency is often not as effective as it is with other forms of GH deficiency. Their growth response may be blunted while their skeletal maturation is accelerated.[134] Thyroid-stimulating hormone and ACTH secretion are much less frequently involved. The incidence of gonadotropin deficiency is less well defined because the children studied have often not reached pubertal years. Studies of adult subjects, however, have shown that gonadotropin function may be disturbed as well. By releasing-factor testing procedures, it has been determined that the hypothalamus rather than the pituitary is the primary site of disordered function. In some cases of thyroid dysfunction following irradiation, it has been shown that the thyroid gland itself has been damaged by irradiation and may undergo malignant degeneration. Other harmful effects of radiation include the possible induction of malignancy in the pituitary following large doses of irradiation.[135]

Miscellaneous Causes.   *Vascular Disturbances.*   Hypofunction of the pituitary-hypothalamic system may result from vascular disturbances. These include malformation of the arteriovenous system[136] and infarction of the pituitary-hypothalamic area. Pituitary necrosis such as occurs postpartum (Sheehan syndrome) is rare in the pediatric age group.

Trauma.   Hypopituitarism may be caused by trauma.[137] Fracture of the sella turcica and other forms of cerebral injury may lead to impairment of function of either the anterior pituitary, the posterior pituitary, or both. The role of trauma to the brain during the perinatal period in the production of hypopituitarism has already been discussed. Another important circumstance in which trauma plays a role is in *child abuse.*[138] In another section of this chapter, the syndrome of deprivation dwarfism is discussed, in which growth retardation occurs but true GH deficiency is generally absent. Children with environmental deprivation may show inadequate responses to GH-releasing stimuli such as insulin or arginine, but they resume normal growth without administration of GH if transferred to a favorable environment. In the syndrome of child abuse, trauma to the brain with subdural hematomas and cerebral contusion may lead to permanent organic hypopituitarism.

Inflammatory Disease.   Impairment of pituitary function may be caused by inflammatory disease of the pituitary and hypothalamus of various kinds.[139] Growth hormone deficiency has occurred in individuals who have had acute bacterial or viral infections, tuberculous meningoencephalitis, syphilis, and granulomatous diseases of various types. The association in some instances may be coincidental. From time to time reports have appeared of granulomatous lymphadenoid hypophysitis leading to hypopituitarism.[140,141] Associated with this, antibodies to pituitary proteins are found in the serum by immunofluorescent techniques. Moreover, subjects with polyglandular autoimmune disease of peripheral endocrine organs may also occasionally develop antibodies to pituitary cells. Thus, hypopituitarism may also occur in the complex of disorders characterized by autoimmune thyroiditis, adrenalitis, parathyroiditis, and so on and mucocutaneous candidiasis. Rare cases of idiopathic hypothalamic atrophy have been described.[142]

Sarcoidosis.[143]   The pituitary or hypothalamus as well as the optic nerves may be affected by sarcoidosis. A variety of deficiencies of the anterior pituitary have been described, including deficiency of GH, TSH, ACTH, and gonadotropins. Sarcoid may involve the neurohypophysis, leading to impairment of normal water metabolism.

Empty Sella Syndrome.   The empty sella syndrome is one in which the sella turcica is completely or partially filled with cerebrospinal fluid on radiologic examination. In the absence of surgical or other trauma the condition is considered as primary and is apparently due to incompetence of the sellar diaphragm. In the majority of adults with an empty sella there is no evidence of pituitary dysfunction. Children undergo radiographic studies of the sella most frequently as part of the investigation of growth disorders, and in them as many as one fourth were found to have an empty sella.[144] In the author's clinic the prevalence of empty sella detected by computed tomography in children with GH deficiency is considerably lower. In children with empty sella syndrome abnormalities of pituitary function are common—in one series, 13 of 19 cases.[145] The abnormality most frequently seen is GH deficiency, but others, such as diabetes insipidus, sexual precocity, hyperprolactinemia, and panhypopituitarism, may occur.

Peripheral Resistance to Growth Hormone.[146–148]   The majority of children with growth failure do not have GH deficiency.

Growth hormone–releasing tests show normal responses, and it is assumed that growth retardation is caused by factors other than impairment of GH secretion. In some, the reason for growth impairment is obvious. For example, in achondroplasia, an intrinsic defect in the bones exists that impairs the ability of the bones to grow normally even though they are exposed to normal amounts of GH.

The concept of true growth hormone resistance is reserved for a disorder described by Laron and his associates in which the typical somatic abnormalities occurring with GH deficiency are found (growth failure, truncal obesity, micropenis, protrusion of the frontal bones, and so on) in association with high circulating levels of GH. It has been suggested that the defect in this disorder may be a failure of generation of somatomedin C in response to action of GH. Increases in somatomedin C activity normally seen following administration of GH do not occur in these Laron-type dwarfs, possibly because of a diminution of GH binding by receptors in the liver.[148] There is a possibility, however, that the deficiency is due to lack of action of GH itself on target tissues.[101]

The subjects with Laron-type dwarfism have a delay of skeletal maturation, increased subcutaneous fat, small hands and feet, small face and mandible, protuberant frontal bones, hypoplastic nasal bridge, delayed dentition, and high-pitched voice, and males have hypoplastic external genitals. Growth hormone–releasing tests such as insulin hypoglycemia show unusually high levels of GH in the blood, generally between 50 and 100 ng/ml. The GH produced by these subjects is biologically active and binds normally to GH receptors. Administration of GH does not lead to enhanced growth, increased nitrogen excretion, or other effects of GH seen in normal or GH-deficient individuals. Also, there is little if any increase in somatomedin C levels in the blood. Subjects with Laron-type dwarfism may experience hypoglycemia, may show increased insulin sensitivity, and often have glucose intolerance. Puberty is delayed and testicular enlargement generally does not begin until age 12 to 14. Menarche is delayed until age 13 or 14. The patients are presumably fertile, and thus far two Laron-type dwarfs, one male and one female, have had children. Growth delay is extreme, however, and the final height reached is rarely in excess of 130 cm.

The disease occurs largely in Jewish families of oriental origin in Israel. Both sexes are affected. The parents are usually of normal height, and it would appear that the condition is transmitted as a recessive trait.

Aside from the conditions listed above reports have been published of the occurrence of GH deficiency in subjects who have other diseases. The list includes α_1-antitrypsin deficiency, chromosome abnormalities not involving chromosome 17, immunoglobulin deficiency, cystic fibrosis of the pancreas, microcephaly, orocraniodigital syndrome, ectodermal dysplasia, Russell-Silver syndrome, congenital rubella, Rieger syndrome. Down syndrome, fetal alcohol syndrome, and "CHARGE" syndrome. There is no good evidence yet that this association can be attributed to anything but chance.

Tests for Growth Hormone Deficiency[149–154]

Deficiency of GH is characterized by well-defined characteristics present in a minority of children with growth retardation. Testing for GH deficiency is not carried out routinely on all subjects with short stature. The diagnostic approach in growth deficiency is described elsewhere in this chapter, including the reasoning leading to a decision to undertake testing for GH deficiency (pp. 51–52).

Growth hormone concentrations in the plasma of normal individuals are often low and may be undetectable by current assay procedures. Random sampling of the blood for measurement of GH levels is therefore of little value. Growth hormone levels should be measured after appropriate stimuli are given for secretion. Because a number of stimuli increase GH secretion (L-dopa, propranolol, estrogens, glucagon, exercise, insulin, arginine, and so on), it is to be expected that considerable variation will occur among endocrinologists in the methods used for growth hormone testing.

Growth hormone is generally measured by immunoassay; that is, its concentration in serum is quantitated by methods that depend on the use of antibodies developed against GH. Depending on the nature of the antibody and its specificity, however, the concentrations reported may vary considerably.[155] Newer methods of radioimmunoassay employ monoclonal antibodies specifically directed against different parts of the GH molecule. Immunoradiometric assays (IRMAs) use two separate antibodies in a single assay, and since they are directed at different parts of the GH molecule they are much more specific and tend to give much lower results. In order to interpret results of an assay correctly it is necessary to know the normal range of responses to a stimulation test or other methods of testing of the laboratory. In the study reported by Reiter et al. the IRMA assay gave results that were about 65 per cent of those given by standard radioimmunoassays.[155]

Testing is often divided into screening tests and definitive tests. Establishing the existence of GH deficiency is most important because, at present, GH with rare exceptions is available only for treatment of subjects with deficiency. To establish the existence of GH deficiency beyond reasonable doubt, injections of insulin and arginine have been used most frequently. Even with this combination of agents, however, children with normal GH reserve occasionally fail to respond normally by increasing their GH concentration to normal levels. In order to obviate the necessity for repeated testing, therefore, endocrinologists have added an additional stimulating factor, estrogen administration, to minimize the number of subnormal responses in normal subjects.

The insulin-arginine-estrogen test requires induction of hypoglycemia, and blood sampling over 2.5 hours. Accordingly, efforts have been made to develop simpler screening tests that, if they show normal GH hormone responses, eliminate the need for the insulin-arginine-estrogen tests. Utilization has been made of the fact that exercise, sleep, or administration of glucagon, L-dopa, clonidine, or propranolol enhance GH secretion.

A screening test that has been widely used for GH deficiency is the measurement of GH in the plasma after exercise. Because the amount of exercise performed has varied, experience with the test has been disappointing and doubt cast on its reliability. In the recent past the amount of exercise performed has been standardized by the use of bicycle ergometers and this has led to greater reliance on the test.[156] If the exercise test is to be used, the subjects must achieve the energy expenditure essential for adequate secretion of GH. Exercise has been combined with other stimuli of GH secretion, such as L-dopa, in order to achieve maximal GH secretion.

In recent years the use of clonidine, an α_2-adrenergic receptor agonist, for the diagnosis of GH deficiency has become increasingly widespread. The test is relatively easy to perform and it is apparently as reliable as most other screening tests.[81,157] A single oral dose of clonidine is administered, approximately 100 μg/sq m of body surface area, and a single sample of blood is collected after 60 min for measurement of GH. The test is relatively free of side effects, but occasionally somnolence may occur and it is important that the subject be recumbent during the test and not be permitted to ambulate until fully recovered. Somnolence is particularly likely to occur when the clonidine test is done after other procedures, such as sampling for 24 hours for the diagnosis of GH deficiency. The low dose of 100 μg/sq m is unlikely to result in low concentrations of cortisol in the blood, but the possibility of this occurrence must be kept in mind.

The screening test most frequently used in the author's clinic is a combination of administration of L-dopa and propranolol; its use is based on the findings of others that these two agents effectively stimulate GH secretion in a large proportion of normal subjects.[152] After an overnight fast, the subject ingests L-dopa (125 mg if the subject's weight is less than 10 kg, 250 mg if between 10 and 30 kg, and 500 mg if greater than 30 kg) and propranolol (0.75 mg/kg up to a maximum dose of 40 mg). Two samples of blood are drawn, one at 60 and the other at 90 min after ingestion of the stimulating agents. If either sample has a concentration of GH in excess of 7 ng/ml, the subject is considered to have normal GH secretory reserve. Some nausea and vomiting are not infrequent during the test, and the subjects are advised to lie down quietly during the test. If vomiting does occur, it is usually 30 to 40 min after ingestion of the stimulating agents and after they have been absorbed. Blood should still be obtained on schedule because normal levels of GH are achieved despite the vomiting. On rare occasions marked hypoglycemia has occurred with this test; in our experience, it has developed in less than 1 per cent of tested subjects. Nevertheless, it is prudent to have glucose available for oral and, very rarely, intravenous administration. This test will eliminate over 90 per cent of children with normal GH reserve. A

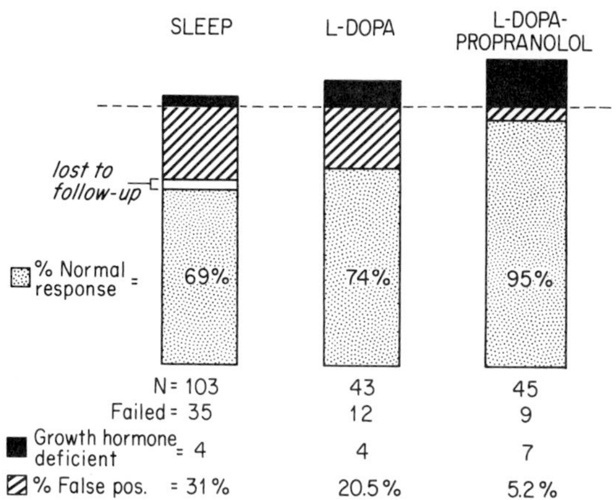

FIGURE 1–19. Growth hormone concentrations in the plasma during three screening tests: sleep, levodopa, and levodopa plus propranolol (see text). Solid area above the broken line indicates the proportion of patients subsequently proven to have GH deficiency. The stippled areas indicate the proportion of subjects in whom GH deficiency was excluded by the screening test. The hatched area shows the percentage of patients in whom the screening test suggested deficiency of GH but in whom the estrogen-insulin-arginine combination of stimuli produced normal secretion of growth hormone. (From Fass B, Lippe BM, Kaplan SA: Relative usefulness of three growth hormone stimulation screening tests. Am J Dis Child 133:931, 1979. Copyright 1979, American Medical Association.)

high proportion of those who fail this test are subsequently shown to have GH deficiency (Fig. 1–19). To increase the accuracy of the screening test, other stimuli have been added, such as estrogens. The value of these additions has not yet been determined. Patients with asthma, previous hypoglycemia, and certain cardiocirculatory disorders should not receive propranolol.

If the screening test shows that the subject does not achieve a level of 7 ng/ml in the plasma, a combined estrogen-insulin-arginine test is done. The method described here is the one carried out in the author's clinic. Other endocrinologists use a test similar to that described by Penny et al.[150] The test in our clinic is performed as follows. Premarin is taken for 3 days prior to the test in a dosage of 5 mg daily if the subject weighs less than 30 kg and 5 mg twice daily if the weight is more than 30 kg. The patient is admitted to the hospital overnight for testing in the morning. No food is administered before the test. Regular insulin is administered intravenously in a dosage of 0.05 to 0.1 unit/kg. The dose of insulin should be sufficient to produce a fall in blood glucose of 40 per cent of the preinjection concentration. Generally we administer smaller doses to subjects who we believe are likely to have GH deficiency and therefore will show excessive sensitivity to insulin. The patient is observed closely, especially for the first hour of the test, and glucose is given intravenously if profound hypoglycemia occurs. However, this rarely occurs. Blood is obtained every 15 min beginning immediately for 2.5 hours. All samples are analyzed for GH concentration, and two samples (the one drawn immediately before the insulin injection and the one drawn 60 min later) are also analyzed for cortisol. Beginning 1 hour after the insulin injection, arginine hydrochloride, 10 per cent in aqueous solution, is infused intravenously over a 45-min period in a dosage of 0.5 gm/kg body weight (Fig. 1–20).

If levels of GH in excess of 10 ng/ml are achieved, the patient is considered to have normal GH reserve. If the level is less than 7 ng/ml, the patient is considered to have GH deficiency. On rare occasions when the highest value reached is between 7 and 10 ng/ml, the patient is considered to have partial GH deficiency. These subjects are also considered candidates for therapy with GH (Fig. 1–21).

The test is useful also for determining the presence of ACTH deficiency, since insulin-induced hypoglycemia is also a potent stimulus for secretion of ACTH. Ordinarily, if plasma cortisol levels in excess of 20 µg/ml are reached, the subject is considered to have normal ACTH reserve. Administration of estrogen for three days, however, causes considerable increase in levels of corticosteroid-binding globulins in the plasma, and under these circumstances higher levels, as much as 35 µg/dl, may have to be reached

if the test is to be interpreted as indicating normal ACTH reserve. It is not feasible to carry out a metyrapone stimulation test in a subject, who has ingested estrogen in the doses necessary for the test because metyrapone is rapidly metabolized and excreted under these conditions.

Despite these disadvantages, we continue to use Premarin in combination with insulin and arginine because its use appears to diminish substantially the need for repeating tests in subjects who may fail the test if given insulin and arginine alone.

A necessary precondition for this test, as for all tests of GH reserve (screening or definitive), is normal thyroid function. If testing has shown that the individual is hypothyroid, thyroid medication must be given in adequate dosage for 3 to 4 weeks before testing for GH reserve is undertaken.

In an effort to reduce the number of false-positive responses, several stimuli here are used in combination, e.g., estrogen, insulin, and arginine. This has given rise to concerns in the minds of some that subjects with partial GH deficiency or diminished reserve may not have such a deficiency detected because of the potency of the combination of agents used for the test. This concern is legitimate, but at present no substantial evidence exists that subjects with GH deficiency are going undetected with the use of these combined testing procedures.

It has been suggested that the results of stimulation tests to induce GH secretion do not necessarily provide an accurate assessment of an individual's ability to secrete GH. For example, if a subject secretes GH in response to insulin-induced hypoglycemia, it may not necessarily follow that in the

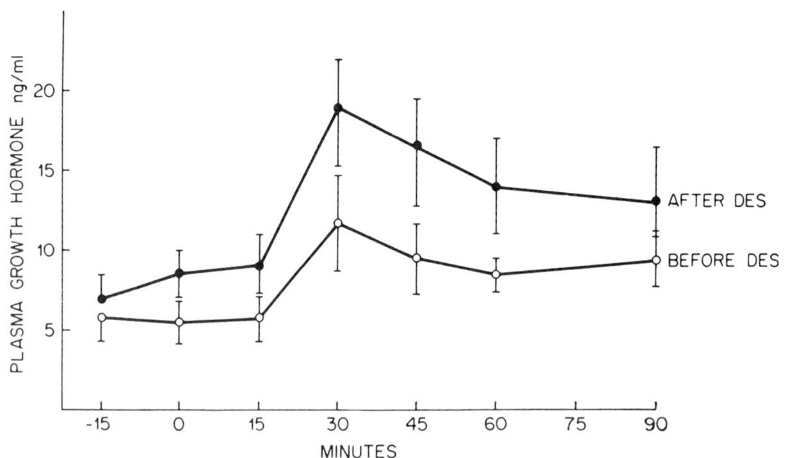

FIGURE 1–20. Growth hormone concentrations in the plasma following insulin hypoglycemia. When diethylstilbestrol was administered as described in the text, the GH response was significantly augmented. Currently Premarin is used instead of diethylstilbestrol. (From Lippe B, Wong S-LR, Kaplan SA: Simultaneous assessment of growth hormone and ACTH reserve in children pretreated with diethylstilbestrol. J Clin Endocrinol Metab 33:949, 1971.)

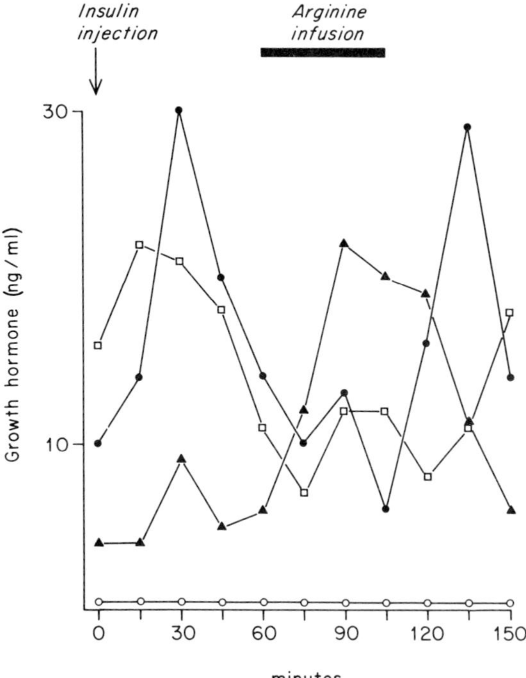

FIGURE 1–21. Growth hormone levels in the plasma of three prepubertal subjects with short stature during estrogen-insulin-arginine stimulation test. Variation in response to insulin and arginine is evident.

normal course of events (that do not include the daily occurrence of hypoglycemia) GH would be secreted in amounts sufficient to effect normal growth. Bercu et al.[158] and Chalew et al.[159] found a poor correlation between "provocative" testing and measurement of GH concentrations in the serum following repeated sampling every 20 min or by a constant withdrawal technique over 24 hours. The term *neurosecretory dysfunction* has been coined to describe the condition in patients who respond normally to "provocative" testing but show subnormal endogenous levels of secretion over prolonged periods of testing. There is no general agreement regarding the diagnostic criteria to establish the presence of this condition, however. These vary from investigator to investigator according the conditions of testing. Factors that complicate the problem are the variations in the concentration of GH arrived at by different methods of assay (discussed elsewhere in this chapter) and differences in integrated levels of 24-hour secretion with age.[160] For example, in one study a mean concentration of GH of less than 2.5 ng/ml was regarded as compatible with the diagnosis of GH neurose-

cretory dysfunction.[161] In another report the mean concentration in normally growing children ranged from 0.5 to 5.6 ng/ml with an average of 1.6.[162] As would be expected from what is known about the effects of estrogens and androgens on the secretion of GH, the integrated levels are significantly increased with the onset and progression of puberty. Another cause for concern in regard to the use of secretory profiles for the diagnosis of GH deficiency is the reproducibility of the assay procedure. Subjects studied on successive nights may experience a doubling or more of the pooled GH concentration between the two sets of observations.[163] While there may be merit in doing GH testing under normal, everyday conditions, proof that subjects with "neurosecretory dysfunction" have GH deficiency must depend on the evidence that their growth rates are substantially improved by therapy with GH. The problem is complicated because evidence is beginning to accumulate that children who do not have GH deficiency may experience at least a temporary acceleration of growth when they receive treatment with GH. The reasons for this observation are not understood but they may be related to the fact that the dosage of GH used for treatment leads to higher concentrations of GH in the plasma than are found under normal circumstances. While children with GH deficiency generally experience sustained growth after many years of treatment, it is not known how long subjects who do not have GH deficiency will continue to respond to treatment with GH. Twenty-four–hour studies of GH secretory patterns do not appear to have much value in predicting the growth response to GH treatment even after short periods of treatment.[162]

Similar data have been published by Rose et al.[164] They studied 54 prepubertal children with short stature, including 23 with GH deficiency identified by provocative tests. Nearly half of the children with GH deficiency had normal spontaneous GH secretion. On the other hand, no child with normal stimulated GH levels had diminished levels of spontaneously secreted GH.

The enthusiasm for the concept of neurosecretory dysfunction and the necessity for measuring endogenous secretion of GH in order to make the diagnosis of GH deficiency appears to have to abated somewhat at the time of this writing. The current consensus appears to be that "provocative" testing is the best method for establishing the diagnosis.

Aside from the above considerations a major disadvantage of the use of endogenous secretion to establish the diagnosis of GH deficiency is the necessity for withdrawal of blood every 20 or 30 min over the day or night. A possible solution to this part of the problem is to measure GH in the urine collected over a 24-hour period. Using highly sensitive immunoassays Albini et al.[165] and Sukegawa et al.[166] have found that GH secretion rates in the urine correlate well with information obtained from sampling of the blood. Because normal children may excrete very small quantities of GH in the urine and the lower limit of the normal range may be difficult to define, it remains to be seen if this method can be used as a discriminator for the diagnosis of GH deficiency.

Treatment of Growth Hormone Deficiency (Fig. 1–22)

Unlike other protein hormones, GH exhibits a remarkable degree of species specificity, and only human GH can produce significant growth in humans. (An exception to this rule is the GH of certain anthropoid species, but this is not a practical source of GH for clinical use.) Growth hormone produced from human pituitaries has always been in short supply because of the problems associated with obtaining sufficient material from which to extract the hormone. A search for synthetic means to produce GH was begun many years ago, and when recombinant DNA technology became available GH was one of the first proteins to be synthesized by this method. The original approach used is standard for many of the peptides synthesized by this technique. Messenger RNA is isolated from pituitary cells grown in tissue culture and is used as a template for the synthesis of a complementary strand of DNA (cDNA), which is then subjected to further chemical manipulation to form a double strand of DNA. This double strand, representing the GH gene, is inserted into a plasmid that is, in turn, inserted into *Escherichia coli*, the bacterium used for the synthesis of GH. Other microorganisms, such as yeast, may also be used for this purpose. A molecule of methionine was included originally because the amino acid was used as a start signal for the transcription of the DNA template. The GH that

was made available for clinical use contained the extra amino acid and is referred to as methionyl-GH. This preparation was as effective in promoting growth as extracted GH. A question has arisen as to whether it is more likely to induce antibody production because it is different from the native hormone. There are no clear answers to this question at present. Antibodies do develop following injection of methionyl-GH, but they also occur following the use of natural (extracted) GH as is described elsewhere in this chapter. In any case recent developments in the field of molecular biology have made it possible for GH to be produced without the extra methionine, and synthetic GH is now available that is identical to the naturally produced human GH. When it became evident that GH extracted from pituitary glands carried the risk of Creutzfeldt-Jakob syndrome this source of GH was virtually eliminated, and recombinant DNA GH is virtually the only form used at present.[167–169]

It has been known for some time that GH therapy was effective in the treatment of GH deficiency, and until synthetic GH became available its use was restricted largely to subjects with proven GH deficiency. At present, the increased availability of GH has permitted its use, at least experimentally, in the treatment of subjects who are not deficient in GH, such as girls with Turner syndrome (see Chapter 9), children and adolescents with chronic renal failure, and children with intrauterine growth retardation. Early results in these experimental trials appear encouraging. There is no proof yet that GH treatment of these subjects will produce long-term benefits sufficient to warrant its use, however. For the present, then, use of GH for treatment of subjects who are not GH deficient must be considered as experimental. Growth hormone is very expensive and the cost has not diminished since the synthetic form became available.

The dose of GH is expressed in milligrams or international units. Growth hormone of the highest purity extracted from pituitary glands had an equivalence of nearly 2 IU/mg. The starting dose is generally 0.1 IU (0.05 mg/kg) three times weekly. Initially, GH was administered by the intramuscular route, because of concern that subcutaneous administration would lead to excessive formation of antibodies to GH.[170] Russo and Moore[171] have shown, however, that sub-

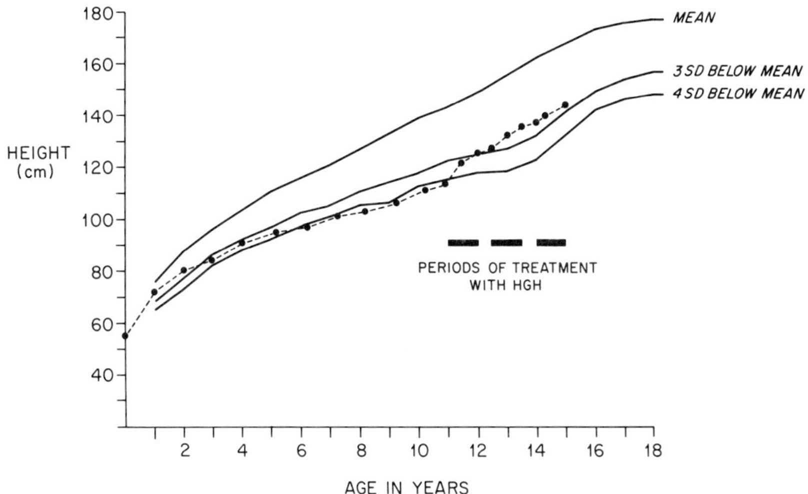

FIGURE 1–22.   Growth chart of a boy with isolated GH deficiency. Treatment with GH resulted in acceleration of growth. Temporary discontinuation of therapy was accompanied by deceleration of growth.

cutaneous administration of the newer, more purified preparations is not more prone to lead to antibody formation, nor is there any diminution in peak levels of GH attained in the plasma or generation of somatomedin C. Since injections of GH are much less painful by the subcutaneous route this has been recommended as the preferred method of injection.[171]

Administration of GH to subjects with GH deficiency leads to acceleration of growth velocity, usually to rates in excess of the normal for age. With the passage of time, however, the response tends to diminish in magnitude and the growth rate in the second year of treatment is usually much less than in the first year. As long as the growth rate does not fall below the expected normal for age as treatment progresses many endocrinologists are content not to increase the dose of GH. If the growth rate is considered inadequate the dose may be increased to 0.1 mg (0.2 IU)/kg three times weekly. With the advent of synthetic GH and increased availability of the agent higher doses have been administered, but the safety and efficacy of such dosage has not been established. A limiting factor is the cost of GH, which at the time of this writing (1988) is about $25/IU or $50/mg. Treatment of children with GH may cost tens of thousands of dollars yearly.

If treatment with GH is not followed by a satisfactory response some have advocated the use of anabolic steroids in combination with GH therapy. The regimens used are similar to those used for the treatment of

growth retardation discussed later in this chapter. While treatment with GH alone rarely leads to excessive advancement of skeletal age, when anabolic steroids are used the skeletal age must be carefully monitored, as it should be whenever these agents are used for the treatment of short stature.

Following a single injection of GH intramuscularly, plasma levels increase to 100 ng/ml or more over the first 6 hours and then gradually decline over the next 6 hours to less than 10 ng/ml.[172] Although concentrations in the plasma are undetectable by radioimmunoassay subsequent to this, the effects of GH are sustained, and most regimens consist of injections three times weekly.

Prior to the availability of synthetic GH dose-response curves for GH treatment were reported in a collaborative study. In the first year of treatment the growth rate in centimeters averaged 5.58 when the dose used per injection was 0.03 IU/kg, 7.31 when the dose was 0.06 IU/kg, 7.22 when the dose was 0.08 IU/kg, and 8.19 when the dose was 0.1 IU/kg.[173]

Advancement in longitudinal growth with GH therapy is usually accompanied by an equivalent degree of advancement of skeletal maturation. It would be expected, therefore, that children treated with GH should achieve statures consistent with their genetic potential. These expectations are generally not fulfilled. Burns et al.[174] found that the final height of children with idiopathic GH deficiency treated with GH for 2 to 15 years (mean 5.4 years) averaged 2.3 standard deviations below the mean for the population and 2.0 standard deviations below their calculated midparental mean. On the other hand, untreated patients achieved adult heights about 6 standard deviations below the mean.

Administration of GH is attended with very few significant side effects. Measurable alterations in carbohydrate tolerance occur, but these do not produce adverse effects in the treated subject. Local tenderness and allergic reactions have been reported but these are rare. Approximately 50 per cent of children treated with extracted GH prior to 1976 developed measurable titers of antibodies to GH in their serum.[175] The reason for development of antibodies is unknown, but it has been attributed to aggregates or impurities contaminating the administered GH. It had been thought that only one region of the GH molecule was the antigenic site, but with the use of monoclonal antibodies it has been shown that at least five different sites are antigenic and these sites behave independently in eliciting the antibody response.[176] While subjects with the highest titers of antibodies may be resistant to GH therapy, in general the titer of antibodies cannot be used as an index of resistance. The reason for development of antibodies even to the newer, purer, synthetic forms of GH is not known, but the possibility exists that small amounts of aggregations or impurities may still be sufficient to lead to antibody formation. According to the manufacturer, administration of methionyl-GH has led to development of persistent antibodies to GH in approximately 40 per cent of subjects who had not been previously treated with GH. However, only 1 of 84 subjects who had been treated with methionyl-GH over 6 to 36 months developed resistance to the treatment. It is evident, then, that antibodies are not a frequent cause of treatment failure. The prevalence of antibodies in subjects who receive GH that is identical to natural GH (i.e., without the extra amino acid) is said to be less than in subjects receiving methionyl-GH, but the clinical significance of this finding may be moot since antibody formation apparently rarely results in resistance to GH therapy and since different methods are used in different laboratories to measure antibody titers. The occurrence of antibodies in the sera of children with GH gene dele-

tions after treatment is initiated is discussed elsewhere in this chapter (p. 33). Another reason for growth failure in hypopituitary subjects receiving GH treatment is induction of hypothyroidism in some subjects.[177] Hypopituitary subjects with normal TSH function may suffer temporary TSH deficiency as a consequence of GH therapy. This deficiency may disappear when therapy is discontinued. The mechanism of production of this deficiency of TSH is not known. However, it is important to remember that thyroid function must be monitored in subjects receiving GH if the growth response is unsatisfactory.

Treatment of hypothyroidism in hypopituitary patients with TSH deficiency is carried out according to the principles followed in the treatment of hypothyroidism irrespective of its etiology (see Chapter 3). The agent of choice is levo-thyroxine, and the dosage must be adequate to maintain the level of thyroxine in the blood within the normal range. The skeletal age must be carefully monitored. Treatment with thyroid as well as GH may accelerate skeletal development more rapidly than longitudinal growth.

If the subject also has ACTH deficiency, treatment with glucocorticoids may be necessary. Even small doses of glucocorticoids, as little as 10 mg cortisone/day by mouth, however, may impair the effects of GH treatment. Accordingly, glucocorticoid therapy is sometimes withheld or the dosage reduced, unless the subject shows evidence of glucocorticoid deficiency such as hypoglycemia. Mineralocorticoid deficiency is virtually unknown in children with ACTH deficiency, and salt-losing crises rarely, if ever, occur.

A controversial issue in regard to GH treatment is whether it enhances the growth of tumors in subjects undergoing therapy. Growth hormone has been used extensively for the treatment of patients who have undergone partial resection of craniopharyngiomas and less often in patients who have other kinds of tumors. Thus far, no compelling evidence has been produced that GH treatment enhances the growth of these tumors.[178] At the time of this writing concern has arisen that individuals treated with GH (extracted or synthetic) may conceivably be at risk for leukemia. In a workshop held by the Lawson Wilkins Pediatric Endocrine Society and the Human Growth Foundation in May 1988, the risk was estimated to be about twice that in the general population. This estimate, which does not imply a greatly increased risk, may be changed when more data are available.

Growth hormone therapy is particularly effective in the first year of treatment and, in general, the growth spurt induced is greater in younger children. With each successive year of treatment the magnitude of the response tends to diminish. To counter this the dose of GH may be increased, but while experimental studies of doses in excess of 0.1 mg/kg three times weekly are being carried out, at this time they cannot be recommended for general use. Increasing the frequency of injections to six or seven times weekly without changing the total dose administered may lead to greater increases in growth velocity.[179] It has been suggested that administration of anabolic steroids in combination with GH may enhance responsiveness in growth. Fluoxymesterone, 2.5 mg/sq m/day, has been used for this purpose.[180] Whenever anabolic steroids are used careful attention must be paid to the rate of skeletal maturation, and treatment must be modified or discontinued if there is excessive advancement.

Human GH was first extracted from pituitaries for use in subjects with GH deficiency in 1958.[61] In 1985, three treated subjects, in their 20s and 30s, developed symptoms of a neurologic disorder characterized by weakness, muscular incoordination, slurred speech, failing vision, muscle jerking, and rigidity, and subsequent progressive memory loss, inappropriate behavior, confusion, and dementia.[181] The disorder was determined to be Creutzfeldt-Jakob syndrome (CJS), a very rare disorder occurring about once in 1 million individuals worldwide. By early 1988 two more cases were reported in America, bringing the total in this country to five. One other patient has been reported who received GH prepared in Britain and another from New Zealand who received GH prepared in the United States. The etiologic agent responsible for the disease has not been identified, but there is evidence to support the fact that it is a particle smaller than a virus, referred to as a prion. The disease is similar to scrapie, which occurs in nonhuman species. Progress in the purification of scrapie led to the identification of an associated protein with a molecular weight of about 30,000, designated as PrP27. This protein has been identified in the brains of subjects dying of

the disease and is the most definitive diagnostic feature of the presence of the disease on examination of the brain at autopsy. The brain is atrophic and histologic examination shows spongiosis, consisting of small vacuoles in the neuropil between the nerve cell bodies.[182] Shortly after the first cases were identified the distribution of extracted GH was discontinued in the United States and most of the world.

Beginning in 1977 the method used to extract GH from pituitary glands was changed to remove impurities that were present in material extracted previously. There is no assurance that the newer method removes the agent responsible for CJS, but all five people in the United States who developed CJS received GH that was processed before 1977. There is no evidence and it is highly unlikely that GH produced by recombinant DNA methodology carries a risk for CJS. Over the years approximately 7000 Americans received the preparation extracted from pituitary glands and thus far there have been only five reported cases of the tragic occurrence of CJS. Aside from these there are recent reports of two patients who have signs of unexplained cerebellar disease, in whom the diagnosis of CJS is as yet uncertain. The troubling aspect of these newer cases is that they received GH processed by the new method and if they do, indeed, show evidence of CJS in the future there is the possibility that a significant number of additional cases will occur.[183] With the passage of time the number of cases of CJS has not increased as fast as was once feared, and the likelihood of an iatrogenic epidemic of CJS appears to have diminished. A "reasonable guess" is that the number of cases will not exceed 20.[183] Time will tell.

Idiopathic (Constitutional) Growth Delay[184,185]

Falling into this category are the majority of children with growth impairment in whom physical examination is normal (except for short stature) and in whom skeletal age is delayed. At the Johns Hopkins Pediatric Endocrine Clinic between 1965 and 1972, 35 per cent of all children with short stature were diagnosed as having this type of growth disorder. Experience in the author's clinic matches these statistics. Characteristically, the infants are of normal length and weight at birth and generally they grow normally for a few months, perhaps even for 1 or 2 years. Then, inexplicably, the growth rate decelerates, for a short period of time, perhaps 2 or 3 years, and the child's height and weight measurements decrease to near or below the 5th centile on the standard growth curves. Skeletal age decelerates in a parallel fashion and usually is equivalent to the height age, i.e., the age at which the height of the child would be at or near the 50th centile. Subsequently, growth resumes at a normal rate and annual increments of more than 5 cm occur. The child is in good health and whatever testing may be carried out fails to yield abnormal results. Puberty develops when the bone age reaches about 10½ years in girls and 11 to 11½ years in boys. Thus sexual maturation begins at a later chronologic age. Growth continues until the epiphyses fuse. Normally this occurs around the age of 18 in boys and 15 in girls, but in this condition growth may continue into the early 20s in males and late teens in females. Puberty is normal except for the delayed timing, and sexual maturation and longevity are unimpaired. Adult height is normal.

There is often a history of occurrence of similar growth patterns in the family. Careful questioning regarding the time of achievement of adult height in the father, mother, and other members of the family may reveal that the pattern in the child is a repetition of that previously noted in either parent. Menarche in the mother or other females in the family may have been delayed to a significant degree. From time to time, reports of abnormal endocrine function in this syndrome have appeared, but the aggregate of experience among pediatric endocrinologists is that endocrine function is appropriate for the bone age.

In children with this disorder, skeletal age may not always be delayed to a degree equivalent to the somatic growth delay. This requires that some children with so-called constitutional growth delay be subclassified as having an element of primary skeletal growth impairment. Little is known about the cause of either pure constitutional growth delay or the variant in which skeletal age is not delayed as much as height age.

Depending on the social circumstances and pressures from peers and family, moderate or serious psychological disturbances can occur because of shortness of stature. In many instances, reassurance that there is no abnormality and that ultimate growth and development will be normal is all that is necessary. The role of the parents in providing adequate psychological support for the individual is critical, and their attitudes may determine how well the child adjusts to the problem. Children with this syndrome are often considered candidates for therapy with anabolic steroids. A discussion of the use of such agents in the treatment of short stature is presented elsewhere in this chapter. If a decision is made to treat with anabolic steroids because of significant psychologic symptoms, x-rays must be taken at frequent intervals to determine if skeletal age is being significantly advanced and if treatment should be discontinued. Whether treatment with GH is justified for this condition is not known. Trials of GH treatment are being carried out at the time of this writing.

THE DIAGNOSTIC APPROACH TO GROWTH DEFICIENCY (Fig. 1–23)

That a growth problem may exist is first perceived by the child, parent, guardian, or physician. The first question that needs to be settled is whether the child is abnormally small and not growing adequately. This is done by careful measurement of the child and by plotting the height and weight on the growth chart. If the height is below the 5th centile, the adjusted midparental height is obtained (p. 1) and the growth of the child is projected parallel to the 5th centile line to age 18. If the projected height is close to the adjusted height of the parents, it is likely that the short stature is genetic. If it is more than 5 cm below the midparental height, it is unlikely that the short stature is genetic. The heights of the parents should be inquired into and also the times at which they achieved adult stature. If more than one height measurement is available, the growth rate should be calculated. If it is less than 5 cm/year (calculated if necessary from measurements over a fraction of a year) and the subject is between the ages of 4 and 10 years, the likelihood that abnormality exists is heightened. Below the age of 4, growth rates are normally considerably in excess of 5 cm, as is discussed on page 1. Normal growth rate between any two ages can be calculated simply by measuring the increment of the 50th centile line. For example, from a growth chart it is evident that the normal growth increment of boys between ages 8 and 9 is from 127 to 132 cm. If a boy at

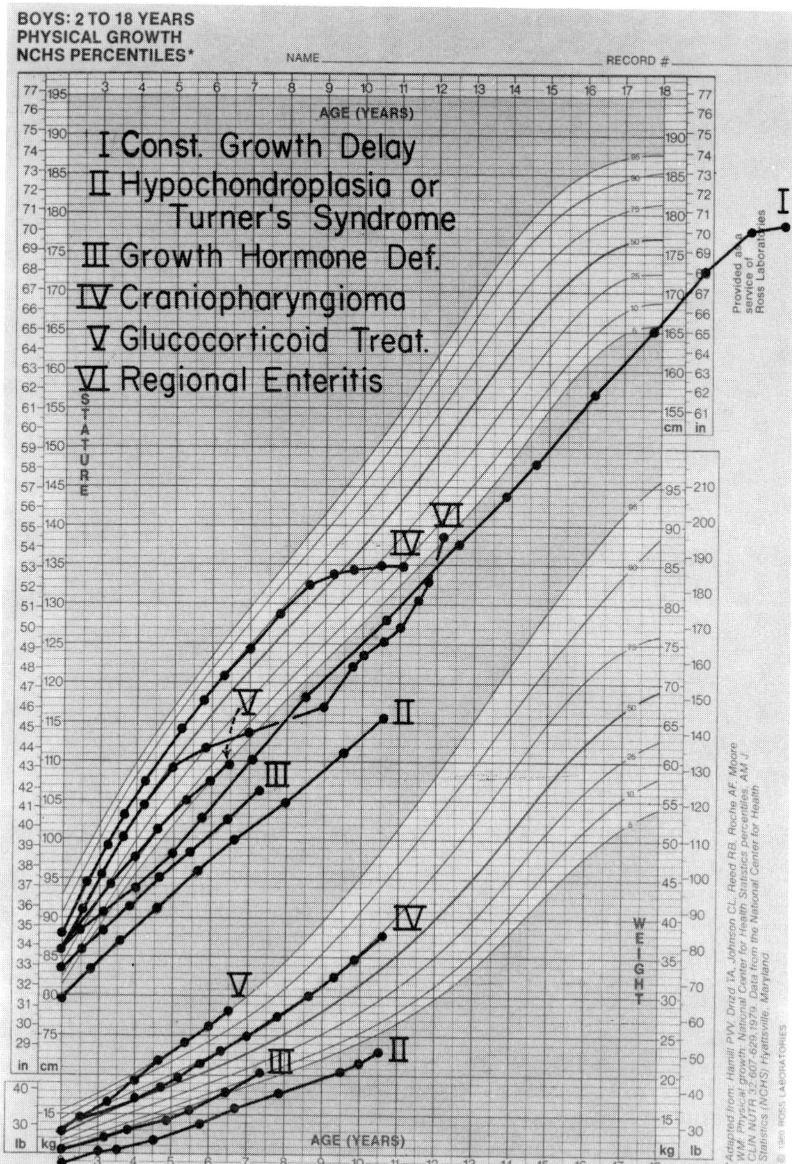

FIGURE 1–23. Growth patterns in children with short stature associated with six different causes. I, Growth curve of a child with idiopathic or constitutional growth delay with normal birth length and weight and deceleration of growth during infancy. After the fifth year of life, growth increments were normal. Because skeletal age is delayed, growth continues into the third decade and adult height is normal. II, Typical growth pattern of a child with hypochondroplasia. Annual growth increments are subnormal. III, In children with GH deficiency, birth weight and growth during infancy are often normal. Velocity of growth is often subnormal after the years of infancy. The weight is close to the 5th centile while the height curve steadily falls away from the 5th centile. The subject is relatively obese. IV, In a patient with craniopharyngioma growth is often normal for several years and then undergoes deceleration. V, With excessive glucocorticoid treatment, linear growth is retarded but weight increments may be normal or even increased. VI, In patients with regional enteritis, growth rate often decelerates but may resume normal velocity if the disease is satisfactorily controlled.

this age is not growing this much in length, irrespective of his actual height, the possibility exists that he has an active growth disorder.

A careful history should be obtained with specific questions directed to elicit symptoms of disorders of all of the organ systems of the body. In no field of medicine is the taking of a careful history more important. A child who is not growing normally because of craniopharyngioma may have no symptoms other than headache. A child with hypothyroidism may have only subtle symptoms of the disorder, such as dry skin or constipation. Answers to questions regarding the age at which deciduous teeth erupted or loosened and the time of appearance of permanent teeth are most important indicators of whether dental age (and therefore, possibly, skeletal age) is delayed. The history is followed by a careful and complete physical examination. If possible, upper and lower segment measurements should be made. A routine blood count and urinalysis are often done at this time.

If the nature of the problem is not evident at this time, the next step should be an x-ray of the hand and wrist for skeletal age. This often permits a classification of the growth retardation into primary or secondary. Lack of delay of skeletal maturation with marked short stature generally excludes secondary causes of growth retardation. Marked growth retardation without bone age delay is not characteristic of GH deficiency or hypothyroidism. In that case, a search for skeletal dysplasia or cause for intrauterine growth retardation represents a more logical approach. One exception to this rule is the recent onset of a disorder. It is conceivable that recent expansion or growth of a symptomless craniopharyngioma may impair growth without having had sufficient time to produce significant delay of skeletal age.

If skeletal age is delayed and the cause is not evident, one should consider the possibility of a silent craniopharyngioma, regional enteritis, hypothyroidism, Turner syndrome, or renal disease. These five disorders may not show the signs and symptoms characteristic of the illness or abnormality and may masquerade as a state of growth retardation. At this stage, one should obtain an x-ray of the skull to look for evidence of a craniopharyngioma and do tests for thyroid function (serum thyroxine and TSH) and kidney disease (serum creatinine and urine pH). Diagnosis of Turner syndrome should also be considered, and a diagnostic approach followed as outlined in Chapter 9. If Crohn disease or celiac disease is suspected, it may be necessary to perform a contrast medium study of the bowel, do an intestinal biopsy, or determine the serum titer of antigliadin antibodies. An indication of the presence of Crohn disease may be a persistently increased erythrocyte sedimentation rate or unexplained anemia.

Only if tests for these disorders are not rewarding should it be necessary to proceed with GH screening and if necessary a definitive test. The procedures used for testing for GH deficiency are described on pages 42–46.

PRINCIPLES OF TREATMENT OF GROWTH RETARDATION

Treatment of growth retardation should be directed at specific causes such as hypothyroidism, GH deficiency, Crohn disease, and so on. If no treatable cause is found, the problem should be discussed with the patient and his or her family, and it should be pointed out that no specific treatment is available. The problem must be handled in a sympathetic and supportive way. Pressures of peers and society often have devastating effects on children who are short, because they may see themselves as handicapped in coping with their problems. A child concerned about his or her short stature may do poorly at school and become withdrawn and depressed. The physician dealing with a child with short stature should point out to the family early on in the management of the case that medical therapy in the form of growth-promoting agents is generally only available if a deficiency or disease exists for which specific therapy is available. Less than one tenth of growth-retarded children attending endocrine clinics can expect such specific assistance.

Most important in such medical management is the discussion of delay in skeletal age if it is present and the growth potential that is increased by such delay. For every year of delay in skeletal age, there is an increase in growth potential of one additional year. Thus, a 10-year-old boy with a height age of 7 years and a skeletal age of 7 years could well be considered to have a normal growth potential. The 3 extra years of growth may be attained after the age of 18, the age at which epiphyses normally fuse, and growth may continue into the late teens or early 20s. Epiphyseal fusion in girls is normally complete at age 15 years, when growth virtually ceases, and in boys at 18 years.

Prediction tables for ultimate height based on skeletal age have been published, but these convey the impression of accuracy far beyond the achievements of the science of growth disorders. The most practical way to make a reasonable prediction is to plot the individual's height on the standard growth curve and then extrapolate the plotted value horizontally to the skeletal age of the individual. The centile at which this horizontal extrapolation interseccts with the skeletal age is then used to estimate mature height. For example, a 10-year-old boy is 120 cm tall and his skeletal age is 7 years. Extrapolation along the 120-cm line on the growth curve to age 7 years indicates that the growth potential is that of an individual around the 40th centile. It is best to confine a prediction in such a case to an estimate that the child's height will be "normal." A rough estimate of the ultimate height can be made by reading the 40th centile height at age 18. In the case under discussion, if the father's height is around 175 cm, a guarded opinion can be given that the child's height will be close to that of the father. This kind of estimation, with careful explanations of how the prediction is being made, is often very reassuring to the child. The knowledge that he or she will probably be normal in height as an adult is often all that is needed to allay extreme anxiety about being a dwarf, a term that carries the connotation of a misshapen, short individual. It is very important, however, not to succumb to the temptation to read a greater delay into a bone age than really exists, in order to allay the fears of a patient and family. In any case such predictions, even when made with great care, may not turn out to be accurate. They are based on the assumption that skeletal age advancement and growth will proceed at an equal pace. This may not happen because of the intrinsic disorder or treatment, which could lead to advancement of skeletal age more rapidly than height age. In the example given above of a 10-year-old boy who is 120 cm tall, if the bone age is minimally delayed, the prediction of adult height would be less than the 5th centile if the skeletal age were 9 years.

In the absence of specific treatment for growth retardation, some physicians have turned to the use of anabolic steroids to promote growth. These drugs are related to testosterone in structure and produce effects similar to testosterone. The goal is to achieve a growth spurt similar to that seen during the adolescent growth spurt of puberty. A variety of agents has been used, and from time to time over the past 30 years claims have appeared that a new agent has

been developed that increases longitudinal growth without a corresponding increase in skeletal age. Such claims are rarely substantiated by double-blind prospective studies with long-term follow-up. It must be recognized that administration of these agents may be attended by signs of virilization as well as advancement of bone age. If bone age is advanced at a rate equivalent to height age and this pattern continues after discontinuation of the medication, then no harm has been done. In this fortunate circumstance, too, the individual may experience considerable psychological improvement in addition to the increase in growth. Because of the dangers of advancing skeletal age unduly, this treatment is rarely used unless there is a substantial delay of skeletal maturation. It is used for short periods of time, and advancement in skeletal age is carefully monitored. However, progressive advancement of skeletal age may continue even after discontinuation of the medication. While this treatment may accelerate growth temporarily, there is no evidence that the ultimate height is increased by such treatment. On the contrary, undue advancement of skeletal age may well lead to a decrease in adult height. Pituitary extracts with little or no pharmacologic potency used in the past are considered by most to have produced an increase in height that is the normal progression of growth in this condition.

In certain instances it is not possible to have the patient or the parents accept the fact that nothing specific is available for treatment of the growth problem. Such individuals often seek the care of physicians who use anabolic steroids in a routine fashion for treatment of constitutional growth delay. If treatment is to be used because of serious symptoms of depression or inadequacy (sometimes threats of suicide have been made), then it should be reserved for older children (age 12 or more) with significant delay in bone age, at least 2 years. Two agents that have been used are oxandrolone (0.1 to 0.25 mg/kg body weight/day) and fluoxymesterone (2 to 5 mg daily). Long-acting testosterone may be given by intramuscular injection in dosage of 50 to 100 mg monthly for limited periods of time. Skeletal age should be monitored every 3 months and therapy discontinued if undesirable effects are seen, including excessive advancement of skeletal age or virilization.

The diagnosis and treatment of delay in

sexual maturation are discussed in Chapters 8 and 10.

EXCESSIVE GROWTH (TALL STATURE)

Causes of Tall Stature

1. Genetic
2. Klinefelter syndrome
3. Marfan syndrome
4. Homocystinuria
5. Growth hormone excess (pituitary gigantism)
6. Cerebral gigantism (Sotos syndrome)
7. Hyperthyroidism
8. Precocious secretion of androgens
9. Precocious secretion of estrogens
10. Obesity
11. Weaver syndrome
12. Pseudoacromegaly

Genetic Tallness

Normal children who are genetically tall constitute the largest number of subjects who seek medical advice for their tallness. Tallness in girls is more likely to produce anxiety than in boys in America, and the vast majority of those who seek medical advice regarding their tall stature are girls. These individuals are usually normal on physical examination and nearly always have very tall parents. Laboratory tests are usually unnecessary, although measurement of skeletal age is often carried out in an effort to make a prediction of ultimate stature. Treatment of this growth pattern is a highly controversial subject. Based on the knowledge that estrogens stimulate growth but also promote rapid epiphyseal fusion, some have advocated that estrogens be used to diminish the final height achieved. If such treatment is to be used, it has to be carried out over a long period of time until the epiphyses fuse. It also has to be started at a relatively young age because treatment of a girl whose skeletal age has reached 12 or 13 and who has only 5 to 10 cm of growth potential cannot be expected to achieve much shortening. Early treatment necessarily leads to early pubertal development. Results of such treatment are not uniform. Double-blind studies have not been done, and estimates of the reduction in stature from the predicted mature height are the only available criteria for success.

The dose of estrogen used has often been far in excess of usual replacement doses, varying from 2.5 to 20 mg/day in the case of conjugated estrogens and from 0.3 to 0.5 mg/day in the case of ethinyl estradiol.[186] The therapy has been continued for 1 to 3 years until epiphyseal fusion has occurred. Estimates of reduction in adult height have varied from 2 to 7 cm in published results. Side effects have included accelerated puberty, nausea, irregular menses, hypertension, and weight gain. Rarely thromboembolism, cystic hyperplasia of the breast, polyps, or endometrial hyperplasia have occurred, but whether their occurrence is coincidental with or related to the treatment is not certain. According to a survey,[186] the vast majority of pediatric endocrinologists in North America, concerned over possible short- and long-term adverse effects of estrogen therapy for tall stature, do not use this treatment for tall girls with genetic tall stature.

Marfan Syndrome[187]

Marfan syndrome or arachnodactyly, is inherited as a dominant trait, although spontaneous mutations are well known. The subjects are tall and thin and the extremities, especially the hands, fingers, feet, and toes, are unusually long. The skull is dolichocephalic, and there are malformations of the external ears and eyes (lens dislocation, coloboma, cataract, and megalocornea). Muscular hypotonia leads to increased flexibility of the joints. As the subjects grow older, kyphosis, scoliosis, cardiac valvular deformities, medionecrosis of the aorta (sometimes with dissection), and other anomalies may appear. No specific treatment of the disorder is available. Patients with *homocystinuria* may have a similar phenotypic appearance to those with arachnodactyly.[188] They are distinguished by the presence of mental retardation in many of the subjects and excretion of large amounts of homocystine in the urine.

Cerebral Gigantism[189]

Cerebral gigantism is a syndrome first described by Sotos et al. in 1964. The features are tall stature, prominent forehead, high arched palate, hypertelorism, dolichocephaly, macrocephaly, antimongoloid slant of the palpebral fissures, and pointed chin. Most subjects are mentally retarded. Skeletal age is usually advanced and because of this the mature height achieved may not be excessive. Endocrine function, including GH secretion, is normal.

Gigantism Caused by Growth Hormone Excess

Increased secretion of GH is typically associated with adenomas of the adenohypophysis, although instances of eosinophilic hyperplasia without adenoma formation have occurred. Because of the difficulty of identifying pituitary cells as eosinophils or chromophobes and because routine histologic staining does not give information on the function of the cell, confusion has arisen regarding the histology of the tumors responsible. In one study of 50 tumors, only 6 were classified as typical eosinophilic adenomas; of the remainder, 22 were classified as chromophobe adneomas.[190]

Typical adenomas are quite small—less than 2 cm in diameter. They usually do not produce visual defects and remain intrasellar in location. Tumors responsible for GH excess may exhibit aggressive enlargement, however, especially in young subjects, and impinge on surrounding structures.

The symptoms and signs of GH excess depend on the age at which excessive secretion of the hormone occurs.[191–193] If this occurs before epiphyseal union, linear growth may be enormous, and some patients have reached a height in excess of 220 cm. The most famous giant, the Alton giant, was about 280 cm at the time of his death at the age of 24 years. The most frequent manifestations of pituitary gigantism are acral enlargement, soft tissue growth, headache, and excessive perspiration. Visual impairment occurs more frequently in gigantism than in acromegaly. The enlargement of the bones and soft tissues gives the individual a characteristic appearance involving prominence of the mandible and supraorbital ridges, large nose, and large hands and feet. Delay or lack of sexual development is common, and other features noted with gigantism include carbohydrate intolerance, galactorrhea, polyuria, and polydipsia. The bones are thick, and joint pains, kyphosis, and osteoporosis occur frequently. Generalized visceral enlargement, hypertension, and heart failure may also occur.

Excessive growth in gigantism generally begins in childhood but may begin in infancy. A delay in epiphyseal closure may prolong the period of growth into the third or fourth decade. Most patients with GH-secreting tumors first show evidence of the tumor between ages 18 and 35. It has been estimated that as many as one sixth of all subjects manifest their earliest signs between ages 10 and 20. However, the diagnosis of GH excess is rare in the pediatric age group.

Radiologic signs of pituitary gigantism include enlargement of the sella turcica and paranasal sinuses and marked elongation of the mandible. Computer tomography or magnetic resonance imaging are most useful for tumor detection. The teeth become separated by large spaces, and malocclusion of the jaws leads to "overbite." Bony overgrowth of the joints of the extremities may lead to distortion of the articular plate and disabling osteoarthritis. "Tufting" of the tips of the terminal phalanges may be seen in radiography. The generalized thickening of connective tissue leads to an increase in the quantity of the soft tissues of the heel, the width of which may be determined by radiographic examination of the foot.

Levels of GH in the plasma may be normal or moderately increased, or may reach extremely high concentrations. Random sampling may show concentrations between 5 and 1000 ng/ml. In some subjects GH concentrations vary little throughout the day; in others peaks and valleys of concentrations are detectable throughout the day. Abnormal GH secretory responses to test agents suggests that the tumors may be under hypothalamic control but the regulatory mechanism is disturbed.[194]

A standard test consists of administration of 75 gm of glucose orally and sampling of blood after 90 min. If the GH concentration at this time is found to be less than 5 ng/ml, the response is considered normal. Concentrations greater than 10 ng/ml are suggestive of a tumor with hypersecretion of GH. Paradoxically, hyperglycemia significantly increases the concentration of GH in the plasma. Another remarkable observation is that administration of L-dopa and bromocriptine, dopamine agonists, often is followed by a significant reduction of concentration of GH in the plasma. Another indication of abnormality in the control of GH secretion is the increase in GH concentration in the plasma after administration of TRH. Somatomedin C levels in the plasma are increased and, because they fluctuate to a lesser degree than GH, the measurement of this growth factor in the plasma may be more useful than the measurement of GH.

Examination of the thyroid often shows it to be enlarged, but the enlargement is due to edema without evidence of hypersecretion. The hypermetabolism, therefore, appears to be ascribable to excess GH rather than hyperthyroidism. Thyroid-stimulating hormone deficiency leading to hypothyroidism may occur late in the disease. Other hormones of the anterior pituitary may also be affected, and deficiency of secretion of ACTH, FSH, and LH may be found in association with delayed pubertal development. Hyperprolactinemia may be found in association with galactorrhea.

Treatment of GH-secreting pituitary tumors is generally carried out with transphenoidal surgery if the tumor is small enough to be approached by this route. If the tumor is large, craniotomy may be necessary. Prognosis for recovery after surgery for such tumors is uncertain because so few have been described in children in recent years, during which major advances have taken place in neurosurgery. Reported cure rates in adults vary depending on the size of the tumor. For "macroadenomas" the cure or remission rates range from 33 to 90 per cent, whereas for "microadenomas" the range is 78 to 97 per cent.[195] Radiation is considered an ancillary form of therapy. Administration of bromocriptine may lead to lessening in severity of the signs and symptoms due to excessive GH secretion but not to a decrease in size of the tumor. Somatostatin analogs, on the other hand, given by injection, have been reported to improve the clinical condition, including shrinking in size of the tumor.[196] Hormonal substitution treatment may be necessary depending on the surviving function of the pituitary.

Pituitary adenomas causing gigantism have occurred together with other intracranial disturbances, including neurofibromatosis, meningiomas and tuberous sclerosis.[197,198] They may also be a component of the syndrome of multiple endocrine adenomatosis (Chapter 7) and polyostotic fibrous dysplasia (Chapter 8).

In a condition known as acromegaloidism a clinical picture virtually indistinguishable from true acromegaly is found. In this syndrome GH concentrations are normal and pituitary tumors do not occur.[199] The cause of the excessive growth is not known but a growth factor has been identified in the plasma of individuals with this syndrome that stimulates colony formation by human erythroid progenitors in vitro.

Accelerated growth occurs in children in whom excessive secretion of *androgens* or *estrogens* occurs prior to puberty. In these cases increased growth rates are accompanied by accelerated rates of epiphyseal maturation. The children do not achieve a taller than normal stature. These disorders are discussed in Chapters 8 and 10. Rarely, increased growth has been associated with *lipodystrophy* and *acanthosis nigricans*.[200] A syndrome of excessive growth associated with accelerated skeletal maturation, unusual facies and camptodactyly has also been described. (Weaver syndrome).[201]

OBESITY AND GROWTH[202]

Idiopathic or exogenous obesity is generally associated with acceleration in growth. Obese children who are tall for their age rarely suffer from an abnormality of the endocrine system. If obesity extends into the second decade, the rule is for obese children to begin puberty early and to have advanced skeletal development. Because of advancement of skeletal age, obese children are generally not taller as adults than would be expected from their genetic potential. Endocrine caues of obesity, on the other hand, are usually associated with growth impairment. Disorders of the endocrine system leading to growth retardation without a commensurate degree of reduction in weight gain or with frank obesity include hypothyroidism, GH deficiency, and adrenocortical excess. Disorders of hypothalamic function, such as may occur with tumors or surgery involving this area, are important causes of progressive and unusual weight gain. Children with pseudohypoparathyroidism also tend to be relatively heavy for their height.

Endocrine disorders are extremely rare causes of obesity, occurring in less than 0.1 per cent of all children who are overweight. Children with obesity must be measured carefully, and their height and weight plotted on growth charts. If the height of the obese child is above the 50th centile for age and if growth increments in the recent past have been normal or in excess of the normal growth rate, it is highly unlikely that investigation of the endocrine system will reveal any abnormality. On the other hand, if the child's height measurement and growth record are below normal, a careful search may have to be made for disease of the thyroid, adrenals, pituitary or hypothalamus.

REFERENCES

1. National Center for Health Statistics: NCHS Growth Charts, 1976. Monthly Vital Statistics Report. Vol 25, No 3, Suppl (HRA) 76-1120. Rockville, MD, Health Resources Administration, June 22, 1976.
2. National Center for Health Statistics: NCHS Growth Curves for Children 0–18 years. United States, Vital and Health Statistics, Series 11, No 165. Washington, DC, Health Resources Administration, US Government Printing Office, 1977.
3. Tanner JM, Davies SWD: Clinical longitudinal standards for height and height velocity for North American children. J Pediatr 107:317, 1985.
4. Villee DB: Human Endocrinology. A Developmental Approach. Philadelphia, WB Saunders Company, pp 319–324.
5. Greulich WW, Pyle SI: Radiographic Atlas of Skeletal Development of the Hand and Wrist. 2nd ed. Stanford, Stanford University Press, 1959.
6. Garn SM, Rohmann CG, Silverman FN: Radiographic standards for postnatal ossification and tooth calcification. Med Radiogr Photogr 43:45, 1967.
7. Tanner JM, Whitehouse RH, Marshall WA, et al: Assessment of Skeletal Maturity and Prediction of Adult Height (TW2 Method). New York, Academic Press, 1975.
8. Bayer LM, Bayley L: Growth Diagnosis. Chicago, University of Chicago Press, 1959, pp 226–231.
9. International nomenclature of constitutional diseases of bone. Committee Report. J Pediatr 93:614, 1978.
10. Horton WA, Rotter JI, Rimoin DL, et al: Standard growth curves for achondroplasia. J Pediatr 93:435, 1978.
11. Horton WA, Hall JG, Scott CI, et al: Growth curves for height for diastrophic dysplasia, spondyloepiphyseal dysplasia congenita, and pseudoachondroplasia. Am J Dis Child 136:316, 1982.
12. Rimoin DL: The chondrodystrophies. In Harris H, Hirschhorn K (eds): Advances in Human Genetics. Vol 5. New York, Plenum, 1975.
13. Warkany J, Monroe BB, Sutherland BS: Intrauterine growth retardation. Am J Dis Child 102:249, 1961.
14. Kaplan SA: Growth Disorders in Children and Adolescents. Springfield, IL, Charles C Thomas, 1964.
15. Clarren SK, Smith DW: The fetal alcohol syndrome. N Engl J Med 298:1063, 1978.
16. Hanson JW, Smith DW: The fetal hydantoin syndrome. J Pediatr 87:285, 1975.
17. Russell AA: A syndrome of "intrauterine" dwarfism recognizable at birth with craniofacial dysostosis, disproportionately short arms and other anomalies (5 examples). Proc R Soc Med 47:1040, 1954.
18. Silver HK: Asymmetry, short stature and variations in sexual development: Syndrome of congenital malformations. Am J Dis Child 107:495, 1964.
19. Migeon CJ, Whitehouse D: Familial occurrence of the somatic phenotype of Turner's syndrome. Johns Hopkins Med J 120:78, 1967.
20. Collins E, Turner G: The Noonan syndrome—a review of the clinical and genetic features of 27 cases. J Pediatr 83:941, 1973.
21. Rosenbloom AL, DeBusk FL: Progeria of Hutchinson-Gilford: A caricature of aging. Am Heart J 82:287, 1971.
22. Bloom D: The syndrome of congenital telangiectatic erythema and stunted growth. J Pediatr 68:103, 1966.
23. Seckel HPG: Bird-Headed Swarfs: Studies in Developmental Anthropology Including Human Proportions. Basel, S Karger, 1960.
24. Rubenstein JH, Taybi H: Broad thumbs and toes and facial abnormalities. A possible mental retardation syndrome. Am J Dis Child 105:588, 1963.
25. Bray GA, Dahms WT, Swerdloff RS, et al: The Prader-Willi syndrome. A study of 40 patients and a review of the literature. Medicine 62:59, 1983.
26. Tanner JM: Genetics of human growth. In Human Growth. Oxford, England, Pergamon, 1960, p 43.
27. Graham GC, Adrianzen T, Rabold J, et al: Later growth of malnourished children. Am J Dis Child 136:348, 1982.
28. Lloyd-Still JD, Hurwitz I, Wolff PH, et al: Intellectual development after severe malnutrition in infancy. Pediatrics 54:306, 1974.
29. Kerpel-Fronius E: Pituitary function in malnutrition. Horm Metab Res 6:82, 1974.
30. Hager A, Thorell JI: Studies on growth hormone secretion in a patient with the diencephalic syndrome of emaciation. Am J Dis Child 126:303, 1973.
31. Edidin DV, Levitsky LL, Schey W, et al: Resurgence of nutritional rickets associated with breast-feeding and special dietary practices. Pediatrics 65:232, 1980.
32. Shull MW, Reed RB, Valadian I, et al: Velocities of growth in vegetarian preschool children. Pediatrics 60:410, 1977.
33. Prasad AS, Schulert AR, Miale A, et al: Zinc and iron deficiencies in male subjects with dwarfism and hypogonadism but without ancylostomiasis, schistosomiasis or severe anemia. Am J Clin Nutr 12:437, 1963.
34. Sobel EH, Silverman FN, Lee CM: Chronic regional enteritis. Am J Dis Child 103:569, 1962.
35. Groll A, Candy DCA, Preece MA, et al: Short stature as the primary manifestation of coeliac disease. Lancet 2:1097, 1980.
36. West CD, Smith WC: An attempt to elucidate the cause of growth retardation in renal disease. Am J Dis Child 91:460, 1956.
37. Bergstrom WH, DeLeon AS, Van Gemund JJ: Growth aberrations in renal disease. Pediatr Clin North Am 11:563, 1964.
38. McSherry E, Morris RC: Attainment and maintenance of normal stature with alkali therapy in infants and children with classic renal tubular acidosis. J Clin Invest 61:509, 1978.
39. Inglefinger JR, Grupe WE, Harmon WE, et al:

Growth acceleration following renal transplantation in children less than 7 years of age. Pediatrics 68:255, 1981.

40. Koch VH, Lippe BM, Sherman BM, Fine RN: Accelerated growth following recombinant human growth hormone therapy in children with chronic renal failure (abstract). Pediatr Res 23:541a, 1988.

41. Mehrizi A, Drash A: Growth disturbance in congenital heart disease. J Pediatr 61:418, 1962.

42. Umansky R, Hauck AJ: Factors in the growth of children with patent ductus arteriosus. Pediatrics 30:540, 1962.

43. Feldt RH, Stickler GB, Weidman WH: Growth of children with congenital heart disease. Am J Dis Child 117:573, 1969.

44. Strangeway A, Fowler R, Cunningham MA, et al: Diet and growth in congenital heart disease. Pediatrics 57:75, 1976.

45. Patton RG, Gardner LI: Growth Failure in Maternal Deprivation. Springfield, IL, Charles C Thomas, 1963.

46. Silver HK, Finklestein M: Deprivation dwarfism. J Pediatr 70:317, 1967.

47. Powell GF, Brasel JA, Blizzard RM: Emotional deprivation and growth retardation simulating idiopathic hypopituitarism. N Engl J Med 276:1271, 1967.

48. Sills RH: Failure to thrive. Am J Dis Child 132:967, 1978.

49. Fine RN, Frasier SD, Donnell GN: Growth in glycogen-storage disease type I. Am J Dis Child 117:169, 1969.

50. Infections as deterrents of child growth. Nutr Rev 39:328, 1981.

51. Payne NR, Hays NT, Regelman WE, et al: Growth in patients with chronic granulomatous disease. J Pediatr 102:397, 1983.

52. Roche AF, Lipman RS, Overall JE, Hung W: The effects of stimulant medication on the growth of hyperkinetic children. Pediatrics 63:847, 1979.

53. Griffin NK, Wadsworth J: Effect of treatment of malignant disease on growth in children. Arch Dis Child 55:600, 1980.

54. Stevens MCG, Maude GH, Cupidore L, et al: Prepubertal growth and skeletal maturation in children with sickle cell disease. Pediatrics 78:124, 1986.

55. Brook CDE, Thompson EN, Marshall WC, Whitehouse RH: Growth in children with thalassaemia major and effect of two different transfusion regimens. Arch Dis Child 44:612, 1969.

56. Costin G, Kogut MD, Hyman CB, Ortega JA: Endocrine abnormalities in thalassemia major. Am J Dis Child 133:497, 1979.

57. Martin AJ, Landau LI, Phelan PD: The effect on growth of childhood asthma. Acta Paediatr Scand 70:683, 1981.

58. Blodgett FM, Burgin L, Iezzoni D, et al: Effects of prolonged cortisone therapy on the statural growth, skeletal maturation and metabolic status of children. N Engl J Med 254:636, 1956.

59. Landon C, Rosenfeld RG: Short stature and pubertal delay in male adolescents with cystic fibrosis. Am J Dis Child 138:388, 1984.

60. Niall HD: Revised primary structure for human growth hormone. Nature New Biol 230:90, 1971.

61. Raben MS: Human growth hormone. Recent Prog Horm Res 15:71, 1959.

62. Martial JA, Hallewell RA, Baxter JD, et al: Human growth hormone: Complementary DNA cloning and expression in bacteria. Science 205:602, 1980.

63. Everitt BJ, Meister B, Hokfelt T, et al: The hypothalamic arcuate nucleus–median eminence complex: Immunohistochemistry of transmitter, peptides and DARP-32 with special reference to the coexistence in dopamine neurons. Brain Res 396:98, 1986.

64. Lechan RM: Neurology of pituitary hormone regulation. In Molich ME, (ed): Pituitary Tumors: Diagnosis and Management. Endocrinology and Metabolism Clinics of North America. Vol 16. Philadelphia, WB Saunders Company, 1987, p 503.

65. Krieger DT: The hypothalamus and neuroendocrinology. In Krieger DT, Hughes JC (eds): Neuroendocrinology. Sunderland, MA, Sinauer Associates, 1980.

66. Guillemin R: Hypothalamic hormones: Releasing and inhibiting factors. In Krieger DT, Hughes JC (eds): Neuroendocrinology. Sunderland, MA, Sinauer Associates, 1980.

67. Stolar MW, Amburn K, Baumann G: Plasma "Big" and "Big-Big" growth hormone (GH) in man: An oligomeric series composed of structurally diverse GH monomers. J Clin Endocrinol Metab 59:212, 1984.

68. Baumann G, Stolar MW, Amburn K, et al: A specific growth hormone-binding protein in human plasma: Initial characterization. J Clin Endocrinol Metab 62:134, 1986.

69. Baumann G, Shaw MA, Winter RJ: Absence of the plasma growth hormone-binding protein in Laron-type dwarfism. J Clin Endocrinol Metab 65:814, 1987.

70. Martin JB: Brain regulation of growth hormone secretion. In Martini L, Ganong WF (eds): Frontiers in Neuroendocrinology. Vol 4, New York, Raven Press, 1976.

71. Sassin JF, Parker DC, Mace JW, et al: Human growth hormone release. Relation to slow-wave sleep and sleep-waking cycles. Science 165:513, 1969.

72. Esch FS, Bohlen P, Ling NC, et al: Primary structures of three human pancreas peptides with growth hormone releasing activity. J Biol Chem 258:1806, 1983.

73. Losa M, Bock L, Schopohl J, et al: Growth hormone releasing factor infusion does not sustain elevated GH levels in normal subjects. Acta Endocrinol 107:462, 1984.

74. GHRH European Multicenter Study Group: Growth hormone (GH) response to a single injection of synthetic GH-releasing hormone in prepubertal children with growth failure. J Clin Endocrinol 65:387, 1987.

75. Chihara K, Kashio Y, Abe H, et al: Idiopathic growth hormone (GH) deficiency, and GH deficiency secondary to hypothalamic germinoma: Effect of single and repeated administration of human GH-releasing factor (hGRF) on plasma GH level and endogenous hGRF-like immunoreactivity level in cerebro-spinal fluid. J Clin Endocrinol Metab 60:269, 1985.

76. Schriock EA, Hulse JA, Harris DA, et al: Evaluation of hypothalamic dysfunction in growth hormone (GH)-deficient patients using single versus multiple doses of GH-releasing hormone (GHRH-44) and evidence for diurnal variation in

somatotroph responsiveness to GHRH in GH-deficient patients. J Clin Endocrinol Metab 65:1177, 1987.

77. Thorner MO, Reschke J, Chitwood J, et al: Acceleration of growth in two children treated with human growth hormone-releasing factor. N Engl J Med 312:4, 1985.

78. Thorner MO, Rogol AD, Blizzard RM, et al: Acceleration of growth rate in growth hormone-deficient children treated with human growth hormone-releasing hormone. Pediatr Res 24:145, 1988.

79. Reichlin S: Somatostatin. N Engl J Med 309:1495, 1556, 1983.

80. Frohman LA: Neurotransmitters as regulators of endocrine function. In Krieger DT, Hughes JC (eds): Neuroendocrinology. Sunderland, MA, Sinauer Associates, 1980.

81. Laron Z, Gil-Ad I, Topper E, et al: Low dose clonidine: An effective screening test for growth hormone deficiency. Acta Paediatr Scand 71:847, 1982.

82. Mendelson WB, Lantigua RA, Wyatt J, et al: Piperidine enhances sleep-related and insulin-induced growth hormone secretion: Further evidence for a cholinergic secretory mechanism. J Clin Endocrinol Metab 52:409, 1981.

83. Schalch DS: The influence of physical stress and exercise on growth hormone and insulin secretion in man. J Lab Clin Med 69:256, 1967.

84. Root AW: Human Pituitary Growth Hormone. Springfield, IL, Charles C Thomas, 1972.

85. Frantz AG, Rabkin MT: Human growth hormone. Clinical measurement, response to hypoglycemia and suppression by corticosteroids. N Engl J Med 271:1375, 1964.

86. Deller JJ, Plunket DC, Forsham PH: Growth hormone studies in growth retardation· Therapeutic response to administration of androgen. Calif Med 104:359, 1966.

87. Katz HP, Youlton R, Kaplan SL, et al: Growth and growth hormone. III. Growth hormone release in children with primary hypothyroidism and thyrotoxicosis. J Clin Endocrinol Metab 29:346, 1969.

88. Novak LP, Hayles AB, Cloutier MD: Effect of HGH on body composition of hypopituitary dwarfs. Mayo Clin Proc 47:241, 1972.

89. Carey DE, Goldberg B, Ratzan SK, et al: Radioimmunoassay for type 1 procollagen in growth hormone-deficient children before and during treatment with growth hormone. Pediatr Res 19:8, 1984.

90. Linderkamp O, Butenandt O, Mader T, et al: The effect of growth hormone deficiency and of growth hormone substitution on blood volume and red cell parameters. J Pediatr Res 11:885, 1977.

91. Rapaport R, Oleske J, Ahdieh H, et al: Suppression of immune function in growth hormone-deficient children during treatment with human growth hormone. J Pediatr 109:434, 1986.

92. Lippe BM, Kaplan SA, Golden MP, et al: Carbohydrate tolerance and insulin receptor binding in children with hypopituitarism: Responses following acute and chronic growth hormone administration. J Clin Endocrinol Metab 53:507, 1981.

93. Phillips LS, Vassilopoulou-Sellin R: Somatomedins. N Engl J Med 302:371, 1980.

94. Van Wyk JJ, Underwood LE: Relation between growth hormone and somatomedin. Annu Rev Med 26:427, 1975.

95. Daughaday WH, Garland JT: The sulfation factor hypothesis: Recent observations. In Pecile A, Muller EE (eds): Growth and Growth Hormone. Amsterdam, Excerpta Medica, 1972.

96. Froesch ER, Schmid C, Schwander J, Zapf J: Actions of insulin-like growth factors. Annu Rev Physiol 47:443, 1985.

97. Rinderknecht E, Humbel RE: The amino acid sequence of human insulin-like growth factor-1 and its structural homology with proinsulin. J Biol Chem 253:2769, 1978.

98. Sherman BM, Frane J, Hintz RL, et al: IGF-1 measurement in growth hormone deficiency: The clinical relevance and dependence on method (abstract). Pediatr Res 23:286A, 1988.

99. Kogut MD, Kaplan SA: Growth retardation: Use of sulfation factor as a bioassay for growth hormone. Pediatrics, 31:538, 1963.

100. Bala RM, Lopatka AL, McCoy E, McArthur RG: Serum immunoreactive somatomedin levels in normal adults, pregnant women at term, children at various ages, and children with constitutionally delayed growth. J Clin Endocrin Metab 52:508, 1981.

101. Golde DW, Bersch N, KaplanSA, et al: Peripheral unresponsiveness to human growth hormone in Laron dwarfism. N Engl J Med 303:1156, 1980.

102. Isaksson OGP, Eden S, Jansson J-O: Mode of action of pituitary growth hormone on target cells. Annu Rev Physiol 47:483, 1985.

103. Pankin JM: Incidence of growth hormone deficiency. Arch Dis Child 49:905, 1974.

104. Rona RJ, Tanner JM: Aetiology of idiopathic growth hormone deficiency in England and Wales. Arch Dis Child 52:197, 1977.

105. Craft WH, Underwood LE, Van Wyk JJ: High incidence of perinatal insult in children with panhypopituitarism. J Pediatr 96:397, 1980.

106. Miller WL, Eberhardt NL: Structure and evaluation of the growth hormone gene family. Annu Rev Med 34:519, 1983.

107. Phillips JA, Hjell BL, Seeburg PH, et al: Molecular basis for familial isolated growth hormone deficiency. Proc Natl Acad Sci (USA) 78:6372, 1981.

108. Illig R, Prader A, Ferrandez A, et al: Hereditary prenatal growth hormone deficiency with increased tendency to growth hormone antibody formation ("A-type" of isolated growth hormone deficiency). Acta Paediatr Scand 60:607, 1971.

109. Phillips JA: Genetic diagnosis: Differentiating growth disorders. Hosp Pract 20:85, 1985.

110. Lindsay AN, MacGillivray MH, Voorhess ML: Growth hormone deficiency in twins. Three cases with normal co-twins. Pediatrics 69:486, 1982.

111. Rimoin DL, Schechter JE: Histological and ultrastructural studies in isolated growth hormone deficiency. J Clin Endocrinol Metab 37:725, 1980.

112. Costom BH, Grumbach MM, Kaplan SL: Effect of thyrotropin releasing factor on serum thyroid-stimulating hormone. J Clin Invest 50:2219, 1971.

113. Brasel JA, Wright JC, Wilkins L, et al: An eval-

uation of 75 patients with hypopituitarism beginning in childhood. Am J Med 38:484, 1965.

114. Goodman HG, Grumbach MM, Kaplan SL: Growth and growth hormone. II. A comparison of isolated growth hormone deficiency and multiple pituitary-hormone deficiencies in 35 patients with idiopathic hypopituitary dwarfism. N Engl J Med 278:57, 1968.

115. Herber SM, Milner RDG: Growth hormone deficiency presenting under age 2 years. Arch Dis Child 59:557, 1984.

116. Fisher RL, Di Chiro G: The small sella turcica. Am J Roentgenol Rad Ther Nuc Med 91:996, 1964.

117. Menkes JH: Textbook of Child Neurology. 2nd ed. Philadelphia, Lea & Febiger, 1980, pp 517–523.

118. Bringas B, Wolter M: Das kraniopharyngiom. Fortschr Neurol Psychiatr 36:117, 1968.

119. Jenkins JS, Gilbert CJ, Ang V: Hypothalamic-pituitary function in patients with craniopharyngiomas. J Clin Endocrinol Metab 43:394, 1976.

120. Wolpert SM: The radiology of pituitary adenomas. *In* Molich ME (ed): Pituitary Tumors: Diagnosis and Management. Endocrinology and Metabolism Clinics of North America. Vol 16. WB Saunders Company, 1987, p 553.

121. Thomsett MJ, Conte FA, Kaplan SL, et al: Endocrine and neurologic outcome in childhood craniopharyngioma. Review of effect of treatment in 42 patients. J Pediatr 97:728, 1980.

122. Patel H, Tze WJ, Crichton JU, et al: Optic nerve hypoplasia with hypopituitarism. Am J Dis Child 129:175, 1975.

123. Huseman CA, Kelch RP, Hopwood NJ, et al: Sexual precocity in association with septo-optic dysplasia and hypothalamic hypopituitarism. J Pediatr 92:748, 1978.

124. Hoyt WF, Kaplan SL, Grumbach MM, et al: Septo-optic dysplasia with pituitary dwarfism. Lancet 893, 1970.

125. Lieblich JM, Rosen SW, Guyda H, et al: The syndrome of basal encephalocele and hypothalamic pituitary dysfunction. Ann Intern Med 89:910, 1978.

126. Hintz RL, Menking M, Sotos JF: Familial holoprosencephaly with endocrine dysgenesis. J Pediatr 72:81, 1968.

127. Roitman A, Laron Z: Hypothalamo-pituitary hormone insufficiency associated with cleft lip and palate. Arch Dis Child 53:952, 1978.

128. Leiken S: The histiocytoses. Pediatr Ann 4:35, 1975.

129. Braunstein GD, Kohler PO: Pituitary function in Hand-Schüller-Christian disease. Evidence for deficient growth hormone release in patients with short stature. N Engl J Med 286:1225, 1972.

130. Richards GE, Wara WM, Grumbach MM, et al: Delayed onset of hypopituitarism: Sequelae of therapeutic irradiation of central nervous system, eye and middle ear tumors. J Pediatr 89:553, 1976.

131. Samaan NA, Bakdash MM, Caderao JB, et al: Hypopituitarism after external irradiation: Evidence for both hypothalamic and pituitary origin. Ann Intern Med 83:771, 1975.

132. Oberfield SE, Allen JC, Pollack J, et al: Long term endocrine sequelae after treatment of medulloblastoma: Prospective study of growth and thyroid function. J Pediatr 108:219, 1986.

133. Shalett SM, Beardwell CG, Morris-Jones PH, et al: Growth hormone deficiency after treatment of acute leukemia in children. Arch Dis Child 51:489, 1976.

134. Winter RJ, Green OC: Irradiation-induced growth hormone deficiency: Blunted growth response and accelerated skeletal maturation to growth hormone therapy. J Pediatr 106:609, 1985.

135. Greenhouse AH: Pituitary sarcoma: A possible consequence of radiation. JAMA 190:269, 1964.

136. Russell JD, Wise PH, Rischbieth HG: Vascular malformation of the hypothalamus: A cause of isolated growth hormone deficiency. Pediatrics 66:306, 1980.

137. Kanade A, Ruiz AE, Tornyos K, et al: Panhypopituitarism and anemia secondary to traumatic fracture of the sella turcica. J Endocrinol Invest 1:263, 1978.

138. Miller WL, Kaplan SL, Grumbach MM: Child abuse as a cause of post-traumatic hypopituitarism. N Engl J Med 302:724, 1980.

139. Bartsocas CS, Pantelakis SN: Human growth hormone therapy in hypopituitarism due to tuberculous meningitis. Acta Pediatr Scand 62:304, 1973.

140. Arvanitakis C, Knouss RF: Selective hypopituitarism. Impaired cell immunity and chronic mucocutaneous candidiasis. JAMA 255:1492, 1973.

141. Mayfield RK, Levine JH, Gordon L, et al: Lymphadenoid hypophysitis presenting as a pituitary tumor. Am J Med 69:619, 1980.

142. Hendricks SA, Lippe BM, Kaplan SA, et al: Hypothalamic atrophy with progressive hypopituitarism in an adolescent girl. J Clin Endocrinol Metab 52:562, 1981.

143. Stuart CA, Neelon FA, Lebovitz HE: Hypothalamic insufficiency: The cause of hypopituitarism in sarcoidosis. Ann Intern Med 88:589, 1978.

144. Shulman DI, Martinez CR, Bercu BB, Root AW: Hypothalamic dysfunction in primary empty sella syndrome in childhood. J Pediatr 108:540, 1986.

145. Costigan DC, Daneman D, Harwood-Nash D, et al: The "empty sella" in childhood. Clin Pediatr 23:427, 1984.

146. New MI, Schwartz E, Parks GA, et al: Pseudohypopituitary dwarfism with normal plasma growth hormone and low serum sulfation factor. J Pediatr 80:620, 1972.

147. Laron Z, Sarel R, Pertzelan A: Puberty in Laron-type dwarfism. Eur J Pediatr 134:79, 1980.

148. Eshet R, Laron Z, Pertzelan A, et al: Defect of human growth hormone receptors in the liver of two with Laron-type dwarfism. Isr J Med 20:8, 1984.

149. Frasier SD: A review of growth hormone stimulation tests in children. Pediatrics 53:929, 1974.

150. Penny R, Blizzard RM, Davis WT: Sequential arginine and insulin tolerance tests on the same day. J Clin Endocrinol Metab 29:1499, 1969.

151. Lippe BM, Wong S-LR, Kaplan SA: Simultaneous assessment of growth hormone and ACTH reserve in children pre-treated with diethylstilbestrol. J Clin Endocrinol Metab 33:949, 1971.

152. Fass B, Lippe BM, Kaplan SA: Relative usefulness of three growth hormone stimulation screening tests. Am J Dis Child 133:931, 1979.

153. Collu R, Leboeuf G, Letarte J: Stimulation of growth hormone secretion by Levo-dopa pro-

pranolol in children and adolescents. Pediatrics 56:262, 1975.

154. Weldon VV, Gupta SK, Klingensmith G: Evaluation of growth hormone release in children using arginine and L-dopa in combination. J Pediatr 87:540, 1975.

155. Reiter EO, Morris AH, MacGillivray MH, Weber DA: Variable estimates of serum growth hormone concentrations by different radioassay systems. J Clin Endocrinol Metab 66:68, 1988.

156. Nicoll AG, Smail PJ, Forsyth CC: Exercise test for growth hormone deficiency. Arch Dis Child 59:1177, 1984.

157. Lanes R, Recker B, Fort P, et al: Low dose oral clonidine. A simple and reliable growth hormone screening test for children. Am J Dis Child 139:87, 1985.

158. Bercu BB, Shulman D, Root AW, Spiliotis BE: Growth hormone (GH) provocative testing frequently does not reflect endogenous GH secretion. J Clin Endocrinol Metab 63:709, 1986.

159. Chalew SA, Raiti S, Armour KM, Kowarski A: Therapy in short children with subnormal concentrations of growth hormone. Am J Dis Child 141:1195, 1987.

160. Zadik Z, Chalew SA, McCarter RJ, et al: The influence of age on the 24-hour integrated concentrations of growth hormone in normal individuals. J Clin Endocrinol Metab 60:153, 1985.

161. Schwartz ID, Hu C-S, Shulman, et al: Relationship of endogenous GH secretion to linear growth response after exogenous GH treatment in short stature (abstract). Pediatr Res 23:286A, 1988.

162. Lin T-H, Kirkland RT, Sherman BM, Kirkland JL: Twenty-four hour studies of growth hormone secretion in normal and short children and their lack of predictive value in growth hormone therapy (abstract). Pediatr Res 23:280A, 1988.

163. Donaldson DL, Hollowell JG, Pan FP, Moore WV: Growth hormone secretory profiles: Significant variation on consecutive nights (abstract). Pediatr Res 23:276A, 1988.

164. Rose SR, Ross JL, Uriarte M, et al: The advantage of stimulated versus spontaneous growth hormone levels in the diagnosis of growth hormone deficiency. N Engl J Med 319:201, 1988.

165. Albini CH, Quattrin T, Vandlen RL, MacGillivray MH: Quantitation of urinary growth hormone in children with normal and abnormal growth. Pediatr Res 23:89, 1988.

166. Sukegawa I, Hizuka N, Takano K, et al: Urinary growth hormone (GH) measurements are useful for evaluating endogenous GH secretion. J Clin Endocrinol Metabol 66:1119, 1988.

167. Rosenfeld RG, Aggarwal BB, Hintz RL, et al: Recombinant DNA-derived methionyl growth hormone is similar in membrane binding properties to human pituitary growth hormone. Biochem Biophys Res Commun 106:202, 1982.

168. Hintz RL, Rosenfeld RG: Clinical uses of synthetic growth hormone. Hosp Pract 18:115, 1983.

169. Kaplan SL, Underwood LE, August GP, et al: Clinical studies with recombinant-DNA-derived methionyl human growth hormone in growth hormone deficient children. Lancet 1:697, 1986.

170. Underwood LE, Viona S, Van Wyk JJ: Restoration of growth by human growth hormone (Roos) in hypopituitary dwarfs immunized by other human growth hormone preparations: Clinical and immunological studies. J Clin Endocrinol Metab 38:288, 1974.

171. Russo L, Moore WV: A comparison of subcutaneous and intramuscular administration of human growth hormone in the therapy of growth hormone deficiency. J Clin Endocrinol Metab 55:1003, 1982.

172. Frasier SD, Costin G, Ling SM, Kaplan SA: Plasma growth hormone concentration after a single intramuscular injection of growth hormone. Pediatr Res 3:557, 1969.

173. Frasier SD, Costin G, Lippe BM, et al: A dose-response curve for human growth hormone. J Clin Endocrinol Metab 53:1213, 1981.

174. Burns EC, Tanner JM, Preece MA, Cameron N: Final height and pubertal development in 55 children with idiopathic growth hormone deficiency, treated for between 2 and 15 years with human growth hormone. Eur J Pediatr 137:155, 1981.

175. Moore WV, Leppert P: Role of aggregated human growth hormone (hGH) in development of antibodies to hGH. J Clin Endocrinol Metab 51:691, 1980.

176. Retegui LA, Masson PL, Paladini AC: Specificities of antibodies to human growth hormone (hGH) in patients treated with hGH: Longitudinal study and comparison with the specificities of animal antisera. J Clin Endocrinol Metab 60:184, 1985.

177. Lippe BM, van Herle AJ, LaFranchi SH, et al: Reversible hypothyroidism in growth hormone-deficient children treated with human growth hormone. J Clin Endocrinol Metab 40:612, 1975.

178. Clayton PE, Shalet SM, Gattamaneni HR, Price DA: Does growth hormone cause relapse of brain tumors? Lancet 1:711, 1987.

179. Bundak R, Hindmarsh PC, Smith PJ, Brook CGD: Long term auxologic effects of human growth hormone. J Pediatr 112:875, 1988.

180. MacGillivray MH, Kolotkin M, Munschauer RW: Enhanced linear growth responses in hypopituitary dwarfs treated with growth hormone plus androgen versus growth hormone alone. Pediatr Res 8:103, 1974.

181. Human Growth Hormone and Creutzfeldt-Jakob Disease. U.S. Department of Health and Human Services, National Institutes of Health Publication No 88-2793. Washington, DC, U.S. Government Printing Office, 1987.

182. Gibbs CJ, Joy A, Heffner R, et al: Clinical and pathological features and laboratory confirmation of Creutzfeldt-Jakob disease in a recipient of pituitary-derived human growth hormone. N Engl J Med 313:734, 1985.

183. Brown P: Human growth hormone therapy and Creutzfeldt-Jakob disease: A drama in three acts. Pediatrics 81:85, 1988.

184. Brasel JA, Blizzard RM: The influence of endocrine glands on growth and development. *In* Williams RH (ed): Textbook of Endocrinology. 2nd ed. Philadelphia, WB Saunders Company, 1974.

185. Kaplan SL, Abrams CAL, Bell JJ, et al: Growth and growth hormone. Changes in serum level of growth hormone following hypoglycemia in 134 children with growth retardation. Pediatr Res 2:43, 1968.

186. Conte FA, Grumbach MM: Estrogen use in chil-

dren and adolescents: A survey. Pediatrics 62:1091, 1978.

187. Smith DW: Recognizable Patterns of Human Malformation. 3rd ed. Philadelphia, WB Saunders Company, 1982, p 350.

188. McKusick V: Heritable Diseases of Connective Tissue, 4th ed. St. Louis, CV Mosby, 1972, p 224.

189. Sotos JF, Cutler EA: Cerebral gigantism. Am J Dis Child 131:627, 1977.

190. Young DG, Bahn RC, Randall RV: Pituitary tumors associated with acromegaly. J Clin Endocrinol 25:249, 1965.

191. Spence HJ, Trias EP, Raiti S: Acromegaly in a 9½-year-old boy. Am J Dis Child 123:504, 1972.

192. AvRuskin TW, Sau K, Tang S, et al: Childhood acromegaly: Successful therapy with conventional radiation and effects of chlorpromazine on growth hormone and prolactin secretion. J Clin Endocrinol Metab 37:380, 1973.

193. DeMajo SF, Onativia A: Acromegaly and gigantism in a boy: Comparison with three overgrown non-acromegalic children. J Pediatr 57:382, 1960.

194. Daughaday WH, Cryer PE: Growth hormone secretion and acromegaly. *In* Krieger DT, Hughes JC (eds): Neuroendocrinology. Sunderland, MA, Sinauer Associates, 1980.

195. Baumann G: Acromegaly. *In* Molitch ME (ed): Pituitary Tumors: Diagnosis and Management. Endocrinology and Metabolism Clinics of North America. Vol 16. Philadelphia, WB Saunders Company, 1987, p 685.

196. Geffner ME, Nagel RA, Dietrich RB, Kaplan SA: Treatment of acromegaly with a somatostatin analog in a patient with McCune-Albright syndrome. J Pediatr 111:740, 1987.

197. Hoffman WH, Perrin JS, Halac E, et al: Acromegalic gigantism and tuberous sclerosis. J Pediatr 93:478, 1978.

198. Bunick EM: Association of acromegaly and meningiomas. JAMA 240:1267, 1978.

199. Ashcraft MW, Hartzband PI, van Herle AJ, et al: A unique factor in patients with acromegaloidism. J Clin Endocrinol Metab 57:272, 1983.

200. Seip M: Lipodystrophy and gigantism with associated endocrine manifestations. A new diencephalic syndrome? Acta Pediatr 48:555, 1959.

201. Weaver DD, Graham B, Thomas IT, et al: A new overgrowth syndrome with accelerated skeletal maturation, unusual facies and camptodactyly. J Pediatr 84:547, 1974.

202. Forbes GB: Nutrition and growth. J Pediatr 91:40, 1977.

2

DISORDERS OF THE POSTERIOR PITUITARY

Hans Henning Bode

Neuroendocrine function of the posterior pituitary was suggested less than 100 years ago when investigators recognized the pituitary to be composed of neuronal tissue and found that an extract prepared from it exhibited vasopressin, oxytocic, galactogogue, and antidiuretic activity.[1-4] The demonstration of an antidiuresis following posterior pituitary extract injection in patients with diabetes insipidus also suggested that the neurohypophysis was involved in the etiology of this clinical entity.[5] Attempts to separate and purify the hormonally active components culminated in the successful structure analysis and synthesis of vasopressin and oxytocin by du Vigneaud in the 1950s.[6,7]

Both oxytocin and vasopressin are synthesized in the hypothalamic nuclei and transported along the neurohypophyseal tract to the posterior pituitary, where they are stored and released under central control.[8,9]

Oxytocin causes uterine contraction and milk ejection and is used clinically for the induction of labor and for maintenance of postpartum uterine tonicity. However, it is not essential for the process of labor and delivery. Very high concentrations of oxytocin in the fetal circulation at the time of delivery have led to speculation that the fetus has a role in determining the onset of labor.[10] Diseases attributed to anomalies in oxytocin secretion have not been observed.

Arginine vasopressin (antidiuretic hormone, ADH) induces membrane permeability for water and urea in the renal collecting tubules. Through modulation of vasopressin secretion, free water losses in the urine can be varied over a 25-fold range. Vasopressin deficiency is clinically expressed as diabetes insipidus, and excess secretion leads to hyponatremia and water intoxication. The postulated influence of vasopressin on unrelated brain function such as memory is not mediated through the posterior pituitary.[11-13]

The aim of this chapter is to review the physiologic and pathophysiologic aspects of the posterior pituitary that relate to the clinical care of children with hypothalamic disease and anomalous regulation of fluid metabolism.

PHYSIOLOGY OF THE POSTERIOR PITUITARY

Anatomy

The posterior pituitary is formed by the evagination of neuronal tissue from the floor of the third ventricle. After its downward migration, it is encapsulated together with the ascending ectodermal cells of Rathke's pouch, which form the anterior pituitary. Both are embedded in the developing sphenoid bone, forming the sella turcica. By the end of the first trimester this development is completed, and vasopressin and oxytocin can be detected in neurohypophyseal tissue.[14] Incomplete descent of neuronal tissue and formation of an ectopic neurohypophysis at the infundibulum is associated with the absence of the pituitary stalk. In contrast to the anterior pituitary, the posterior pituitary has no hormone-synthesizing capabilities, but represents the distal termination of neurons originating in the supraoptic and paraventricular nuclei of the anterior hypothalamus.[15] These nuclei are paired structures easily recognizable with specific staining because of their magnicellular neurons containing microvesicles with dense core granules (Fig. 2–1). The su-

"

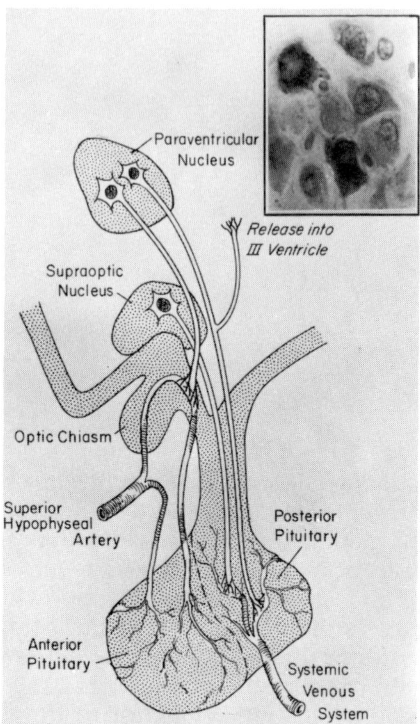

FIGURE 2–1. Schematic diagram of the neurohypophyseal system. Vasopressin and oxytocin are synthesized in the supraoptic and paraventricular nuclei. These are paired magnicellular structures, projected here on the midline from their parasagittal position. Bound to neurophysins, the hormones are transported along the unmyelinated axons to the posterior pituitary. Separate neurons transport neurohypophyseal hormones to the median eminence and the wall of the third ventricle. Destruction of the supraoptic nucleus and section of the neuronal axons above the median eminence prevent hormone delivery into the systemic circulation. The inset depicts a Gomori stain of the large cells in the supraoptic nucleus containing microvesicles with hormone granules.

praoptic nuclei lie just above the optic chiasm; the paraventricular nuclei are located ventral to the thalamus and adjacent to the third ventricle. Their unmyelinated axons traverse the basal hypothalamus, form the neural stalk, and terminate in the posterior lobe of the pituitary. Shorter axons from the paraventricular nuclei terminate at the floor of the third ventricle and in the median eminence.

Both hypothalamic nuclei are under the influence of multiple neuronal stimuli from other centers of the brain. They are surrounded by neuroendocrine cells controlling anterior pituitary hormone secretion and have a very close anatomic and functional relation to the area mediating thirst. Osmoreceptors controlling thirst and vasopressin secretion are apparently located in

the supraoptic nucleus and in the organum vasculosum laminae terminalis anteriorly to the paraventricular nuclei.[16,17] Destruction of this area attenuates secretion of vasopressin and drinking in response to hypertonic saline and angiotensin II but not the response to hemorrhage. Located slightly more to the posterior are the areas controlling hunger and satiety. These anatomic considerations are of clinical importance and explain the variable symptoms and signs associated with diabetes insipidus due to hypothalamic disease or tumor.

Hormone Biosynthesis

Vasopressin and oxytocin are synthesized as large prehormones by separate cells of the supraoptic and paraventricular nuclei.[18] Immediately after synthesis the hormones are cleaved from the large protein molecule, bound at the NH_2-terminal to smaller proteins (the neurophysins), and transported along the neurohypophyseal tract to the posterior pituitary. Neurophysins are also nerve cell products of the supraoptic and paraventricular nuclei and may represent another fraction of the prehormones.[19,20] They play a role as hormone carriers during the transport and storage in the posterior pituitary. Vasopressin neurophysin (neurophysin I) binds and is concurrently secreted with vasopressin.[21] Oxytocin and its neurophysin (neurophysin II) are produced also in equimolar quantities and independently of vasopressin. After release from the posterior pituitary, the hormones and their neurophysins circulate in blood in free form; different half-lives explain why serum concentrations do not remain equimolar. Neurophysins have no proven biologic activity in blood.

Hormone Structure

Vasopressin and oxytocin are very similar nonapeptides containing a disulfide link and a terminal amide group (Fig. 2–2). The difference in biologic activity is based on the amino acids in postions 3 and 8. Oxytocin has no antidiuretic activity at physiologic concentrations,[22] whereas arginine vasopressin, the antidiuretic hormone of humans and most mammals, does not influence milk ejection or uterine contractions unless injected in pharmacologic amounts.[23] The vasoconstrictive effects of vasopressin are also observed only in high

FIGURE 2–2. Structure and activities of neurohypophyseal hormones.[22] Lysine vasopressin, the antidiuretic hormone of the pig family, is available for treatment as a nasal spray (Lypressin). Deamination of cysteine in position 1 of vasopressin and substitution of L-arginine with the D-isomer causes reduction in vasoconstrictive action and provides the long-acting, potent antidiuretic analog, 1-desamino-8-D-arginine vasopressin (DDAVP).

doses. Lysine vasopressin, the antidiuretic hormone of the pig family, has a biologic activity of approximately one third of human ADH. Synthetic lysine vasopressin is available as a short-acting ADH for the treatment of diabetes insipidus.

The synthesis of vasopressin and oxytocin analogs has permitted the evaluation of the biologic importance of each amino acid in the molecule. These studies have also provided analogs with more selective and higher biologic activity. One of these products, 1-desamino-8-D-arginine vasopressin (DDAVP), proved to be ideally suited for the treatment of vasopressin deficiency. This analog has a very low affinity for V_1 receptors, the predominant receptors in the central nervous and cardiovascular systems, and exerts its antidiuretic action through V_2 receptors in the kidney.[24] Thus, DDAVP is a selective and potent ADH that is resistant to rapid degradation and free of most the systemic side effects of arginine vasopressin.

Plasma concentration of vasopressin and oxytocin can be measured by radioimmunoassay and by bioassay.[25] Determination of serum or urine vasopressin concentrations is not considered essential for the diagnosis of all cases of diabetes insipidus, but it may be useful in patients with mild vasopressin deficiency.[26]

Neurophysin I and II

Neurophysin levels can be determined accurately by radioimmunoassay.[25] The measurements may reflect concentrations of vasopressin and oxytocin in the plasma. Neurophysin I concentrations increase in response to nicotine stimulation and hemorrhage; a specific stimulus for neurophysin II and oxytocin is estrogen administration.[19]

In certain clinical situations, however, the levels of neurohypophyseal hormones do not correlate with those of their neurophysins. In the genetic form of diabetes insipidus of the Brattleboro rat, neurophysin I release is normal and vasopressin synthesis does not occur. In certain tumors with ectopic vasopressin production, on the other hand, there is no evidence of concurrent synthesis of neurophysin.

Neurophysins are present in the posterior pituitary extracts (Pitressin) available for therapy of diabetes insipidus and may be responsible for the allergic reactions occasionally observed.

Regulation of Hormone Secretion

Vasopressin secretion is influenced by a multitude of stimuli (Table 2–1). All initiate pituitary release of the hormone through depolarization of the neurohypophyseal neurons.[27] An important and sensitive control is mediated through the osmoreceptors, cells located in the supraoptic nucleus and organum vasculosum laminae terminalis and stimulated by hyperosmolality and angiotensin II.[16,17] The antidiuretic, but not the polydipsic response to increased plasma tonicity, remains intact even after surgical separation of the hypothalamus from the rest of the brain.[28] The simultaneous stimulation of drinking and ADH secretion provides the kidney with an optimal hormonal and fluid environment to maintain systemic tonicity and hydration in a very narrow range. In his now classic experiments Verney showed that increasing serum osmotic pressure by only 1 or 2 per cent resulted in vasopressin release and increased urine concentration.[29]

An almost linear relationship exists between plasma vasopressin and serum osmolality (Fig. 2–3). The slope and the X-intercept provide a measure of the sensitivity

TABLE 2–1. FACTORS INFLUENCING VASOPRESSIN SECRETION

Factor	Increased Secretion	Decreased Secretion
Physiologic	Hypovolemia Hyperosmolality Upright position Central hyperthermia	Hypervolemia Hypo-osmolality Recumbent position Central hypothermia
Pathologic	Cerebral disease Chest disease Malignancies Adrenal insufficiency	Diabetes insipidus
Pharmacologic	Carbamazepine, clofibrate Nicotine, angiotensin II Cholinergic drugs Morphine, barbiturates	Alcohol Dilantin Anticholinergic agents

and threshold of the system. Hyperglycemia and hypocalcemia suppress the sensitivity of vasopressin release to hyperosmolality, whereas it is increased during hypoglycemia and hypercalcemia.[30]

The threshold for ADH secretion is influenced by intravascular volume.[31,32] Acute hemorrhage causes greater vasopressin secretion than dehydration and the rise in plasma vasopressin appears to be exponential.[22,23] Stretch receptors in the left atrium inhibit vasopressin release during hyper-volemia, and baroreceptors located in the carotid sinus stimulate ADH release during hypotension. Baroreceptor signals are mediated through the vagus nerve. In addition, vasopressin secretion is inhibited centrally by cardiac release of atrial natriuretic factor (ANF) during blood volume expansion and atrial stretch.[34] The simultaneous stimulation of thirst and vasopressin secretion during hypovolemia is independent of a functioning organum vasculosum laminae terminalis. However, the destruction of the latter inhibits drinking and ADH secretion in response to hypertonic saline and angiotensin II.[16]

Baroreceptors are responsible for the physiologic increase in serum vasopressin that occurs upon assuming the upright position. Clinically, baroreceptor-stimulated ADH secretion can be of importance when "effective" blood volume is shifted to the dependent body portion, for example, in chronically ill, bedridden patients, rendering them susceptible to water intoxication. When hypovolemia is associated with salt loss, as is typically observed after excessive sweating or adrenal insufficiency, thirst is associated with salt hunger, and drinking behavior will be sustained only if salt and water are provided simultaneously.[35] Premature cessation of drinking and suppression of ADH secretion, even prior to fluid absorption, has also been observed when water is offered after solute-induced hyperosmolality[36] or when iced water was provided.[37] Presumably these effects are transmitted through oropharyngeal receptors. These sensors may be responsible for the preference for cold water observed in patients with diabetes insipidus. The anti-

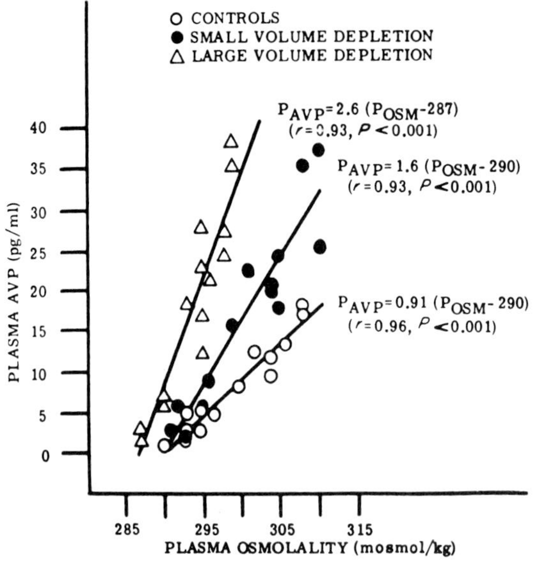

FIGURE 2–3. Progressive hypovolemia increases the sensitivity of osmoreceptor-dependent vasopressin release. Regression lines in the hypovolemic groups are significantly different from those of controls. (From Dunn FL et al: The role of blood osmolality and volume in regulating vasopressin secretion in the rat. J Clin Invest 52:3212, 1973.)

diuresis and polydipsia observed during febrile illness are under direct hypothalamic control. Isolated warming of the anterior hypothalamus in experimental animals is associated with thirst and vasopressin secretion.

Stimulation of vasopressin secretion from the brain cortex was documented early by Verney, who observed antidiuresis during emotional and physical stress.[29] However, the renal response to vasopressin in this situation is of much lesser importance than that of the anterior pituitary. Recent observations[38,39] have provided strong evidence to suggest that vasopressin is the hypothalamic hormone primarily responsible for inducing pituitary adrenocorticotropic hormone (ACTH) release during stress and insulin-induced hypoglycemia, while corticotropin-releasing hormone (CRH) plays only a permissive role in this process. These studies provide a rational explanation for the well-known clinical observation of a rise in plasma cortisol to normal levels in some patients with anterior pituitary insufficiency during an insulin tolerance test or after pyrogen injection.[40]

Mechanisms controlling the secretion of oxytocin have not been equally well documented. As is the case with vasopressin, oxytocin is released in response to insulin-induced hypoglycemia.[41] Oxytocin release in response to tactile stimulation of the nipple is a typical example of a neurohumoral reflex mechanism, as is its increased secretion during sexual arousal.[42] During nursing and estrogen administration a sharp increase occurs in plasma concentrations of oxytocin and its neurophysin, but not of vasopressin.[19,25] Increasing quantities of oxytocin are secreted during pregnancy and parturition, and there is no doubt that oxytocin participates in the process of delivery. Cervical and vaginal dilation by the fetus during labor has been postulated to further augment oxytocin release.[43] The physiologic importance of oxytocin in the process of labor is, however, unclear, and evidence suggests that parturition will proceed even in the absence of this hormone.

Vasopressin and oxytocin release into the third ventricle occurs with circadian rhythmicity and is independent of hormone secretion into the systemic circulation.[44] Vasopressin delivered into the median eminence is taken up by the portal circulation and apparently modulates anterior pituitary function.

Hormone Distribution and Metabolism

Once secreted, vasopressin and oxytocin are distributed in unbound form in the plasma. Metabolic degradation takes place in the liver and kidney. Reports on the half-life of vasopressin in blood vary greatly but it is generally agreed to be less than 10 min. Vasopressin degradation is enhanced during dehydration and inhibited during overhydration.[25] In pregnant women placental vasopressinase enhances the degradation. According to Robertson et al.[45] plasma levels of vasopressin average 2.7 ± 1.4 pg/ml in recumbent persons whose plasma osmolality is 287 ± 2.1 mOsm/kg. Antidiuretic hormone levels decline to 1.4 ± 0.8 pg/ml during overhydration and rise to 5.4 ± 3.4 pg/ml after prolonged water deprivation with concurrent increases in plasma osmolality to 292 mOsm/kg (vasopressin 1 pg = 0.4 μU) These changes in circulating levels of ADH in response to alterations in plasma osmotic pressure are surprisingly small. A wider range of vasopressin levels is observed with alteration in blood volume (Fig. 2–3). Under certain clinical conditions associated with water retention and hypoproteinemia, baroreceptor-mediated stimulation of vasopressin excretion will override the inhibitory effect of systemic hypoosmolality and thus exaggerate fluid accumulation.

Oxytocin has a distribution space and metabolism similar to that of vasopressin. Its half-life is approximately 5 to 17 min (mean = 10.3 ± 1.6 min).[46]

Mechanism of Vasopressin Action

The ability to dilute and concentrate urine is unique to the mammalian kidney. The formation of dilute urine is achieved by the phylogenetically new architecture of the renal medulla, in which the loops of Henle function as a countercurrent multiplier system.[47,48]

Approximately 80 to 90 per cent of the isosmotic glomerular filtrate is reabsorbed in the proximal tubule. The remaining filtrate enters the descending limb of Henle's loop and equilibrates with the increasingly hypertonic interstitium of the renal medulla through passive reabsorption of water. The osmolar concentration at the tip of the loop in the renal papilla can be as high as 1200 mOsm/kg. During the passage through the ascending limb of Henle's loop urine osmolality declines and reaches greater dilution than the corresponding interstitial environment through active chloride and sodium removal in the thick section of the limb, which is less permeable to water. Urine delivered to the distal convoluted tubule is therefore always dilute. The active chloride pump in the ascending loop is the source for the concentrating gradient in the renal medulla. Active sodium chloride transport in the medullary portion of the loop is enhanced by vasopressin in several species, but this hormone has no effect on salt transport in the cortical part of the ascending loop.[49] The U-shaped vasa recta are in osmotic equilibrium with the interstitial environment. They function as highly efficient countercurrent exchangers and allow removal of reabsorbed solute and water. The efficiency of this countercurrent gradient system is dependent on normal urine flow and kidney perfusion.

In the absence of vasopressin, the collecting duct and distal cortical nephron are impermeable and prevent bulk flow of water into the hypertonic renal medullary interstitium. The dilute urine of the distal convoluted tubule can be changed only minimally in volume and tonicity at the tip of the renal papilla, where reabsorption can occur even in the absence of vasopressin. Urine volume in severe diabetes insipidus can be as high as 10 per cent of the total glomerular filtrate. In the presence of vasopressin the collecting duct becomes permeable, allowing passive bulk flow of water to equilibrate with the surrounding interstitium. Urine volume markedly decreases and osmolality exceeds 1000 mOsm/kg.

Vasopressin evokes specific cell responses via two separate receptors and second-messenger systems.[24] The antidiuretic action of vasopressin is mediated via V_2 receptor–adenylate cyclase interaction at the capillary membrane of the tubular cells. This system is dependent on a hyperosmolar environment in the kidney. The vasopressin-receptor interaction leads to greater permeability and increased water and urea flux through the intercellular spaces of the tubular system.[50] Extrarenal V_2 receptors mediate the DDAVP-induced decrease in blood pressure, increase in plasma renin activity, and stimulation of factor VIIIc release.[51] Vasopressin interaction with V_1 receptors involves calcium as a second-messenger system. V_1 receptors do not bind DDAVP, but account for the vascular and

central nervous system effects of vasopressin. In the kidney V_1 receptors promote cell contraction and prostaglandin synthesis in three sites: glomerular mesangial cells, vascular smooth muscle, and the renomedullary interstitial cells. V_1 receptor activation may also indirectly alter urinary concentrating ability through prostaglandin synthesis, which affects medullary blood flow and solute transport into the medullary interstitium and thus modulates the hydroosmotic vasopressin action. Inhibition of prostaglandin synthesis by indomethacin results in increased urinary concentration and papillary solute content.[52]

Interrelationship of Vasopressin and Oxytocin With Other Hormones

The secretion, action, and degradation of the posterior pituitary hormones are well known to be modified by other endocrine systems. Estrogen administration stimulates oxytocin secretion and plasma levels rise progressively during pregnancy. On the other hand, there is decreased sensitivity to both oxytocin and vasopressin during pregnancy, probably as a result of increased placental production of oxytocinase and vasopressinase. Nursing is accompanied by pituitary release of oxytocin, but not of vasopressin. The antidiuresis observed during lactation is believed to be induced by a direct, vasopressin-independent effect of prolactin on kidney function. Oxytocin has a very mild antidiuretic action, and administration of pharmacologic doses has been shown to inhibit renal vasopressin sensitivity, presumably through competition at the receptor site.[53]

Panhypopituitarism ameliorates symptoms of diabetes insipidus, and isolated anterior pituitary insufficiency increases the susceptibility to water intoxication. The latter phenomenon is probably caused by ACTH deficiency and decreased production of cortisol, which is instrumental in suppression of ADH secretion during systemic hypotonicity.[54] Hypothyroidism is a frequent cause of hyponatremia and water retention. Afflicted patients respond suboptimally to both water deprivation and loading. Excessive production of ADH seems to play a lesser role in the development of the phenomenon than the decreased glomerular filtration rate and slow tubular urine flow.[55] Hyperthyroidism, on the other hand, is associated with polyuria and decreased response to exogenous vasopressin. Symptoms are ameliorated by β-adrenergic blockade, again suggesting that blood and urine flow, and not deficient ADH secretion or concurrent hypercalciuria, contribute to the polyuria.

As a consequence of hypovolemia in adrenal insufficiency, the excretion of a water load is delayed and ADH levels in plasma are elevated. Saline infusion or steroid replacement will correct water retention and suppress vasopressin secretion. In Brattleboro rats with diabetes insipidus, adrenalectomy decreases urine flow rate and dilution ability following a water load.[56] Glucocorticoid replacement corrects rate of urine flow, but mineralocorticoid treatment is required to restore the capacity for urine dilution. It is likely that the mineralocorticoid action under this particular circumstance is unrelated to ADH and that correction of sodium deficiency by saline infusion is equally efficient.[57] Aldosterone excess can cause vasopressin-resistant polyuria if associated hypokalemia exists. Similar circumstances exist during hypercalcemia.

The catecholamines influence thirst, ADH secretion, and renal ADH response. Epinephrine inhibits ADH release centrally, whereas norepinephrine interferes with vasopressin action on the kidney.[58] The latter is corrected by simultaneous administration of α-adrenergic blocking agents.[59]

PATHOPHYSIOLOGY OF THE POSTERIOR PITUITARY

The principal endocrine diseases involving the neurohypophysis are limited to those presenting with deficient or excessive ADH secretion. Primary abnormalities in drinking behavior are frequently associated with defective vasopressin response because of the close anatomic relation and functional interdependence of hypothalamic nuclei mediating thirst with those elaborating vasopressin. Abnormalities of oxytocin secretion have not been recognized as clinical entities.

Central Diabetes Insipidus

Diabetes insipidus includes all conditions presenting with an inability to form concentrated urine in spite of a normally operative countercurrent gradient system. In its severest form the urine volume and tonicity will only be changed minimally in the distal tubule and collection duct. Urinary losses will therefore apporach 10 per cent of glomerular filtrate, and osmolalities will be 100 mOsm/kg or less. This is observed after complete destruction of the supraoptic nuclei or after interruption of the supraoptic-hypophyseal tract above the median eminence, preventing vasopressin delivery into the systemic circulation. Less severe disturbance of function can be expected when the division occurs within the median eminence, allowing at least some vasopressin to pass outside the blood-brain barrier. Stalk section below the median eminence or surgical removal of the posterior pituitary will cause only transient diabetes insipidus, and thereafter a mild, asymptomatic concentration defect. Associated with the recovery of vasopressin secretion after trauma is the formation of a new ectopic neurohypophysis just proximal to the severed pituitary stalk. Such an event has been documented clinically with magnetic resonance imaging,[60] a technique that lends itself equally well to the demonstration of developmental errors during the formation of the neuroadenohypophysis (Fig. 2–4).

In experimental animals as well as in humans the surgical interruption of the supraoptic-neurohypophyseal tract may be followed acutely by a triphasic pattern of vasopressin secretion (Fig. 2–5).[61,62] Immediately after dissection, diabetes insipidus is clinically evident. This stage lasts for approximately 3 to 5 days and is followed by the *interphase*, an antidiuretic period resulting from vasopressin "leakage" from the degenerating posterior pituitary lobe. During this period circulating vasopressin levels are functionally independent, and failure to recognize this phenomenon in patients after hypothalamic tumor removal or trauma can have hazardous consequences. The interphase usually lasts for several days, and depending on extent and location of the division is followed either by permanent diabetes insipidus or by complete recovery with resumption of normal fluid homeostasis. This triphasic response is not observed when the posterior pituitary is removed simultaneously with the dissection of the neurohypophyseal tract.[62]

Etiology

The various clinical entities leading to diabetes insipidus are listed in Table 2–2. In

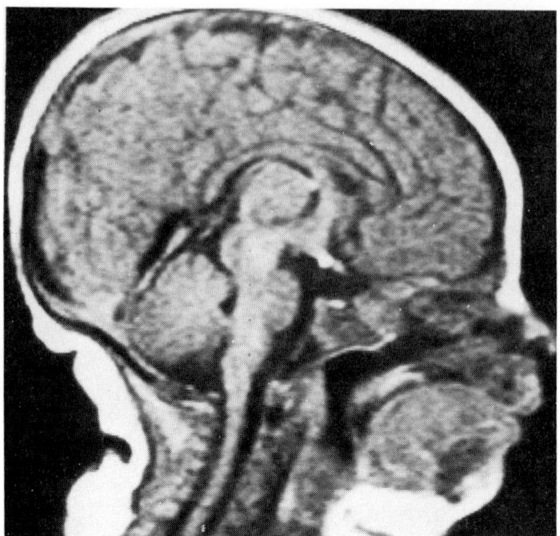

FIGURE 2–4. Ecctopic posterior pituitary in a newborn with anterior pituitary deficiency due to migrational arrest and nonfusion of the neuro- and adenohypophysis. Increased MRI signal intensity in the infundibulum represents neurohypophyseal tissue while the signal along the floor of the sella originates from hypotrophic adenohypophysial cells. The lower portion of the infundibulum and the pituitary stalk are not developed. Magnetic resonance imaging results analogous to these have been observed in patients with pituitary stalk sectioning whose diabetes insipidus subsided with a neoformation of an ectopic neurohypophysis proximal to the injury.[60]

older series before advanced laboratory techniques and computed tomography were readily available, idiopathic diabetes insipidus comprised a large percentage. Those patients in whom no etiology can be found initially, however, will later often either prove to have genetic disease as manifested by similarly affected offspring or show ad-

ditional symptoms leading to tumor recognition.

Trauma represents a major cause of diabetes insipidus. It is frequently surgically induced during removal of tumors in the hypothalamic area. In transsphenoidal hypophysectomy, polydipsia and polyuria often are transient. In contrast to the case in adults, accidental trauma is still a relatively rare cause of permanent vasopressin deficiency in children.

In our series of patients with diabetes insipidus, tumor is the most frequent cause. Craniopharyngiomas are the most common; however, polydipsia and polyuria are very rarely the initial complaints and often appear only after surgery. Diencephalic gliomas, hamartomas, and germinomas as well as infiltrative diseases such as histiocytosis, sarcoidosis, and leukemia are also associated with diabetes insipidus. In histiocytosis, polyuria is often the presenting symptom.[63] Diabetes insipidus may also occur in patients who have septo-optic dysplasia (see Chapter 1).

In inflammatory processes diabetes insipidus is a relatively rare complication but, when present, is often associated with anterior pituitary disease. Autoimmune neurohypophysitis has been suggested to be a possible etiology in several patients with idiopathic diabetes insipidus. Scherbaum et al.[64] found evidence of other autoimmune disease and circulating vasopressin cell antibodies far more frequently in patients with idiopathic diabetes insipidus than in those with vasopressin deficiency due to known causes. Among the degenerative diseases of the central nervous system associated with

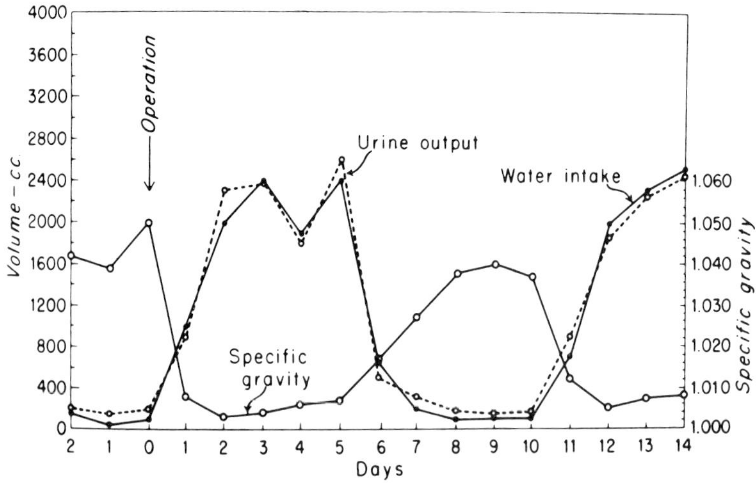

FIGURE 2–5. Typical triphasic pattern of urine excretion following section of the pituitary stalk and damage to the median eminence. Polyuria was interrupted by the *interphase* from day 6 to day 11. During this antidiuretic period, administration of fluid and solute has to be adjusted to avoid dilutional hyponatremia. (From Hollinshead WH: The interphase of diabetes insipidus. Proc Staff Meet Mayo Clin 39:92, 1964, reproduced with permission.)

TABLE 2–2. ETIOLOGIES OF VASOPRESSIN DEFICIENCY

Primary	Defective synthesis (genetic, new mutation)
	Idiopathic
Secondary	Tumors of the hypothalamus (germinoma, glioma, craniopharyngioma, cysts, and so on)
	Histiocytosis
	Granulomatous disease (sarcoidosis, tuberculosis, Wegener syndrome)
	Inflammatory (encephalitis, meningitis, etc.)
	Autoimmune neurohypophysitis
	Vascular (aneurysm, thrombosis, embolus)
	Trauma (neurosurgical, accidental)
	Congenital malformations (septo-optic dysplasia, etc.)

diabetes insipidus, the syndrome presenting with vasopressin deficiency, optic atrophy, nerve deafness, and juvenile diabetes mellitus is of particular interest. Diabetes mellitus often precedes the symptoms of intracranial disease, but the sequence of the development of the various features is variable. Family studies indicate that this syndrome has autosomal-recessive inheritance.[65] Other forms of familial diabetes insipidus are discussed separately later in this chapter.

Clinical Manifestations

The symptomatology in children with diabetes insipidus varies and is influenced not only by the extent of vasopressin deficiency but also by diet, renal function, preservation of thirst, and anterior pituitary integrity. More than two thirds of the patients give a history of abrupt onset. Nocturia and enuresis in a previously toilet-trained child often leads to the initial visit to the physician. A careful history elicits additional symptoms that set the child apart from those with bed-wetting or excess fluid intake. Children often prefer iced water, are thirsty during the night, and become irritable and inconsolable when fluid is withheld. Their urine color is described as clear even upon awakening. Poor weight gain can usually be documented, and deficient growth should suggest coexisting anterior pituitary disease. A history of additional symptoms such as recent onset of strabismus, double vision, or precocious puberty should prompt a search for a hypothalamic tumor.

In uncomplicated diabetes insipidus the physical findings may be limited to signs of mild dehydration, but unless the patient is examined immediately after voiding, a large, distended bladder can often be palpated. Visual field restriction, blindness, and optic atrophy suggest the presence of a suprasellar tumor. Midbrain lesions can produce nystagmus, abnormal pupillary responses, and paralysis of upward gaze. In advanced disease due to tumors, headaches and vomiting may occur. Skull films may show calcification, especially in craniopharyngiomas, or an abnormal sella turcica (see Chapter 1).

Diagnosis

The diagnosis of diabetes insipidus is confirmed when, in the presence of serum hypertonicity, inappropriately dilute urine is excreted. Central nervous system disease is implicated when this defect can be corrected with vasopressin administration. Initial screening studies should be undertaken. After fluid is withheld overnight, a normal child will concentrate urine to at least 800 mOsm/kg or to a specific gravity of 1.018. Depriving a child of water overnight may be hazardous, however, and it is better to do the test as described below. Random serum sodium concentrations and osmolalities in diabetes insipidus tend to be in the high normal or hypertonic range. Low serum sodium concentrations suggest that the polyuria is secondary to excess fluid intake or renal tubular disease. The presence of hypokalemia, hypercalcemia, and azotemia should be excluded before specific testing is initiated.

Water Deprivation Test. This test is begun in the morning. Breakfast is withheld, the patient is weighed, and 500 ml/m^2 of water is given by mouth. Thereafter, hourly weights and urine volumes are recorded, and the patient is given water in amounts equal to urine volumes. When a steady diuresis is established, initial blood samples are drawn for measurement of serum sodium, osmolality, and vasopressin. Thereafter, fluids are withheld for 6 hours. Urine volumes and osmolalities and the patient's weights are recorded hourly. At the termination of the test blood and urine samples for sodium, osmolality, and vasopressin determinations are obtained.

The persistent excretion of dilute urine with osmolalities less than that of the plasma, a rise in serum sodium (>145 mEq/ L) and serum osmolality (>290 mOsm/kg), and a weight loss of 3 to 5 per cent suggest the presence of diabetes insipidus. Antidiuretic hormone deficiency is established when the patient responds to vasopressin with a rise in urine tonicity to at least 100 mOsm/kg beyond the maximal concentration during water deprivation. Hourly weight loss should be compared with urine volumes to exclude surreptitious fluid intake. Urine sodium concentration at the termination of the test should be less than 20 mEq/L, in spite of coexisting hypernatremia. High urine sodium losses suggest the presence of renal disease with loss of the sodium-conserving mechanism during hypovolemia. In infants and small children 6 hours of water deprivation is not always necessary, and the test should be interrupted as soon as serum hypertonicity has been established. In older children, if prolongation of the test is necessary, the subject must be kept under close observation and the test terminated as soon as possible. Measurements of serum vasopressin at the end of the test will confirm the diagnosis in most patients.

Water deprivation with ensuing systemic hyperosmolality and fluid loss should lead to vasopressin release by both osmoreceptor and volume receptor mechanisms. When diabetes insipidus is due to an isolated osmoreceptor deficiency, but the response to hypovolemia is normal, the water deprivation test will provide inconclusive results. Therefore, urine concentration ability must be tested by increasing plasma osmolality while normal blood volume is maintained.

Hypertonic Saline Infusion Test.[66] Fasting in the morning, the patient is given 20 ml/kg of 2.5 per cent glucose water intravenously over a period of 1 hour. Hydration may be alternatively accomplished with water by mouth, 500 ml/m²/hour until steady diuresis is observed. Thereafter, hypertonic sodium chloride solution (2.5 per cent) is infused intravenously at a rate of 0.25 ml/kg body weight/minute for 45 min. Urine volume and osmolality are determined every 15 min, and serum sodium and osmolality are measured before and at the end of the hypertonic infusion.

Normal subjects will respond with an antidiuresis within 30 min after saline infusion is initiated. Patients with diabetes insipidus will show an increase in urine volume and a fall in urine osmolality. This test should

never be performed in children unless vasopressin sensitivity has been documented. In renal diabetes insipidus severe hypernatremia may ensue, which then requires large amounts of solute-free water for correction.

Other Diagnostic Tests. Other diagnostic tests are very rarely needed to establish the presence of vasopressin deficiency. The injection of nicotine causes a direct central stimulation of vasopressin release and a subsequent antidiuresis for about 30 min.[67] The side effects of this test outweigh the diagnostic advantages for routine clinical use. In all patients in whom a specific etiology for vasopressin is not readily apparent, magnetic resonance imaging (MRI) and computed tomography (CT) of the pituitary-hypothalamic region should be obtained. We consider the former technique especially well suited for the demonstration of neurohypophyseal tissue, which provides increased signal intensity because of its lipoid content (Fig. 2–4).

Familial Vasopressin-Sensitive Diabetes Insipidus

The familial occurrence of diabetes insipidus has been well recognized ever since the first description by Lacombe in 1841.[68] While there is variation in severity of the disorder from one pedigree to another, most affected members show some evidence of residual vasopressin secretion and are relatively asymptomatic until after infancy. There are no other neurosecretory anomalies or physical stigmata associated with this disease, and the radiologic search for gross anatomic malformation has been fruitless. In two families Martin showed residual vasopressin secretion after nicotine injection, but a failure to achieve antidiuresis when the serum was hypertonic.[69] These findings led him to suggest an inherited defect in osmoreceptors in these subjects. Development of slight antidiuresis during water deprivation and failure to decrease the volume of urine formed during hypertonic saline infusion (Hickey-Hare test) are in keeping with the defective osmoreceptor theory and suggest a qualitatively normal response to the volume receptor (Fig. 2–6).

Genetics. Review of reported pedigrees and the author's own experience suggest that this clinical entity can be caused by a variety of single gene defects. Both autosomal-dominant and X-linked inheritance

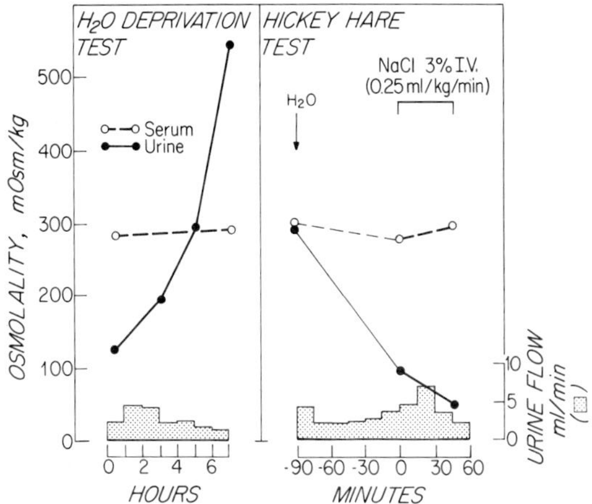

FIGURE 2–6. Familial diabetes insipidus due to abnormal osmoregulation of vasopressin secretion. During fluid restriction antidiuresis was observed, but urine osmolality (548 mOsm/kg) was inappropriately low for coexisting hemoconcentration (plasma osmolality 296 mOsm/kg). After water deprivation, urine sodium concentration was 4 mEq/L, indicating normal renal sodium conservation during hypovolemia. After fluid restriction overnight, plasma hypertonicity and isosthenuria were observed. Dehydration was corrected before hypertonic saline was infused. In response to the induced plasma hyperosmolality and blood volume expansion, diuresis and greater urine dilution were documented. Fluid deprivation caused a qualitatively normal response, but the Hickey-Hare test[66] was diagnostic for deficient vasopressin secretion.

have been described. Autosomal-dominant inheritance was strongly suggested in a large pedigree described by three generations of physicians.[70–72] Males and females were equally affected in number and severity, and male-to-male inheritance was observed on several occasions. Later Forssman[73] reported two pedigrees, one with an autosomal-dominant and the other with an X-linked mode of inheritance. He suggested that the X-linked–inherited disease was also present in those previously reported families in which females had been described as having less severe symptoms than males. The autosomal inheritance pattern is far more frequently observed than the defect on the X chromosome. We have observed apparent new mutations in two males previously diagnosed as idiopathic diabetes insipidus who fathered equally affected sons.

Clinical Manifestations. Many patients come to medical attention only years after the symptoms of polyuria and polydipsia are first observed. The stoic acceptance of "water drinking" as a family habit often prevents affected individuals from seeking medical advice, and even after the estab-

lishment of the diagnosis there is reluctance, especially among adults, to accept the need for therapy. Younger children are often brought to the physician because of persistent bed-wetting. Severe symptoms during infancy are rare and often develop only at the time of puberty.

Diagnosis. The diagnosis depends on the documentation of vasopressin responsiveness and familial occurrence. With primary osmoreceptor anomalies the hypertonic saline infusion test is necessary for diagnosis. The prompt cessation of polydipsia and polyuria after vasopressin administration confirms the diagnosis. For distinction among the various subgroups we have routinely employed short-term therapy with chlorpropamide, 125 mg/m² body surface, and found it to be a valuable tool in defining the nature and severity of the defect in families with clinically similar presentations. For chronic therapy we consider long-acting nasal vasopressin spray the preferred treatment; however, in most patients there is a slight delay after beginning treatment before maximal antidiuresis is achieved.

Prognosis. The prognosis for all patients should be excellent even without treatment. Chronic severe hypernatremia is rarely found in these patients, and we have also not encountered the difficulties during infancy that are so characteristic of nephrogenic diabetes insipidus. Unfortunately, the most frequent complications observed among our cases were iatrogenic and occurred when patients were hospitalized for unrelated disease and were unable to convince physicians of their special need for free water.

Differential Diagnosis

The differential diagnosis of diabetes insipidus includes all conditions associated with polyuria (Table 2–3). These can be divided into two categories. In the first there is physiologic suppression of vasopressin secretion during excess water intake. In the second group there is an inability of the kidney to elaborate concentrated urine despite vasopressin stimulation.

Primary organic hyperdipsia is extremely rare, but has been reported with tumors and hypothalamic infiltrative disease.[74] Drug-induced thirst can be excluded by the medical history. Psychogenic polydipsia is seldom seen in childhood. Characteristically, compulsive water drinkers deny the classi-

TABLE 2–3. POLYURIC CONDITIONS MIMICKING VASOPRESSIN DEFICIENCY

Physiologic suppression of vasopressin secretion
  Psychogenic polydipsia
  Organic polydipsia (hypothalamic disease)
  Drug-induced polydipsia (thioridazine, tricyclics)
Reduced renal responsiveness to vasopressin
  Genetic: Nephrogenic diabetes insipidus
             Medullary cystic disease
  Pharmacologic: Lithium, demeclocycline,
                   penthrane, diuretics
  Osmotic diuresis: Diabetes mellitus
                      Reduced nephron population
  Electrolyte disturbance: Hypercalcemia
                             Hypokalemia
  Renal disease: Postobstructive diuresis
                   Renal tubular acidosis
                   Pyelonephritis, papillary necrosis
                   Sickle cell disease
  Hemodynamic: Hyperthyroidism

cal history found in most patients with diabetes insipidus, such as sudden onset of symptoms, persistent need to drink during the night and preference for iced water. Their serum sodium and osmolality are usually in the low-normal range even upon awakening.[75] Occasionally these patients may be difficult to distinguish from those with primary vasopressin deficiency because chronic excess water consumption may have "washed out" the renal concentration gradient so that urine concentration after water deprivation will initially be suboptimal. When given vasopressin, compulsive water drinkers continue their habit and invariably become water intoxicated. A less dramatic, but equally sensitive diagnostic distinction can be accomplished by short-term treatment with chlorpropamide (see later in this chapter). If this drug causes amelioration of polydipsia, psychogenic water drinking is excluded and vasopressin deficiency is the likely diagnosis. In young children excessive drinking and urination is not an infrequent parental complaint. It usually reflects the child's preference for milk, juice, and soda over eating solid food, or it reflects parentally induced polydipsia. In the former, urine volume will be markedly reduced when fluid intake is limited to plain water, whereas marked differences in fluid volume between day and night collections will be apparent in parentally induced high fluid turnover.

Polyuria and polydipsia due to renal unresponsiveness to vasopressin is far more common than primary polydipsia. In all af-

fected patients there is a higher urinary osmolality after water deprivation and dehydration than after vasopressin administration and unrestricted fluid intake. Vasopressin resistance is most severely expressed in inherited X-linked nephrogenic diabetes insipidus. The typical history permits easy differentiation. Also, severe symptoms may follow treatment with lithium or demethylchlortetracycline. These drugs selectively interfere with the vasopressin-cell interaction in the renal tubules. In other forms of renal diabetes insipidus the symptoms are milder. Daily urine volumes rarely exceed 2.5 L/m^2 body surface.

Metabolic disease such as diabetes mellitus does not present a diagnostic problem. Hypercalcemia and hypokalemia both damage the renal tubular cells, but this is usually reversible when the underlying abnormality is corrected. Typically, the polyuria is of sudden onset and, in the case of hypokalemia, is associated with alkalosis and glucose intolerance. Thyrotoxicosis is associated with rapid tubular urine flow and increased renal perfusion. The resulting diuresis is always relatively minor.

Most patients with primary renal disease have isosthenuria and can be easily distinguished from those with diabetes insipidus by history, physical findings, and appropriate laboratory tests. Both homozygous and heterozygous patients with sickle cell disorder have a concentrating defect, which in young children can be corrected with blood transfusion. The defect is presumably caused by the hypertonicity of the renal medulla, which precipitates formation of sickle-shaped erythrocytes, and this leads to obstruction of vasa recta and papillary edema. The massive diuresis that follows the relief of urinary tract obstruction presents more of a therapeutic than a diagnostic problem. In these patients bicarbonate and sodium wasting occur, but urinary losses of potassium and phosphate are minimal.

Treatment of Diabetes Insipidus

Isolated vasopressin deficiency is not a life-threatening disease in patients who have a normal sensation of thirst and adjust their fluid intake accordingly. Three conceptually different therapeutic approaches permit a choice of regimen that is the most appropriate for each individual patient:

1. Hormone replacement will establish a persistent antidiuresis throughout the duration of action of the particular vasopressin preparation employed.

2. Certain nonhormonal drugs will stimulate a secretion of or potentiate the renal medullary response to residual vasopressin in patients with incomplete diabetes insipidus.

3. The combined therapy of diet and saluretic agents will reduce fluid requirements in all patients with diabetes insipidus, but this treatment is best suited for infants with vasopressin deficiency and patients with nephrogenic diabetes insipidus and will be discussed in that section of this chapter.

Hormone Replacement Therapy. The drug of choice for hormone replacement is DDAVP, a synthetic analog that differs from arginine vasopressin by the deamination of cysteine in the 1 position and substitution of L-arginine in the 8 position with the D isomer (Fig. 2–2). DDAVP is a pure V_2 receptor agonist and thus free of vasopressor effects occasionally encountered when aqueous vasopressin is administered in high doses. A second advantage of this analog is its very delayed breakdown. The duration of action varies between 8 and 24 hours and is dependent on the patients's state of hydration.[76,77] Nasal insufflation of DDAVP, 2.5 to 10 µg (25 to 100 µl) once or twice daily, will usually restore the fluid requirements and volume of urine to normal. The antidiuretic response occurs rapidly and its decline is similarly abrupt (Fig. 2–7).

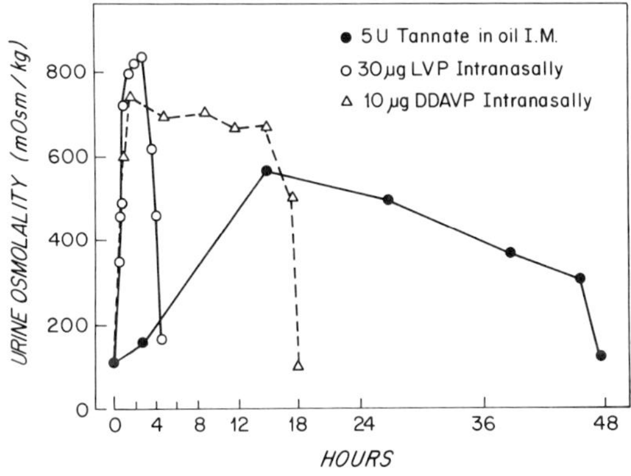

FIGURE 2–7. Antidiuretic response to single doses of Pitressin in oil, lysine vasopressin, and DDAVP. Note the rapid onset and abrupt decline of antidiuresis during DDAVP theray. Higher doses will prolong action but not increase the intensity of antidiuresis.

Nonhormonal Therapy. Among the "hormone amplifiers"[78] chlorpropamide is the most effective and frequently prescribed. This hypoglycemic agent effectively reduces polyuria by enhancing the medullary adenylate cyclase response to vasopressin through inhibition of prostaglandin action.[79,80] The recommended dose of 150 mg/m^2 of body surface should be given once daily. The drug causes a simultaneous stimulation of insulin secretion, but symptomatic hypoglycemia is rarely observed unless the dosage is excessive or there is coexisting anterior pituitary deficiency. The treatment reduces daily fluid turnover, but does not produce the high daily urine concentrations observed following vasopressin administration. It does lead to better fluid homeostasis and tolerance of variation in fluid intake (see Fig. 2–8). Excess drinking that consistently leads to water intoxication in vasopressin-treated patients usually is accompanied by greater dilution of urine. However, occasionally insufficient adaptation occurs and symptomatic hyponatremia develops.[81] Another advantage of chlorpropamide therapy is that the drug appears to stimulate the thirst mechanism.[82,83] It is therefore especially well suited for the therapy of patients who have diabetes insipidus complicated by hypodipsia.

Occasionally diabetes insipidus will be responsive to treatment with acetaminophen and aminopyrine, drugs assumed to have a similar mode of action to sulfonylureas such as chlorpropamide. While less toxic, they are also less effective in reducing urine volume and are limited in their clinical applicability. The use of indomethacin, a potent prostaglandin inhibitor, is mainly reserved for treatment of nephrogenic diabetes insipidus.

Several other pharmacologic agents have been reported to reduce polyuria by central stimulation of vasopressin secretion.[84] The most prominent among them is clofibrate, which was marketed originally for its cholesterol-suppressing properties. It will cause amelioration of mild vasopressin deficiency in some but not all patients responsive to chlorpropamide. The recommended dose is 45 mg/kg/day. Side effects of clofibrate such as abdominal pain and diarrhea may be observed early in the course of therapy. Vasopressin release can also be elicited with carbamazepine.[85] The mechanism for initiating ADH release is different from that of clofibrate. Selective responses to either

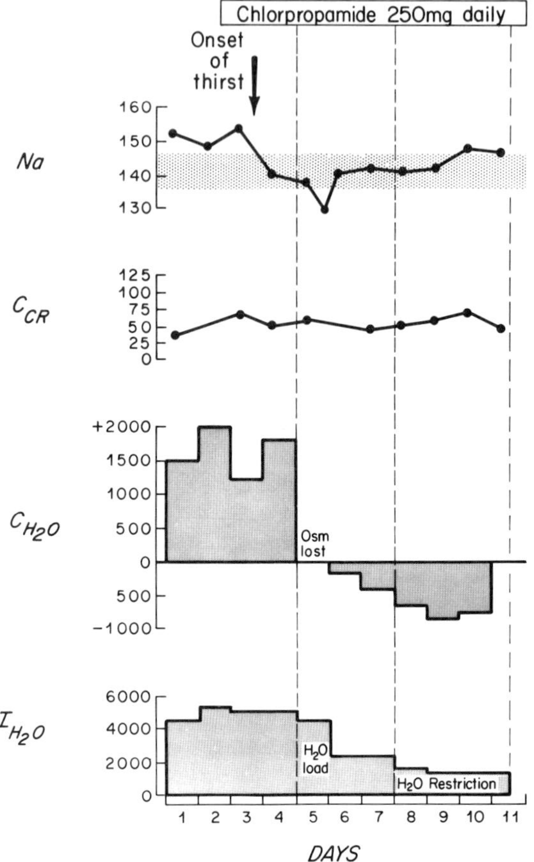

FIGURE 2–8. Chlorpropamide-induced restoration of normal drinking behavior and fluid homeostasis in a patient with diabetes insipidus, chronic hypernatremia, and adipsia. Previous chronic therapy with vasopressin had decreased urine volumes but failed to correct hypernatremia because of the patient's persistent refusal to drink. While off antidiuretic therapy hypernatremia persisted in spite of forced fluid intake. Within 36 hours after initiation of chlorpropamide therapy the patient demanded water and 2 days later appropriately refused to drink when hyponatremia developed during water loading. Restriction of fluid intake was accompanied by antidiuresis and renewed sensation of thirst.[83]

one of the agents have been observed, and combined therapy is associated with an additive antidiuretic effect.[86] We consider carbamazepine too toxic for routine clinical use in the treatment of central diabetes insipidus.

Special Therapeutic Considerations. The therapy of diabetes insipidus has to be adjusted under those conditions that either demand high fluid intake for coverage of caloric need, as in the newborn, or prohibit drinking entirely, as in the postoperative period.

Management of Diabetes Insipidus in Infancy. The treatment of diabetes insipidus in infants is particularly problematic and requires review of some physiologic aspects germane to this age group.[87] All formula- and breast-fed infants have obligatory hyposthenuria to compensate for excess free water intake until feedings are spaced more than 4 hours apart. Vasopressin administration has therefore to be coupled with limitation of food intake to avoid water intoxication. In young infants the daily solute load presented to the kidney varies from 250 to 500 mOsm/m² body surface. In untreated diabetes insipidus the excretion of this solute requires a daily fluid intake of approximately 3.1 to 5.6 L/m² body surface, assuming that urine osmolality will be close to 100 mOsm/kg and insensible water loss 600 ml/m²/day. Even if the fluid needs are further reduced by providing a very-low-solute formula and a humid environment, the infant will require feeding at least every 2 hours to prevent intermittent dehydration. The opposite approach (i.e., therapy with a high-solute diet and vasopressin in doses sufficient to maintain antidiuresis) limits fluid tolerance at most to 1.4 L/m²/day and prevents provision of sufficient calories. Intermittent administration of vasopressin, allowing polyuria to recur, is equally unsatisfactory, since it is accompanied by large fluctuations in serum osmolar and sodium concentration. An additional problem with DDAVP therapy in infancy is drug administration and failure to achieve consistently reproducible results. Intranasal administration of a very small dose (10 μl or 1 μg) may induce antidiuresis extending beyond 10 hours or may not be absorbed in sufficient amounts to affect urine osmolality. This unpredictable response can have dire consequences since food intake needs to be curtailed for the length of the expected antidiuresis. Parenteral DDAVP injection of 0.02 ml (0.08 μg)/kg body weight will induce antidiuresis for approximately 12 hours. This maneuver is particularly well suited for diagnostic testing as long as fluids are curtailed simultaneously. However, hunger-induced irritability should be expected during this limited time interval.

We have found that provision of a low-dietary-solute load and large water intake combined with administration of thiazides is the safest approach to therapy in infancy. This therapy is described in detail under the section dealing with nephrogenic diabetes insipidus. In those infants with a normal thirst mechanism and central diabetes insipidus the addition of a single dose of short-acting intranasal lysine vasopressin at bedtime will further reduce oral fluid needs and allow infants and parents at least a short interval of uninterrupted sleep. In a relatively large number of affected newborns diabetes insipidus is complicated by coexisting brain damage and hypodipsia. These infants require nasogastric or gastrostomy tube feeding to maintain adequate hydration.

Treatment during Parenteral Fluid Therapy. All patients with diabetes insipidus will need adjustment of therapy when intravenous fluid administration is the sole source of water intake. This occurs most often in the perioperative period and with acute gastrointestinal disease. The therapeutic options are again to maintain antidiuresis or to eliminate vasopressin treatment entirely. We prefer therapy designed to produce constant antidiuresis, which can be induced with DDAVP administered in 8- to 12-hour intervals, with daily injections of Pitressin in oil, or with intravenous infusion of aqueous vasopressin, 0.03 mU (75 pg or 6.7 fmol)/kg body weight/minute.[88] This dose is within the range required to produce antidiuresis in normal subjects. The volume of intravenous fluids should initially be reduced to approximately 600 ml/m^2 and thereafter be adjusted according to observed changes in urine and serum osmolar and sodium concentrations. Osmolality and sodium concentrations are determined for blood and urine at 12-hour intervals. With insufficient fluid administration patients will complain of thirst, and sodium levels in their concentrated urine will fall below 20 mEq/L before a significant rise in serum osmolality and sodium content is observed. When fluid is infused in excess of needs, clinical symptoms will initially be absent but urine sodium losses exceeding 70 mEq/L will signal incipient water intoxication. This regimen is especially attractive in the management of unconscious or neurosurgical patients, who are very sensitive to overhydration. The therapy will eliminate complications associated with sudden endogenous vasopressin release during the interphase (Fig. 2–5) and enable the maintenance of serum tonicity and sodium levels within a very narrow range. In children it is superior to the regimen involving omission of hormone therapy and hourly adjustment of intravenous fluid replacement in amounts sufficient to cover preceding urinary and insensible water losses. The latter therapy requires catheterization of the bladder and intensive nursing care, and will cause hyperglycemia and wide fluctuations in serum sodium and osmolar concentration.

Nephrogenic Diabetes Insipidus

Nephrogenic diabetes insipidus was first described by Waring et al.[89] who observed six male infants presenting with failure to thrive, intermittent fever without evidence of infection, hypertonic dehydration, constipation, and excretion of hypotonic urine. Two of the patients were brothers, which led the authors to postulate the possibility of a congenital familial disease. The inability of these patients to form concentrated urine even after vasopressin infusion in doses sufficient to cause systemic side effects led Williams and Henry[90] to propose a target organ resistance to ADH. The presence of biologically active hormone has since been demonstrated by several authors.[91,92] However, the renal and extrarenal unresponsiveness to DDAVP but persistent V_1 receptor sensitivity to arginine vasopressin suggest a defect within the V_2 receptor–adenylate cylase unit.[51,93,94] In mice with nephrogenic diabetes insipidus the defect is due to an abnormally rapid cAMP catabolism in the collecting tubules. In vitro studies have demonstrated excessive phosphodiesterase activity that prevents effective intracellular cAMP accumulation.[95]

Genetics

Many of the patients suffering from this disorder in North America are descendants of the so-called Ulster Scot, who settled in Nova Scotia during the 18th century. Their folklore account of the "water drinkers' curse" dates back to more than a century before Gregor Mendel proposed his laws of heredity in 1865, and gives an accurate description of the X-linked pattern of inheritance[96]:

A gypsy woman and her son were traveling the road and became thirsty. Pausing at a well in front of the next house, the gypsy requested water for her son; the housewife refused, whereupon, the gypsy woman cast upon her a curse. Henceforth, the story goes, the woman's sons would be afflicted with a craving for water. The curse would be passed on by her daughters and revisited upon their sons for generations to come.

In all reported pedigrees this mode of inheritance was documented. Even Cannon's[97] large Mormon family conforms to X-linked transmission when we disregard those instances of male-to-male inheritance in early generations in which he had to rely on historical data for diagnosis as well as for exclusion of consanguinity.[98]

Most female heterozygotes manifest a partial concentration defect (Fig. 2–9) and will give a history of greater water turnover after puberty and especially during pregnancy. Only rarely will a heterozygous female exhibit excess polyuria and seek medical advice.

We have encountered authentic nephrogenic diabetes insipidus in five boys whose families were free of the disease and whose ethnic background excluded a relation to the Ulster Scot. These boys are still too young to have their own progeny, and dependence of their symptoms on a mutant gene of the X chromosome has not been established.

Recent studies suggest that the gene is located in the Xq28 region.[99] Previous linkage studies have shown no association with known X-linked markers.[100] Coexisting color blindness has not been found in any patient with nephrogenic diabetes insipi-

dus, which may suggest close linkage of the two genes on the X chromosome.

Clinical Presentation

Affected boys with nephrogenic diabetes insipidus show initial symptoms within the first 3 weeks of life, but unless anticipated through the family's awareness of the genetic defect, the diagnosis is often delayed. Increased urinary frequency and polyuria are rarely recognized in the diaper stage, and failure to thrive is usually the most apparent clinical finding. The infants are irritable and cry constantly. They suck eagerly, but frequently vomit unless prefed with water. A history of constipation with passage of very firm stools and erratic intermittent fevers can nearly always be elicited.

By the time the diagnosis is made, the infants are usually severely malnourished, their skin is doughy and dry, and there is absence of tears and perspiration. When recognition of the disease is delayed, bouts of severe hypertonic dehydration may be complicated by seizures and even death. Mental retardation is a frequent consequence of these episodes of dehydration, but can be

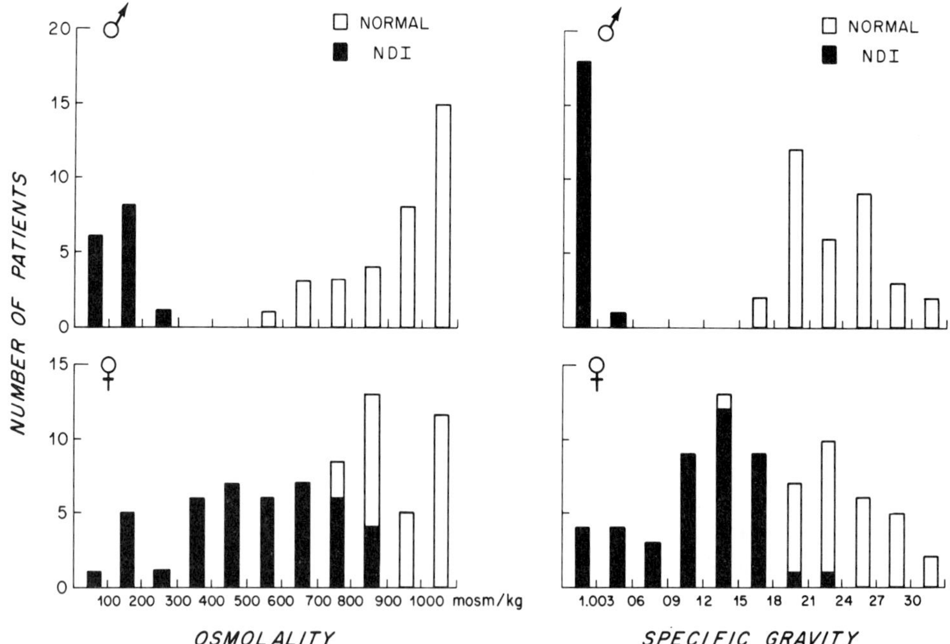

FIGURE 2–9. Urine osmolality and specific gravity in families with nephrogenic diabetes insipidus.[96] Urine was collected after water restriction overnight or for as long as tolerated. Dark columns indicate gene carriers; white columns, unaffected family members and spouses. Neither urine osmolality nor specific gravity clearly separated the female heterozygotes from the normal controls.

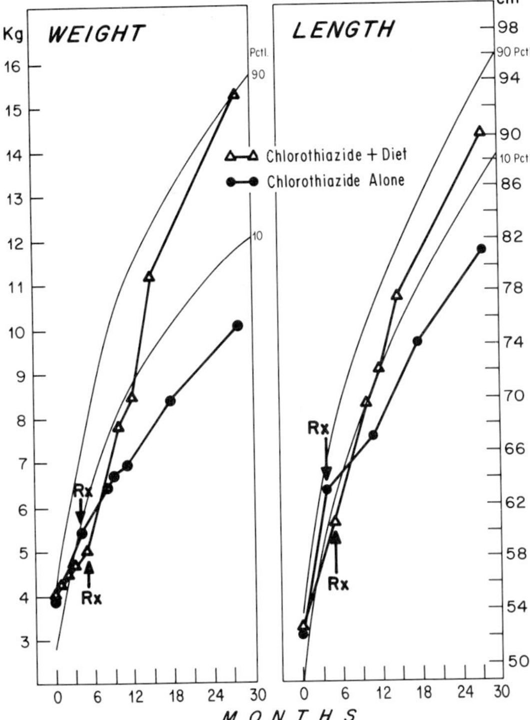

FIGURE 2–10. The importance of diet in the management of nephrogenic diabetes insipidus is reflected in the growth curves of affected cousins. Both received chlorothiazide therapy, but the mother of one did not adhere to the prescribed diet low in sodium and solute residue. He remained hypernatremic and did not improve in growth and weight gain.[98]

prevented by liberal and frequent feeding of free water.[101] Even after the diagnosis is established, infants often show poor growth as a result of either chronic serum hypertonicity or poor caloric intake as a consequence of the large water consumption and avoidance of protein and salt (see Fig. 2–10). Many patients will remain chronically hypernatremic and exhibit elevated serum uric acid concentrations; however, gouty arthritis is only observed during adulthood.[102]

Once the patient has reached an age when water is readily obtainable, acute complications and exacerbations occur rarely and only with infections or conditions restricting oral fluid consumption.

The ever-present thirst and increased urinary frequency consume much of the daily activity of these patients and lead to frequent interruption of sleep.[103] Short attention span and poor scholastic performance are often found in these patients. Early in childhood asymptomatic bladder and ureter

dilation may be observed.[104] Radiologic findings may be similar to those of chronic bladder outlet obstruction. Extensive urologic and radiologic evaluation will invariably fail to document an anatomic defect in the urethra, and neither bladder neck dilation nor uretostomy will result in improvement in symptoms. In the presence of ureteral reflux, surgical therapy should always be preceded by gas cystometry and antegrade pyelography with pressure profiles. In very severe cases irreversible fibrosis of the bladder wall with loss of muscle tone and structure has been documented.[105]

Diagnosis

The diagnosis of nephrogenic diabetes insipidus is now rarely delayed beyond the age of 3 months. The disease should be suspected in all infants presenting with hypernatremia and failure to thrive. Documentation of normal kidney function, serum hyperosmolality, and continuous excretion of dilute urine even after vasopressin administration will establish the diagnosis. Small infants may be exquisitely sensitive to aqueous vasopressin and may show no antidiuretic response even when systemic side effects are apparent and normal renal vasopressin sensitivity is maintained. We therefore recommend a single parenteral injection of DDAVP 0.08 μg (0.02 ml)/kg body weight as the definite diagnostic test. Documentation of elevated plasma vasopressin concentration is equally useful for the diagnosis but rarely required.

In boys, the defect is complete, and a water deprivation test need not be extended beyond 4 hours. A hypertonic saline infusion test should be avoided, since severe hypernatremia may ensue and restoration of sodium concentration to normal may require many hours, if not days.

A careful family history may disclose similarly affected relatives. Most mothers can be identified as carriers by measurement of urine osmolality after a 12-hour period of fluid restriction overnight (see Fig. 2–9).

Treatment

The therapy of nephrogenic diabetes insipidus should be directed toward prevention of hypertonic dehydration and reduction of urine volume. However, a high water intake with frequent feeding, even during the night, will always be required. The diet should be restricted in salt and protein since both sodium and urea enhance obligatory water secretion. When the daily intake of sodium is restricted to less than 0.7 mEq/kg body weight and that of protein to less than 1 gm/kg body weight, a reduction in urine volume and serum osmolality will invariably be observed. Breast milk, with its lower renal osmolar load, is preferable to formula, and baby food should be carefully screened for sodium content. To secure adequate caloric intake sugar can be added to the water fed between and before meals.

The most dramatic improvement in management of these patients was provided by Crawford and Kennedy in 1959 with the introduction of chlorothiazide therapy.[106] These saluretic agents (chlorothiazide 30 mg/kg in three divided doses or hydrochlorothiazide 3 mg/kg daily) decrease sodium reabsorption in the cortical diluting segment, increase urinary sodium loss, and cause plasma volume contraction, which in turn leads to enhanced proximal tubular reabsorption of fluid from the glomerular filtrate. Thiazide therapy is ineffective when simultaneous dietary sodium intake is insufficiently restricted to keep serum sodium concentration below the normal range (Fig. 2–8). Careful monitoring of serum sodium and potassium should be undertaken, especially initially when the dose is being adjusted so that serum sodium concentrations range between 133 and 137 mEq/L. Almost invariably a rise in serum uric acid concentration will be observed initially that may exceed 10 mg/dl if not monitored carefully. The dietary potassium intake should be sufficient to prevent hypokalemia. Under optimal conditions urine volume can be decreased by as much as 40 per cent.

More recently indomethacin has been introduced to the therapy of nephrogenic diabetes insipidus. This prostaglandin synthesis inhibitor has been shown to increase the concentrations of sodium and chloride in the renal medulla.[52] In most boys with nephrogenic diabetes insipidus, indomethacin in doses of 1.5 to 3.0 mg/kg body weight reduces urine flow and has an additive effect to that of chlorothiazide.[107] It is thought that indomethacin causes an antidiuretic effect by enhancing proximal tubular reabsorption of the glomerular filtrate. We have not employed this drug in the treatment of infants. However, a therapeutic trial may be warranted when chlorothiazide-induced hyperuricacidemia cannot be avoided.

Present treatment of nephrogenic diabetes insipidus is still symptomatic and cumbersome. Nevertheless, normal growth and weight gain can be achieved. Recurrent episodes of hypertonic dehydration can be avoided, and the prognosis for normal intellectual develoment is no longer dismal.

Neurogenic Hypernatremia

Neurogenic hypernatremia is a relatively rare syndrome observed primarily in the young and very old. Chronically affected patients have serum sodium concentrations constantly above 145 mEq/l and intermittently show rises to above 180 mEq/l without experiencing the desire to correct the systemic hypertonicity with increased water intake. Unless dehydrated, the children show remarkably few symptoms. They often have coexisting severe neurologic and hypothalamic disease or a history of extensive neurosurgical procedures. Symptomatic diabetes insipidus is present in approximately half of the patients, but all patients show maximal antidiuresis only when very high plasma osmolalities and sodium concentrations have been reached. Plasma vasopressin concentrations are usually measurable but low for the degree of hyperosmolality. One recent study[88] suggested that increased renal sensitivity to vasopressin was present in some of the patients.

The primary cause of this disease entity is a defective thirst mechanism and thus loss of an integral part of the regulatory system maintaining fluid homeostasis. Studies of drinking behavior and fluid and electrolyte metabolism have shown a defect in osmoreceptor-mediated thirst and vasopressin secretion in several patients with normal volume receptor function. Several authors have therefore suggested that these patients have reached a new "set-point" for serum osmolality at which vasopressin secretion and thirst sensation are initiated.[108–111]

For the clinical management of these patients we consider it helpful to separate patients with neurogenic hypernatremia into groups according to their defect and adjust therapy accordingly (Table 2–4). Clear separation will not always be possible and overlap will occur between the groups. The response to challenges such as fluid restriction, hypertonic saline infusion, and water loading should be examined in each patient. Before each test patients should be well hydrated; elevated plasma renin activ-

TABLE 2–4. DIFFERENTIAL DIAGNOSIS OF NEUROGENIC HYPERNATREMIA

| Clinical Disorder | Defect | Qualitative Response To | | | Improvement with ADH Therapy | Recommended Therapy |
		H_2O Deprivation	3% Saline	H_2O Load		
Nephrogenic diabetes insipidus	Adjustment to chronic hypernatremia	Abnormal	Abnormal	Normal	No	Chlorothiazides NaCl restriction
Essential hypernatremia	Abnormal osmo-regulation of thirst and ADH	Normal	Abnormal	Often abnormal	No	Chlorpropamide or Chlorothiazides
Diabetes insipidus with hypodipsia	Vasopressin deficiency and hypodipsia	Abnormal	Abnormal	Normal or delayed	Partial, no thirst	Chlorpropamide (vasopressin)
Primary hypodipsia	Abnormal thirst normal ADH	Normal	Normal	Normal	No	Fluid intake of >1.5 L/m²/day

ity and uric acid concentrations indicate poor renal perfusion and hypovolemia.

The untreated child with nephrogenic diabetes insipidus, listed as the first category of Table 2–4, is forced to accept a new set-point for thirst during infancy when fluids are not readily available. Serum sodium concentrations in this group of patients vary from 144 to 152 mEq/L. The patients experience normal thirst during water deprivation and systemic hypertonicity. In response to a water load they excrete dilute urine rapidly and show a slow decline in plasma sodium levels. Their kidneys exhibit normal sodium-conserving mechanisms when overhydrated for a prolonged time. Hyponatremia does not, therefore, occur acutely.

A second group of hypernatremic children are those with abnormal thirst and vasopressin release in response to changes in plasma osmolality. They usually have normal baroreceptor-mediated vasopressin release and are not polyuric. Urine osmolality may reach 1000 mOsm/kg during prolonged water deprivation when hypovolemia and hypernatremia ensue. Antidiuresis also occurs when a baroreceptor response is elicited pharmacologically by vasodilation or by placing the patient on a tilting table.[108,109] However, deficient vasopressin release can be shown after infusion of hypertonic saline when the hypovolemic stimulus is eliminated. Some of these patients will also show abnormal suppression of ADH and develop hyponatremia after a water load is administered. Studies by Dunger et al.[88] suggested that the latter phenomenon may be

a consequence of increased renal sensitivity to vasopressin. When their patients were treated with a pure V_2 receptor agonist, such as DDAVP, the condition improved. However, this has not been observed in most of the patients reported by others. Thirst stimulation with chlorpropamide should be tried. The patients will respond to salt restriction and chlorothiazide therapy since this will induce mild hypovolemia.

The entity of diabetes insipidus and hypodipsia is seen most often in patients with extensive hypothalamic damage. They experience polyuria and usually concentrate their urine to less than 800 mOsm/kg during dehydration and severe hyperosmolality. During treatment with long-acting vasopressin preparations, they show wide fluctuation in serum osmolality, even if fluid intake is carefully regulated. Many of these patients will respond to chlorpropamide therapy with both antidiuresis and improvement of thirst sensation (Fig. 2–8).[82,83]

Primary hypodipsia is very rarely seen and can be caused by anomalies of the thirst center or by interruption of pathways relating to the limbic system. These patients have normal vasopressin regulation and will respond normally to all three challenge tests. Hypernatremia can be avoided by securing an adequate daily fluid intake.

On rare occasions hypernatremia is observed in patients with chronic upper airway obstruction and hypoventilation due to obesity. These children have a hypoventilatory response to carbon dioxide stimulation and may have chronic or intermittent hypernatremia.[112] Restoration of normal weight or removal of the upper airway obstruction will cure abnormal ventilation and hypernatremic episodes.[113] It is unclear whether this anomaly is caused by carbon dioxide inhibition of vasopressin secretion or by severe fluid losses from excessive perspiration.

Excessive Secretion of Vasopressin

When healthy subjects are exposed chronically to exogenous vasopressin, water retention, weight gain, and dilutional hyponatremia will be observed within 48 hours. The extracellular fluid expansion and hypervolemia cause increased glomerular filtration, decreased proximal tubular reabsorption of sodium, and suppression of aldosterone secretion. Very high urinary sodium losses ensue and further aggravate systemic hypotonicity and hyponatremia.[114] None of these changes is observed when fluid intake is restricted during vasopressin administration, indicating that the thirst center is very weak in suppressing customary drinking behavior.

Clinical findings very similar to those produced by continuous vasopressin administration were observed by Schwartz et al[115] in two patients with bronchogenic carcinomas. Both patients presented with dilutional hyponatremia and sodium diuresis. They had no evidence of renal, cardiac, or adrenal disease. The authors postulated that these manifestations were produced by endogenous vasopressin production inappropriate with respect to serum osmolality. Their hypothesis was supported by subsequent documentation of high plasma vasopressin levels in patients with pulmonary malignancies and ADH production by the tumor tissue.[116,117] Since then the condition has been referred to as the syndrome of inappropriate ADH secretion (SIADH) or the Schwartz-Bartter syndrome.

A great variety of clinical conditions has been associated with excess vasopressin production (see Table 2–1).[118,119] The ectopic production of vasopressin has been noted in association with many types of tumors. In children it is less frequently observed with tumors than with pulmonary and cerebral abnormalities. Nonmalignant lung tissue is capable of vasopressin synthesis. In pulmonary tuberculosis infected lung tissue has a high vasopressin content.[120] In viral and bacterial pneumonia, particularly in infections with *Staphylococcus aureus*, symptoms of SIADH are frequently observed.

Intracranial diseases due to tumor, infection, inflammation, trauma, and hemorrhage are often associated with excessive vasopressin secretion. Antidiuresis during emotional stress and pain was observed in early experiments by Verney.[29] In intensive-care nurseries, SIADH occurs often in newborns treated with positive-pressure breathing[121] and in infants with bronchopulmonary dysplasia.[122]

Drug-induced vasopressin secretion ocurs with administration of chlorpropamide, carbamazepine, analgesics, barbiturates, and, more importantly for the pediatric population, with chemotherapeutic agents such as vincristine and cytoxan. The antidiuresis following cytoxan administration is so frequent that fluid loading to prevent chemical cystitis should be undertaken with isotonic solutions.

In myxedema and cardiac disease, hyponatremia and fluid retention are related to the decreased delivery of glomerular filtrate to the diluting segment of the nephron.[55] In adrenal insufficiency, SIADH is induced by failure of cortisol-dependent ADH suppression.

The symptoms of SIADH include weight gain, weakness, anorexia, and lethargy. In severe cases confusion, convulsions, and coma can occur. Laboratory findings include low serum concentration of urea, creatinine, uric acid, and albumin. Hyponatremia is accompanied by high urine sodium losses. Only in severely hyponatremic children does urine sodium concentration fall as low as 30 mEq/L. In adrenal insufficiency, hyponatremia and sodium diuresis are also observed, but these patients usually have a history of weight loss and demonstrate hyperkalemia and low plasma cortisol concentrations.

Treatment

SIADH should be treated with fluid restriction.[118,119] This will be accompanied by loss of body weight and a steady rise in serum sodium and osmolality. Only if severe symptoms and signs develop is more aggressive therapy indicated. Slow intravenous administration of 3 per cent saline, 5 ml/kg, should be combined with furosemide therapy to minimize further expansion of intravascular volume. No attempt should be made to correct the hyponatremia rapidly, since central pontine myelinolysis has been produced with this maneuver in experimental models.[123] Drug therapy inducing either vasopressin resistance at the renal medulla or vasopressin suppression is rarely used in children. Lithium salts may cause renal diabetes insipidus, but this therapy is generally too toxic. Demethylchlortetracycline causes vasopressin resistance but is effective only after more than 24 hours of treatment and is not recommended for children under the age of 8 years.[124] It has been used for long-term treatment of chronic SIADH. Alcohol suppresses pituitary ADH secretion but not ectopic vasopressin production. It has no place in the therapy of SIADH in children. Treatment with vasopressin receptor antagonists may hold promise for the future.[125]

More important than therapy is the prevention of SIADH. The physician should become aware that this syndrome is one of the most frequent iatrogenic diseases seen in hospitalized children receiving intravenous therapy.

REFERENCES

1. Oliver G, Schafer EA: On the physiological action of extracts of pituitary body and certain other glandular organs. J Physiol 18:277, 1895.
2. Dale HH: On some physiological actions of ergot. J Physiol 34:163, 1906.
3. Ott I, Scott JC: The action of infundibulin upon the mammary secretion. Proc Soc Exp Biol Med 8:48, 1910.
4. von den Velden R: Die Nierenwirkung von Hypophysenextrakten beim Menschen. Berl Klin Wochenschr 50:2083, 1913.
5. Farmi F: Über Diabetes Insipidus und Hypophysistherapie. Wien Klin Wochenschr 26:1867, 1913.
6. du Vigneaud V, Ressler C, Swan JM, et al: The synthesis of an octapeptide amide with the hormonal activity of oxytocin. J Am Chem Soc 75:4879, 1954.
7. du Vigneaud V, Gish DT, Kaisoyannis PG, et al: Synthesis of the pressor-antidiuretic hormone, arginine-vasopressin. J Am Chem Soc 80:3355, 1958.
8. Bargmann W, Scharrer I: The site of origin of the hormones of the posterior pituitary. Am Sci 39:255, 1951.
9. Hayward JN: The amygdaloid nuclear complex and mechanisms of release of vasopressin from the neurohypophysis. In Eleftheriou BE (ed): Neurobiology of the Amygdala. New York, Plenum Press, 1972, p 685.
10. Dawood MY, Wang CF, Gupta R, et al: Fetal contribution to oxytocin in human labor. Obstet Gynecol 52:205, 1978.
11. De Wied D, Versteeg DH: Neurohypophyseal principles and memory. Fed Proc 38:2348, 1979.
12. Weingartner H, Gold P, Ballenger JC, et al: Effects of vasopressin on human memory functions. Science 211:601, 1981.
13. Van Ree JM, Bohus B, Versteeg DH, et al: Neurohypophyseal principles and memory processes. Biochem Pharmacol 27:1793, 1978.
14. Skowsky WR, Fisher DA: Fetal neurohypophyseal arginine vasopressin and arginine vasotocin in man and sheep. Pediatr Res 11:627, 1977.
15. Sawyer WH: Evolution of antidiuretic hormones and their functions. Am J Med 42:678, 1967.
16. Thrasher TN, Keil LC: Regulation of drinking and vasopressin secretion: Role of organum vasculosum laminae terminalis. Am J Physiol 253:R108, 1987.
17. Gross PM, Sposito NM, Pettersen SE, Fenstermacher JD: Differences in function and structure of the capillary endothelium in the supraoptic nucleus and pituitary neural lobe of rats: Evidence for the supraoptic nucleus as an osmometer. Neuroendocrinology 44:401, 1986.
18. Sachs H, Takabataki Y: Evidence for a precursor in vasopressin biosynthesis. Endocrinology 75:943, 1964.
19. Robinson AG: Neurophysins and their physiologic significance. In Krieger DT, Hughes JC (eds): Neuroendocrinology. A Hospital Practice Book. Sunderland, MA, Sinauer Associates, 1980.
20. Chard T: The posterior pituitary gland. Clin Endocrinol 4:89, 1975.
21. Cheung KW, Friesen HG: Physiological factors regulating secretion of neurophysin. Metabolism 19:876, 1970.
22. Sawyer WH: Neurohypophysial hormones. Pharmacol Rev 13:225, 1961.
23. Sala NL: Milk-ejecting effect induced by various octapeptides in human beings. Acta Physiol Lat Am 15:191, 1965.
24. Ausiello A, Shorecki KL, Verkman AS, Bonventre JV: Vasopressin signaling in the kidney. Kidney Int 31:521, 1987.
25. Robinson AG, Frantz AG: Radioimmunoassay of posterior pituitary peptides: A review. Metabolism 22:1047, 1973.
26. Robertson GL: Diagnosis of diabetes insipidus. In Czernichow P, Robinson AG (eds): Diabetes Insipidus in Man. Frontiers in Hormone Research. Vol 13. Basel, S Karger, 1985, p 176.
27. Martin JB, Reichlin S, Brown GM: Clinical Neuroendocrinology. Contemporary Neurology Series. Philadelphia, FA Davis, 1977.
28. Bard P, Woods JW, Bleier R: The locus and functional capacity of the osmoreceptors in the deafferented hypothalamus. Trans Assoc Am Phys 79:107, 1966.
29. Verney EG: Croonian Lecture: Antidiuretic hormone and factors which determine its release. Proc R Soc Med B 135:25, 1947.
30. Robertson GL: Physiology of ADH release. Kidney Int 31:S20, 1987.
31. Share L, Claybaugh JR: Regulation of body fluids. Annu Rev Physiol 334:235, 1972.
32. Johnson JA, Zehr JE, Moore VW: Effects of separate and concurrent osmotic and volume stimuli on plasma ADH in sheep. Am J Physiol 281:1273, 1970.
33. Daniel AR, Lederis K: Effects of ether anaesthesia and haemorrhage on hormone storage and ul-

trastructure of the rat neurohypophysis. J Endocrinology 34:91, 1966.

34. Lee J, Malvin RL, Claybaugh JR, Huang BS: Atrial natriuretic factor inhibits vasopressin secretion in conscious sheep. Proc Soc Exp Biol Med 185:272, 1987.

35. Adolph EF, Basker JP, Hoy PA: Multiple factors in thirst. Am J Physiol 178:538, 1954.

36. Thompson CJ, Burd JM, Baylis PH: Acute suppression of plasma vasopressin and thirst after drinking in hypernatremic humans. Am J Physiol 252:R1138, 1987.

37. Salata RA, Verbalis JG, Robinson AG: Cold water stimulation of oropharyngeal receptors in man inhibits release of vasopressin. J Clin Endocrinol Metab 64:561, 1987.

38. Plotzky PM, Bruhm TO, Vale W: Evidence for multifactor regulation of the adenocorticotropin secretory response to hemodynamic stimuli. Endocrinology 116:633, 1985.

39. Plotzky PM, Bruhm TO, Vale W: Hypophysiotropic regulation of ACTH secretion in response to insulin-induced hypoglycemia. Endocrinology 117:323, 1985.

40. van Wyk JJ, Dugger GS, Newsome JF, Thomas PZ: The effect of pituitary stalk section on the adrenal function of women with cancer of the breast. J Clin Endocrinol Metab 20:157, 1960.

41. Fischer BM, Baylis PH, Frier BM: Plasma oxytocin, arginine vasopressin and atrial natriuretic peptide responses during insulin-induced hypoglycemia. Clin Endocrinology 26:179, 1987.

42. Carmichael MS, Humbert R, Dixen J, Palmisano G, Greenleaf W, Davidson JM: Plasma oxytocin increase in the human sexual response. J Clin Endocrinol Metab 64:27, 1987.

43. Ferguson JKW: A study of the motility of the intact uterus at term. Surg Gynecol Obstet 73:359, 1941.

44. Reppert SM, Artman HG, Swaminathan S, et al: Vasopressin exhibits a rhythmic daily pattern in cerebral spinal fluid but not in blood. Science 213:1256, 1981.

45. Robertson GL, Mahr EA, Athar S, et al: Development and clinical application of a new method for the radioimmunoassay of arginine vasopressin in human plasma. J Clin Invest 52:2340, 1973.

46. Dawood MY, Ylikorkala O, Trivedi D, et al: Oxytocin levels and disappearance rate and plasma follicle-stimulating hormone and luteinizing hormone after oxytocin infusion in man. J Clin Endocrinol Metab 50:397, 1980.

47. Wirz H, Hargitay B, Kuhn W: Lokalisation des konzentrierungsprozesses in der niere durch direkte kryoskopie. Helv Physiol Pharmacol Acta 9:196, 1951.

48. Kokko JP, Rector FC Jr: Countercurrent multiplication system without active transport in inner medulla. Kidney Int 2:214, 1972.

49. Herbert SC, Reeves WB, Malong DA, Andreoli TE: The medullary thick limb: Function and modulation of the single-effect multiplier. Kidney Int 31:580, 1987.

50. Strange K, Spring KR: Absence of significant cellular dilution during ADH stimulated water resorption. Science 235:1068, 1987.

51. Bichet DG, Razi M, Lonergan M, Arthus MF, Papukna V, Kortas C, Barjon JN: Hemodynamic and coagulation responses to DDAVP in patients with congenital nephrogenic diabetes insipidus. N Engl J Med 318:881, 1988.

52. Ganguli M, Tobian L, Azar S, O'Donell M: Evidence that prostaglandin synthesis inhibitors increase the concentration of sodium and chloride in the rat medulla. Circ Res 40:1135, 1977.

53. Sawyer WH, Valtin H: Antidiuretic responses of rats with hereditary hypothalamic diabetes insipidus to vasopressin, oxytocin and nicotine. Endocrinology 80:207, 1967.

54. Agus ZS, Goldberg M: Role of antidiuretic hormone in the abnormal water diuresis of anterior hypopituitarism in man. J Clin Invest 50:1478, 1971.

55. deRubertis FR, Michelis MF, Gloom MF, et al: Impaired water excretion in myxedema. Am J Med 51:41, 1971.

56. Green HH, Harrington AR, Valtin H: On the role of antidiuretic hormone in the inhibition of acute water diuresis in adrenal insufficiency and the effects of gluco- and mineralocorticoids in reversing the inhibition. J Clin Invest 49:1724, 1970.

57. Ufferman RC, Schrier RW: Importance of sodium intake and mineralocorticoid hormone in the impaired water excretion in adrenal insufficiency. J Clin Invest 51:1639, 1972.

58. Abrahams VC, Pickford M: Observation on a central antagonism between adrenaline and acetylcholine. J Physiol 131:712, 1956.

59. Fisher DA: Norepinephrine inhibition of vasopressin antidiuresis. J Clin Invest 47:540, 1968.

60. Kikuchi K, Fujifawa I, Momoi P, Yamaraka C, Kaji M, Nakano Y, Konishi J, Mikawa H, Sudo M: Hypothalamic-pituitary function in growth hormone-deficient patients with pituitary stalk transection. J Clin Endocrinol Metab 67:817, 1988.

61. Randall RV, Clark EC, Dodge JW Jr, et al: Polyuria after operation for tumors in the region of the hypophysis and hypothalamus. J Clin Endocrin 20:1614, 1960.

62. Hollinshead WH: The interphase of diabetes insipidus. Proc Staff Meet Mayo Clin 39:92, 1964.

63. Atkinson FRB: Schüller-Christian's disease. Br J Child Dis 34:28, 1937.

64. Scherbaum WA, Bottazzo GF, Gzernichow P, Wass JAH, Doniach D: Role of autoimmunity in central diabetes insipidus. In Czernichow P, Robinson AG (eds): Diabetes Insipidus in Man. Frontiers in Hormone Research. Vol 13. Basel, S Karger, 1985, p 232.

65. Nagi NA: Diabetes insipidus, diabetes mellitus, optic atrophy and deafness. A clinical and genetic study. Postgrad Med J 55:377, 1979.

66. Hickey RC, Hare K: The renal excretion of chloride and water in diabetes insipidus. J Clin Invest 23:768, 1944.

67. Gates JE, Garrod O: The effect of nicotine on urinary flow in diabetes insipidus. Clin Sci 10:145, 1951.

68. Lacombe LU: De la polydipsia. L'experience. J Med Chir 7:309, 1841.

69. Martin FIR: Familial diabetes insipidus. Q J Med 28:573, 1959.

70. Weil A: Über die hereditäre Form des Diabetes Insipidus. Virchows Arch Path Anat 95:70, 1881.

71. Weil A: Über die hereditäre Form des Diabetes Insipidus. Arch Klin Med Leipzig 93:180, 1908.

72. Just G: Ein Wort zu Weils Diabetes Insipidus-stammbaum. Arch Rassenk 16:312, 1924.

73. Forssman H: On hereditary diabetes insipidus. With special reference to a sex-linked form. Acta Med Scand 121(Suppl 159):1, 1945.

74. Stuart CA, Neelon FA, Lebovitz HE: Disordered control of thirst in hypothalamic-pituitary sarcoidosis. N Engl J Med 303:1078, 1980.

75. Barlow ED, de Wardener HE: Compulsive water drinking. Q J Med 28:235, 1959.

76. Vavra I, Machova A, Holecek F, et al: Effect of a synthetic analogue of vasopressin in animals and in patients with diabetes insipidus. Lancet 1:948, 1968.

77. Robinson AG: DDAVP in the treatment of central diabetes insipidus. N Engl J Med 294:507, 1976.

78. Crawford JD, Bode HH: Diabetes and the amplifier hypothesis. N Engl J Med 282:635, 1970.

79. Ozer A, Sharp GWG: Modulation of adenyl cyclase action in toad bladder by chlorpropamide: Antagonism to prostaglandin E. Eur J Pharmacol 22:227, 1973.

80. Bode HH, Meara P, Jones HS, et al: Sulfonylureas inhibit prostaglandin E. Pediatr Res 7:385, 1973.

81. Hayes JS, Kaye M: Inappropriate secretion of antidiuretic hormone induced by chlorpropamide. Am J Med Sci 263:137, 1972.

82. Mahoney JH, Goodman DA: Hypernatremia due to hypodipsia and elevated threshold for vasopressin release. Effects of treatment with hydrochlorothiazide, chlorpropamide and tolbutamide. N Engl J Med 279:1191, 1968.

83. Bode HH, Harley BM, Crawford JD: Restoration of normal drinking behavior by chlorpropamide in patients with hypodipsia and diabetes insipidus. Am J Med 51:304, 1971.

84. Moses AM, Howanitz J, van Gemert M, et al: Clofibrate induced antidiuresis. J Clin Invest 52:535, 1973.

85. Kimura T, Matsui K, Sato T, et al: Mechanism of carbamazepine (Tegretol)-induced antidiuresis: Evidence for release of antidiuretic hormone and impaired secretion of a water load. J Clin Endocrinol Metab 38:356, 1974.

86. Muhlendahl KF, Manz F: Treatment of pitressin-sensitive diabetes insipidus in children with clofibrate and carbmazepine. Z Kinder 115:83, 1973.

87. Crigler JF: Commentary: On the use of pitressin in infants with neurogenic diabetes insipidus. J Pediatr 88:295, 1976.

88. Dunger DB, Seckl JR, Lightman SL: Increased renal sensitivity to vasopressin in two patients with essential hypernatremia. J Clin Endocrinol Metab 64:185, 1987.

89. Waring AG, Kajdi L, Tappan F: A congenital defect of water metabolism. AMA J Dis Child 69:323, 1945.

90. Williams RH, Henry C: Nephrogenic diabetes insipidus transmitted by females and appearing during infancy in males. Ann Intern Med 27:84, 1947.

91. Dancis J, Birmingham JR, Leslie SH: Congenital diabetes insipidus resistant to treatment with pitressin. AMA J Dis Child 75:316, 1948.

92. Holliday MA, Burstin C, Hurrak J: Evidence that the antidiuretic substance in the plasma of children with nephrogenic diabetes insipidus is ADH. Pediatrics 32:384, 1963.

93. Fichman MP, Brooker G: Deficient renal cyclic adenosine 3',5'-monophosphate production in nephrogenic diabetes insipidus. J Clin Endocrinol Metab 35:35, 1972.

94. Bell MH, Clark CM Jr, Avery S, et al: Demonstration of a defect in the formation of adenosine 3',5'-monophosphate in vasopressin resistant diabetes insipidus. Pediatr Res 8:223, 1974.

95. Gapstur S, Hemma S, Coffey A, Valtin H, Dousa TP: Abnormal cAMP catabolism in collecting tubules of mice with hereditary nephrogenic diabetes insipidus. (abstr). Kidney Int 33:264, 1988.

96. Bode HH, Crawford JD: Nephrogenic diabetes insipidus in North America: The Hopewell hypothesis. N Engl J Med 280:750, 1969.

97. Cannon JF: Diabetes insipidus: Clinical and experimental studies with consideration of genetic relationships. AMA Arch Intern Med 96:215, 1955.

98. Crawford JD, Bode HH: Disorders of the posterior pituitary in children. *In* Gardner LJ (ed): Endocrine and Genetic Diseases of Childhood. Philadelphia, WB Saunders Company, 1975, p 126.

99. Kambouris M, Dlouhy SR, Trofattaer JA, Conneally PM, Hodes ME: Localization of the gene for X-linked nephrogenic diabetes insipidus to Xq28. Am J Med Genet 29:239, 1988.

100. Bode HH, Miettinen OS: Nephrogenic diabetes insipidus: Absence of close linkage with Xg. Am J Hum Genet 22:221, 1970.

101. Ruess AI, Rosenthal IM: Intelligence in nephrogenic diabetes insipidus. Am J Dis Child 105:358, 1963.

102. Gordon P, Robertson GL, Seegmiller JE: Hyperuricemia, a concomitant of congenital vasopressin-resistant diabetes insipidus in the adult. N Engl J Med 281:1057, 1971.

103. Hillman DA, Neyzi O, Porter P, et al: Renal (vasopressin resistant) diabetes insipidus: Definition of the effects of a homeostatic limitation in capacity to conserve water on the physical, intellectual and emotional development of a child. Pediatrics 21:430, 1958.

104. Vest M, Talbot NB, Crawford JD: Hypocaloric dwarfism and hydronephrosis in diabetes insipidus. Am J Dis Child 105:175, 1963.

105. Carter RC, Goldman AD: Nephrogenic diabetes insipidus accompanied by massive dilation of the kidneys, ureters and bladder. J Urology 89:366, 1963.

106. Crawford JD, Kennedy GC: Chlorothiazide in diabetes insipidus. Nature 183:891, 1959.

107. Niaudet P, Dechaux M, Leroy D, Broyer M: Nephrogenic diabetes insipidus in children. *In* Czernichow P, Robinson AG (eds): Diabetes Insipidus in Man. Frontiers in Hormone Research. Vol 13. Basel, S Karger, 1985, p 224.

108. DeRubertis FR, Michelis MS, Beck N, et al: "Essential" hypernatremia due to ineffective osmotic and intact volume regulation of vasopressin secretion. J Clin Invest 50:97, 1971.

109. Halter BH, Goldberg AP, Robertson GL, et al: Selective osmoreceptor dysfunction in the syndrome of chronic hypernatremia. J Clin Endocrinol Metab 44:609, 1977.

110. Brezis M, Weiler-Ravell D: Hypernatremia, hypodipsia and partial diabetes insipidus: A model

for defective osmoregulation. Am J Med Sci 279:37, 1980.

111. Sridhar CB, Calvert GD, Ibbertson HK: Syndrome of hypernatremia, hypodipsia and partial diabetes insipidus: A new interpretation. J Clin Endocrinol 38:890, 1974.

112. Moskowitz MA, Fisher JN, Simpser MD, et al: Periodic apnea, exercise hypoventilation and hypothalamic dysfunction. Ann Intern Med 84:171, 1976.

113. Schaad U, Vassella F, Zuppinger K, et al: Hypodipsia-hypernatraemia syndrome. Helv Paediatr Acta 34:63, 1979.

114. Leaf A, Bartter FC, Santos RF, et al: Evidence in man that urinary electrolyte loss induced by pitressin is a function of water retention. J Clin Invest 32:868, 1953.

115. Schwartz WB, Bennett W, Curelop M, et al: A syndrome of renal sodium loss and hyponatremia, probably resulting from inappropriate secretion of antidiuretic hormone. Am J Med 23:529, 1957.

116. George JM, Capen CC, Phillips AS: Biosynthesis of vasopressin in vitro and ultrastructure of a bronchogenic carcinoma. Patient with the syndrome of inappropriate secretion of antidiuretic hormone. J Clin Invest 512:141, 1972.

117. Vorherr V, Vorherr UF, McConnell TS, et al: Localization and origin of antidiuretic principle in para-endocrine active malignant tumors. Oncology 29:201, 1974.

118. Mendoza SA: Syndrome of inappropriate antidiuretic hormone secretion (SIADH). Pediatr Clin North Am 23:681, 1976.

119. Friedman AL, Segal WE: Antidiuretic hormone excess. J Pediatr 94:521, 1979.

120. Vorherr H, Masry SG, Fallet R, et al: Antidiuretic principle in tuberculous lung tissue of a patient with pulmonary tuberculosis and hyponatremia. Ann Intern Med 72:383, 1970.

121. Paxton CL, Stoerner JW, Denson SE, et al: Syndrome of inappropriate antidiuretic hormone secretion in neonates with pneumothorax or atelectasis. J Pediatr 91:459, 1977.

122. Rao M, Eid N, Herrod L, Parekh A, Steiner P: Antidiuretic hormone response in children with bronchopulmonary dysplasia during episodes of acute respiratory distress. Am J Dis Child 140:825, 1986.

123. Kleinschmidt-De Masters BK, Norenberg MD: Rapid correction of hyponatremia causes demyelination: Relation to central pontine myelinolysis. Science 211:1068, 1981.

124. Forrest JN Jr, Cox M, Hong C, et al: Superiority of demeclocycline over lithium in the treatment of chronic syndrome of inappropriate secretion of antidiuretic hormone. N Engl J Med 298:173, 1978.

125. Hofbauer KG, Mah SC: Vasopressin antagonists: Present and future. Kidney Int 31:521, 1987.

3

THE THYROID

Delbert A. Fisher

Thyroid hormones exert important effects on energy metabolism and the metabolism of nutrients and inorganic ions, and these actions are qualitatively similar in children and in adults. Thyroid hormones also exert important effects on growth and development, and these developmental actions are uniquely manifested during the first two decades of life.[1-3] In addition, embryologic and genetic abnormalities involving thyroid hormone production or action are prominent during childhood. In the present chapter we review thyroid hormone physiology and pharmacology and the congenital and acquired disorders of thyroid function with which the pediatric endocrinologist must be familiar.

SYNTHESIS OF THYROID HORMONES

The function of the thyroid gland is to concentrate iodide from the blood and return it to peripheral tissues in a hormonally active form. The major substrates for thyroid hormone synthesis are iodide and tyrosine.[1,2] Tyrosine is not rate limiting even in individuals with phenylketonuria, in whom tyrosine becomes an essential amino acid. Iodine, by contrast, is a trace element that can be rate limiting in thyroid hormone synthesis. The thyroid follicular cell membrane contains a mechanism for transporting iodide from plasma against a concentration gradient. This iodine concentrating mechanism, sometimes referred to as the iodide pump, confers on the gland its ability to concentrate iodide to many times its level in plasma and to maintain thyroid hormone synthesis in the face of relative or absolute iodine deficiency.

The transport of iodide across the thyroid cell membrane is the first and rate-limiting step in thyroid hormone biosynthesis[1-3] (Fig. 3–1). This transport is a potassium- and energy-requiring process, but the molecular structure and mechanism of the iodide transporter are not yet clear.[3] Normally the thyroid follicular cell generates a thyroid-serum (T:S ratio) concentration gradient of 30- to 40-fold. This gradient increases markedly when stimulated by a low-iodine diet, by thyroid-stimulating hormone (TSH), by thyroid-stimulating immunoglobulins (TSI), or by drugs that impair the efficiency of hormone synthesis. The salivary glands, gastric mucosa, uterus, mammary glands, small intestine, and placenta also are able to concentrate iodide; however, they are not capable of iodothyronine synthesis. Several anions are capable of competitively inhibiting iodide transport. These include bromide (Br^-), nitrite (NO_2), thiocyanate (SCN^-), perchlorate (ClO_4), and technetium (TcO_4).

The oxidation of iodide to an active intermediate is followed by iodination of thyroglobulin-bound tyrosyl residues to form monoiodotyrosine (MIT) and diiodotyrosine (DIT).[1,2] Both iodide oxidation and organification are catalyzed by thyroid peroxidase. Iodination also requires generation of peroxide (H_2O_2). Thyroglobulin (TG), which provides the tyrosyl residues for iodotyrosine synthesis, is an iodinated glycoprotein with a molecular weight approximating 660,000 and a sedimentation coefficient of 19.4 (19S).[4] It is composed of two 12S subunits each of which is comprised of two to four peptide chains. Monoiodotyrosine, diiodotyrosine, triiodothyronine (T_3), and thyroxine (T_4) are present within TG as iodoaminoacyl residues that can be cleaved by proteolytic enzymes. The tyrosyl residues, which are the iodine acceptors of TG, comprise about 3 per cent of the weight of the protein, and about two thirds of these are spatially oriented to be susceptible to iodi-

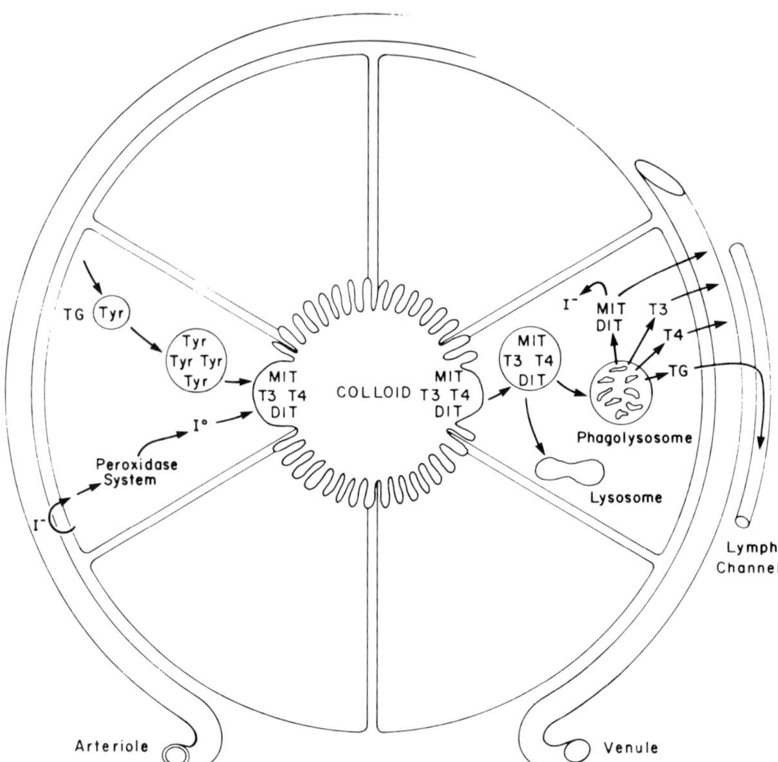

FIGURE 3–1. Thyroid hormone synthesis and secretion by thyroid follicular cells. Synthesis and secretion are shown separately, but occur in the same cell. The thyroid follicular cells form spherules with a storage pool of colloid in the center; this drawing shows a cross-section of a spheroid follicle (TG, thyroglobulin; I⁻, iodide; I°, oxidized, reactive iodine; Tyr, tyrosine; MIT, monoiodotyrosine; DIT, diiodotyrosine; T_3, triiodothyronine; T_4, thyroxine). Thyroglobulin containing tyrosine residues is synthesized within the cell and transported to the luminal membrane, where it is exposed to oxidized, reactive iodine. The exposed tyrosine molecules within the TG are iodinated to MIT or DIT and those MIT and DIT molecules are spatially oriented for coupling to form T_3 or T_4 molecules. The iodinated thyroglobulin is stored as colloid. Activation of secretion by TSH stimulates colloid endocytosis. Infolding colloid droplets fuse with cell lysosomes to form phagolysosomes within which thyroglobulin is degraded to release iodotyrosines T_3 and T_4. Some thyroglobulin escapes from the cell to the circulation, predominantly via lymphatics.

nation. The thyroid gland normally contains 50 to 100 mg TG for every 1 gm of gland.

In addition to catalyzing the iodination of tyrosines, thyroid peroxidase catalyzes the coupling of iodotyrosines within the TG molecule to form T_3 and T_4. Coupling efficiency also is dependent on TSH. The relative proportions of T_3 and T_4 formed depend on the amount of available iodide, the extent of TG iodination, and the level of TSH stimulation. Low-iodine diets increase the MIT:DIT ratio, increase T_3 synthesis, and increase the TG T_3:T_4 ratio. High-iodine diets decrease the MIT:DIT ratio and favor T_4 synthesis. In the absence of iodine deficiency, about 30 per cent of the iodoprotein is iodothyronine, with a T_4:T_3 ratio of 10:1 to 20:1.

The first step in thyroid hormone release is the endocytosis of stored colloid (Fig. 3–1). Within a few minutes after administration of TSH or other thyroid stimulators apical cell membrane pseudopods are formed at the luminal surface of the thyroid follicular cell. The pseudopods enlarge to become intracellular colloid droplets (a process of pinocytosis) and these fuse with proteolytic enzyme–containing lysosomes to form phagolysosomes, wherein TG hydrolysis occurs.[1,2] Digestion of TG involves reduction of the disulfide bonds followed by proteolysis and release of free iodothyronines into the cytoplasm. The free iodothyronines diffuse down the concentration gradient into blood (Fig. 3–1).

The thyroid gland, like other tissues, contains an outer ring iodothyronine deiodinase that monodeiodinates T_4 to T_3.[5] The enzyme activity is stimulated by TSH with the result that the ratio of T_3 to T_4 secreted from the thyroid gland increases with increasing TSH stimulation. Thyroid-stimulating immunoglobulins in Graves disease probably produce a similar effect, accounting, at least in part, for the increased $T_3:T_4$ secretion ratio in Graves hyperthyroidism.

The MIT and DIT released during hydrolysis of TG are largely deiodinated under the influence of a thyroid iodotyrosine deiodinase.[1,2] The free iodide formed enters the intracellular iodide pool and is reutilized for new hormone synthesis. Nonthyroidal tissues also are capable of deiodinating iodotyrosines and presumably contain similar iodotyrosine deiodinating enzymes. A defect in thyroid iodotyrosine deiodinase leads to release of intact iodotyrosines into the circulation and their excretion in urine. The loss of this normally recycled iodine, amounting to 70 to 80 per cent of the daily thyroidal iodine supply, can lead to significant iodine deficiency.

Some TG escapes degradation in thyroid phagolysosomes and appears in serum in association with secreted iodothyronines.[1,4] There is good evidence that TG reaches the general circulation via thyroidal lymphatics (Fig. 3–1). The role of TG in serum or plasma is not known. Circulating TG concentrations in normal children range from <1 to 80 ng/ml.[6,7] Values increase after TSH administration and decrease during thyroid hormone administration. Circulating TG levels are high in newborn infants, especially premature infants, during the first weeks of life, and concentrations decrease with age throughout infancy and childhood. Thyroglobulin concentrations are elevated in patients with a variety of thyroid disorders reflecting thyroidal hyperactivity, including endemic goiter, subacute thyroiditis, Graves disease, and toxic multinodular goiter.[4,6,7] Serum TG concentrations also are increased, often markedly, in patients with thyroid adenoma and papillary-follicular carcinoma, although not in those with anaplastic or medullary carcinoma.[4]

REGULATION OF THYROID FUNCTION

Thyroid function is regulated by circulating TSH and iodide levels.[1–3,8] Thyroid-stimulating hormone binding to the plasma membrane TSH receptor of the thyroid follicular cell stimulates production and accumulation of intracellular cyclic AMP (cAMP) which, in turn, stimulates iodide trapping, iodothyronine synthesis, TG synthesis, glucose oxidation, colloid pinocytosis, thyroid hormone release, and thyroid growth.[1,2,8] Human chorionic gonadotropin (hCG) in patients with choriocarcinoma and TSI in patients with Graves disease compete with TSH for receptors on thyroid follicular cells and stimulate thyroid function. Thyroid-stimulating hormone also stimulates phosphoinositol turnover in thyroid follicular cell membranes as well as transmembrane calcium flux, and recent evidence suggests that growth of thyroid cells may be stimulated by immunoglobulins from patients with autoimmune thyroid disease separately from the effects on thyroid hormone metabolism.[9–11] It has been proposed that these actions are subserved by different types of TSH receptors or different intracellular signals, but this is not yet clear.

Variation in iodine intake in the physiologic range modulates thyroid membrane iodide trapping. As plasma iodide levels fall iodide transport intracellularly is stimulated. High plasma iodide levels reduce iodide transport and iodide uptake. This adaptation to a change in mean iodide intake requires 2 to 4 weeks. In pharmacologic doses iodide can impair the peroxidase enzyme system and inhibit organification (the Wolff-Chaikoff effect); TG synthesis and hormone release also are impaired by high intrathyroidal iodide levels.[1] At least one important mechanism for these latter effects is the inhibitory action of iodide on the stimulation of cAMP formation by TSH.

Thyroid-stimulating hormone functions as a trophic hormone, and removal of the pituitary gland reduces thyroid cell function to a basal level.[8] Thyroid-stimulating hormone secretion is modulated by thyrotropin-releasing hormone (TRH), a tripeptide synthesized in the hypothalamus and secreted into the pituitary portal vascular system for transport to the anterior pituitary thyrotroph cell[8,12,13] (Fig. 3–2). Thyrotropin-releasing hormone production is modulated by environmental temperature via both peripheral and central (hypothalamic) thermal receptors, which in turn modulate neuronal output to the hypothalamic centers regulating TRH secretion (Fig. 3–2). Decreasing environmental and body temperature increases TRH release and increases the tonic level of TSH secretion. Thyroid hormone feedback modulation of TSH release occurs at both the pituitary and the hypothalamic levels[8,14,15]; T_3 modulates hy-

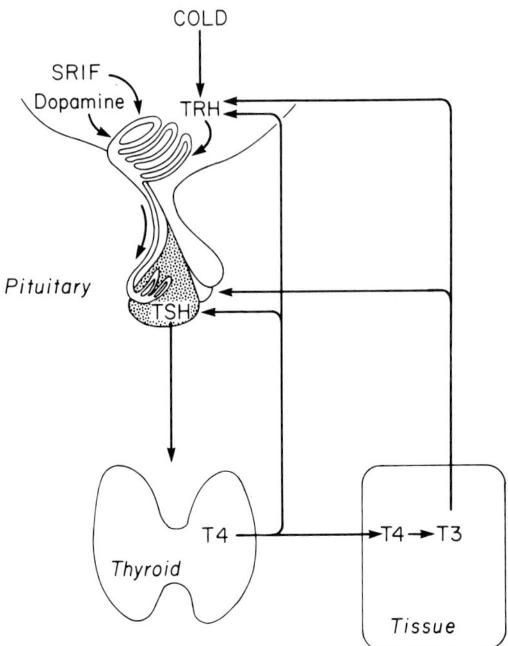

FIGURE 3–2. Regulation of TSH secretion. Pituitary TSH synthesis and release are modulated by hypothalamic thyrotropin-releasing hormone (TRH), which is transported to the anterior pituitary gland via the pituitary portal vascular system. Thyrotropin-releasing hormone synthesis and release are modulated, in turn, via anterior hypothalamic thermal receptors and by input from peripheral thermal receptors. Body cooling stimulates TRH release. Thyroid hormone feedback to the hypothalamus also modulates TRH synthesis; decreased thyroid hormone stimulates and increased hormone inhibits TRH synthesis. Thyrotropin-releasing hormone acts via receptors in the pituitary thyrotropic cells to stimulate synthesis and release of TSH. Thyroid hormone feedback at the pituitary cell modulates the TRH effect by modulating TRH receptor binding and modulating TSH synthesis. As a result decreased thyroid hormone increases, and increased hormone inhibits pituitary TSH secretion. Somatostatin (SRIF) and dopamine can inhibit TSH release.

pothalamic TRH synthesis and in addition modulates pituitary TSH release by inhibiting pituitary cell membrane TRH receptor binding and TRH-mediated TSH release.[8,9,12–15]

Somatostatin (somatotropin release–inhibiting factors; SRIF) and dopamine can inhibit pituitary TSH release and contribute to central nervous system control of TSH release. Norepinephrine and serotonin can inhibit TSH release, but their significance is not clear.[8] There is a diurnal pattern of TSH secretion with peak values at night. Glucocorticoids appear to be involved in modulation of this diurnal TSH release pattern with both effects at the hypothalamic level to inhibit TRH release and a direct action

on the pituitary to regulate the TSH response to TRH.[8]

METABOLISM OF THYROID HORMONES

The thyroid gland is the sole source of T_4. By contrast, most of the T_3 in blood is derived from nonglandular sources via monodeiodination of T_4 in peripheral tissues.[1,16–19] Both hormones in blood are associated with plasma proteins. These include thyroxine-binding globulin (TBG), thyroxine-binding prealbumin (TBPA), and albumin.[1,17] Thyroxine-binding globulin is the most important carrier protein for T_4; TBPA has lesser, but significant T_4 binding affinity. Thyroxine-binding globulin binds T_3 with much lower affinity than T_4. Albumin also is important, but T_3 does not bind to TBPA. The binding affinities and protein concentrations are such that the binding reactions are nearly complete, so that the euthyroid steady-state concentrations of free T_4 and free T_3 approximate 0.03 and 0.30 per cent, respectively, of the total hormone concentrations. Absolute mean free T_4 and T_3 concentrations approximate 3.0 and 0.5 ng/dl, respectively. Thyroxine-binding globulin levels are higher in children than in adults and decrease progressively to adult levels during adolescence. Thyroxine-binding prealbumin concentrations are low in childhood and increase during adolescence.

There are at least two major extravascular pools of thyroid hormones, one in which plasma-tissue interchange is rapid (chiefly liver, kidney, and lung) and one in which exchange is slow (chiefly skeletal muscle and skin).[17] An additional pool, chiefly in gut and bone, with an intermediate exchange rate has been suggested. Peak T_4 concentrations after single-pulse doses of labeled hormone occur in these "pools" in minutes, hours, and days, respectively. In adults it has been estimated that about 20 per cent of T_4 is present in plasma, 30 per cent in fast tissues, 45 per cent in slow tissues, and about 5 per cent in intermediate tissues.

Deiodination is the major pathway of thyroid hormone metabolism in man (Fig. 3–3). The first step in T_4 metabolism in conversion either to T_3 or to reverse T_3 (rT_3).[16–19] Monodeiodination of the outer (hydroxyl) iodothyronine ring produces T_3, which has three to four times the metabolic

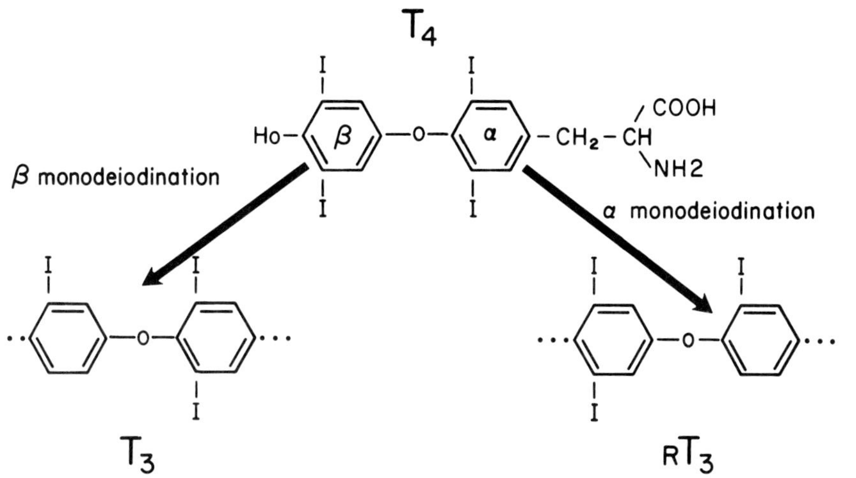

FIGURE 3–3. Patterns of monodeiodination of thyroxine. Thyroxine (T$_4$) is monodeiodinated by one of two enzyme-mediated pathways. Monodeiodination of the β or hydroxyl ring (5′-monodeiodination) produces 3,5,3′-triiodothyronine (T$_3$), which has three to four times the metabolic potency of T$_4$ via its higher affinity for nuclear thyroid receptors. Monodeiodination of the α or alanine ring (5-monodeiodination) produces reverse T$_3$ (rT$_3$), which is metabolically inactive. Further progressive monodeiodination produces deiodinated thyronine.

potency of T$_4$. Monodeiodination of the inner (alanine) ring produces rT$_3$, which is metabolically inactive. From 70 to 90 per cent of circulating T$_3$ is derived from peripheral conversion and 10 to 25 per cent from the thyroid gland. For rT$_3$ the values are 96 to 98 per cent and 2 to 4 per cent, respectively. Progressive tissue monodeiodination reactions degrade T$_3$ and rT$_3$ to diiodo-, monoiodo-, and noniodinated thyronine, all of which are biologically inactive.[16–18]

The alanine side chain of the inner ring of the iodothyronine hormones also is subject to degradative reactions, including transamination, deamination, and decarboxylation.[19] Acetic acid analogs are produced and have biologic activity in vitro. However, they are degraded rapidly and have little in vivo activity. Pyruvic acid analogs and small amounts of lactic acid analogs have been observed in urine and bile; these, too, have minimal biological activity. The extent of side chain cleavage reactions, relative to deiodination, has not been adequately quantified. Thyroid hormones are excreted in urine and stool in both free and conjugated forms. The conjugation reactions, which also inactivate the iodothyronines, involve both glucuronide and sulfoconjugation.[1,19] Conjugated analogs are excreted in bile and appear in the gut. Some of the conjugated hormone in gut is hydrolyzed and reabsorbed. Fecal excretion of thyroid hormones is somewhat variable, but in general

0 to 15 per cent of T$_3$ or T$_4$ is excreted via the gut in conjugated form.

THYROID HORMONE EFFECTS

Thyroid hormones penetrate the cell membrane and bind to a specific nuclear, nonhistone receptor protein.[20] (Fig. 3–4). These receptors have significant homology with glucocorticoid receptors.[21,22] At least two human thyroid receptor genes have been characterized. One appears to be expressed predominantly in the brain and to a lesser extent in several other tissues, with low expression in the liver; a second receptor is expressed in placenta and other tissues, including the liver.[23,24] There may be other thyroid hormone receptor genes in the human genome but the significance of these is not yet clear.[21]

Triiodothyronine binds to the nuclear receptors with 10 times the affinity of T$_4$. It also binds to plasma membrane and mitochondrial receptors, but the major effects of thyroid hormones appear to be mediated via the nuclear T$_3$ receptors.[1,20] Triiodothyronine receptor binding modulates gene transcription and synthesis of messenger RNA and cytoplasmic proteins (Fig. 3–4). Various tissues and cell functions are modified via varying patterns of genome activation and protein and receptor synthesis to account for the multiple physiologic actions of thyroid hormones. In addition to calorigenesis,

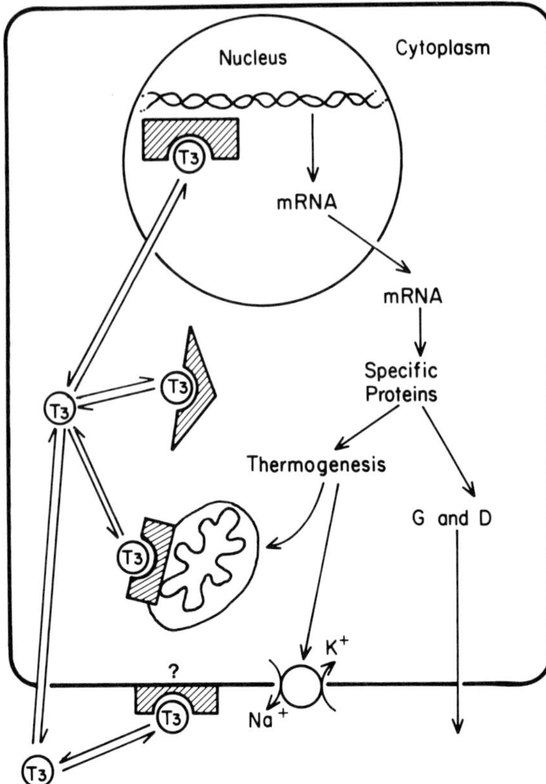

FIGURE 3–4. Thyroid hormone binding and action. Thyroid hormones exert their actions at the cell level by binding to one of several T_3 receptors. The most important is the nuclear receptor, a member of the steroid receptor family, which has a predominant affinity for T_3. The T_3-receptor complex activates gene transcription, mRNA synthesis, and protein synthesis. In general thyroid hormones stimulate growth and development (G and D), which involve a variety of protein species, and thermogenesis, which involves production of mitochondrial proteins and membrane Na^+/K^+ pumps. However, the pattern of protein synthesis and the thyroid hormone effects will depend on the cell type involved (see text for details). Triiodothyronine receptors also have been identified on the cell plasma membrane and on the inner mitochondrial membrane. The significance of these receptors is not clear. Cytoplasmic T_3 binding proteins have been described but are of relatively low affinity.

these include stimulation of water and ion transport, acceleration of substrate turnover (including cholesterol) and amino acid and lipid metabolism, and stimulation of growth and development of various tissues at critical periods, including the central nervous system and skeleton.[1,20,25,26]

Thyroid hormone–dependent effects known to be mediated by stimulation and accumulation of mRNAs coding for specific proteins include growth hormone (GH) synthesis in pituitary cells, selected enzymes and proteins in liver (including malic en-

zyme), β-myosin heavy chain synthesis in cardiac tissue, Na^+/K^+-ATPase in a variety of tissues, epidermal growth factor in salivary gland and kidney, epidermal growth factor receptors in liver, and uncoupling protein (thermogenin) in brown adipose tissue.[20,25–30] Thyroid hormones have been shown to inhibit the expression of other genes, including pituitary thyrotropin (TSH) and the myosin heavy chain in cardiac tissue.[25,26,31]

Thyroid hormones have important effects on other cell functions, although the mechanisms are not yet clear. They stimulate thermogenesis in most body cells, and this effect is associated with increases in mitochondrial RNA polymerase and α-glycerophosphate dehydrogenase.[20,32,33] It has been proposed that thyroid hormone–stimulated calorigenesis might be due to parallel enhancement of membrane Na^+/K^+-ATPase and mitochondrial α-glycerophosphate dehydrogenase activities coupling the augmented ADP production by Na^+/K^+-ATPase stimulation to increased mitochondrial ATP production.[34] Oppenheimer and colleagues have shown that thyroid hormone stimulates S14 mRNA in brown adipose tissue (BAT) in association with a marked and proportional increase in BAT lipogenesis.[20] They proposed that thyroid hormone–stimulated fatty acid synthesis in BAT with cycling and oxidative degradation in liver could account, at least in part, for thyroid-stimulated thermogenesis. Thyroid hormone modulation of BAT thermogenesis may be mediated by modulation of BAT uncoupling protein.

Thyroid hormones also potentiate the actions of catecholamines; increased catecholamine effects are prominent manifestations of the hyperthyroid state.[1,35] These effects are mediated via increased β-adrenergic receptor binding as well as postreceptor responsiveness, and are manifest in the face of normal or lowered circulating concentrations of catecholamines.[1,35] Brown adipose tissue thermogenesis is stimulated by catecholamines via β receptors and the response is conditioned via thyroid hormone modulation of thermogenin. The β-adrenergic effects, such as tachycardia, tremor, and lid lag, can be blocked in hyperthyroid subjects by propranolol, a β receptor–blocking agent, but propranolol does not alter thyroid function or the basal level of cellular activity.[1]

DEVELOPMENTAL ASPECTS OF THYROID FUNCTION

The fetal pituitary-thyroid axis develops autonomously of the maternal system.[36,37] The placenta is impermeable to TSH and relatively impermeable to T_4 and T_3; in addition, placental tissue contains an active inner ring iodothyronine deiodinase that deiodinates T_4 to inactive rT_3 and deiodinates T_3 to inactive T_2.[38] Thus, in sheep and probably humans little active maternal hormone is transferred to the fetus. In the rat, small amounts of T_4 have been shown to cross the placenta and to provide substrate for deiodination to T_3 in fetal brain.[39] The fetal pituitary and thyroid glands are well formed by 10 to 12 weeks but are relatively inactive at this time. Between 18 and 24 weeks there is a progressive increase in pituitary TSH content and concentration and a progressive increase in fetal serum TSH concentration with a parallel increase in fetal thyroid radioiodine uptake. This stimulation of TSH synthesis and secretion at midgestation probably correlates with maturation of the hypothalamic-pituitary portal blood vascular system. Thyrotropin-releasing hormone synthesis in the fetus occurs in pancreas, gut, and placental tissues during midgestation. Levels increase in the hypothalamus during the third trimester. Extra-hypothalamic TRH may play a role in maintaining the high TSH levels in the midgestation fetus. Between midgestation and term, fetal serum TSH concentrations remain relatively high and there is a progressive increase in fetal serum T_4 and free T_4 concentrations. These data suggest a progressive increase in fetal T_4 secretion during the last trimester of pregnancy.

Fetal serum T_3 concentrations are low throughout gestation (Fig. 3–5). Studies in fetal sheep have shown a low T_3 production rate and high $T_4:T_3$ and $rT_3:T_3$ production ratios.[36,37] The low fetal T_3 production rate

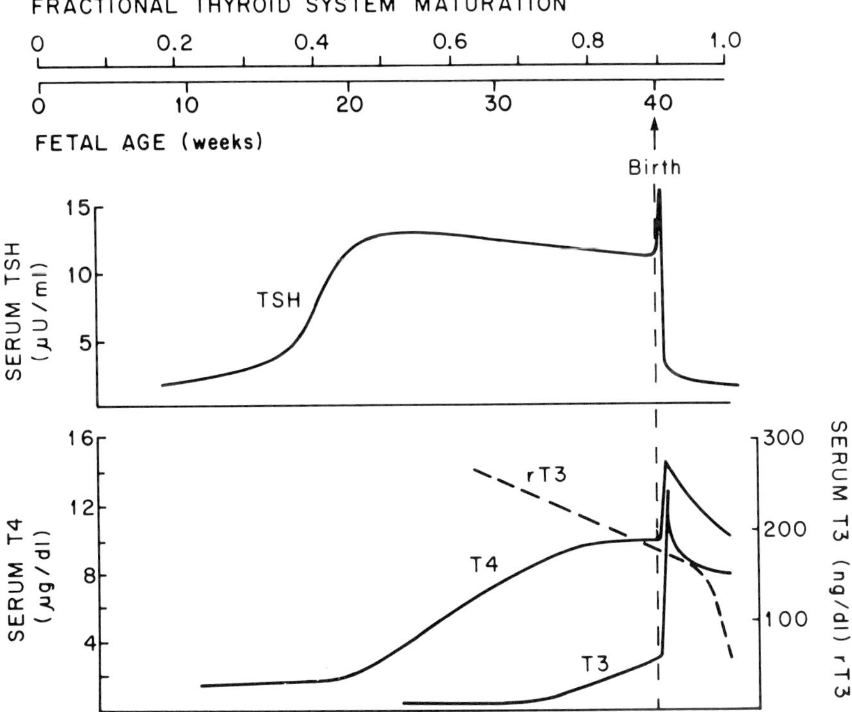

FIGURE 3–5. Pattern of thyroid system maturation in the human fetus and neonate. Fetal age is shown in weeks with thyroid maturation time shown fractionally. Maturation is complete by about 4 weeks of postnatal age. Serum TSH increases at midgestation, followed by a progressive increase in serum T_4 as a result of a progressive increase in the level of TBG. Free T_4 also increases progressively as a result of TSH stimulation of thyroid secretion and progressive maturation of thyroid responsiveness. Fetal T_4 is monodeiodinated predominantly to reverse T_3 (rT_3), which is biologically inactive. Active T_3 begins to increase near term. At birth the TSH surge (peaking at 30 min and due to extrauterine cooling) stimulates acute increases in T_4 and T_3 secretion by the thyroid gland. In addition, augmented T_4-to-T_3 conversion in liver and other tissues, perhaps including brown fat, maintains the much higher serum T_3 level after birth. Production of rT_3 progressively declines and serum levels approximate adult values by 3 to 4 weeks.

is associated with low levels of outer ring iodothyronine deiodinase activity in fetal liver and probably other tissues.[37] Human fetal blood rT_3 levels are high by 20 to 24 weeks and fall thereafter to term. However, levels at term are still quite high. Reverse T_3 also is produced in the placenta, but the failure of rT_3 levels to fall in the early neonatal period suggests that most of the circulating rT_3 in the fetus is derived from fetal tissues.[38] Thyroxine to rT_3 conversion is quite active in liver and probably accounts for most of the fetal rT_3 production. Fetal pituitary, brain, and BAT contain active outer ring iodothyronine deiodinases capable of local T_3 production from T_4.[16,40] This T_3 production may be important in fetal brain development, particularly in the hypothyroid fetus.

Near-term fetal serum T_3 levels increase modestly, from 15 to about 50 ng/dl.[37] Data in sheep suggest that this near-term increase in fetal serum T_3 levels is mediated by an increase in fetal cortisol secretion; cortisol increases fetal serum T_3 levels by increasing the capacity of fetal liver to convert T_4 to T_3. Immediately after delivery there is an abrupt (1- to 4-hour) increase in T_3 levels in newborn serum that is largely due to the marked postnatal TSH surge; newborn TSH levels peak at 30 min in the range of 70 to 100 μU/ml, probably stimulated by cooling of the neonate in the extrauterine environment[37,41] (Fig. 3–5). In response, both T_4 and T_3 secretion from the thyroid gland are stimulated, and serum T_4 and T_3 concentrations increase briskly.[37,41] Between 4 and 24 hours a further progressive increase in serum T_3 levels occurs as a result of augmented conversion of T_4 to T_3 in neonatal tissues. Both liver and BAT may be involved. Thyroid T_3 secretion also continues.

Serum TBG concentrations remain unchanged at levels approximating 2.5 mg/dl so that serum free T_4 and free T_3 levels abruptly increase. The high levels of serum rT_3 only gradually decrease to adult values during the first 2 to 3 weeks. The physiologic significance of the neonatal hyperthyroid state remains speculative, but it has been shown that the increased thyroid hormone levels stimulate catecholamine-mediated BAT thermogenesis and mobilization of fatty acid from body fat stores as well as catecholamine-mediated nonshivering thermogenesis.[42] Other catecholamine-mediated as well as noncatecholamine effects of thyroid hormones also may be stimulated.

During childhood there is a progressive decrease in oxygen consumption with age, a decrease in per cent labeled thyroid hormone appearing in plasma 24 hours after administration of a tracer dose of radioiodine, a decreasing serum TG concentration, and a decreasing T_4 degradation rate expressed as fraction of the extrathyroidal T_4 pool degraded daily[43–45] (Fig. 3–6). The serum TBG concentration falls with age to nadir

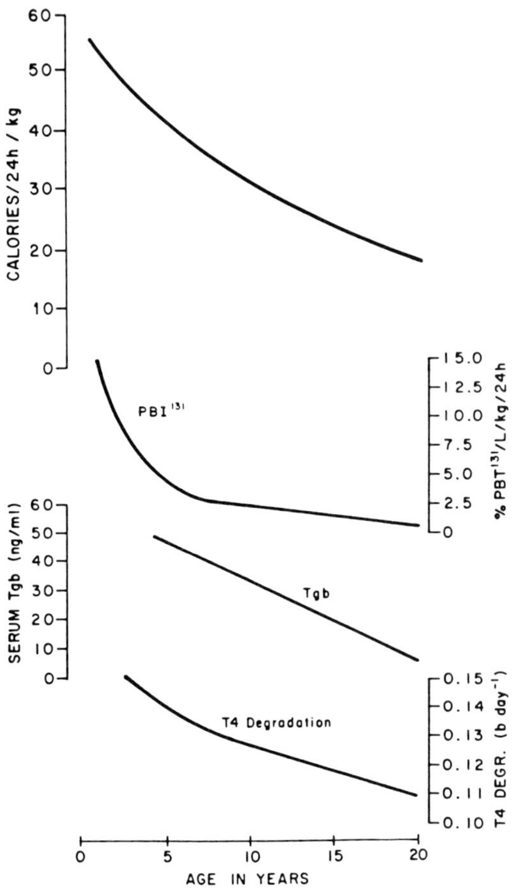

FIGURE 3–6. Changes in thyroid function during childhood. During the first two decades of life there is a progressive decrease in metabolic activity manifest as a decrease in calories expended per kilogram body mass. This decrease is shown at the top of the figure. Thyroid gland activity also decreases. This is shown as a decrease in serum protein-bound ^{131}I (^{131}PBI) concentration after a dose of radioiodine (^{131}I). The percentage of the ^{131}I dose appearing per liter of serum per kilogram per 24 hours reflects the activity of the thyroid gland in organifying and secreting the ^{131}I label as hormone. This decreasing hormone secretion with age also is reflected in a decrease in T_4 degradation rate, shown as fraction of the extrathyroidal T_4 pool cleared per day (b day^{-1}). The progressive fall in serum thyroglobulin (Tgb) concentration probably also reflects the decreased glandular activity.

values during adolescence.[46,47] There is a reciprocal change in TBPA levels.[47] These changes are mediated in part by gonadal steroids, but an age-dependent decrease in TBG also is involved prior to puberty. The change in TBG is associated with corresponding decreases in serum T_4 and T_3 concentrations.[46] Recent limited data suggest a progressive fall in serum TSH concentrations in euthyroid children between 7 and 17 years of age.[44] These several changes in thyroid function with age reflect a gradual decrease in thyroid hormone utilization with increasing age, and account for the progressive decrease of the thyroid replacement dose from 10 to 15 µg/kg/day during the first year of life to 2 to 4 µg/kg/day during adolescence. Serum T_4 and T_3 levels also decrease progressively with age. These changes are summarized in Table 3–1.

Thyroid hormone actions also vary with age. Thyroid hormone deficiency during human fetal life has minimal untoward effects. Somatic growth and development and linear bone growth proceed normally in the athyroid fetus and bone maturation is normal or minimally (3 to 6 weeks) retarded.[48–50] Brain growth, as assessed by head circumference measurements, is not abnormal, and IQ measurements in athyroid children at 6 to 8 years of age are normal with early and adequate postnatal thyroid hormone replacement.[51–54] The reason(s) for the relative lack of thyroid hormone effect in the fetus is not clear. There is no deficiency of T_3 receptors; available data indicate an early appearance of nuclear thyroid receptors in human fetal tissues.[55,56] More likely explanations include low levels of active thyroid hormone in fetal serum and tissues and/or immaturity of thyroid hormone receptor responsiveness at the transcription, translation, or action levels.[57]

The developmental effects of thyroid hormones are most obvious during infancy and early childhood. Somatic growth, bone growth and maturation, and tooth development and eruption are thyroid dependent. In addition, 60 to 70 per cent of postnatal brain growth and differentiation occurs during the first 2 years of life; and it is during this period that the thyroid dependency of brain is manifest.[58] After 3 to 4 years of age thyroid hormone deficiency is not associated with mental retardation, but delayed somatic and linear bone growth and delayed eruption of permanent dentition are prominent. Bone maturation, measured as bone age, also is delayed, diaphyseal bone growth is reduced, and epiphyseal growth and mineralization largely cease.[54–61]

Hypothalamic anterior pituitary function also may be abnormal in hypothyroid children. Although in most children thyroid hormone deficiency leads to delayed sexual development, an occasion hypothyroid child manifests precocious sexual maturation with increased levels of circulating gonadotropins.[62–65] In females, serum prolactin levels also tend to be increased, and galactorrhea may occur if serum estrogen levels are high enough to permit breast development and milk production. Increased TRH secretion could account for the prolactin hypersecretion, but the mechanism of the precocious sexual maturation and gonadotropin

TABLE 3–1.   NORMAL VALUES (AND RANGES) FOR SERUM THYROID FUNCTION PARAMETERS VERSUS AGE

Age	T_4 (µg/dl)	T_3 (ng/dl)	rT_3 (ng/dl)	TBG (mg/dl)	TG (ng/dl)
Birth	10.8 (6.5–17.5)	50 (15–85)	220 (100–500)	2.7 (0.7–4.7)	24 (5–54)
1–4 weeks	13 (8.0–17.0)	175 (100–300)	90 (25–300)	2.5 (0.5–4.5)	50 (5–140)
1–12 months	11 (7.0–15.5)	175 (100–260)	40 (40–130)	2.6 (1.6–3.6)	—
1–5 years	10.5 (7.0–15.0)	165 (95–250)	35 (15–70)	2.1 (1.3–2.8)	—
6–10 years	9.3 (6.5–13.5)	150 (95–240)	35 (15–70)	2.0 (1.4–2.6)	35 (5–65)
11–15 years	8.1 (5.0–11.8)	133 (80–215)	40 (20–80)	2.0 (1.4–2.6)	18 (3–36)
16–20 years	8.0 (4.5–11.7)	130 (80–210)	40 (20–80)	2.0 (1.4–2.6)	4 (0.5–15)

release is not clear. These changes seem to occur in children with high serum TSH levels, and enlargement of the sella turcica has been observed.

During childhood and adolescence and until epiphyseal closure, thyroid hormone deficiency leads to reduced somatic growth, reduced linear bone growth, and delayed bone maturation. In addition, epiphyseal dysgenesis is commonly observed.[66] Delay in eruption of second dentition may occur. Abnormalities of hypothalamic-pituitary function secondary to hypothyroidism are common in adolescence. Puberty often is delayed or incomplete. In normal females, menstrual cycles commonly are nonovulatory and bleeding may be irregular. This pattern usually is more prolonged in hypothyroid female adolescents. In addition, menorrhagia or hypomenorrhea may occur.

MECHANISMS OF THYROID HORMONE ACTIONS ON GROWTH AND DEVELOPMENT

The effects of thyroid hormones on somatic and skeletal growth are mediated, at least in part, by stimulation of GH and somatomedin synthesis and action[67]; GH synthesis by pituitary cells is known to be thyroid hormone dependent.[67–71] The growth effects of GH are mediated, at least in part, by the somatomedins, a family of insulin-line hormones under GH control.[72] Growth hormone binding to liver and other cells stimulates somatomedin production, and somatomedins in turn stimulate growth effects, particularly in bone and muscle tissues.[72–77] Thyroxine also has been shown to increase serum somatomedin activity in hypopituitary mice that are incapable of synthesizing GH.[75] Combined T_3 and GH therapy of hypophysectomized rats is necessary to normalize growth as well as serum somatomedin levels.[75,78] In addition, there is evidence to suggest that thyroid hormones potentiate the actions of somatomedin on cartilage growth.[74]

The precise mechanism of T_4 dependency of other growth processes is not so clear. Other peptide growth factors may mediate the thyroid hormone effects on specific target tissues. In the mouse the epidermal growth factor (EGF) content of various tissues has been shown to be thyroid hormone responsive,[79–82] and exogenous EGF has been shown to stimulate T_4-dependent eye opening and incisor eruption in hypothyroid neonatal mice.[81] Thyroxine also increases EGF receptor binding in selected tissues.[29,83] Erythropoietin synthesis by the kidney is known to be thyroid hormone responsive, and there are known correlations between circulating erythropoietin levels, erythrocyte production, and hemoglobin concentrations in hypo- and hyperthyroidism.[67] Nerve growth factor (NGF) contents of various tissues of the mouse also are thyroid hormone responsive, and sympathetic nervous system development is known to be both thyroid hormone and NGF dependent.[67,84,85] Nerve growth factor has been suggested to mediate the effects of thyroid hormone on sympathetic nervous system development. These observations have suggested the hypothesis that thyroid hormones exert their developmental effects, at least in part, via stimulation of the production and/or effect of various tissue-specific growth factors. The extent and significance of these pathways, however, remain to be clarified.

THYROID DYSFUNCTION SYNDROMES IN THE PREMATURE INFANT

Transient Hypothyroxinemia

Serum T_4 concentrations increase progressively with gestational age. Most term infants have serum T_4 concentrations above 6.5 µg/dl; only 2 to 3 per cent have serum T_4 levels below this level. In contrast, some 50 per cent of premature infants delivered before 30 weeks' gestation have serum T_4 values below 6.5 µg/dl.[37,86,87] Infants with hypothyroxinemia also have relatively low levels of free T_4. These levels are not in the low range of neonates with congenital hypothyroidism; rather, they are similar to the levels in adults. The relatively low free T_4 levels in premature infants are associated with normal or even low basal serum TSH values and normal TSH and T_4 responses to TRH, the latter indicating responsive pituitary and thyroid glands. The hypothyroxinemia is transient, correcting spontaneously (over 4 to 8 weeks) with progressive maturation.[86] Postnatal growth and development of these infants is normal so that they do not require treatment and treatment does not increase growth rate.[86,88] Thus, such infants appear to manifest a state of hypothalamic (or tertiary) hypothyroidism or immaturity that represents a normal stage of thyroid system development.

Transient Primary Hypothyroidism

Transient hypothyroidism in the neonate, characterized by low serum T_4 and high TSH concentrations, is more common in Europe than in America, and the prevalence varies geographically relative to iodine intake.[89–91] The prevalence of transient hypothyroidism in Belgium approximately 20 per cent of premature infants, the incidence increasing with decreasing gestational age. Cord blood T_4 and TSH values in these infants usually are in the normal range for premature infants. However, premature infants require higher iodine intake levels than term infants to maintain a positive iodine balance in the extrauterine environment, and in iodine-deficient geographic areas they may develop neonatal iodine deficiency. The primary hypothyroid state develops during the first 1 to 2 weeks of extrauterine life and often is superimposed on the transient hypothyroxinemia characteristic of prematurity. Urinary iodine and thyroid iodine contents are reduced. The hypothyroidism is transient but may persist for 2 to 3 months so that treatment is recommended; T_4 or T_3 can be prescribed. The average time to recovery of function and discontinuation of treatment in Belgium was 50 days. Iodine treatment also corrects the primary hypothyroid state.

Premature infants also are particularly susceptible to transient, *iodine-induced* hypothyroidism.[90,91] The mechanism for thyroid cell membrane inhibition of iodide transport in response to increased plasma iodide levels matures near term.[92] Thus, either in utero or in the postnatal period, administration of iodide or iodine-containing drugs to the mother or amniotic injection of radiographic contrast agents for amniofetography has induced hypothyroidism. Premature infants are more susceptible, but term infants also can develop iodide-induced hypothyroidism. The dose of iodine required approximates 50 to 100 $\mu g/kg/day$. Urine iodine levels in iodine-induced hypothyroid infants usually exceed 1 mg/L. The hypothyroidism, with or without goiter, is characterized by low serum total T_4 and free T_4 concentrations and high levels of TSH. Treatment of these infants at birth is indicated.

Transient Hyperthyrotropinemia

Idiopathic hyperthyrotropinemia is a rare disorder. The serum TSH concentration is increased, often markedly, but other thyroid function parameters are normal and the infants are euthyroid. In Japan the prevalence is 1:15,000 to 20,000 newborns; the prevalence in Europe and America is not precisely known, but is much lower.[37,93] The serum TSH concentration remains elevated for as long as 9 months before spontaneously normalizing. Affected infants do not require treatment, but prolonged follow-up is necessary to exclude the possibility of a permanent disorder, such as an ectopic thyroid gland, an inborn defect in thyroid hormonogenesis, or a thyroid hormone resistance syndrome. Transient hyperthyrotropinemia without hypothyroxinemia in the newborn also may occur in response to intrauterine antithyroid drug exposure or intrauterine iodine excess or deficiency, and has been recorded as a TSH assay artifact. The mechanism of transient idiopathic hyperthyrotropinemia is not clear. Delayed maturation of thyroid responsiveness to TSH, immature feedback control of pituitary TSH secretion or TSH receptor antibody may be involved.

Low T_3 Syndrome in Premature Infants

In the preterm infant the changes in thyroid function parameters during neonatal adaptation are qualitatively similar to those in term infants, but are quantitatively obtunded.[37] The neonatal TSH surge and the neonatal T_4 peak decrease in amplitude with decreasing gestational age; the neonatal T_3 peak also is obtunded. This transient low T_3 state probably is related to the state of relative undernutrition in the neonatal period. Premature infants have an increase susceptibility to neonatal morbidity, including respiratory distress, and premature infants have an increased risk of birth trauma, vascular accidents, hypoxia, hypoglycemia, hypocalcemia, and infection superimposed on relative malnutrition.[37,90,94,95] All of these factors tend to inhibit T_4 to T_3 conversion in the neonatal period and aggravate the extent of the low T_3 state characteristic of prematurity. Serum T_3 values may remain low in these infants for 1 to 2 months.

Features of the low T_3 syndrome in premature infants include a low serum T_3 concentration secondary to a decreased rate of conversion of T_4 to T_3, variable but usually elevated serum rT_3 levels, and normal or low total serum T_4 concentrations.[37,90,94,95] Free T_4 levels usually are in the range of values for healthy premature infants of matched gestational age and weight. In some infants serum TBG levels are low, and there may be an inhibitor of T_4 binding to TBG as described in adults with the low T_3 syndrome. Serum TSH concentrations are normal, indicating a euthyroid state.

CONGENITAL HYPOTHYROIDISM

Thyroid Dysgenesis

The term *thyroid dysgenesis* describes infants with ectopic or hypoplastic thyroid glands (or both) as well as those with total thyroid agenesis.[96–98] Thyroid dysgenesis is the etiologic factor in most infants with permanent congenital hypothyroidism detected in newborn screening programs. The prevalence approximates 1:4000 newborns worldwide (Table 3–2). Some thyroid tissue probably is present in two thirds of these infants, so that they represent a spectrum of severity of thyroid deficiency. A normal or near-normal circulating level of T_3 in the face of a low T_4 value suggests that presence of residual thyroid tissue, and this can be confirmed by a thyroid scan. A measurable level of serum TG indicates the presence of some thyroid tissue; athyroid infants have no circulating TG.[7]

Thyroid dysgenesis is more prevalent in female than in male infants; the female-to-male ratio approximates 2:1. The disorder has been reported to be less prevalent in black (1:32,000) than in white infants and

TABLE 3–2. THYROID DISORDERS AND THEIR APPROXIMATE PREVALENCES IN THE NEONATAL PERIOD

Thyroid dysgenesis	1:4000
Agenesis	
Hypogenesis	
Ectopia	
Thyroid dyshormonogenesis	1:30,000
TSH receptor defect	
Iodide trapping defect	
Organification defect	
Iodotyrosine deiodinase deficiency	
Defect in thyroglobulin	
Hypothalamic-pituitary hypothyroidism	1:100,000
Hypothalamic-pituitary anomaly	
Panhypopituitarism	
Isolated TSH deficiency	
Transient hypothyroidism	1:40,000
Drug induced	
Maternal antibody induced	
Idiopathic	

may be more frequent (1:2000) in hispanic infants.[99,100] However, the numbers of these minority groups screened in these studies was relatively small. Although thyroid dysgenesis usually is sporadic, rare familial cases have been described and the prevalence is increased in infants with Down syndrome.[101] An increased prevalence of nonthyroid anomalies also has been suggested in infants with congenital hypothyroidism, but this observation remains controversial.[102] A seasonal variation in incidence has been observed in Japan and Australia.[103] In rare instances thyroid dysgenesis has occurred in association with maternal autoimmune thyroiditis. However, this may be coincidence; there usually is no correlation between thyroid dysgenesis and the presence of maternal autoimmune thyroiditis or circulating thyroid antimicrosomal or antithyroglobulin autoantibodies.[104] Immunoglobulins blocking TSH-stimulated thyroid cell growth in tissue culture have been reported in about half of both maternal and newborn blood samples in cases of sporadic congenital hypothyroidism, but a role for such growth-blocking immunoglobulins in the pathogenesis of congenital hypothyroidism has not been established.[105,106]

Most infants with thyroid dysgenesis are asymptomatic, and few have signs of hypothyroidism during the early weeks of life. Consequently, only about 5 per cent of hypothyroid infants are detected by clinical criteria before the chemical screening diagnosis is established.[96–98] Most affected infants have low serum T_4 and high TSH concentrations in cord blood or in filter-paper blood spots collected at 2 to 5 days of age. Ten to 20 per cent of hypothyroid infants have T_4 levels in the low-normal range with increased TSH values. These infants usually have ectopic thyroid tissue on scanning and have significant residual functioning thyroid tissue and significant levels of circulating thyroglobulin.

Hypothalamic Pituitary Defects

Congenital hypothyroidism due to decreased effective TSH stimulation of thyroid hormone secretion can result from a variety of abnormalities in TSH synthesis and metabolism[2,96,107,108]: anomalous hypothalamic or pituitary development; an isolated, sporadic, or familial deficiency in TRH or TSH secretion; or TSH deficiency in association with other pituitary hormone deficiencies. Abnormal TSH is a theoretical possibility not yet described clinically. Several TSH deficiency syndromes have been described: hypothalamic hypothyroidism with TRH deficiency or insensitivity (or both); isolated TSH deficiency; familial panhypopituitarism; congenital absence of the pituitary; and panhypopituitarism with absence of the sella turcica.[2] The combined prevalence of these abnormalities associated with congenital hypothyroidism approximates 1:60,000 to 140,000 births.[96,109]

Inborn Defects of Thyroid Hormone Production

Infants with inborn defects in thyroid metabolism comprise about 10 per cent of newborns with congenital nonendemic hypothyroidism[96,109–111] (Table 3–2). The defects in such patients include (1) a decreased thyroid response to TSH; (2) decreased thyroid iodide trapping; (3) defective organification of trapped iodide; (4) decresed capacity for deiodinating iodotyrosines; and (5) abnormalities in thyroglobulin synthesis, storage, or release.[2,3,112] These disorders usually are transmitted as autosomal-recessive traits.[2,3,112] Except for the familial incidence and tendency for affected individuals to develop goiter, the clinical manifestations of congenital hypothyroidism due to a biochemical defect are similar to those in infants with thyroid dysgenesis.[2,110–112] Thyroid enlargement may be manifest at birth, but in many patients development of the goiter is delayed.

Decreased TSH Responsiveness

Only a few such patients have been reported.[2,112] Consanguinity has been common. The patients had low T_4 and high TSH levels with small thyroid glands, low-normal radioiodine uptake, and no radioiodine uptake response to TSH. The TSH has been bioactive when tested. In one patient with normal TSH receptor binding there was no thyroid cAMP response to TSH, whereas the cAMP response to fluoride was intact. A defect in TSH receptor–adenylate cyclase coupling was postulated. In another patient TSH receptor binding was present but there was no cAMP response to TSH or fluoride. Impaired generation of cyclic AMP was postulated.

Failure to Concentrate Iodide

Several patients have been described with hyperplastic thyroid glands and minimal uptake of radioactive iodine.[2,3,112] The thyroid glands in these patients were enlarged two to four times and all infants were hypothyroid. Salivary glands and gastric mucosa also failed to concentrate iodide from the circulation. Several patients have been reported with a partial defect in iodide trapping. Thyroid radioiodine uptake was decreased but not absent in these patients and did not respond to TSH. These patients also manifested the defect in salivary and gastric tissues; the saliva-plasma ratio of radioiodine was reduced but measurable. Lugol's solution ameliorates the hypothyroidism by increasing the intrathyroidal inorganic iodide concentration via diffusion, but the molecular defect is not known.

Iodide Organification Defects

The first patient with an inborn defect in thyroid hormonogenesis described by Stanbury in 1950 had an absent or deficient peroxidase enzyme for oxidizing thyroidal iodide to reactive iodine.[2] The administration of thiocyanate or perchlorate to such patients within 2 hours after administration of a test dose of radioiodine is followed by a precipitous fall in thyroid radioactivity sometimes involving 50 to 90 per cent of the trapped radioactivity; normal subjects have less than a 10 per cent discharge of thyroidal radioiodine after perchlorate administration. Patients with complete peroxidase enzyme defects usually present with congenital hypothyroidism. Diagnosis is confirmed by measuring low or absent levels of thyroid peroxidase activity in thyroid tissue obtained by biopsy.

Several patients have been described who were euthyroid or only mildly hypothyroid but manifested goiter and *partial* perchlorate-induced discharge of radioiodine. During studies of thyroid gland tissue homogenates obtained by biopsy, defects in hematin (enzyme cofactor) binding to apoenzyme, or defects in thyroid H_2O_2 generation due to defective biosynthesis of FAD from riboflavin have been postulated.[2,112]

Pendred in 1896 described two sisters with deafness and goiter and hypothyroidism living in a nonendemic goiter area, and many similar patients with the so-called

Pendred syndrome have been described.[2,112] The prevalence has been estimated to be 1.5 to 3 cases per 100,000 school children. Pendred syndrome includes high tone or complete deafness, goiter, and mild hypothyroidism. About one third of patients have the complete syndrome; others present without hearing loss or with a small euthyroid goiter. Most patients have a positive perchlorate discharge test indicating a defect in the thyroid peroxidase enzyme system, but patients with a negative test result have been described. The biochemical defect in Pendred syndrome is not clear; thyroid peroxidase activity is normal. The cause of deafness is not known.

Iodotyrosine Deiodinase Defect

Deficiency of thyroid iodotyrosine deiodinase can be associated with congenital hypothyroidism or with a less severe form of familial goiter.[2,112] Failure to deiodinate thyroid MIT and DIT as they are released from thyroglobulin leads to severe iodine wastage, since these nondeiodinated iodotyrosines diffuse out of the thyroid to be excreted in urine. The first patients described were hypothyroid with goiters present at birth or during infancy. Iodotyrosine deiodinases also are present in peripheral tissues, and abnormalities involving both thyroidal and peripheral iodotyrosine deiodinase systems have been described. Several patients have been reported with euthyroid goiter and partial defects in deiodination of iodotyrosine (1) in both thyroid and peripheral tissues, (2) in peripheral tissues only, or (3) in thyroid tissue only.

Defects in TG Synthesis or Transport

Thyroglobulin synthesis, transport, and processing represent a series of complex events involving thyroid hormone synthesis and storage.[2,112] Patients with defects in TG metabolism present with familial hypothyroidism and goiter associated with circulating nonthyroglobulin iodoprotein. In patients unable to synthesize TG there will be absent or low levels of TG in serum by radioimmunoassay.[7] In the absence of TG substrate for hormone synthesis and iodine fixation, thyroid proteins, such as albumin, are iodinated and escape into the circulation. These proteins can be detected as butanol-insoluble radioiodoprotein after administration of radioiodine. Patients may have a positive perchlorate discharge test and may excrete abnormal quantities of iodohistidine in their urine, presumably as degradation products of the iodinated albumin. Patients reported to date can be classified as having (1) impaired TG synthesis, (2) impaired TG transport (to colloid), or (3) structurally abnormal TG. Definitive diagnosis requires biochemical and immunohistochemical studies of thyroid biopsy material. The human TG gene has been cloned and molecular studies of TG synthesis can be conducted in vitro.

Transient Congenital Hypothyroidism

Congenital hypothyroidism may occur as a transient defect persisting for a variable period after birth.[90,96] Usually transient neonatal hypothyroidism is caused by maternal ingestion of goitrogenic substances that reach the fetus via placental transfer. The most frequently ingested goitrogenic drug is iodide prescribed in expectorants for treatment of asthma or as treatment for maternal thyrotoxicosis. The mothers of these children often have taken large doses of iodide for many years without developing large goiters and have been euthyroid during pregnancy. The fetus is unusually sensitive to iodide-induced hypothyroidism because of immaturity of the mechanism(s) for decreasing thyroid iodide uptake to compensate for high plasma iodide levels.[92] Urine iodine concentrations in these infants usually exceed 1 mg/L.

Other goitrogens that have caused neonatal goiter include the thioureas, sulfonamides, and hematinic preparations containing cobalt. Neonatal goiters resulting from antithyroid drug administration are uncommon unless large doses of the drugs are given to the mother (more than 150 mg/day propylthiouracil or equivalent near term). Amniotic injection of radiographic contrast agents for amniofetography also can lead to transient congenital hypothyroidism.

Maternal-to-fetal transfer of TSH receptor–blocking antibodies also can lead to transient perinatal hypothyroidism.[90,106,113–115] This condition is rare, but has been reported in the neonates of women with euthyroid or hypothyroid autoimmune thyroid disease. In such infants TSH-receptor autoantibodies are detectable in maternal and cord blood. These antibodies can be measured either as TSH-binding–inhibiting immunoglobulins (TBII) or TSH (cAMP)–

blocking antibodies (TBA). The duration of the hypothyroid state in the newborn is directly correlated with the initial titer of blocking antibody and the duration of its presence in newborn blood. Transient congenital hypothyroidism must be differentiated from transient hyperthyrotropinemia.

Diagnosis and Management

Infants with congenital hypothyroidism are born with little or no clinical evidence of thyroid hormone deficiency. Thus, detection based on signs and symptoms usually is delayed 6 to 12 weeks or longer. Early clinical diagnosis must be based on a high index of suspicion regarding nonspecific symptoms and signs. The diagnosis should be considered in any infant exhibiting prolonged physiologic jaundice, transient hypothermia, an enlarged (greater than 1 cm) posterior fontanel, failure to feed properly, or respiratory distress with feeding.

The *classic* signs evolve during the first weeks after birth.[96–98] There is a progressive accumulation of myxedema in the subcutaneous tissues and in the tongue. The thickened tongue becomes protuberant, and the infant develops increasing difficulty in nursing and handling salivary secretion. The cry is hoarse because of myxedema of the vocal cords. There is marked muscular hypotonia,

an umbilical hernia, constipation, and bradycardia and the extremities are cool and may exhibit extreme pallor and circulatory mottling. The cardiac silhouette may be enlarged, and the electrocardiogram shows low voltage and a prolonged conduction time. Many of the signs and symptoms are present by 6 to 12 weeks, especially lethargy, constipation, and the umbilical hernia. The cretinoid facies and growth retardation become progressively more obvious over the first several months of life (Fig. 3–7).

Newborn screening for congenital hypothyroidism now is routine in most industrialized areas of the world and is conducted either by combined T_4 and TSH testing or by TSH testing alone.[96,109,116,117] Screening data confirm that serum T_4 values are low and TSH concentrations high in most newborns with primary hypothyroidism. However, 10 to 20 per cent of infants with congenital hypothyroidism have T_4 values in the low-normal range (7 to 11 ng/dl), and programs using T_4 followed by TSH screening now measure TSH in all samples with T_4 concentrations at or below the 10th percentile level to avoid missing these infants. Eight to 10 per cent of infants with congenital hypothyroidism will have a screening TSH values less than 50 μU/ml, and 1:12 to 24 hypothyroid infants (1:50,000 to 1:100,000 newborns) will have a screening

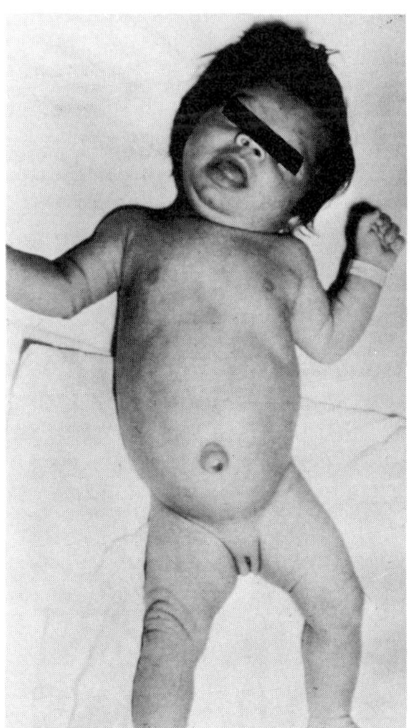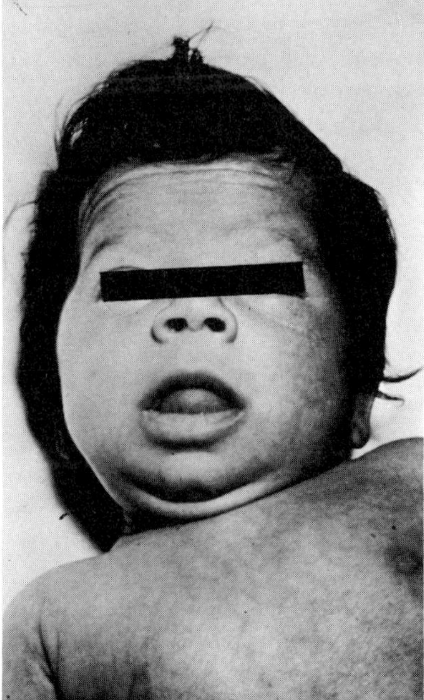

FIGURE 3–7. A 3½-month-old-infant with congenital hypothyroidism illustrates the hypotonic flexion posture, protuberant abdomen, and umbilical hernia (left); and puffy facies, a large, protruding tongue, and mottled skin (right).

TSH level less than 20 μU/ml with a delayed postnatal rise to hypothyroid levels.[96,106,118–120] Infants with TSH deficiency are not detected by newborn screening. Also infants with congenital hypothyroidism can escape detection because of errors in sample collection or laboratory routine. For all of these reasons, it is important to remember that an occasional infant with congenital hypothyroidism will escape detection in any newborn screening program and that these infants must be diagnosed on clinical grounds. It has been estimated that 5 to 10 per cent of infants might be missed.[109,118–120]

Congenital hypothyroidism is diagnosed by a low serum T_4 and high TSH concentration in individual cord blood or neonatal blood samples. A cord serum T_4 of 6.0 μg/dl or less with a TSH in excess of 80 μU/ml suggests hypothyroidism. At 3 to 5 days of age, a serum T_4 less than 7 μg/dl with a serum TSH in excess of 20 μU/ml suggests hypothyroidism. During the first 24 to 48 hours of life serum TSH levels are elevated as a result of the neonatal TSH surge. Sampling infants during this time increases the number of false-positive results, but infants with congenital hypothyroidism are not usually missed. The diagnosis of congenital hypothyroidism must be confirmed by measurement of serum T_4 and TSH concentrations in any infant with suspicious screening or neonatal sampling results. After 7 days of age a serum T_4 less than 6 μg/dl with a TSH greater than 50 μU/ml indicates primary hypothyroidism. A serum T_4 less than 10 μg/dl with a TSH in the 20- to 50-μU/ml range is suggestive and repeat testing is necessary.

Hypothalamic-pituitary hypothyroidism is more difficult to diagnose.[96,107,108] The disorder is characterized by a low serum T_4 concentration with a normal range TSH value. The low T_4–low TSH pattern most commonly reflects prematurity or a low TBG concentration. Measurements of serum TBG and/or free T_4 concentrations will distinguish these possibilities. An infant or child with a low free T_4 concentration and low TSH level should be carefully examined for evidence of hypothyroidism and other tests of pituitary function should be conducted. A subnormal TSH response to TRH confirms a diagnosis of pituitary TSH deficiency. If the peak level of TSH is normal and/or prolonged, hypothalamic TSH deficiency can be inferred. The TSH deficiency may be isolated or associated with other pituitary hormone deficiencies. In these infants treatment with T_4 raises the serum T_4 and free T_4 to normal levels.

The treatment of hypothyroidism is accomplished with exogenous thyroid hormone. Sodium-*l*-thyroxine (NaT_4) is the drug of choice because of its uniform potency and reliable absorption: approximate doses of synthetic T_4 also produce normal serum levels of T_3 via peripheral conversion.[96,121,122] The best guide to adequacy of therapy is periodic measurement of circulating levels of T_4 and TSH; during the initial stages of treatment a T_3 determination also may be of value. The history and physical examination are important in follow-up, but mild hypothyroidism or hyperthyroidism cannot always be excluded on clinical grounds. Using NaT_4 for treatment, the serum T_4 should be adjusted to the upper-normal range (10 to 16 μg/dl), at which time serum T_3 levels should be normal (70 to 220 ng/dl).

Serum TSH levels may be normal or elevated in adequately treated patients. The thyroid hormone–pituitary feedback set-point seems to be altered in about half of the infants with congenital hypothyroidism, and in such infants the serum TSH concentration remains elevated in the face of a normal or even elevated serum T_4 level.[123–125] The usual starting dose of NaT_4 for hypothyroid infants is 10 to 15 μg/kg/day; we routinely begin treatment in term infants with a 50-μg T_4 tablet daily crushed and given orally in a small amount of liquid.[126] This dose normalizes the serum T_4 value (to greater than 10 μg/dl) within 30 days. The dose of T_4 can be adjusted after 3 to 4 weeks to maintain the (corrected) T_4 in the 10- to 16-μg/dl range.

Infants with presumably transient hypothyroidism caused by maternal goitrogenic drugs need not be treated unless the low serum T_4 and elevated TSH levels persist beyond 2 weeks. Therapy usually can be discontinued after 8 to 12 weeks. Hyperthyroid mothers on antithyroid drugs may breast-feed their infants, since the concentrations of drug in breast milk are very low. Infants with hypothyroidism induced by TSH receptor–blocking antibody may require treatment for 2 to 5 months.

Adequate dosage of T_4 in the first year ordinarily ranges between 25 and 50 μg daily.[126] The growth rate should accelerate after initiation of therapy, and any growth deficit is restored within a few months.

Bone age is a sensitive index of thyroid deficiency, and delayed bone maturation suggests inadequate dosage even when other signs of hypothyroidism have been ameliorated. Overtreatment can induce tachycardia, excessive nervousness, disturbed sleep patterns, and other findings suggesting thyrotoxicosis. Excessive thyroxine administered over a long period can produce premature synostosis of cranial sutures and undue advancement of bone age.[126] In infants with cranial synostosis the dose of thyroid hormone has exceeded 200 µg daily.[126]

ACQUIRED HYPOTHYROIDISM

Hypothyroidism may develop at any age in previously normal individuals. The onset usually is insidious. Many children with acquired hypothyroidism have circulating antithyroid antibodies and autoimmune thyroiditis. In others, acquired juvenile hypothyroidism may be due to exposure to goitrogenic agents, the late manifestation of thyroid dysgenesis, late onset of hypothyroidism secondary to an inborn error of thyroid hormone biosynthesis, thyroid hormone resistance, acquired hypothalamic or pituitary hypothyroidism, or endemic goitrogens (Table 3–3).

Causes of Acquired Hypothyroidism

Exposure to Goitrogenic Agents

Any food or drug that interferes with thyroid hormone synthesis is a potential cause of goiter and hypothyroidism. These include selected anions such as iodide, perchlorate, and thiocyanate; cations such as cobalt, arsenic, and lithium; antithyroid drugs, including the thioureylene drugs; amino-

TABLE 3–3. CAUSES OF ACQUIRED HYPOTHYROIDISM IN CHILDREN

Autoimmune thyroid disease
Late-onset thyroid dysgenesis
Late-onset thyroid dyshormonogenesis
Decreased responsiveness to thyroid hormones
TSH deficiency
Drug induced
Iatrogenic
Endemic iodine deficiency
Miscellaneous
    Chromosomal disorders
    Cystinosis

salicylic acid, aminoglutethimide, and phenylbutazone; and a variety of naturally occurring goitrogens that may be difficult to identify.[127] Goitrins may appear in the milk of cows fed crops of the genus *Brassica*. Goiter in school children in the Appalachian mountains of the eastern United States seems to be, at least in part, due to the presence of unidentified goitrogens in ground water. There is also a high prevalence of antithyroid antibodies in Appalachian children, so that both environmental (region-specific) and genetic factors may play a role in the same population.[128,129]

Thyroid Dysgenesis

Ectopic thyroid glands in children may present as an enlarging mass at the base of the tongue or along the course of the thyroglossal duct. Generally only one sibling is affected, but rare familial instances have been reported. Various degrees of hypothyroidism from barely detectable to severe have been described. The term cryptothyroidism has been applied in such instances by analogy with cryptorchidism.[130] Children with unilateral thyroid aplasia have presented with an enlarged functional hemithyroid gland. Such patients may be diagnosed as having a functioning thyroid nodule. An occasional patient may be missed in a newborn screening program and present with hypothyroidism during late infancy or childhood. Severe hypothyroidism also may occur after surgical removal of a presumed thyroglossal duct cyst; seemingly isolated masses in the neck may prove to be the only functional thyroid tissue in such patients.

Autoimmune (Hashimoto) Thyroiditis

Hashimoto thyroiditis (chronic lymphocytic thyroiditis or autoimmune thyroiditis) was described by Hashimoto in 1912 in four patients with goiter. The thyroid glands were infiltrated with plasma cells and lymphocytes and demonstrated fibrosis, parenchymal atrophy, and eosinophilic degeneration in some of the acini. It is the most common cause of acquired hypothyroidism in nonendemic goiter areas.[131–134] The disease occurs in a genetically predisposed population; there is a family history of thyroid disease in 30 to 40 per cent of patients. The disease has a marked predilection for females. The onset of the disorder usually is insidious. Most children present with a small goiter with or without mild hypothyroidism.[133–137] Five to 10 per cent of patients, particularly those in adolescence, may present with tachycardia, nervousness, and other signs suggestive of thyrotoxicosis.[138] The course of Hashimoto thyroiditis is variable. Usually the gland undergoes progressive atrophy, and the patient presents with acquired hypothyroidism. In adult populations the yearly incidence of hypothyroidism among patients with subclinical Hashimoto thyroiditis is 5 to 7 per cent.[139,140] Spontaneous remission has been reported to occur in some 30 per cent of adolescent patients.[133]

The spectrum of the disease in children includes euthyroid goiter, hypothyroid goiter, thyrotoxicosis, nodular goiter, thyroid antigen-antibody nephritis, and multiple endocrine deficiency disease[131,138,141–145] (Table 3–4). The latter includes diabetes mellitus, adrenal insufficiency, hypoparathyrodism, moniliasis, and less commonly pernicious anemia and thrombocytopenia.[142,143] The commonest clinical association is Hashimoto thyroiditis and diabetes mellitus with or without adrenal cortical insufficiency, sometimes referred to as Schmidt syndrome. Recent studies have shown a prevalence of thyroid autoantibodies of 30 per cent in children with type I diabetes mellitus and a prevalence of elevated serum TSH levels approximating 10 per cent.[141,142] All children with diabetes mellitus should be screened for autoimmune thyroid disease.

Primary myxedema represents "burned out" hypothyroidism. These patients may still have significant antithyroid antibody levels and other autoimmune manifestations. The disorder is common in adults and uncommon in children.[138] Fibrous or Riedel thyroiditis is a rapidly progressing variant of autoimmune thyroiditis associated with a marked perithyroidal fibrosis. It is uncommon in adults and rare in children. These patients tend to have elevated titers of collagen-stimulating antibody. Thyroid lymphoma is increased in prevalence in patients with autoimmune thyroiditis, but this manifestation also is rare in children.[138]

The histology of Hashimoto thyroiditis includes prominent lymphoid and plasma cell infiltration with varying degrees of thyroid cell atrophy and fibrosis[134,136,137] (Fig. 3–8). Most patients have detectable circulating levels of antithyroid antibodies. These include antithyroglobulin, antimicrosomal, antiperoxidase, TSH receptor–blocking, TSH receptor–stimulating, thyroid growth–inhibiting, thyroid growth–stimulating, collagen-stimulating and non-TG (anticolloid II) antibodies[131,132,146,147] (Table 3–5). Antithyroglobulin and antimicrosomal antibodies are most useful in diagnosis. The prevalence of such antibodies measured by sensitive methods such as radioimmunoassay in patients with Hashimoto thyroiditis approaches 95 per cent. The presence of these antibodies, however, is not pathognomonic; significant antibody titers occur in 10 to 15 per cent of patients without thyroiditis. At least some of these subjects represent genetically predisposed individuals who have not yet developed thyroiditis. The familial prevalence of antithyroid antibody serves to identify the familial predisposition to autoimmune thyroid disease. Perhaps 10 per cent of children with Hashimoto thyroiditis will develop significant titers of TSH receptor–stimulating antibody and develop mild to moderate hyperthyroidism. The combined disorder has been referred to as "Hashitoxicosis."

A genetically determined defect in the immune surveillance system has been postulated as the basic defect in patients with autoimmune thyroid disease.[131,132,147]

TABLE 3–4. CLINICAL SPECTRUM OF AUTOIMMUNE THYROID DISEASE

Thyroid disorders
  Hashimoto thyroiditis
  Primary myxedema
  Fibrous thyroiditis
  Thyroid lymphoma
  Hashitoxicosis
  Graves disease
Autoimmune polyglandular disease, type II*
  Diabetes mellitus
  Addison disease
  Hypoparathyroidism
Associated autoimmune disorders
  Idiopathic thrombocytopenia
  Thyroid antigen/antibody nephritis
Pregnancy-associated thyroid disorders
  Transient postpartum hypothyroidism
  Transient postpartum hyperthyroidism
  Transient congenital hypothyroidism
  Neonatal Graves disease
Nontoxic goiter
  Simple adolescent goiter
  Adult multinodular goiter
Sporadic cretinism

*May include ovarian failure, pernicious anemia, myasthenia gravis, vitiligo, and alopecia.

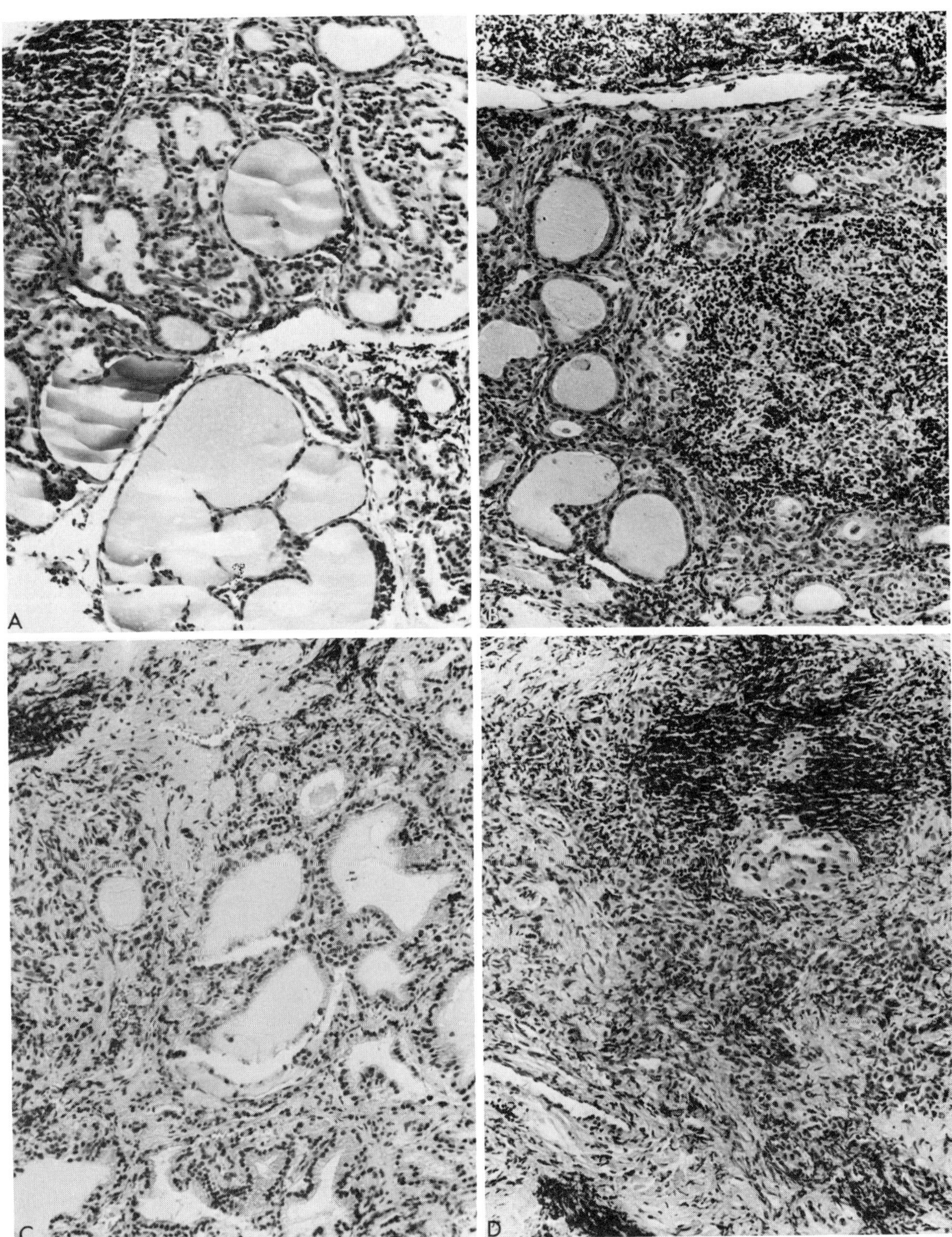

FIGURE 3–8. Progression in severity of chronic lymphocytic thyroiditis as demonstrated by the degree of loss of parenchymal tissue, replacement by lymphocytic diseases. *A*, Variable size of follicles and height of acinar epithelium with focal lymphocytic infiltrations. *B*, Moderate disease: more generalized lymphocytic infiltration with lymphoid follicle and formation of germinal center. *C*, Advanced disease: interstitial fibrosis and variable degree of lymphocytic infiltration. *D*, Severe disease: fibrous variant with dense fibrous tissue, extensive lymphocytic infiltration and scanty, small thyroid follicles. (From Ling SM, Kaplan SA, Weitzman JJ, Reed, GB, Costin G, Landing BH: Euthyroid goiters in children: Correlation of needle biopsy with other clinical and laboratory findings in chronic lymphocytic thyroiditis and simple goiter. Pediatrics 44:695–708, 1969, with permission from the American Academy of Pediatrics, Evanston, Illinois.)

TABLE 3–5. THYROID AUTOANTIBODIES IN HUMAN SUBJECTS

Antithyroglobulin
Antimicrosomal
Antiperoxidase
TSH receptor antibodies
  Stimulating
  Blocking
TSH binding inhibiting
Thyroid growth stimulating
Thyroid growth blocking
Collagen stimulating
Anticolloid II (nonthyroglobulin)

Unsuppressed clones of T lymphocytes sensitized against thyroidal components could explain the cell-mediated immune response as well as the presence of humoral antibodies directed at various thyroid and other tissue components. The humoral antibodies are produced by B lymphocytes. T helper and T suppressor cells as well as antiidiotypic antibodies are involved in the control of immunoglobulin in production by B cells. In autoimmune thyroid disease this complex control system also is abnormal.

Compensated Defect in Thyroid Hormone Biosynthesis

Most cases of hypothyroidism due to defective hormone synthesis present as congenital hypothyroidism. However, infants with a compensated defect and normal T_4 and/or TSH values may escape detection in a neonatal T_4 screening program. The goiter in these patients also may be delayed in appearance or detection.[2,112] Thus, children with a goiter and compensated or partially compensated hypothyroidism may develop clinical hypothyroidism late in infancy or during childhood.

Decreased Responsiveness to Thyroid Hormones

Refetoff and associates in 1967 described a familial syndrome in three siblings with deaf-mutism, stippled epiphyses, retarded skeletal age, goiter, elevated levels of serum free T_4 and free T_3, and normal plasma TSH concentrations.[148] Growth rate, metabolic rate, and intelligence were normal. The thyroid glands of these children were secreting five times the normal amount of T_4 daily. Administration of 1000 µg/day of T_4 or 375 µg/day of T_3 produced few if any metabolic effects. As the patients matured, the plasma T_4 tended to return to normal levels, the epiphyses closed, and the goiters disappeared. The pituitary gland in these patients shares the TSH resistance, and there is a normal TSH response to TRH despite three-fold-elevated serum free T_4 and free T_3 levels.

Several other patients have been described with variable degrees of thyroid hormone unresponsiveness and goiter.[148–152] Both autosomal-recessive and autosomal-dominant inheritance patterns have been suggested.[148,149] The youngest patient reported was diagnosed at 6 months with regurgitation and failure to thrive.[150] Studies of nuclear T_3 receptor binding in lymphocytes and fibroblasts usually have yielded variable results, suggesting defects at the receptor or postreceptor levels.[148–152] However, decreased T_3 receptor binding affinity has been observed.[149] Several T_3 nuclear receptor genes have been cloned. Relative fragment length polymorphism (RFLP) studies conducted in three children in one family tested for polymorphisms of the β-receptor gene showed that two were heterozygous and one was homozygous for one of the polymorphic alleles.[153] This supports a receptor gene defect. The variable pattern of affected tissues from one kindred to another also is consistent with a genetic abnormality in one of several T_3 nuclear receptor gene products.[149]

Acquired Hypothalamic Pituitary Hypothyroidism

Hypothalamic or pituitary disorders may be acquired secondary to head trauma, tumors including craniopharyngiomas, granulomatous disease, meningitis, head irradiation, or rare vascular accidents. Growth failure due to GH and/or TSH deficiency usually is the earliest manifestation of pituitary hypofunction, but other signs and symptoms related to the primary disease, neurologic disorder, and/or hypothalamic dysfunction may occur. Mild to moderate TSH deficiency hypothyroidism also may occur as a result of treatment of GH-deficient children with exogenous GH.[154] The mechanism is unclear; an inhibitory effect of GH on the pituitary-thyroid axis has been postulated.[155]

Endemic Goiter and Hypothyroidism

Endemic goiter is the commonest thyroid disease worldwide; some 300 million people are affected.[156-158] Iodine deficiency is the most important etiologic factor, but a variety of environmental agents and genetic factors may play a role. In some areas of the world vegetables of the *Brassicae* family, and particularly cassava, potentiate the effects of iodine deficiency. The goitrogenic action of cassava results from the release of cyanide from linamarin, a glycoside present in large amounts in cassava, and the conversion of cyanide to thiocyanate, which blocks iodide organification. Iodine deficiency, with or without the added effect of a goitrogen, impairs thyroid hormone production, which leads to increased TSH secretion, increased iodide trapping, and goiter. These adaptive responses compensate to a variable extent for the impaired hormone biosynthetic capacity and a spectrum of clinical manifestations occurs, ranging from cretinism to goitrous hypothyroidism to euthyroidism with goiter. The prevalence of endemic cretinism may be as high as 5 to 8 per cent of the population in areas of severe iodine deficiency.

Endemic goiter largely due to iodine deficiency still is prevalent in several areas of Europe and the Middle East, although the prevalence is decreasing.[159] The areas of highest prevalence include West Germany, Switzerland, Austria, Spain, Italy, Greece, Lebanon, and Iraq.[159] Effective iodization programs are being introduced gradually to these areas and endemic cretinism is no longer a problem.[90,91] The iodine deficiency is associated with transient neonatal hypothyroidism, especially in premature infants.[90,91]

Miscellaneous Causes

There is an increased frequency of hypothyroidism in patients with abnormal chromosome karyotypes, including Turner syndrome, Down syndrome, Klinefelter syndrome, and Noonan syndrome.[101,160,161] In Down syndrome there is an increased prevalence of thyroid dysgenesis. Autoimmune thyroiditis has been said to be more prevalent in all of these disorders. Compensated hypothyroidism occurs frequently and early in children with nephropathic cystinosis, and some children with the disorder will manifest overt hypothyroidism.[162] The thyroid glands show extensive destruction and infiltration of the epithelium with cystine crystals.

TABLE 3–6. MANIFESTATIONS OF ACQUIRED HYPOTHYROIDISM UNIQUE TO CHILDHOOD

Growth retardation
Bone age retardation
Muscle hypertrophy (pseudodystrophy)
Sexual disorders
   Delayed puberty
   Precocious puberty

Diagnosis of Acquired Hypothyroidism

The clinical manifestations of acquired hypothyroidism in childhood differ from those in the adult (Table 3–6). The classic manifestations that occur in the adult also may occur in children. These include decreased appetite, lethargy, constipation, bradycardia, dry skin and hair, prolonged reflex relaxation time, decreased metabolic rate, hypercholesterolemia, and reduced glomerular filtration rate. However, these manifestations are not prominent. Instead the most important sign of acquired hypothyroidism in childhood is growth failure. Usually a number of years elapse between the onset of hypothyroidism and the emergence of classic signs of myxedema. However, if growth records are available, the onset of hypothyroidism can be documented as the beginning of a progressive downward deviation from a previously normal linear growth pattern. Weight tends to increase modestly, and in most instances weight for age is proportionately greater than height for age. The retardation of bone age in hypothyroidism usually equals or exceeds the retardation in linear growth, but bone age retardation also is present in other forms of dwarfism and is not pathognomonic of hypothyroidism. Other signs of hypothyroidism and varying clinical manifestations of myxedema related to organ hypofunction (cardiac, gut, skin, renal, etc.) usually occur and are helpful in differential diagnosis. However, in some children the predominant manifestation is growth retardation, which makes it difficult to distinguish acquired hypothyroidism from primary hypopituitarism.[163] Muscle weakness is observed in 30 to 40 per cent of children with hypothyroidism. Muscle bulk usually is normal or increased, but atrophy may occur.[164]

Muscular hypertrophy may be marked in hypothyroid children, and this phenomenon has been referred to as the Kocher-Debré-Sémélaigne syndrome.[165] Creatinine phosphokinase levels may be elevated.[164] The proximal musculature of the pelvic and shoulder girdles is primarily affected, but hypertrophy may involve the calves, thighs, hands, neck, tongue, and facial muscles.[164,165] As in adults, the prolongation of muscle contraction produces the characteristic slow relaxation phase of the tendon reflex reaction. Muscle dysfunction resembling dermatomyositis or polymyositis also has been described.[164] The mechanism is not clear.

Sexual development usually is delayed in hypothyroid children in proportion to the retardation of skeletal age. However, some children with hypothyroidism present with manifestations of sexual precocity.[166,167] In females this includes precocious menstruation, breast development, and galactorrhea. Males show excessive enlargement of the penis and testes. Most of these patients lack sexual hair, and bone age is retarded in keeping with the duration of the hypothyroid state. The sella turcica may be enlarged and serum gonadotropin and prolactin levels are elevated.[168,169] The increased serum prolactin may be explained by the fact that TRH directly stimulates both TSH and prolactin release from the pituitary. Other non-TSH pituitary hormone secretion may be due to paracrine effects of TRH-stimulated second messenger in pituitary tissue. With treatment the manifestations of sexual precocity regress and normal puberty ensues at the appropriate time relative to maturity.

The diagnosis of *Hashimoto thyroiditis* in euthyroid patients is based on a series of five characteristic findings[170]: (1) the thyroid gland is moderately enlarged, firm, and bosselated in 80 to 90 per cent of patients; (2) the thyroid scan shows a spotty pattern of radioiodine uptake in 60 to 70 per cent of patients; (3) 90 to 95 per cent of patients have increased titers of antithyroglobulin and/or antimicrosomal or antiperoxidase antibody; (4) 60 to 70 per cent of patients manifest a defect in organification of iodide within the thyroid demonstrable by an abnormal discharge of radioactivity following oral administration of potassium perchlorate (positive perchlorate discharge test); and (5) 30 to 40 per cent of patients have compensated hypothyroidism associated with a low serum T_4 concentration, a normal or near-normal serum T_3 concentration, an elevated TSH level, and/or an augmented TSH response to TRH. The presence of two of these five markers provides a presumptive diagnosis; three of five positive criteria support the diagnosis with 85 to 90 per cent reliability. A presumptive diagnosis of Hashimoto thyroiditis is warranted in an overtly hypothyroid patient with elevated antithyroid antibody titers. In addition to antithyroglobulin, antimicrosomal, and antiperoxidase antibodies, these patients may manifest significant titers of TSH receptor–blocking antibodies, thyroid growth-stimulating antibodies, anticolloid III antibodies, and collagen-stimulating antibodies.[138] The positive perchlorate discharge test probably is due to the antiperoxidase antibody.

The diagnosis should be supported by objective test criteria before treatment is instituted. Minimal documentation should include measurement of serum T_4 and TSH levels. In children without thyroid autoantibodies a thyroid scan is useful to exclude thyroid dysgenesis or thyroid hemiagenesis. An elevated blood TSH level establishes that the disease originates in the thyroid rather than the pituitary gland. A low serum T_4 (and free T_4) with a low serum TSH level implies a hypothalamic or pituitary defect. A normal (or prolonged) TSH response to TRH in such a child indicates hypothalamic TRH deficiency; a low or absent TSH response indicates pituitary TSH deficiency. Whenever TSH deficiency is suspected, other pituitary hormone deficiencies should be identified by pituitary function studies, including provocative tests of adrenocorticotropic hormone (ACTH) and GH secretion. Appropriate neurologic and specialized studies should be carried out to exclude a pituitary tumor in patients with acquired TSH deficiency.

Treatment of Acquired Hypothyroidism

The treatment of children with hypothyroidism should be accomplished with NaT_4 in a dose approximating 100 $\mu g/m^2$ body surface daily.[171,172] This usually amounts to a dose of 2 to 7 $\mu g/kg/day$ and a total dose of 50 to 300 $\mu g/day$ (Table 3–7). Treatment of patients with compensated hypothyroidism due to autoimmune thyroiditis is indicated. Treatment of such patients during the euthyroid phase of the disease is controversial. Thyroid hormone therapy prevents the development of mild and subtle hypothyroidism and may suppress autoantibody titers somewhat. However, there is no evidence that the natural progression of the disease is altered.[133] Treated children resume growth

TABLE 3–7. REPLACEMENT DOSAGE OF NaT$_4$ IN INFANCY AND CHILDHOOD

Age	Dose of NaT$_4$	
	μg/day	μg/kg/day
1–12 months	25–50	10–15
1–15 years	50–100	5–7
5–10 years	100–150	3–5
10–20 years	100–300	2–4

TABLE 3–8. SUBCLASSES OF NONTHYROIDAL ILLNESS

Subclasses	Serum Concentration*			
	T_4	T_3	rT_3	TSH
Low T_3 syndrome	N	D	N or I	N
Low T_4 syndrome	D	D	N or I	N
High T_4 syndrome	I	D	N or I	N

* D, decreased; N, normal; I, increased.

at a rate greater than normal, the period of transient catch-up growth. This catch-up growth usually is adequate to compensate the preexistant growth retardation and normalize predicted adult height. In children in whom treatment is delayed, catch-up growth may be inadequate to normalize predicted adult height.[173] Excessive T_4 dosage may accelerate bone maturation disproportionately and reduce adult stature. In patients with pituitary TSH deficiency or deficiency of other anterior pituitary hormones, treatment with adrenal glucocorticoids and/or GH should be provided as necessary.

NONTHYROIDAL ILLNESS (THE LOW T$_3$ SYNDROME)

Sullivan et al. in 1973 first described a selective deficiency of serum and tissue T_3 in patients dying with severe prolonged illness.[174–176] They referred to these patients as the "euthyroid sick." More recently other terms, including the *low T_3 syndrome* and *nonthyroidal illness* (NTI), have been applied. The syndrome includes low total and free serum T_3; normal, low, or high total serum T_4 with normal to high free T_4 levels; and normal serum TSH concentrations. The disorder occurs in premature neonates, patients with protein-calorie malnutrition or anorexia nervosa, fasting subjects, postoperative patients, and patients with a variety of severe acute and chronic illness. The latter have included patients with diabetic ketoacidosis, severe trauma, burns, febrile states, hepatic cirrhosis, and renal failure. In addition, a number of drugs produce a similar syndrome of selective T_3 deficiency; these drugs include dexamethasone, selected radiographic contrast agents, propylthiouracil propranolol, and amiodarone.

Three patterns of change in thyroid hormone levels have been described (Table 3–8): low T_4, normal T_4, and high T_4 NTI syndromes. The low serum T_3 level in this syndrome occurs as a result of inhibition of iodothyronine β ring monodeiodinase activity and a decreased rate of T_3 production from T_4.[174,175] Alpha ring monodeiodination is not impaired, so that rT_3 production is not reduced. Moreover, rT_3 degradation is decreased because the conversion of rT_3 to DIT is impaired. Thus, serum T_3 levels fall and rT_3 levels tend to remain normal or increase. In some patients serum T_4 levels also fall. Thyroid-binding globulin levels may be reduced in such patients, and a tissue-derived inhibitor of T_4 binding to TBG has been described in the serum of such patients.[177] The high T_4 NTI syndrome probably involves one or more induced abnormalities in the disposal pathways of T_4.[174] There is no beneficial effect of treatment with thyroid hormone, either T_4 or T_3, in NTI.[88,178] Treatment is directed to the primary systemic illness.

DIFFUSE NONTOXIC GOITER (SIMPLE COLLOID GOITER; ADOLESCENT GOITER)

A syndrome of euthyroid diffuse goiter has been described during adolescence in nonendemic goiter areas. Many such patients represent Hashimoto thyroiditis. Others, however, have no evidence of thyroid lymphocytic infiltration and are described as having adolescent goiter. A common finding in such patients is a family history of goiter, but detailed tests of thyroid function fail to reveal identifiable defects.[179,180] The genetic pattern in such families is suggestive of an autosomal-dominant mode of transmission, with greater expression in the female.[180] The goitrous adolescent may manifest circulating non-T_4 iodine (a protein-bound iodine–T_4 iodine difference that exceeds 2 μg/dl), but other thyroid function tests are normal and thyroid biopsy reveals only "colloid goiter." The thyroid enlargement often will regress spontaneously, but many patients who develop nodular goiters in the third, fourth, and fifth decades have a history of mild diffuse thyroid enlargement during childhood or adolescence.[180,181] There is increasing evidence for the presence of thyroid growth-stimulating immunoglobulins in the sera of such patients so that simple goiter of adolescence may represent a mild form of autoimmune thyroid disease.[10,11,106,138,182]

SUBACUTE THYROIDITIS

Subacute thyroiditis is a self-limited inflammation of the thyroid that follows or is associated with an upper respiratory illness.[183,184] Patients have been identified with evidence of associated mumps virus infection and others with cat-scratch fever. It is likely that a variety of viral agents may be responsible for this condition. The incidence is similar in males and females. Patients present with fever and pain that may be local or referred to the angles of the jaw. The thyroid gland usually is tender and may be exquisitely so.

Characteristically there is an increase in serum T_4 and T_3 levels as a result of release of stored hormone, and signs and symptoms of hyperthyroidism develop. Thyroidal radioiodine uptake at this time is low or absent, indicating thyroid cell damage. Signs and symptoms of hyperthyroidism usually persist for 1 to 4 weeks. After this time there is a period of transient hypothyroidism as the thyroid gland recovers. The total course runs 2 to 9 months.[183,184] A syndrome of painless (subacute) thyroiditis also has been described with a similar pattern of transient hyperthyroidism associated with a low thyroid radioiodine uptake. This "painless thyroiditis" syndrome, however, resembles Hashimoto thyroiditis histologically and often occurs in the postpartum period in women with a history of autoimmune thyroid disease.[147] This syndrome has not yet been described in children.

Treatment of subacute, painful (viral) thyroiditis includes acetylsalicylic acid or other antiflammatory drugs; in severe cases, adrenal corticosteroid medication may be helpful. Most patients do not develop antithyroid antibodies and recover with no residual defect in thyroid function. Subacute thyroiditis may be difficult to distinguish from acute purulent thyroiditis, but the latter condition now is rare.

ACUTE SUPPURATIVE THYROIDITIS

There is an inherent resistance of the thyroid gland to local infection, perhaps related to the high levels of iodine in the gland. Also, it is completely encapsulated and protected to some degree from direct extension of infection in neighboring tissues. Thus, bacterial infection of the thyroid gland is rare, but does occur.[185,186] It is characterized by fever, dysphagia, a hoarse voice, a painful, tender mass in the anterior neck, severe pain with neck extension, and a rapid progression to abscess formation. The left lobe of the thyroid is involved more frequently than the right. Leukocytosis is increased and acute-phase reactant tests are positive. Thyroid function tests usually are normal, but the thyroid scan shows diminished activity over the affected area of gland. Streptococcus, staphylococcus, and pneumococcus have been reported, as well as a predominance of anaerobic bacteria such as *Bacteroides*, *Peptostreptococcus*, and *Peptococcus*, in recent reports.[185,186] Antibiotic therapy must, therefore, be individualized. In many patients and in most of those with recurrent suppurative thyroiditis, barium meals have revealed a sinus tract from the pyriform sinus of the pharynx to the thyroid, usually on the left side. A child with acute suppurative thyroiditis, particularly involving the left lobe and associated with an anaerobic organism, should be investigated to rule out a congenital pharyngeal sinus tract.

GRAVES DISEASE

Pathogenesis

Thyrotoxicosis in childhood and adolescence usually is caused by Graves disease, a multisystem disorder involving hyperthyroidism, eye manifestations, and dermopathy.[187–193] Graves disease is an autoimmune disorder, and like Hashimoto thyroiditis occurs in a genetically predisposed population. The disease may occur in preschool children and rarely may begin in infancy, but there is a sharp increase in incidence as children approach adolescence.

Girls are afflicted six to eight times more often than boys. A high proportion of patients have a family history positive for goiter, hyperthyroidism, and hypothyroidism.

Among the thyroid system–directed autoimmune antibodies in patients with Graves disease are immunoglobulins with thyroid-stimulating activity (TSA). The first TSA described was referred to as the long-acting thyroid stimulator (LATS) because of its prolonged action in bioassay mice. More recently other immunoglobulins with human thyroid-stimulating activity have been identified by bioassay and receptor assay techniques.[147] TSA stimulates cAMP production in thyroid cell membranes in a manner similar to TSH. TSA also displaces radiolabeled TSH from thyroid membrane TSH receptors; TSA measured in this way is referred to as TSH-binding–inhibiting immunoglobulin (TBII). It is possible that TSH receptor–directed antibodies displace TSH but fail to stimulate cAMP. Such "blocking antibodies" have been reported, but are not common in patients with Graves disease.

Ophthalmopathy in Graves disease often is associated with the presence of collagen-stimulating antibodies.[138] Other antibodies include thyroid growth-stimulating antibody, which seems to correlate with large goiters. Antimicrosomal and antithyroglobulin antibodies also are present, but usually in lesser titers than in patients with Hashimoto thyroiditis.[138]

Clinical Features

Children with thyrotoxicosis present with nervousness, palpitations, increased apetite, and muscle weakness (Table 3–9). Marked weight loss may occur. Except for the eye signs, the symptoms of thyrotoxicosis are nonspecific. Behavior abnormalities and declining school performance may dominate the clinical picture. In other patients cardiovascular signs are more prominent. Fatigability and objective muscle weakness occur in 60 to 70 per cent of patients. The disease may occur in association with myasthenia gravis or periodic paralysis. Many of the signs and symptoms of Graves disease are due to hyperactivity of the sympathetic nervous system. Tachycardia, a widened pulse pressure and an overactive precordium are common signs; others include tremor, excessive perspiration,

TABLE 3–9. CLINICAL MANIFESTATIONS OF GRAVES DISEASE IN CHILDHOOD*

Clinical Sign/Symptom	Prevalence (%)
Goiter	100
Prominence of eyes	100
Tachycardia	95
Nervousness	80
Exophthalmos	75
Increased appetite	70
Weight loss	65
Emotional lability	40
Heat tolerance	40
Frequent stools	20

* From Saxena KM, Crawford JD, Talbot NB: Childhood thyrotoxicosis, a long term perspective.

shortened tendon reflex relaxation time, and emotional lability.

The size of the thyroid gland is highly variable, and the goiter may escape notice in a patient whose gland is only slightly enlarged. Careful thyroid examination is essential. The eye signs of Graves disease also are variable. However, severe Graves ophthalmopathy is uncommon in children and malignant exophthalmos is virtually unknown. Some of the eye findings are secondary to the sympathetic hyperactivity. There is a stare, owing to retraction of the upper lid and a wide palpebral aperture, and a lag in the descent of the upper lid on looking downward (lid lag). These latter findings improve with propranolol treatment, and disappear as the patient is rendered euthyroid. By contrast, manifestations of the inherent autoimmune ophthalmopathy often persist for months or years. The accumulation of mucopolysaccharides in skin and subcutaneous tissues (Graves dermopathy) is rare in children.

Graves disease and Hashimoto thyroiditis occasionally are encountered in the same patient.[138] Such children have clinical and laboratory features of Hashimoto thyroiditis, and in addition exhibit thyrotoxicosis. In these patients, a thyroid-stimulating antibody develops among the spectrum of autoimmune antibodies, and if the titer is high enough clinical thyrotoxicosis develops. The thyrotoxic state may occur at any time in a patient with autoimmune thyroiditis as long as the thyroid gland is still TSH responsive. The term *Hashitoxicosis* has been applied to this condition. These patients may be difficult to distinguish from the routine patient with Graves disease.

Diagnosis and Management

Initial laboratory tests should include measurements of serum T_4, including an assessment of free T_4 (the free T_4 index), and a sensitive serum TSH measurement to rule out TSH-dependent hyperthyroidism. A measurement of serum T_3 concentration is particularly useful since it usually is increased more markedly than the T_4 concentration. The free T_4 and free T_3 levels are elevated and the TSH concentration is depressed below the normal range. Patients with thyrotoxicosis also have an absent or depressed TSH response to TRH. Thyroid radioactive iodine uptake assessment is not usually necessary. Measurements of serum levels of thyroid-stimulating antibodies may be very helpful in confirming the diagnosis in selected patients.

Treatment of thyrotoxicosis is directed to reducing the secretory rate of thyroid hormones and blunting their effects. Three principal methods are available for reducing thyroid hormone secretion: antithyroid drug treatment, subtotal thyroidectomy, and radioactive iodine. *Antithyroid drug treatment* is most commonly employed,[187-193] and the thioureylene drugs are most effective. These drugs, which inhibit thyroid hormone synthesis via a thiocarbamide group $(S=C-N)$, include thiourea, thiouracil, methylthiouracil, propylthiouracil, methimazole, and carbimazole.[194] The drugs currently used include propylithiouracil (PTU), methimazole (MMI), and carbimazole (CBI). Carbimazole acts by conversion to MMI. The thioureylene drugs act by inhibiting the organification of iodine via inhibition of thyroid peroxidase activity.[194,195] Inhibition of hormone synthesis results in depletion of the thyroid stores of iodinated thyroglobulin and a progressive decrease in thyroid hormone secretion from the thyroid gland. In addition to blocking hormone synthesis, PTU inhibits the peripheral conversion of T_4 to T_3; MMI does not share this action.[194] Effective amounts of the drugs are absorbed within 30 to 60 min after an oral dose. The half-life of PTU in plasma approximates 2 hours, and that for MMI or CBI 6 to 13 hours. The drugs are concentrated within the thyroid and metabolites are excreted largely in urine. They cross the placenta and appear in breast milk.

There always is a lag time between institution of drug treatment and achievement of a euthyroid state, since the biosynthetic block is not complete and the stores of preformed hormone must first be discharged. The rapidity of response to therapy correlates best with the initial size of the thyroid gland. Those patients with a small gland usually exhibit improvement in a few weeks, whereas those with very large glands may not respond for 2 to 3 months. The initial dosage of PTU varies from 300 to 600 mg daily (175 mg/m^2 or 4 to 6 mg/kg) in dosages spaced at 6- or 8-hour intervals. The dosage of MMI or CBI is about one-tenth that of PTU.

There is a significant incidence of toxic reactions to all thioureylene drugs.[194] The most common minor reaction is a purpuric, papular rash that usually is mild and subsides spontaneously. Other minor reactions include nausea, headache, paresthesias, hair loss, and joint pain and stiffness. Agranulocytosis, the most serious reaction, is observed in 1:500 to 1:1000 cases. It usually develops during the first few months of treatment and may develop rapidly. Mild granulocytopenia can be due to thyrotoxicosis or may be an early sign of serious drug toxicity. Drug fever, hepatitis, nephritis, and a lupus-like reaction are rare complications.

A drug rash, if persistent, can be managed by substituting another thioureylene drug since cross-sensitivity is not common. Should granulocytopenia be observed, frequent leukocyte counts are indicated to rule out serious drug toxicity. Routine blood counts in all patients are not necessary since agranulocytosis can develop after several months and may appear rapidly. Patients should be instructed to report development of sore throat or fever, which may herald agranulocytosis. Persistent neutropenia requires discontinuing drug treatment. Agranulocytosis usually reverses spontaneously but intensive transient supportive treatment may be required if severe.

Sodium ipodate or iopanoate are *iodinated organic radiographic contrast agents* that have been shown to be effective antithyroid drugs.[196-199] They inhibit the enzymatic monodeiodination of T_4 to T_3 and produce a rapid reduction in serum T_3 concentrations.[196,197] In addition, they inhibit thyroid hormone secretion from the thyroid gland so that serum T_4 levels also fall.[196-200] Chronic treatment (6 to 12 months) has been successful in from 50 to more than 90 per cent of patients with Graves disease.[196-198] Sodium ipodate may be more effective than sodium iopanoic acid, but data to date are limited in this regard.[197,198] Sodium ipodate has been used successfully in an infant with neonatal Graves disease.[199] No serious side effects have been observed to date, but experience is limited. Interestingly, in contrast to the situation with iodide, prolonged blockade of thyroid function does not occur and radioiodine treatment has been applied within 2 to 4 weeks of discontinuing sodium ipodate therapy.[197] These agents may be very useful for treatment of patients who develop toxicity to thioureylene drugs. Also, they may be useful adjuncts to other antithyroid drug regimens and may be helpful in short-term preoperative or preradioiodine treatment of severe thyrotoxicosis.

Iodide is the oldest antithyroid drug. In large doses (more than 0.1 mg/kg/day) it inhibits thyroid iodide transport, iodothyronine synthesis, and thyroid hormone release.[201] As a result there is a rapid fall in serum thyroid hormone levels that may persist several weeks. Eventually there is an "escape" from the thyroid iodide blockade mediated in part by the inhibition of thyroid cell membrane iodide transport and a reduction in intrathyroidal iodide concentrations. Thus, iodide usually is restricted to short-term therapy (several weeks). Iodide treatment has been used in the immediate preoperative period to prepare patients for thyroidectomy and for treatment of severe thyrotoxicosis or thyroid crisis in conjunction with thioureylene drugs.

Toxic reactions to iodide are observed occasionally.[201] Acute life-threatening angioedema and laryngeal edema may occur with or without a cutaneous hemorrhagic rash. Serum sickness–like manifestations also have been observed, with fever, arthralgia, eosinophilia, and lymphadenopathy. Chronic intoxication (iodism) also is described, including soreness of the teeth and gums, increased salivation, nasal irritation, swelling of the eyes, headache, and chronic cough. Acneiform skin lesions, gastric irritation, and diarrhea may occur. These signs and symptoms disappear within a few days after discontinuing iodide ingestion. Iodide preparations include strong iodine solution (Lugol's solution) for oral use and sodium iodide for intravenous use. Lugol's solution is formulated as 5 per cent iodine and 10 per cent potassium iodide. The iodine is reduced to iodide in the intestine before absorption. Intravenous sodium iodide is available as a 10 per cent solution.

β-Adrenergic blocking drugs are useful to control the sympathetic hyperactivity. These drugs also have proven life saving in critically ill patients in thyroid storm, but cannot be relied upon as the only therapy in such patients. β receptor blockade is potentially dangerous in patients with cardiac failure or arrhythmias.

Surgery offers the most rapid resolution of thyrotoxicosis. With proper surgical management most patients achieve satisfactory remission, and requirements for intensive medical follow-up are less rigorous than in those patients treated exclusively with drugs.[188,193,202] The availability of an experienced thyroid surgeon is an important criterion for successful surgical treatment. With proper preparation of the patient for surgical thyroidectomy, the immediate operative mortality approximates that for other major surgical procedures.

In several series of reported cases of surgical treatment of juvenile Graves disease totaling 411 cases there was only one surgical death.[202] Loss of one recurrent laryngeal nerve occurred in 1 per cent of the children; there were no instances of bilateral loss. Permanent hypoparathyroidism occurred in 2 per cent of the 411 patients. Forty-nine of the 411 patients were treated by total thyroidectomy and 362 by subtotal thyroidectomy; 45 per cent became hypothyroid and required replacement therapy.[202] Of 186 patients followed for an average of 10 years, 10 per cent developed recurrent thyrotoxicosis.[202]

In terms of ease, cost, efficacy, and short-term safety, treatment with radioiodine is superior.[203] However, this approach has not been extensively used in childhood and adolescence because of the high prevalence of posttreatment hypothyroidism and concern about radiation oncogenesis and genetic damage. Late development of primary hypothyroidism after ^{131}I therapy has occurred in every series of patients studied, regardless of the dosage of radioiodine employed. Approximately 10 to 20 per cent of patients treated with radioiodine are hypothyroid within 1 year, and the incidence of hypothyroidism is 3 to 5 per cent per year thereafter. The concern about inducing leukemia and thyroid carcinoma in adult patients with radioiodine treatment has been largely alleviated.[204] However, the thyroid glands of young animals are much more susceptible to induction of thyroid carcinoma by ionizing radiation than those of older animals, and radiation has been incriminated as an important cause of thyroid cancer in children.[204]

Thus, it has been the practice in most clinics to reserve the use of radioiodine for treatment of thyrotoxicosis in older adolescents who fail to follow a medical regimen and who cannot be adequately prepared for surgical thyroidectomy. However, the recent report by Hamburger of the successful treatment of 191 children and adolescents with radioiodine over a 23-year period suggests that this approach may be safe enough to consider as initial treatment in some patients.[203] In Hamburger's series one dose of radioiodine provided effective treatment in 85 per cent of cases.

The choice of therapy in thyrotoxicosis must be individualized, taking into consideration any illness, the quality of surgery available, and the socioeconomic factors that condition the success of a prolonged medical regimen. In most instances treatment is begun with an antithyroid drug and a decision regarding continuing drug therapy, surgery, or radioiodine is made when the patient becomes euthyroid. Usually it is necessary to continue drug therapy for a minimum of 1 to 2 years, and in many instances treatment has been continued for 3 to 6 years before the gland has lost its hyperplastic character. The best clinical prognostic guide is the size of the thyroid gland. Most patients with continued thyroid enlargement will relapse if antithyroid drugs are discontinued early. It is also possible to monitor the level of circulating TSA. When circulating TSA disappears in a patient in clinical remission on drug treatment, a permanent remission off treatment is likely. Probably, antithyroid drugs have no influence on the fundamental disease process. However, drug treatment does permit the patient to remain euthyroid and in good health until such time as the disease has spontaneously run its course.

Neonatal Thyrotoxicosis

Neonatal Graves disease is rare, probably because of the low incidence of thyrotoxicosis in pregnancy (1 to 2 cases per 1000 pregnancies) and the fact that the neonatal disease occurs only in about 1:70 cases of thyrotoxic pregnancy.[205,206] In most cases the disease is due to transplacental passage of TSA from a mother with active or inactive Graves disease or Hashimoto thyroiditis.[199,207–212] Thus, prediction of neonatal Graves disease from the maternal clinical status is not always possible. However, it is possible to predict neonatal disease in offspring of women with high TSA titers. In a recent report all women with TSA titers (measured by stimulation of cAMP in human thyroid slices) exceeding 500 per cent of control values delivered thyrotoxic infants, whereas those with lower titers delivered euthyroid infants.[213] In some infants both TSH receptor–stimulating and TSH receptor–blocking antibodies are acquired from the mother, and the blocking antibodies have been reported to block the effect of the stimulating antibodies for 4 to 6 weeks, such that the infant develops late-onset neonatal Graves disease.[209]

Graves disease in the newborn is manifested by irritability, flushing, tachycardia, hypertension, poor weight gain, thyroid enlargement, and exophthalmos. Thrombocytopenia, hepatosplenomegaly, jaundice, and hypoprothrombinemia also have been observed. Arrhythmias, cardiac failure, and death may occur if the thyrotoxicity is severe and the treatment is inadequate. Mortality approaches 25 per cent in disease severe enough to be diagnosed. In some infants the onset of symptoms and signs in the newborn may be delayed as long as 8 to 9 days. This is because of the postnatal depletion of transplacentally acquired blocking doses of antithyroid drugs, and the fact that there is an abrupt increase in conversion of T_4 to active T_3 shortly after birth. The diagnosis is confirmed by measuring high levels of T_4, free T_4, and T_3 is postnatal blood.[199,208] Cord blood values may be normal or near-normal while levels at 2 to 5 days may be markedly increased; the serum TSH is low. Neonatal Graves disease resolves spontaneously as maternal TSA in the newborn is degraded: the half-life approximates 12 days. The usual clinical course of neonatal Graves disease extends 3 to 12 weeks.[199]

The treatment of hyperthyroidism in the newborn includes sedatives and digitalization as necessary. Iodide or antithyroid drugs are administered to decrease thyroid hormone secretion.[207] These drugs have additive effects with regard to inhibition of hormone synthesis; in addition, iodide will rapidly inhibit hormone release. Lugol's solution (126 mg of iodine/ml) is given in doses of one drop (about 8 mg) three times daily. Methimazole, CBI, or PTU is administered in doses of 0.5 to 1 mg, 0.5 to 1 mg, or 5 to

10 mg, respectively, per kilogram daily in divided doses at 8-hour intervals. A therapeutic response should be observed within 24 to 36 hours. If a satisfactory response is not observed, the dose of antithyroid drug and iodide can be increased by 50 per cent. Adrenal corticosteroids in anti-inflammatory dosage and propranolol (1 to 2 mg/kg/day) also may be helpful. Radiographic contrast agents also may be useful in treatment (100 mg/day or 5.5 gm every 3 days) either alone or in conjunction with antithyroid drug treatment.[199]

THYROTROPIN-DEPENDENT HYPERTHYROIDISM

Rarely, hyperthyroidism is due to hypersecretion of TSH. Two syndromes have been described; TSH-dependent hyperthyroidism due to a pituitary TSH-secreting tumor, and nonneoplastic hypersecretion of TSH associated with abnormal pituitary feedback control of TSH secretion by thyroid hormones.[214,215] Both disorders are associated with goiter and clinical hyperthyroidism, and one of these disorders should be suspected in any child who presents with goitrous hyperthyroidism and hyperthyroxinemia in whom the serum TSH concentration is not suppressed and autoantibodies are not present.

Pituitary Tumors

Thyroid-stimulating hormone–secreting pituitary tumors associated with clinical hyperthyroidism are quite rare, but have been reported in children as well as adults.[214,215] Most have been chromophobe or basophilic adenomas. Local manifestations of the tumor are prominent, including visual changes, optic atrophy, hydrocephalus, and amaurosis. Children with hyperthyroidism should be examined for evidence of neurologic dysfunction and visual abnormalities; and skull roentgenograms for careful evaluation of the sella turcica are indicated if this evaluation arouses suspicion or if the serum TSH concentration is elevated. A mass lesion in the pituitary usually can be demonstrated and the circulating level of TSH α subunit is elevated. The serum TSH level fails to respond to exogenous TRH.

Abnormal Pituitary Feedback: Selected Pituitary T₃ Resistance

Hyperthyroidism with diffuse goiter and elevated serum TSH levels has been reported in several patients without pituitary enlargement.[215,216] These patients manifest resistance to the feedback effect of T_3 on TSH release and represent cases of selective pituitary resistance to thyroid hormone. Features of thyroid autoimmune disease are absent and the serum TSH level is inappropriately elevated in relation to the serum T_4 and T_3 concentrations. In contrast to patients with pituitary TSH-secreting tumors, the TSH α subunit level is not elevated and the TSH response to TRH is increased. Treatment of the disorder is difficult. Thyroid ablation controls the hyperthyroidism but aggravates the TSH hypersecretion and increases the risk of development of a pituitary adenoma. Suppression of TSH by exogenous thyroid hormone may aggravate the hyperthyroidism. However, this approach has been successful[217,218] and treatment with 3,4,3′-triiodothyroacetic acid (TRIAC) or long-acting somatostatin has been proposed.[218,219] Both of these latter agents are experimental drugs.

AUTONOMOUS (NODULAR) HYPERTHYROIDISM

Autonomous-functioning thyroid nodules are uncommon in childhood and adolescence. Thyroid function in patients with a thyroid nodule is variable; most patients are euthyroid. Rarely, single or multiple autonomously functioning nodules may be associated with clinical hyperthyroidism.[1,220,221] Such nodules are true follicular adenomas and nearly always are benign; the incidence of thyroid carcinoma in functioning nodules is less than 1 per cent. Generally, function in a thyroid nodule excludes a diagnosis of thyroid carcinoma. Small functional nodules usually do not produce clinical thyrotoxicosis; large nodules (in excess of 3 cm in diameter) are more likely to do so.

Nodular autonomy usually is determined by thyroid radioiodine scan. A nodule clearly is autonomous if it is the only thyroid tissue showing uptake. If the nodule shows increased radioiodine uptake but the remaining thyroid tissue is still visible on scan, autonomy is likely. Autonomy is confirmed if the serum TSH concentration measured by a highly sensitive method is suppressed, and/or is unresponsive to TRH stimulation.[220,221] The absence of clinical thyrotoxicosis and the presence of normal-range serum T_4 and T_3 concentrations still is compatible with a blunted TSH response to TRH. Thyroxine or T_3 suppression testing also has been used to confirm autonomy; radioiodine uptake in autonomous nodules is not suppressible by exogenous thyroid hormone.

The natural history of functioning thyroid nodules in the individual patient is variable. Most likely, if euthyroid, such patients will remain euthyroid, but there may be a gradual increase in autonomous thyroid hormone production with development of clinical evidence of hyperthyroidism. Functioning nodules producing clinical and chemical thyrotoxicosis require surgical removal. Complete lobectomy with removal of pericapsular lymph nodes and preservation of the recurrent laryngeal nerve is the most desirable procedure.

THYROID NEOPLASIA

A solitary thyroid mass with a consistency differing from that of the rest of the thyroid gland suggests neoplasia.[222,223] The prevalence of malignancy in adult thyroid nodules approximates 4 per cent.[223] In children with thyroid nodules the current prevalence has been estimated to be 15 to 20 per cent.[224] Nodular enlargement in the male is somewhat more likely to be cancerous than in the female, and the female-to-male ratio among children with thyroid cancer is 2:1. External radiation therapy to the head and neck during infancy and childhood has been shown to predispose to thyroid cancer. In a series of children reported in the 1950s with thyroid cancer, 80 per cent had a history of prior head and neck radiotherapy.[225,226] The average time between the irradiation and the recognition of the tumor was 10 years. However, the etiology of most childhood thyroid carcinoma now remains obscure since head and neck irradiation is no longer administered for benign disease in children.

Primary thyroid neoplasia in children includes follicular adenoma, follicular, papillary, or mixed carcinoma, medullary carcinoma, and rarely teratoma, lymphoma, anaplastic carcinoma, or metastatic tumor. Fifty per cent or more of solitary thyroid nodules during childhood prove to be cystic lesions or benign adenomas. Hyperfunctioning adenomas are rare the first two decades of life. Well-differentiated thyroid follicular carcinomas account for over 90 percent of the malignant lesions in this age group.[222] Well-differentiated carcinomas are further classified into papillary and follicular adenocarcinomas. If sufficient tissue sections are examined, most well-differentiated carcinomas will contain both cell patterns, and management and prognosis are similar for both tumor types.

Medullary thyroid carcinoma (MTC) arises from the parafollicular C cells of the thyroid gland, and these tumors comprise 4 to 10 per cent of thyroid carcinomas.[227] The histologic picture includes large deposits of amyloid situated among sheets of pleomorphic epithelial cells. Both sporadic and familial cases of MTC have been described. The familial cases seem to be transmitted as an autosomal-dominant trait, and many are associated with multiple endocrine neoplasia (MEN). Thus, MTC is part of a MEN syndrome (MEN II) that can be distinguished from MEN I (with parathyroid, pituitary, and pancreatic tumors). MEN IIa includes MTC, pheochromocytomas, and hyperparathyroidism; MEN IIb includes MTC, pheochromocytomas, and multiple mucosal neuromata. MEN IIb is also referred to as MEN III (see chapter 7). The common feature of all those tumors is a neuroectodermal origin. Patients with mucosal neuromas usually have a distinctive appearance, with protruding, thick, often bumpy lips, occasional prognathism, and a Marfanoid habitus.

Medullary thyroid carcinoma is associated with excessive secretion of calcitonin.[227] Other substances, including ACTH, melanocyte-stimulating hormone (MSH), histaminase, serotonin, prostaglandins, somatostatin, and β-endorphin, may be produced. Calcitonin levels are invariably elevated in patients with palpable tumors. Subclinical tumors can be detected in children before development of palpable mass by serum calcitonin measurement before and/or after simulation tests (administration of intravenous calcium or pentagastrin). Testing can be carried out at regular intervals (1 to 2 years) on all children of affected families. Such testing allows detection of MTC in prepubertal children and removal of the thyroid at a time when the tumor is only a few millimeters in size.

Diagnosis and Management

A scan of the neck following administration of radioiodine or technetium can be helpful in the diagnosis of thyroid nodules during childhood. If the nodule concentrates iodide, carcinoma is unlikely. If there is associated Hashimoto thyroiditis, carcinoma is unlikely; 10 to 15 per cent of such patients present with thyroid nodules that are lymphoid in type or represent areas of thyroid hyperplasia.[170] Scanning the neck with ultrasound can identify cystic lesions that are likely to be benign. However, small-needle biopsy of the nodule is now considered the procedure of choice in the management of a thyroid nodule. If the nodule is large enough and accessible, small-needle aspiration allows diagnosis of cystic nodules and allows differentiation of malignant and benign lesions.[223,228] The presence of colloid and benign follicular cells in the needle aspirate indicates a pseudonodule or adenoma. The absence of colloid and the presence of cellular malignancy criteria suggest papillary-follicular carcinoma or medullary carcinoma.

Surgery is recommended for a cold nodule in an otherwise normal thyroid gland if malignancy criteria are present. These include a history of radiation to the head or neck; rapid growth of a nodule that is very firm or hard; satellite lymph nodes; hoarseness or dysphagia; or evidence for distant metastases. When there are no malignancy criteria and the nodule is large enough, management is based on results of the needle biopsy. A negative biopsy allows thyroid suppression treatment with observation. Surgery is indicated if the biopsy is positive or suspicious. The initial approach to surgery is simple removal of the affected lobe. No further surgery is necessary if the mass proves to be a cystic lesion or benign adenoma. If frozen section reveals carcinoma, total lobectomy should be carried out on the side of origin, and as much of the contralateral lobe should be excised as is compatible with preservation of the parathyroid glands and recurrent laryngeal nerves.

Although accessible regional nodes should be removal, a mutilating neck dissection is not warranted.[223] Routine radioiodine treatment following surgery is of questionable benefit in a child with a small (less than 2 cm), well-differentiated thyroid carcinoma and no evidence of metastases. In patients with large tumors, multiple tumors, lymph node involvement, or distant metastases postoperative radioiodine should be given to ablate any residual functioning thyroid tissue and identifiable metastatic loci. Patients then are followed after surgery and radioiodine treatment by measurement of serum TG concentrations as a reliable tumor marker. Serum TG levels of less than 1 ng/ml on T_4 suppression treatment or less than 10 ng/ml off T_4 suppression indicate remission; higher values suggest the presence of metastases. Metastatic disease usually is treated with high-dose radioiodine. Following surgery or surgery and radioiodine all patients should be maintained on a suppressive dose of exogenous thyroid hormone to avoid stimulation of tumor growth by endogenous TSH.[223] The dose should be adjusted to maintain the serum TSH level below 0.2 μU/ml with a sensitive assay system while avoiding clinical evidence of hyperthyroidism.

The prognosis in children with metastatic well-differentiated thyroid follicular cell carcinoma is good.[229] Life expectancy in such patients is similar to that in a normal population of similar age. The course usually is an indolent one, with long periods in which there is little progression. Mortality in thyroid carcinoma during childhood and adolescence is primarily accounted for by the relatively uncommon instances of medullary carcinoma and undifferentiated carcinoma.[230] In these cases more radical surgery combined with radiation or cancer chemotherapy is fully justified.

DISORDERS OF THYROID HORMONE CARRIER PROTEINS

The major determinants of the levels of circulating thyroid hormones are the concentrations of thyroid hormone binding proteins. Thyroxine-binding globulin, TBPA, and albumin all participate as thyroid hormone carrier proteins. Abnormalities of the levels or patterns of serum albumin concentration have been described. The major categories are dysalbuminemia and analbuminemia. Since albumin usually binds only about 10 per cent of the circulating T_4 and 30 to 50 per cent of T_3 and the concentrations of TBG and TBPA are normal or increased in these disorders, the levels of thyroid hormone in these patients usually are

TABLE 3–10. PATTERNS OF CHANGE IN SERUM THYROID HORMONE LEVELS ASSOCIATED WITH DISORDERS OF THYROID BINDING PROTEINS*

	T_4	T_3	Free T_4	TSH
TBG deficiency	D	D†	N	N
Low TBG	D	D†	N	N
TBG excess	I	I†	N	N
Familial dysalbumin- emic hyperthyroxinemia	I	N	N	N

* D, decreased; N, normal; I, increased.
† Change less than for T_4.

in the normal range.[161,231] No confirmed primary disorder or TBPA-involving abnormalities of thyroid hormone levels has been described to date. Thus the plasma protein disorders associated with abnormal serum T_4 levels include only the variations in TBG and the recently described hyperthyroxinemic state "familial dysalbuminemic hyperthyroxinema" (Table 3–10).

Thyroxine-Binding Globulin Deficiency

Thyroxine-binding globulin deficiency was first described in 1959 in a euthyroid male. Since that time many reports of a familial TBG deficiency have appeared.[161,231–239] The prevalence of the disorder varies from 1:5000 to 1:12,000 newborns and is transmitted as an X-chromosome–linked trait; serum TBG levels measured either by immunoassay or T_4 binding capacity are very low in affected males and approximately half normal in carrier females. In about half the families the TBG level by radioimmunoassay (RIA) is very low; in the other half the defect is partial. Serum T_4 levels vary similarly. Male-to-male transmission has not been observed and there is invariable transmission of the trait from affected males to female offspring. Affected subjects are euthyroid with normal serum TSH responses to exogenous TRH. Treatment is not indicated.

It is now clear that there are a variety of structural defects of the TBG molecule accounting for the defective TBG-T_4 binding. Variants have been reported in Australian aborigenes, American blacks, and families without a particular ethnic origin.[232–236] The precise alterations remain unknown. The inherited defects seem not to be due to large fragment deletions, insertions, or rearrangements, so that RFLP studies have not

been helpful on a limited scale in detection or screening.[238] A single nucleotide substitution, an asparagine for isoleucine at position 96 of the TBG molecule, accounted for the marked reduction of T_4 binding capacity of TBG-Gary.[235] Table 3–11 summarizes the reported properties of several variant TBG molecules recently investigated. Most of these patients with partial TBG deficiency were selected for elevated levels of denatured TBG measured by RIA, and each manifested a defective molecule with reduced stability and decreased binding capacity.[236] Patients with severe TBG deficiency have been postulated to have a defect in hepatic TBG synthesis, but the molecular mechanism remains obscure.[238]

Thyroxine-Binding Globulin Excess

Subjects with increased levels of TBG have increased total serum T_4 concentrations with normal TSH levels.[161,232] Serum T_3 concentrations are increased modestly. In these subjects as in those with low TBG concentrations TBG production rates and serum levels are correlated, suggesting that the mechanism for the high TBG concentrations is increased production, presumably by the liver, but the mechanism(s) have not been defined. Thyroxine-binding globulin levels are increased four- to fivefold in affected individuals, and carrier females have serum concentrations intermediate between normal values and the high levels in affected males. Early reports suggested a dominant mode of inheritance, but subse-

TABLE 3–11. PROPERTIES OF SEVERAL VARIANT TBG MOLECULES*

Type	TBG Concentrations (RIA)		T_4 Concentration	TBG K_a for T_4
	Normal	Denatured		
TBG Normal†	100	100	100	100
TBG-S	88	100	84	100
TBG-A	74	100	58	54
TBG-Quebec	16	260	41	70
TBG-Montreal	14	390	38	<3
TBG-Gary	1	1000	24	<5

* From Takamatsu J, Refetoff S, Charbonneau M, Dussault JH: Two new inherited defects of the thyroxine-binding globulin (TBG) molecule presenting as partial TBG deficiency. J Clin Invest 79:833, 1987; values listed as percent of values in normal subjects.
† Normal values for TBG-normal RIA, 1.1 to 2.1 mg/dl; TBG-denatured RIA, <2 to 8 μg/dl; T_4, 5 to 12 μg/dl; K_a, 0.7 to 1.35 × 10^{-10} M.

quent studies are compatible with an X-linked mode of inheritance.

Familial Dysalbuminemic Hyperthyroxinemia

Several groups of investigators have reported euthyroid subjects with increased serum T_4 concentrations not corrected by the use of the free T_4 index correction and with normal free T_4, total serum T_3, and TSH levels.[232,239–241] There is increased binding of T_4 to albumin, and the albumin in these patients has an affinity for T_4 binding intermediate between TBG and TBPA. Triiodothyronine is less avidly bound, accounting for the preferential increase in serum T_4 concentration. Patients with the disorder are euthyroid with normal thyroid hormone production rates. The abnormal albumin seems to be transmitted as an autosomal dominant trait. There is male-to-male transmission and an affected-to-unaffected ratio of $1:1$ or greater in first-degree relatives.

Diagnosis in these patients is confirmed by protein electrophoresis of serum containing labeled T_4; the fraction of T_4 label associated with TBG, TBPA, or albumin is measured and the albumin-bound T_4 can be calculated and related to normal values. Measurements of TBG and TBPA concentrations also are useful. Therapy is not necessary in these patients but it is important to make the diagnosis to avoid misdiagnosis and treatment of hyperthyroidism.

REFERENCES

1. Ingbar SH: The thyroid gland. *In* Wilson JD, Foster DW (eds): Textbook of Endocrinology. Philadelphia, WB Saunders Company, 1986, pp 682–815.
2. Stanbury JB, Dumont JE: Familial goiter and related disorders. *In* Stanbury JB, et al. (eds): The Metabolic Basis of Inherited Disease. 5th ed. New York, McGraw-Hill, 1983, pp 231–269.
3. Wolff J: Congenital goiter with defective iodine transport. Endocr Rev 4:420, 1983.
4. Van Herle AJ, Vassart G, Dumont JE: Control of thyroglobulin synthesis and secretion. N Engl J Med 301:239, 1979.
5. Wu SY: Thyrotropin mediated induction of thyroidal iodothyronine monodeiodinases in the dog. Endocrinology 112:417, 1983.
6. De Nayer PH, Cornette C, Vandershueren M, Eggermont E, Devlieger H, Jaeken J, Beckers C: Serum thyroglobulin levels in preterm neonates. Clin Endocrinol 21:149, 1984.
7. Fisher DA: Thyroid hormone and thyroglobulin synthesis and secretion. *In* Delange F, Fisher DA, Malvaux P (eds): Pediatric Thyroidology. Basel, Karger, 1985, pp 44–56.
8. Morley JE: Neuroendocrine control of thyrotropin secretion. Endocr Rev 2:326, 1981.
9. Gershengorn MC: Thyrotropin releasing hormone stimulation by pituitary hormone secretion. Annu Rev Physiol 48:515, 1986.
10. Smyth PPA, McMullan NM, Grubek Loebenstein B, O'Donovan DK: Thyroid growth stimulating immunoglobulins in goitrous disease: Relationship to thyroid stimulating immunoglobulins. Acta Endocrinol 111:321, 1986.
11. Karsenty G, Alquier C, Jelsema C, Weintraub BD: Thyrotropin induces growth and iodothyronine production in a human thyroid cell line without affecting adenosine 3',5'-monophosphate production. Endocrinology 123:1977, 1988.
12. Kourides IA, Gurr JA, Wolf O: The regulation and organization of thyroid stimulating hormones genes. Rec Prog Horm Res 40:79, 1984.
13. Lippman SS, Amr S, Weintraub B: Discordant effects of thyrotropin (TSH)-releasing hormone in pre and post translational regulation of TSH biosynthesis in rat pituitary. Endocrinology 119:323, 1986.
14. Hinkle PM, Goh KBC: Regulation of thyrotropin releasing hormone receptors and responses by L-triiodothyronine in dispersed rat pituitary cell cultures. Endocrinology 110:1725, 1982.
15. Segerson TP, Kauer J, Wolfe HC, Mobtaker H, Wu P, Jackson IMD, Lechan RM: Thyroid hormone regulates TRH biosynthesis in the paraventricular nucleus of the rat hypothalamus. Science 238:78, 1987.
16. Kaplan MM: Metabolism of thyroid hormones. *In* Dussault JH, Walker P (eds): New York, Marcel Dekker, 1983, pp 11–35.
17. Di Stefano JJ, Fisher DA: Peripheral distribution and metabolism of the thyroid hormones: A primarily quantitative assessment. *In* Hershman JM, Bray GA (eds): The Thyroid, Physiology and Treatment of Diseases. Oxford, England, Pergamon Press, 1979, pp 47–82.
18. Chopra IJ, Solomon DH, Chopra U, Wu SY, Fisher DA, Nakamura Y: Pathways of metabolism of thyroid hormones. Rec Prog Horm Res 34:521, 1978.
19. Engler D, Burger AG: The deiodination of iodothyronines and of their derivatives in man. Endocr Rev 5:151, 1984.
20. Oppenheimer JH, Schwartz HL, Mariash CN, Kinlaw WB, Wong NCW, Freake HC: Advances in our understanding of thyroid hormone action at the cellular level. Endocr Rev 8:288, 1987.
21. Weinberger C, Thompson CC, Ong ES, Lebo R, Gruol GH, Evans RM: The c-erb A gene encodes a thyroid hormone receptor. Nature 324:641, 1986.
22. Sap J, Munoz A, Damm K, Goldberg Y, Ghysdael J, Leutz A, Beng H, Vennstrom B: The c-erb A protein is a high affinity receptor for thyroid hormone. Nature 324:635, 1986.
23. Thompson CC, Weinberg C, Lebo R, Evans RM: Identification of a novel thyroid hormone receptor expressed in the mammalian central nervous system. Science 237:1610, 1987.
24. Benbrook D, Pfahl M: A novel thyroid hormone

receptor encoded by a cDNA clone from a human testis library. Science 238:788, 1987.

25. Samuels HH, Forman BM, Horowitz D, Ye ZS: Regulation of gene expression by thyroid hormone. J Clin Invest 81:957, 1988.

26. Izumo S, Lompre AM, Matsuoka R, Koren G, Schwartz K, Nadal-Ginard B, Mahdavi V: Myosin heavy chain messenger RNA and protein isoform transitions between hemodynamic and thyroid hormone induced signals. J Clin Invest 79:970, 1987.

27. Chaudhury S, Ismail-Beigi F, Gick GG, Levenson R, Edelman IS: Effect of thyroid hormone on the abundance of Na-K-adenosine triphosphatase alpha subunit messenger ribonucleic acid. Mol Endocrinol 1:83, 1987.

28. Gubits RM, Shaw PA, Gresik EW, Onetti-Muda A, Barka T: Epidermal growth factor gene expression is regulated differently in mouse kidney and submandibular gland. Endocrinology 119:1382, 1986.

29. Mukku VR: Regulation of epidermal growth factor receptor levels by thyroid hormones. J Biol Chem 254:6453, 1984.

30. Bianco AC, Silva JE: Intracellular conversion of thyroxine to triiodothyronine is required for the optimal thermogenic function of brown adipose tissue. J Clin Invest 79:295, 1987.

31. Shupnik MA, Chin WW, Habener JF, Ridgway EC: Transcriptional regulation of the thyrotropin subunit genes by thyroid hormone. J Biol Chem 260:2900, 1985.

32. Barker SB, Klitgaard HM: Metabolism of tissues excised from thyroxine-injected rats. Am J Physiol 170:81, 1952.

33. Martino G, Covello C, DeGiovanni R, Filippelli R, Pitrelli G: Direct in-vitro action of thyroid hormones on mitochondrial RNA-polymerase. Mol Biol Rep 11:205, 1986.

34. Ismail-Beigi F, Edelman IS: Mechanism of thyroid calorigenesis. Role of active sodium transport. Proc Natl Acad Sci (USA) 67:1071, 1970.

35. Stiles G, Caron MG, Lefkowitz RJ: β-adrenergic receptors: Biochemical mechanisms of physiological regulation. Physiol Rev 64:661, 1984.

36. Fisher DA, Dussault JH, Sack J, Chopra IJ: Ontogenesis of hypothalamic pituitary-thyroid function and metabolism in man, sheep and rat. Rec Prog Horm Res 33:59, 1977.

37. Fisher DA, Klein AH: Thyroid development and disorders of thyroid function in the newborn. N Engl J Med 304:702, 1981.

38. Roti E, Gnudi A, Braverman LE: The placental transport, synthesis and metabolism of hormones and drugs which affect thyroid function. Endocr Rev 4:121, 1983.

39. Morreale de Escobar G, Obregon MJ, Ruiz de Ona C, Escobar del Rey F: Transfer of thyroxine from the mother to be rat fetus near term: Effects on brain 3,5,3'-triodothyronine deficiency. Endocrinology 122:1521, 1988.

40. Ferreiro B, Bernal J, Morreale de Escobar G, Porter BJ: Preferential saturation of brain 3,5,3'-triiodothyronine receptor during development in fetal lambs. Endocrinology 122:438, 1988.

41. Polk DH, Wu SY, Fisher DA: Serum thyroid hormone and tissue 5'-monodeiodinase activity in acutely thyroidectomized newborn lambs. Am J Physiol: Endocrinol Metab 14:E151, 1986.

42. Polk DH, Padbury JF, Callegari C, Newnham JP, Reviczky AL, Klein AH, Fisher DA: Effect of fetal thyroidectomy on newborn thermogenesis in lambs. Pediatr Res 21:453, 1987.

43. Fisher DA, Dussault JH: Development of the mammalian thyroid gland. In Greer MA, Solomon DH (eds): Handbook of Physiology, Part III, Endocrinology, Chapter 3, The Thyroid. Washington, DC, American Physiological Society, 1974, pp 143–166.

44. Penny R, Spencer CA, Frasier SD, Nicoloff JT: Thyroid stimulating hormone and thyroglobulin levels decrease with chronological age in children and adolescents. J Clin Endocrinol Metab 56:177, 1983.

45. Oddie TH, Meade JH Jr, Fisher DA: An analysis of published data on thyroxine turnover in human subjects. J Clin Endocrinol Metab 26:425, 1966.

46. Fisher DA, Sack J, Oddie TH, Pekary AE, Hershman JM, Lam RW, Parslow ME: Serum T$_4$, TBG, T$_4$ uptake, T$_3$, reverse T$_3$ and TSH concentrations in children 1 to 15 years of age. J Clin Endocrinol Metabl 45:191, 1977.

47. Braverman LW, Dawber NA, Ingbar SH: Observations concerning the binding of thyroid hormones in sera of normal subjects of varying ages. J Clin Invest 45:1273, 1966.

48. Letarte J, Guyda H, Dussault JH: Clinical, biochemical and radiological features of neonatal hypothyroid infants. In Burrow GN, Dussault JH (eds): Neonatal Thyroid Screening. New York, Raven Press, 1980, pp 225–236.

49. Price DA, Ehrlich RM, Walfish PG: Congenital hypothyroidism, clinical and laboratory characteristics of infants detected by neonatal screening. Arch Dis Child 56:845, 1981.

50. Letarte J, LaFranchi S: Clinical features of congenital hypothyroidism. In Walker P, Dussault JH (eds): Congenital Hypothyroidism. New York, Marcel Dekker, 1983, pp 351–383.

51. Klein AH, Meltzer S, Kenny FN: Improved prognosis of congenital hypothyroidism treated before age 3 months. J Pediatr 81:912, 1972.

52. Raiti S, Newns GA: Cretinism: Early diagnosis and its relation to mental prognosis. Arch Dis Child 46:692, 1971.

53. Glorieux J, Dussault JH, Morissette J, Dejardins M, Letarte J, Guyda H: Follow-up at ages 5 and 7 years on mental development in children with hypothyroidism detected by Quebec screening program. J Pediatr 107:913, 1985.

54. New England Congenital Hypothyroidism Collaborative: Neonatal hypothyroidism screening: Status of patients at 6 years of age. J Pediatr 107:915, 1985.

55. Gonzales LW, Ballard PL: Identification and characterization of nuclear 3,5,3'-Triiodothyronine binding sites in fetal human lung. J Clin Endocrinol Metab 53:21, 1981.

56. Bernal J, Pekonen F. Ontogenesis of nuclear 3,5,3'-triiodothyronine receptor in human fetal brain. Endocrinology 114:677, 1984.

57. Fisher DA: The unique endocrine milieu of the fetus. J Clin Invest 78:603, 1986.

58. Dobbing J: The later growth of the brain and its vulnerability. J Pediatr 53:2, 1974.

59. Pickering DE, Fisher DA: Growth and metabolism following L-thyroxine administration in thyroid ablated infant rhesus monkeys. Am J Dis Child 86:147, 1953.

60. Pickering DE, Fisher DA: Therapeutic concepts relating to hypothyroidism in childhood. J Chronic Dis 7:242, 1958.

61. Andersen JH: Nongoitrous hypothyroidism. *In* Gardner LI (ed): Endocrine and Genetic Diseases of Childhood and Adolescence. Philadelphia, WB Saunders Company, 1975, pp 238–260.

62. Van Wyk JJ, Grumbach MM: Syndrome of precocious menstruation and galactorrhea in juvenile hypothyroidism: An example of hormonal overlap in pituitary feedback. J Pediatr 57:416, 1960.

63. Costin G, Kershnar AK, Kogut MD, Turkington RW: Prolactin activity in juvenile hypothyroidism and precocious puberty. Pediatrics 50:881, 1972.

64. Lee PA, Blizzard RM: Serum gonadotropins in hypothyroid girls with and without sexual precocity. Johns Hopkins Med J 135:55, 1974.

65. Hemady ZS, Siler-Khodr TM, Najjar S: Precocious puberty in juvenile hypothyroidism. J Pediatr 92:55, 1978.

66. Reilly WA, Smyth FS: Cretinoid epiphyseal dysgenesis. J Pediatr 11:786, 1937.

67. Fisher DA, Hoath S, Lakshmanan J: The thyroid hormone effects on growth and development may be mediated by growth factors. Endocrinol Exp 16:259, 1982.

68. Simpson ME, Asling CW, Evans HM: Some endocrine influence in skeletal growth and differentiation. Yale J Biol Med 23:1, 1950.

69. Solomon J, Greep RD: The effect of alterations in thyroid function on the pituitary growth hormone content and acidophil cytology. Endocrinology 68:158, 1959.

70. Samuels HH, Stanley F, Shapiro LE: Dose dependent depletion of nuclear receptors for L-triiodothyronine: Evidence for a role in induction of growth hormone synthesis in cultured GH cells. Proc Natl Acad Sci (USA) 73:3877, 1976.

71. Baxter JD, Eberhardt NL, Apriletti JW, Johnson LK, Ivarie RD, Schachter BS, Morris JA, Seeburg PH, Goodman HM, Latham KR, Polansky JR, Martial JA: Thyroid hormone receptors and responses. Rec Prog Horm Res 35:97, 1979.

72. Van Wyk JJ, Underwood LE, Hintz RL, Clemmons DR, Voina SJ, Weaver RP: The somatomedins: A family of insulin-like hormones under growth hormone control. Rec Prog Horm Res 30:259, 1974.

73. Daughaday WH, Phillips LS, Muller MC: The effect of insulin and growth hormone on the release of somatomedin by the isolated rat liver. Endocrinology 98:1214, 1976.

74. Froesch ER, Zapf J, Audhya TK, Ben Porath E, Segen BJ, Gibson KD: Nonsuppressible insulin-like activity and thyroid hormones: Major pituitary dependent sulfation factors for chick embryo cartilage. Proc Natl Acad Sci (USA) 73:2904, 1976.

75. Holder AT, Wallis M: Actions of growth hormone, prolactin and thyroxine on serum somatomedin-like activity and growth in hypopituitary dwarf mice. J Endocrinol 74:223, 1977.

76. Hughes JP: Identification and characterization of high and low affinity binding sites for growth hormone in rabbit liver. Endocrinology 105:414, 1979.

77. Schalch DS, Udo EH, Drazin B, Johnson CF, Miller LL: role of the liver in regulating somatomedin activity: Hormonal effects on the synthesis and release of insulin-like growth factor and its carrier protein by the isolated perfused rat liver. Endocrinology 104:1143, 1979.

78. Glassock GF, Nicoll CS: Hormonal control of growth in the infant rat. Endocrinology 109:176, 1981.

79. Walker P, Weichel ME Jr, Hoath SB, Poland RE, Fisher DA: Effect of thyroxine, testosterone and corticosterone on nerve growth factor (NGF) and epidermal growth factor (EGF) concentrations in female mouse submaxillary gland. Dissociation of NGF and EGF responses. Endocrinology 109:582, 1981.

80. Hoath S, Lakshmanan J, Scott SM, Fisher DA: Effect of thyroid hormones on epidermal growth factor concentration in neonatal mouse skin. Endocrinology 112:308, 1983.

81. Lakshmanan J, Perheentupa J, Hoath SB, Kim H, Grueters A, Odell C, Fisher DA: Epidermal growth factor in mouse ocular tissue: Effect of thyroxine and exogenous EGF. Pediatric Res 19:315, 1985.

82. Perheentupa J, Lakshmanan J, Fisher DA: Epidermal growth factor in mouse urine: Maturative effect of thyroxine. Pediatric Res 18:1080, 1984.

83. Hoath SB, Lakshmanan J, Fisher DA: Epidermal growth factor binding to neonatal mouse skin explants and membrane preparations effect of triiodothyronine. Pediatric Res 19:277, 1985.

84. Walker P, Weichel ME Jr, Guo SM, Fisher DA, Fisher DA: Radioimmunoassay for mouse nerve growth factor (NGF), effect of thyroxine administration on tissue NGF levels. Brain Res 183:331, 1980.

85. Lakshmanan J, Beri U, Perheentupa J, Grueters A, Kim H, Macaso T, Fisher DA: Acquisition of submandibular gland nerve growth factor responsiveness to thyroxine in neonatal mice. J Neurosci Res 12:71, 1984.

86. Hadeed AJ, Asay LD, Klein AH, Fisher DA: Significance of transient hypothyroxinemia in premature infants with and without respiratory distress syndrome. Pediatr Res 68:494, 1981.

87. Klein AH, Oddie T, Parslow M, Foley TP Jr, Fisher DA: Development changes in pituitary thyroid function in the human fetus and newborn. Early Hum Dev 6:321, 1982.

88. Chowdry P, Scanlon JW, Auerbach R, Abbassi V: Results of controlled double blind study of thyroid replacement in very low birth weight premature infants with hypothyroxinemia. Pediatrics 73:301, 1984.

89. Delange F, Dalhem A, Bourdoux P, Lagasse R, Glinoer D, Fisher DA, Walfish PG, Ermans AM: Increased risk of primary hypothyroidism in preterm infants. J Pediatr 105:462, 1984.

90. Delange F, Bourdoux P, Ermans AM: Transient disorders of thyroid function and regulation in preterm infants. *In* Delange F, Fisher DA, Malvaux P (eds): Pediatric Thyroidology. Basel, Karger, 1985, p 369.

91. Allemand Dl', Grueters A, Beyer P, Weber B: Iodine in contrast agents and skin disinfectants is the major cause for hypothyroidism in premature infants during intensive care. Horm Res 28:42, 1987.

92. Price DJ, Sherwin JR: Autoregulation of iodide transport in the rabbit: Absence of autoregulation in fetal tissue and comparison of maternal

and fetal thyroid iodination products. Endocrinology 119:2547, 1986.

93. Miyai K, Harada T, Nose O, Mizuta H, Amino N, Yabuuchi H: Hyperthyrotropinemia with normal thyroid hormone concentrations in newborn babies. *In* Naruse H, Irie M (eds): Neonatal Screening (International Congress Series 606). Amsterdam, Excerpta Medica, 1983, p 44.

94. Franklin R, O'Grady C: Neonatal thyroid function: Effects of nonthyroidal illness. J Pediatr 107:599, 1985.

95. Fisher DA, Klein AH, Hadeed A: Normal and abnormal thyroid function in premature infants: The low T3 syndrome. *In* Hesch RD (ed): The Low T3 Syndromes. New York, Academic Press, 1986, pp 225–242.

96. Fisher DA: Thyroid development and thyroid disorders in infancy. *In* Van Middlesworth L (ed): The Thyroid Gland, Practical Clinical Treatise. Chicago, Year Book, 1986, pp 111–129.

97. Rochiccioli P: Thyroid dysgenesis. *In* Delange F, Fisher DA, Malvaux P (eds): Pediatric Thyroidology. Basel, Karger, 1985, pp 154–173.

98. Foley TP Jr: Sporadic congenital hypothyroidism. *In* Dussault JH, Walker P (eds): Congenital Hypothyroidism. New York, Marcel Dekker, 1983, pp 231–260.

99. Frasier SD, Penny R, Synder R: Primary congenital hypothyroidism in spanish surnamed infants in Southern California. J Pediatr 101:315, 1982.

100. Brown AL, Fernhoff PM, Milner J, McEwen C, Elsas LS: Racial differences in the incidence of congenital hypothyroidism. J Pediatr 99:934, 1981.

101. Fort P, Lifshitz F, Bellissario R, Davis J, Lanes R, Pugliese M, Richman R, Post EM, David R: Abnormalities of thyroid function in infants with Down's syndrome. J Pediatr 104:545, 1984.

102. Chanoine JP, Bourdoux P, Delange F: Congenital anomalies associated with hypothyroidism. Arch Dis Child 61:1147, 1986.

103. Miyai K, Connelly JF, Foley TP Jr, Irie M, Illig R, Lie SO, Morissette J, Nakajima H, Rochiccioli P, Walfish P: An analysis of the variation of incidence of congenital dysgenetic hypothyroidism in various countries. Endocrinol Jpn 31:77, 1984.

104. Dussault JH, Letarte J, Guyda H, Laberge C: Lack of influence of thyroid antibodies on thyroid function in the newborn infant and on a mass screening program for congenital hypothyroidism. J Pediatr 96:385, 1980.

105. Van Der Gaag RD, Drexhage HA, Dussault JH: Role of maternal immunoglobulins blocking TSH-induced thyroid growth in sporadic forms of congenital hypothyroidism. Lancet 1:246, 1985.

106. Drexhage HA, Bottazzo GF: The thyroid and autoimmunity. *In* Delange F, Fisher DA, Malvaux P (eds): Pediatric Thyroidology. Basel, Karger, 1985, pp 90–105.

107. Foley TP Jr: Congenital hypopituitarism. *In* Dussault JH, Walker P (eds): Congenital Hypothyroidism. New York, Marcel Dekker, 1983, pp 331–350.

108. Miyai K: Defect in hypothalamic-pituitary function. *In* Delange F, Fisher DA, Malvaux P (eds): Pediatric Thyroidology. Basel, Karger, 1985, pp 143–153.

109. La Franchi SH, Hanna CE, Krainz PL, Skeels MR, Miyahara RS, Sesser DE: Screening for congenital hypothyroidism with specimen collection at two time periods: Results of the Northwest Regional Screening Program. Pediatrics 76:734, 1985.

110. Rochiccioli P, Dutau G: Congenital goiter. *In* Dussault JH, Walker P (eds): Congenital Hypothyroidism. New York, Marcel Dekker, 1983, pp 261–274.

111. Foley TP Jr: Familial thyroid dyshormonogenesis. *In* Delange F, Fisher DA, Malvaux P (eds): Pediatric Thyroidology. Basel, Karger, 1985, pp 174–188.

112. Lever EG, Medeiros-Neto GA, DeGroot LJ: Inherited disorders of thyroid metabolism. Endocr Rev 4:213, 1983.

113. Matsuura N, Yamada Y, Nohara Y, Konishi J, Kasagi K, Endo K, Kojima H, Watoya K: Familial neonatal transient hypothyroidism due to maternal TSH binding inhibiting immunoglobulins. N Engl J Med 303:738, 1980.

114. Connors MH, Styne DH: Transient neonatal athyreosis resulting from thyrotropin inhibitory immunoglobulins. Pediatrics 78:287, 1986.

115. Pandian MR, Horlick M, Holm WL, Geffner ME, Fisher DA: TSH receptor blocking antibodies in transient congenital hypothyroidism. J Pediatr (in press).

116. Mitchell ML, Larsen PR: Screening for congenital hypothyroidism: The T4-TSH approach. *In* Dussault JH, Walker P (eds): Congenital Hypothyroidism. New York, Marcel Dekker, 1983, pp 169–178.

117. Illig R: 1983 Primary TSH screening. *In* Dussault JH, Walker P (eds): Congenital Hypothyroidism. New York, Marcel Dekker, 1983, pp 179–188.

118. Fisher DA: Background, strategies and problems of newborn screening for congenital hypothyroidism. *In* Carter TP, Willey AM (eds): Genetic Disease Screening and Management. New York, Alan R. Liss, 1986, pp 233–251.

119. Fisher DA: Effectiveness of newborn screening programs for congenital hypothyroidism: Prevalence of missed cases. Pediatr Clin North Am 34:879, 1987.

120. New England Regional Screening Program and the New England Congenital Hypothyroidism Collaborative: Pitfalls in screening for congenital hypothyroidism. Pediatrics 70:165, 1982.

121. Fisher DA: Hypothyroidism. *In* Nelson NM (ed): Current Therapy in Neonatal Perinatal Medicine. Philadelphia, BC Decker, 1985, pp 223–226.

122. Guyda HJ: Treatment of congenital hypothyroidism. *In* Dussault JH, Walker P (eds): Congenital Hypothyroidism. New York, Marcel Dekker, 1983, pp 385–396.

123. Sato T, Suzuke Y, Taetani T, Ishigura K, Nakajima H: Age related change in the pituitary threshold for TSH release during thyroxine replacement therapy for cretinism. J Clin Endocrinol Metab 44:553, 1977.

124. McCrossin RB, Sheffield LJ, Robertson EF: Persisting abnormality in the pituitary-thyroid axis in congenital hypothyroidism. *In* Nagataki S, Stockigt JHR (eds): Thyroid Research. Vol VIII. Canberra, Australian Academy of Sciences, 1980, pp 37–40.

125. Sack J, Shafrir Y, Urbach D, Amado O: Thyroid stimulating hormone, prolactin, and growth hormone response to thyrotropin releasing hormone in treated children with congenital hypothyroidism. Pediatr Res 19:1037, 1985.

126. Fisher DA, Foley B: Early treatment of congenital hypothyroidism. Pediatrics 83:785, 1988.

127. Vagenakis AG, Braverman LE: Drug induced hypothyroidism. *In* Hershman JM, Bray GA (eds): The Thyroid: Physiology and Treatment of Disease. Oxford, England, Pergamon Press, 1979, pp 389–399.

128. Delange FM, Ermans AM: 1979 Endemic goiter and cretinism. Naturally occurring goitrogens. *In* Hershman JM, Bray GA (eds): The Thyroid: Physiology and Treatment of Disease. Oxford, England, Pergamon Press, 1979, pp 415–452.

129. Gaitan ED, Cooksey RC, Logan JS, Gaitan GS, Montalvo JM, Pino AM: The Kentucky Appalachian goiter revisited. *In* Proceedings of the American Thyroid Association Meeting, Abstract 16, 1984, p T8.

130. Little G, Meador K, Cunningham R, Pittman JA: Cryptothyroidism. The major cause of sporadic athyreotic cretinism. J Clin Endocrinol Metab 25:1529, 1965.

131. Fisher DA, Beall GN: Hashimoto's thyroiditis. Pharmacol Ther 1:445, 1976.

132. Volpe R: Autoimmune thyroiditis. *In* Van Middlesworth L, Givins JR (eds): The Thyroid Gland. Chicago, Year Book, 1986, pp 281–295.

133. Rallison M, Dobyns BM, Keating FR, Rall JE, Tyler FH: Chronic thyroiditis: Occurrence and natural history of chronic lymphocytic thyroiditis in children. J Pediatr 86:675, 1975.

134. Inoue M, Taketani N, Sato, Nakajima H: High incidence of chronic lymphocytic thyroiditis in apparently healthy school children: Epidemiological and clinical study. Endocrinol Jpn 22:483, 1975.

135. Nilsson LR, Doniach D: Autoimmune thyroiditis in children and adolescents, I—clinical studies. Acta Paediatr 53:255, 1964.

136. Ling SM, Kaplan SA, Weitzman JJ, Reed GB, Costin G, Landing BH: Euthyroid goiters in children: Correlation of needle biopsy with other clinical and laboratory findings in chronic lymphocytic thyroiditis and simple goiter. Pediatrics 44:695, 1969.

137. Greenberg AH, Czernichow P, Hung W, Shelley W, Winship T, Blizzard RW: Juvenile chronic lymphocytic thyroiditis: Clinical, laboratory, and histological correlations. J Clin Endocrinol Metab 30:293, 1970.

138. Fisher DA, Pandian MR, Carlton E: Autoimmune thyroid disease: An expanding spectrum. Pediatr Clin North Am 34:907, 1987.

139. Gordin A, Lamberg BA: Spontaneous hypothyroidism in symptomless autoimmune thyroiditis. A long term follow-up study. Clin Endocrinol 15:537, 1981.

140. Hayashi Y, Tamai H, Fukata S, Hirota Y, Katayama S, Kuma K, Kumagai LF, Nagataki S: A long term clinical, immunological and histological follow-up study of patients with goitrous chronic lymphocytic thyroiditis. J Clin Endocrinol Metab 61:1172, 1985.

141. Gilani BB, MacGillivray MH, Voorhees ML, Mills BJ, Riley RJ, Maclaren NK: Thyroid hormone abnormalities in diagnosis of insulin-dependent diabetes mellitus in children. J Pediatr 105:218, 1984.

142. Gray RS, Borsey DQ, Seth J, Herd R, Brown NS, Clarke BF: Prevalence of subclinical thyroid failure in insulin-dependent diabetes. J Clin Endocrinol Metab 50:1034, 1980.

143. Bright GM, Blizzard RM, Kaiser DL, Clarke WL: Organ specific autoantibodies in children with common endocrine diseases. J Pediatr 100:8, 1982.

144. Hymes K, Blum M, Lackner H, Karpatkin S: Easy bruising, thrombocytopenia, and elevated platelet immunoglobulin G in Graves' disease and Hashimoto's thyroiditis. Ann Intern Med 94:27, 1981.

145. Jordan SG, Buckingham B, Sakai R, Olson D: Studies of immune complex glomerulonephritis mediated by human thyroglobulin. N Engl J Med 30:1212, 1981.

146. Portmann L, Hamada N, Heinrich G, Degroot LJ: Antithyroid peroxidase antibody in patients with autoimmune thyroid disease. Possible identity with antimicrosomal antibody. J Clin Endocrinol Metab 61:1001, 1985.

147. Weetman AP, McGregor AM: Autoimmune thyroid disease: Developments in our understanding. Endocr Rev 5:309, 1984.

148. Retetoff S: Syndromes of thyroid hormone resistance. Am J Physiol 243:E88, 1982.

149. Magner JA, Petrick P, Menezes-Ferreira M, Stelling M, Weintraub BD: Familial generalized resistance to thyroid hormones: Report of three kindreds and correlation of patterns of affected tissues with the binding of ^{125}I-triiodothyronine to fibroblast nuclei. J Endocrinol Invest 9:459, 1986.

150. Kaplowitz PB, D'Ercole J, Utiger RD: Peripheral resistance to thyroid hormone in an infant. J Clin Endocrinol Metab 53:958, 1981.

151. Gheri RC, Bianchi R, Mariani G, Toccafondi R, Cappelli G, Brat A, Borghi A, Gusti G, Forti G: A new case of familial partial generalized resistance to thyroid hormones: study of 3,5,3'-triiodothyronine (T_3) binding to lymphocyte and fibroblast nuclei and in vivo conversion of thyroxine to T_3. J Clin Endocrinol Metab 58:563, 1984.

152. DeNayer P, Lambot MP, Desmons MC, Rennotte B, Malvaux P, Beckers C: Sex hormone binding protein in hyperthyroxinemic patients: A discriminator for thyroid status in thyroid hormone resistance and familial dysalbuminemic hyperthyroxinemia. J Clin Endocrinol Metab 62:1309, 1986.

153. Usala SJ, Bale AE, Gesundheit N, Weinberger C, Menezes-Ferreira M, Lash RW, Weintraub BD: The role of human c-erb A-α and c-erb A-β receptor genes in generalized thyroid hormone resistance. Proceedings of The Endocrine Society, Abstract 33, 1988, p 29.

154. Lippe BM, Van Herle AJ, LaFranchi SH, Uller RP, Lavin N, Kaplan SA: Reversible hypothyroidism on growth hormone deficient children treated with human growth hormone. J Clin Endocrinol Metab 40:612, 1975.

155. Root AW, Shulman D, Root J, Diamond F: The interrelationships of hypo and hyperthyroid male rats. *In* Illig R, Visser HKA (eds): Pediatric Endocrinology. Acta Endocrinol [Suppl] (Copenh) 279:367–375, 1986.

156. Delange F, Ermans AM: Endemic goiter and cretinism. Naturally occurring goitrogens. *In* Hershman JM, Bray GA (eds): The Thyroid: Physiology and Treatment of Disease. Oxford, England, Pergamon Press, 1979, pp 415–451.

157. Delange F: Physiopathology of iodine nutrition. *In* Chandra RK (ed): Trace Elements in Nutrition of Children. New York, Raven Press, 1985, pp 291–299.

158. Delange F: Adaptation to iodine deficiency during growth. Etiopathogenesis of endemic goiter and cretinism. *In* Delange F, Fisher DA, Malvaux P (eds): Pediatric Thyroidology. Basel, Karger, 1985, pp 295–326.

159. Koutras DA: Europe and the middle east. *In* Stanbury JB, Hetzel BS (eds): Endemic Goiter and Endemic Cretinism. New York, John Wiley & Sons, 1980, pp 79–100.

160. Pai GS, Leach DC, Weiss L, Wolf C, Van Dyke DL: Thyroid abnormalities in 20 children with Turner syndrome. J Pediatr 91:267, 1977.

161. Fisher DA: Thyroid disorders. *In* Emery AEH, Rimoin PL (eds): The Principles and Practice of Medical Genetics. Edinburgh, Churchill Livingstone, 1983, pp 1152–1163.

162. Lucky AW, Howley PM, Megylesi K, Spielberg SB, Schulman JH: Endocrine studies in cystinosis: Compensated primary hypothyroidism. J Pediatr 91:204, 1977.

163. Raiti S, Trias E, Maclaren NK: Primary hypothyroidism: Differentiation from primary hypopituitarism. Am J Dis Child 129:1397, 1975.

164. Newman AJ, Lee C: Hypothyroidism simulating dermatomyositis. J Pediatr 97:772, 1980.

165. Najjar SS: Muscular hypertrophy in hypothyroid children: The Kocher-Debra-Semelaigne syndrome. J Pediatr 85:236, 1974.

166. Van Wyk JJ, Grumbach MM: Syndrome of precocious menstruation and galactorrhea in juvenile hypothyroidism: an example of hormonal overlap in pituitary feedback. J Pediatr 57:416, 1960.

167. Hemady ZS, Siler-Khodr TM, Najjar S: Precocious puberty in juvenile hypothyroidism. Pediatrics 92:55, 1978.

168. Costin G, Kershnar AK, Kogut MD, Turkington RW: Prolactin activity in juvenile hypothyroidism and precocious puberty. Pediatrics 50:881, 1972.

169. Lee PA, Blizzard RM: Serum gonadotropins in hypothyroid girls with and without sexual precocity. Johns Hopkins Med J 135:55, 1974.

170. Fisher DA, Oddie TH, Johnson DE, Nelson TC: The diagnosis of Hashimoto's thyroiditis. J Clin Endocrinol Metab 40:795, 1975.

171. Abbassi V, Aldige C: Evaluation of sodium *l*-thyroxine requirement in replacement therapy of hypothyroidism. J Pediatr 90:298, 1977.

172. Rezvani I, Di George AM: Reassessment of the daily dose of oral thyroxine for replacement therapy of hypothyroid children. J Pediatr 90:291, 1977.

173. Rivkees SA, Bode HH, Crawford J: Long term growth in juvenile acquired hypothryoidism: the failure to achieve normal adult stature. N Engl J Med 318:599, 1988.

174. Engler D, Burger AG: The deiodination of the iodothyronines and of their derivatives in man. Endocr Rev 5:151, 1984.

175. Brent GA, Hershman JM: Effects of nonthyroidal illness of thyroid function tests. *In* Van Middlesworth L, Givens JR (eds): The Thyroid Gland, A Practical Clinical Treatise. Chicago, Year Book, 1986, pp 83–109.

176. Chopra IJ, Hershman JM, Pardridge WM, Nicoloff JT: Thyroid function in nonthyroidal illness. Ann Intern Med 98:946, 1983.

177. Chopra IJ, Solomon DH, Chua Teco GN, Eisenberg JB: An inhibitor of the binding of thyroid hormones to serum proteins is present in extrathyroidal tissues. Science 215:407, 1982.

178. Brent GA, Hershman JM: Thyroxine therapy in patients with severe nonthyroidal illness and low serum thyroxine concentration. J Clin Endocrinol Metab 63:1, 1986.

179. Ling SM, Kaplan SA, Weitzman JJ, Reed GB, Costin G, Landing BH: Euthyroid goiters in children: Correlation of needle biopsy with other clinical and laboratory findings in chronic lymphocytic thyroiditis and simple goiter. Pediatrics 44:695, 1969.

180. Nilsson LR, Persson PS: Cytological aspiration biopsy in adolescent goitre. Acta Paediatr 53:333, 1964.

181. Studer H, Rameli F: Simple goiter and its variants: Euthyroid and hyperthyroid multinodular goiters. Endocr Rev 3:40, 1982.

182. Drexhage HA, Bottazzo GH, Doniach D, Bitensky L, Chayen J: Evidence for thyroid growth stimulating immunoglobulins in some goitrous thyroid diseases. Lancet 2:287, 1980.

183. Volpe R: Subacute thyroiditis. *In* Delange F, Fisher DA, Malvaux P (eds): Pediatric Thyroidology. Basel, Karger, 1985, pp 252–264.

184. Cassidy CE: Subacute painful thyroiditis. *In* Van Middlesworth L, Givens JR (eds): The Thyroid Gland, A Practical Clinical Treatise. Chicago, Year Book, 1986, pp 363–370.

185. Abe K, Taguchi T, Okuno A, Matsuura N, Sasaki H: Acute suppurative thyroiditis in children. J Pediatr 94:912, 1979.

186. Taguchi T, Okuno A, Fujita K, Sanae N, Azuma H, Yashioka H: Etiologic factors in acute suppurative thyroiditis. J Infect Dis 146:447, 1982.

187. Saxena KM, Crawford JD, Talbot NB: Childhood thyrotoxicosis, a long term perspective. Br Med J 2:1153, 1964.

188. Howard CP, Hayles AB: Hyperthyroidism in childhood. Clin Endocrinol Metab 7:127, 1978.

189. Clayton GW: Thyrotoxicosis in children. *In* Kaplan SA (ed): Clinical Pediatric and Adolescent Endocrinology. Philadelphia, WB Saunders Company, 1982, pp 110–117.

190. Barnes V, Blizzard RM: Antithyroid drug therapy for toxic diffuse goiter (Graves' disease): Thirty years experience in children and adolescent. J Pediatr 91:313, 1977.

191. Maenpaa J, Kuusi A: Children hyperthyroidism. Acta Paediatr Scand 69:137, 1980.

192. Collen RJ, Landau EM, Kaplan SA, Lippe RM: Remission rates of children and adolescents with thyrotoxicosis treated with antithyroid drugs. Pediatrics 65:550, 1980.

193. Zimmerman D, Hayles AB: Hyperthyroidism in children. *In* Delange F, Fisher DA, Malvaux P (eds): Pediatric Thyroidology. Basel, Karger, 1985, pp 223–239.

194. Marchant B, Lees JFH, Alexander WD: Antithyroid drugs. *In* Hershman JD, Bray GA (eds): The Thyroid: Physiology and Treatment of Disease.

Oxford, England, Pergamon Press, 1979, pp 209–252.

195. Engler H, Taurog A, Nakashima T: Mechanism of inactivation of thyroid peroxidase by thioureylene drugs. Biochem Pharmacol 31:3801, 1982.

196. Wu SY, Chopra IJ, Solomon DH, Johnson DE: The effect of repeated administration of ipodate (Orografin) in hyperthyroidism. J Clin Endocrinol Metab 47:1358, 1978.

197. Shen DC, Wu SY, Chopra IJ, Huang HW, Shian LR, Bian TY, Jeng CY, Solomon DH: Long term treatment of Graves' hyperthyroidism with sodium ipodate. J Clin Endocrinol Metab 61:723, 1985.

198. Wang YS, Tsou CT, Lin WH, Hershman JM: Long term treatment of Graves' disease with iopanoic acid (Telepaque). J Clin Endocrinol Metab 65:679, 1987.

199. Karpman BA, Rappoport B, Filetti S, Fisher DA: Treatment of neonatal hyperthyroidism due to Graves' disease with sodium ipodate. J Clin Endocrinol Metab 64:119, 1987.

200. Laurberg P: Multisite inhibitor by ipodate of iodothyronine secretion from perfused dog thyroid lobes. Endocrinology 117:1639, 1985.

201. Haynes RC Jr, Murad F: Thyroid and antithyroid drugs. *In* Goodman LS, Gilman AG, Rall TW, Murad F (eds): The Pharmacological Basis of Therapeutics. 7th ed. New York, Macmillan, 1985, pp 1389–1411.

202. Hayles AB, Zimmerman D: Graves' disease in childhood. *In* Ingbar SH, Braverman LE (eds): The Thyroid. Philadelphia, JB Lippincott, 1986, pp 1412–1426.

203. Hamburger JI: Management of hyperthyroidism in children and adolescents. J Clin Endocrinol Metab 60:1019, 1985.

204. Brill AB, Becker DV: The safety of ^{131}I treatment of hyperthyroidism. *In* Van Middlesworth L, Givins JR (eds): The Thyroid, A Practical Clinical Treatise. Chicago, Year Book, 1986, pp 347–362.

205. Harve P, Francis HH: Pregnancy and thyrotoxicosis. Br Med J 2:817, 1962.

206. Burrow GN: The Thyroid Gland in Pregnancy. Philadelphia, WB Saunders Company, 1974, pp 83–100.

207. McKenzie JM: Neonatal Graves' disease. J Clin Endocrinol Metab 24:660, 1964.

208. Smallridge RC, Wartofsky L, Chopra IJ, Marinelli PV, Broughton RE, Dimond RC, Burman KD: Neonatal thyrotoxicosis: Alterations in serum concentrations of LATS protector, T_4, T_3, reverse T_3 and $3,3'T_2$. J Pediatr 93:118, 1978.

209. Zakarija M, McKenzie JM, Munro DS: Immunoglobulin G inhibitor of thyroid-stimulating antibody is a cause of delay in the onset of neonatal Graves' disease. J Clin Invest 72:1352, 1983.

210. McKenzie JM, Zakarija M: Pathogenesis of neonatal Graves' disease. J Endocrinol Invest 2:183, 1978.

211. Sunshine P, Kusumoto H, Kriss JP: Survival time of circulating long-acting thyroid stimulator in neonatal thyrotoxicosis: Implications for diagnosis and therapy of the disorder. Pediatrics 36:869, 1965.

212. Maisey MN, Stimmler L: The role of long acting thyroid stimulator in neonatal thyrotoxicosis. Clin Endocrinol (Oxf) 1:81, 1972.

213. Zakarija M, McKenzie JM, Hoffman WH: Prediction and therapy of intrauterine and late onset neonatal hyperthyroidism. J Clin Endocrinol Metab 62:368, 1986.

214. Tolis G, Bird C, Bertrand G, McKenzie JM, Ezrin C: Pituitary hyperthyroidism: Case report and review of the literature. Am J Med 64:177, 1978.

215. Weintraub BD, Gershengorn MC, Kourides IA, Fein H: Inappropriate secretion of thyroid stimulating hormone. Ann Intern Med 95:339, 1981.

216. Gershengorn MC, Weintraub BD: Thyrotropin induced hyperthyroidism caused by selective pituitary resistance to thyroid hormone: A new syndrome of inappropriate secretion of TSH. J Clin Invest 56:633, 1975.

217. Rosler A, Litvin Y, Hoge C, Gross J, Cerasi E: Familial hyperthyroidism due to inappropriate thyrotropin secretion successfully treated with triiodothyronine. J Clin Endocrinol Metab 54:76, 1982.

218. Isales CM, Tamborlane W, Gertner JM, Genel M, Insogna KL: Effect of short-term somatostatin and long term triiodothyronine administration to a child with nontumorous inappropriate thyrotropin secretion. J Pediatr 112:51, 1988.

219. Beck Peccoz P, Piscitelli G, Cattaneo MG: Successful treatment of hyperthyroidism due to nonneoplastic pituitary TSH secretion with $3,5,3'$-triiodothyroacetic acid (TRIAC). J Endocrinol Invest 6:217, 1983.

220. Abe K, Konno M, Sato T, Matsuura N: Hyperfunctioning thyroid nodules in children. Am J Dis Child 134:961, 1983.

221. Osburne RC, Goren EN, Bybee DE, Johnsonbaugh RE: Autonomous thyroid nodules in adolescents: clinical characteristics and results of TRH testing. J Pediatr 100:383, 1982.

222. Fisher DA: Thyroid nodules in childhood and their management. J Pediatr 84:866, 1976.

223. Robbins J: Thyroid cancer. *In* Van Middlesworth L, Givens JR (eds): The Thyroid Gland, A Practical Clinical Treatise. Chicago, Year Book, 1986, p 405.

224. Scott MD, Crawford JD: Solitary thyroid nodules in childhood: Is the incidence of thyroid carcinoma declining? Pediatrics 58:521, 1976.

225. Winship T, Rasvoll RV: Thyroid carcinoma in children: Final report and 20 year study. Clin Proc Child Hosp Wash, DC 26:327, 1970.

226. Refetoff S, Harrison J, Karanfilski BT, Kaplan EL, DeGroot LJ, Bekerman C: Continuing occurrence of thyroid carcinoma after irradiation to the neck in infancy and childhood. N Engl J Med 292:171, 1975.

227. Melvin KEW: Familial medullary carcinoma of the thyroid. *In* Van Middlesworth L, Givens JR (eds): The Thyroid Gland, A Practical Clinical Treatise. Chicago, Year Book, 1986, pp 429–447.

228. Miller JM, Kini SR, Hamburger JL: Needle Biopsy of the Thyroid. Traeger, New York, 1983.

229. Ruegemer JJ, Hay ID, Bergstralh EJ, Ryan JJ, Offord KP, Gorman CA: Distant metastases in differentiated thyroid carcinoma: A multivariate analysis of prognostic variables. J Clin Endocrinol Metab 67:501, 1988.

230. Samaan NA, Schultz PN, Hickey RC: Medullary thyroid carcinoma: Prognosis of familial versus sporadic disease and role of radiotherapy. J Clin Endocrinol Metab 67:801, 1988.

231. Hollander CS, Bernstein G, Oppenheimer JH: Abnormalities of thyroxine binding in analbu-

minemia. J Clin Endocrinol Metab 28:1064, 1968.

232. Glinoer D, DeNayer P: Anomalies in thyroid hormone transport proteins. *In* Delange F, Fisher DA, Malvaux P (eds): Pediatric Thyroidology. Basel, Karger, 1985, pp 394–406.

233. Dick M, Watson F: A possible variant of thyroxine-binding globulin in Australian Aborigines. Clin Chem Acta 116:361, 1981.

234. Daiger SP, Rummel DP, Wang L, Cavalli-Sforza LL: Detection of genetic variation of thyroxine-binding globulin (TBG). Am J Hum Genet 33:640, 1981.

235. Takamatsu J, Ando M, Weinberg M, Refetoff S: Isoelectric focusing variant thyroxine-binding globulin in american blacks: Increased heat lability and reduced serum concentration. J Clin Endocrinol Metab 63:80, 1986.

236. Murata Y, Takamatsu J, Refetoff S: Inherited abnormality of thyroxine-binding globulin with no demonstrable thyroxine-binding activity and high serum levels of denatured thyroxine-binding globulin. N Engl J Med 314:694, 1986.

237. Takamatsu J, Refetoff S, Charbonneau M, Dussault JH: Two new inherited defects of the thyroxine-binding globulin (TBG) molecule presenting as partial TBG defiency. J Clin Invest 79:833, 1987.

238. Mori Y, Refetoff S, Flink IL, Charbonneau M, Murata Y, Seo S, Morkin E, Dussault JH: Detection of the thyroxine-binding globulin (TBG) gene in six unrelated families with complete TBG deficiency. J Clin Endocrinol Metab 67:727, 1988.

239. Lee WNP, Golden MP, Van Herle AJ, Lippe BM, Kaplan SA: Inheritied abnormal thyroid hormone binding protein causing selective increase in total serum thyroxine. J Clin Endocrinol Metab 49:292, 1979.

240. Stockigt JR, Topliss DJ, Barlow JW, White EL, Hurley DM, Taft P: Familial euthyroid thyroxine excess: An appropriate response to abnormal thyroxine binding associated with albumin. J Clin Endocrinol Metab 53:353, 1981.

241. Ruiz M, Rajatanavin R, Young RA, Taylor C, Brown R, Braverman LE, Ingbar SH: Familial dysalbuminemic hyperthyroxinemia. N Engl J Med 306:635, 1982.

4

DIABETES MELLITUS

Mark A. Sperling

Diabetes mellitus is a syndrome of disturbed energy metabolism caused by deficiency of insulin secretion, or insulin action at the cellular level, that results in altered fuel homeostasis affecting carbohydrate, protein, and fat. It is the most common endocrine/metabolic disorder of childhood, with important consequences for physical and emotional development. An appreciation of the acute clinical features of this disease requires some understanding of the mechanism responsible for insulin synthesis, secretion, and action.

INSULIN BIOSYNTHESIS

Insulin is synthesized on the ribosomes of pancreatic islet beta cells and released into the circulation as a molecule comprised of two separate straight polypeptide chains linked by disulfide bridges between and within these chains.[1-3] As is apparent from Figure 4–1, the two chains are not separately synthesized but derived from a larger precursor, proinsulin, a single coiled chain in which the NH_2-terminus of the A chain is linked to the COOH-terminus of the B chain by a connecting or C peptide. An even larger precursor, pre-proinsulin, containing an additional peptide chain on the NH_2-terminus of the A chain is first synthesized, but this additional piece, important for initiating synthesis, is rapidly excised. Further processing of proinsulin within the beta cell cleaves the C peptide, consisting of 31 amino acids, from the insulin molecule at the sites indicated in the figure. Defects in these cleavage sites are inherited in an autosomal-dominant manner and result in insulin molecules with less than normal biologic activity that can give rise to two types of familial hyperproinsulinemia.[1,4-7] One defect yields B-C proinsulin, cleaved at site

1 but not site 2 in Figure 4–1; this intermediate has 50 per cent of the biologic activity of insulin, enough to prevent any abnormality in carbohydrate metabolism. The defect at site 1 yields A-C proinsulin, cleaved at site 2 but not site 1, which has inadequate biologic activity to prevent carbohydrate intolerance. A structural mutation in the proinsulin molecule, between the C peptide and insulin, has been confirmed.[5] In addition, a defect in the enzymatic conversion of a normal proinsulin molecule to insulin, yielding hyperproinsulinemia and mild carbohydrate intolerance, also occurs.[6] Native proinsulin has less than 5 per cent, whereas C peptide has none, of the biologic activity of insulin.[3] During synthesis, C peptide's role appears to be the provision of the spatial arrangement necessary for the formation of the disulfide bonds.[1-3] Other defects in insulin biosynthesis involving substitution of amino acids in the B chain that lead to impaired glucose tolerance in the presence of hyperinsulinemia have been described.[4-7] The insulin gene has been cloned and localized to chromosome 11, but genetic defects in insulin synthesis are not commonly associated with diabetes.[8,9]

Under normal circumstances, only small quantities of proinsulin are released into the circulation, amounting to less than 15 per cent of total insulin as measured by radioimmunoassay (RIA). Even smaller quantities of proinsulin intermediates are also released. However, during insulin secretion induced by all stimuli, one molecule of C peptide is released with each molecule of insulin.[1,3] Thus, the plasma of normal individuals contains small amounts of proinsulin, proinsulin intermediates, and almost equimolar amounts of insulin and C peptide. The plasma metabolic half-life of C peptide is, however, longer than that of in-

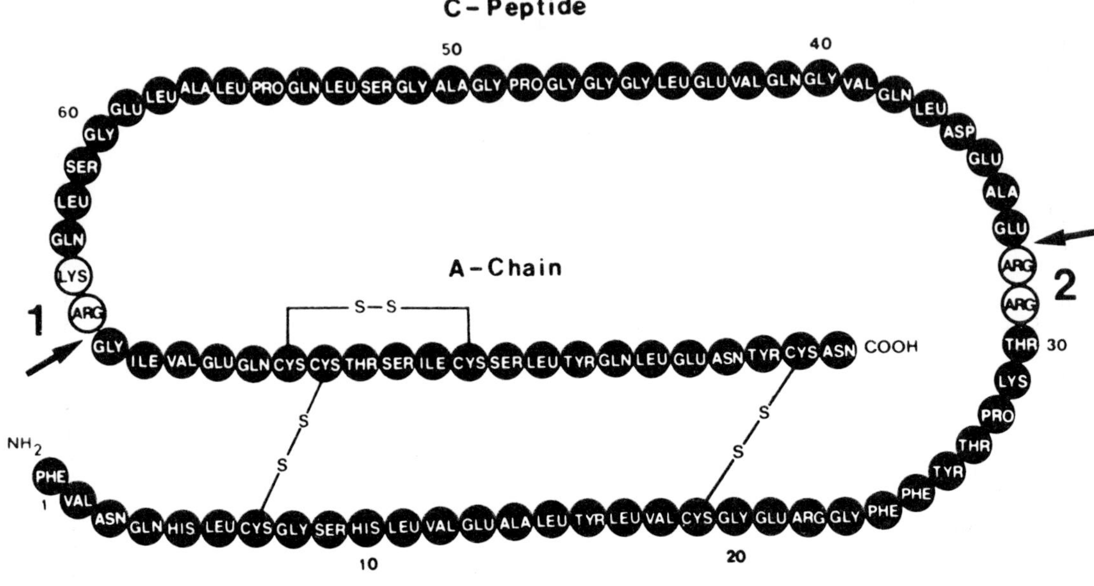

FIGURE 4–1.   Arrows 1 and 2 indicate the two sites of normal cleavage that yield insulin and C peptide when the amino acid residues indicated in the open circles are removed. These cleavage points are known mutation sites, inherited in an autosomal-dominant manner, and can yield two types of familial hyperproinsulinemia (see text for details). During insulin secretion, eqimolar amounts of insulin and C peptide are released.

sulin so that the molar ratio of C peptide to insulin in peripheral plasma is always greater than 1 and the peak of C peptide secretion or the nadir following suppression of release appear to occur later than those of insulin.[1,3] Although standard RIA of insulin will also measure proinsulin, C peptide will not be measured because it is immunologically distinct. Separation of proinsulin from insulin can be achieved by chromatography to separate the larger proinsulin prior to assay, by the use of an enzyme that degrades insulin but not proinsulin, or by the use of a C peptide assay that will also measure proinsulin but not insulin. Because C peptide is immunologically distinct, RIAs for this substance can be used to assess beta cell secretory reserve even in the presence of insulin antibodies formed in response to injections of bovine-porcine insulin. Endogenous insulin secretion is accompanied by C peptide release, whereas exogenous insulin administration suppresses endogenous insulin (and hence C peptide) secretion in all circumstances except insulinoma; results of standard RIA using double antibody precipitation are high in both circumstances.[1,3] Measurements of C peptide kinetics or of urinary excretion of C peptide can be used as an index of endogenous insulin secretion.[10,11]

INSULIN SECRETION

Insulin secretion is governed by the interaction of nutrients, hormones, and the autonomic nervous system.[12] Glucose, as well as certain other sugars that are metabolized by islets, stimulate insulin release. Basal and peak insulin levels are closely related to the glucose concentration, and prolonged fasting will further reduce both glucose and insulin levels, which, however, remain in the measurable range at approximately 5 μU/ml. There is evidence that the beta cell membrane contains a specific receptor for glucose that triggers insulin release independently of glucose utilization. However, there is also evidence that a product or products of glucose metabolism may be involved in maintaining insulin secretion and that sugars not metabolized by islets do not promote insulin release. During glucose infusion, insulin secretion is biphasic, with an initial spike followed by a sustained plateau. It is proposed that the initial spike represents preformed insulin whereas the sustained plateau represents newly synthesized insulin. cAMP is involved in stimulating insulin release, hence agents that inhibit phosphodiesterase and reduce cAMP destruction, such as theophylline, augment insulin release. Translocation of calcium ions into the cytoplasm from the exterior as well as from the intracellular organelles plays a key role in the contractile forces that propel insulin to the cell surface. There, the membrane of the insulin vesicle fuses with the cell membrane, allowing extrusion of insulin granules into the surrounding vascular space, a process known as emiocytosis.[2,12] Other ions, including potassium and magnesium, are involved in insulin secretion. Amino acids also stimulate insulin release, although the potency of individual amino acids varies. A group of amino acids is more potent than any single one and the insulin secretory response is potentiated in the presence of glucose. Free fatty acids and ketone bodies may also stimulate insulin release.

Insulin responses to oral glucose administration are always greater than responses to intravenous glucose administration that results in the same blood glucose profile. This has led to the concept that gut factors modulate insulin secretion and, indeed, a variety of gut hormones participate in promoting insulin release. Of these, gastrointestinal polypeptide hormone (GIP) plays a major role. Somatotropin release–inhibiting factor (SRIF; somatostatin), produced in the delta cells of islets, inhibits insulin and glucagon release and also reduces splanchnic blood flow.[13–15] Pancreatic glucagon and "gut" glucagon also stimulate insulin release. These factors may finely regulate nutrient intake and its disposition and together form an enteroinsular axis for metabolic homeostasis.[14] In addition to these gut hormones, several other hormones modulate insulin secretion. Growth hormone is involved in insulin synthesis and storage; persons with congenital growth hormone deficiency have subnormal basal and stimulated insulin responses, whereas in acromegaly basal and stimulated insulin levels are increased. Human chorionic somatomammotropin (hCS; also known as human placental lactogen, hPL), structurally related to growth hormone, likewise affects insulin release. However, the stimulatory effect of both hormones on insulin secretion are antagonized by their anti-insulin effect at the peripheral level. Similarly, glucocorticoids and estrogens evoke greater insulin secretion while inducing peripheral insulin resistance, in part by decreasing insulin receptors on target cells.[16]

Insulin secretion is constantly modulated by the autonomic nervous system.[15] The parasympathetic arm, via the vagus, directly stimulates insulin release. Modulation of insulin secretion by the sympathetic arm depends on whether α- or β-adrenergic receptors are activated. Activation of β_2 receptors by agents such as isoproterenol stimulates insulin secretion by a process that involves cAMP generation; blockade of β-adrenergic receptors by propranolol blunts basal and stimulated insulin release. Conversely, activation of α-adrenergic receptors blunts insulin secretion and blockade of these receptors by agents like phentolamine augments basal and glucose-stimulated insulin release. Both epinephrine and norepinephrine stimulate predominantly α-adrenergic receptors in islets, resulting in impaired insulin secretion as observed during stress or in patients with pheochromocytoma.

In summary, in normal man, insulin secretion is constantly modulated by the quantity, quality, and frequency of nutrient intake, by the hormonal milieu, and by autonomic impulses.[12,15] The ingestion of nutrients, principally carbohydrate and protein, produces intestinal hormonal signals that prime and initiate insulin release. The interaction of glucose with a specific beta cell receptor may separately induce release of preformed insulin. This sequence involves cAMP, β-adrenergic receptors, and ions, principally calcium. Subsequent glucose metabolism within the beta cell provides energy for further synthesis and release of insulin.

INSULIN ACTION

Insulin action on target cells in tissues such as liver, adipocytes, and muscle begins by binding to specific insulin receptors located on the cell membrane; binding to these receptors is saturable, occurs with a high energy of association (affinity), and is pH and temperature dependent.[16–19] The insulin receptor is a heterodimeric glycoprotein, consisting of two alpha and two beta subunits linked by disulfide bonds. The alpha subunit, with a molecular weight of approximately 125,000, acts as the binding site, while the beta subunit, with a molecular weight of approximately 90,000, possesses tyrosine kinase activity for both endogenous and exogenous substrates.[19] This ability to phosphorylate proteins may underlie some of insulin's manifold actions. Insulin action may also be mediated, in part, by hydrolysis of glycanphosphoinositides in the cell plasma membrane.[19] The insulin receptor gene has been cloned and localized to chromosome 19 while the structurally related insulin-like growth factor I (IGF-I) receptor has been localized to chromosome 15.

Under normal conditions, only a fraction of the total available cell receptors need to be occupied in order to achieve maximal biologic response, so that ordinarily there are spare receptors. Insulin receptors display two phenomena: down-regulation, wherein high ambient insulin concentrations reduce the number of available receptors, and negative cooperativity, wherein the occupancy of a receptor reduces the affinity of adjoining receptor sites. Scatchard analysis of insulin binding data in in vitro systems reveals curvilinear plots that are compatible with negative cooperativity or with two classes of receptors: high affinity–low capacity and low affinity–high capacity. Total receptor number and the affinities of both classes of receptor sites can be calculated from these Scatchard plots.[16–19] Following binding to the cell surface, the receptor-insulin complex is internalized within the cell, processed by lysozomal enzymes with release of free insulin and potential recycling of the receptor back to the cell membrane. Binding of insulin to the cell surface receptor, perhaps with the participation of internalization that permits insulin action at the level of the nucleus, leads to the complex biochemical processes characteristic of insulin action in a given tissue; the ultimate mechanism(s) by which insulin exerts its effects beyond receptor binding and phosphorylation remain unknown.[19] However, assuming postreceptor events to be normal, the biologic response to insulin in a tissue is a function of the number of receptor-insulin complexes formed, which in turn is directly related to the circulating insulin concentration and to the receptor concentration.[16] Thus, a reduction in receptor number could be compensated by an increase in insulin concentration so long as the critical number of receptors necessary to produce maximal biologic response remains. Conversely, reduced insulin concentration could be compensated by an increase in receptor number, providing the minimum amount of insulin necessary to produce a maximal biologic response is present. Clearly, primary defects in insulin receptor number or affinity may produce the same profound derangements in intermediary metabolism as deficient insulin secretion, and similar disturbances may result, despite normal insulin concentration and normal receptor characteristics, if postreceptor steps are defective.[16–19]

Examples of each type of defect in the individual components of this integrated system that comprises insulin biosynthesis, secretion, and action exist and can account for the metabolic abnormalities that characterize diabetes mellitus. An approach based on principles of insulin biosynthesis secretion and action also permits a rational classification of diabetes mellitus.

CLASSIFICATION

Diabetes mellitus is not a single entity but a heterogeneous group of disorders in which there are distinct genetic patterns of inheritance as well as separate etiologic and pathophysiologic mechanisms all leading to impairment of glucose tolerance. The National Diabetes Data Group proposed a classification of diabetes and other categories of glucose intolerance based on contemporary knowledge; this classification has been endorsed and accepted by various diabetes associations throughout the world as well as by pediatric investigators.[20,21] Three major forms of diabetes and several forms of carbohydrate intolerance have been identified (Table 4–1).

Type I Diabetes

This condition is characterized by severe insulinopenia and dependence on injected insulin to prevent ketosis and to preserve life; the condition is therefore called insulin-dependent diabetes mellitus (IDDM). There may, however, be preketotic non-insulin-dependent phases in the natural history of the disease (Fig. 4–2). In the preponderance of cases onset is in youth, but IDDM is not restricted to onset in childhood and may occur at any age. Hence, formerly used terms such as juvenile diabetes, ketosis-prone diabetes, and brittle diabetes have

TABLE 4–1.   SUMMARY OF CLASSIFICATION OF DIABETES MELLITUS IN CHILDREN AND ADOLESCENTS*

Category	Criteria
Diabetes Mellitus	
1. Insulin-dependent (IDDM, type I)	Typical symptoms: glucosuria, ketonuria; random plasma glucose (PG) > 200 mg/dl.
2. Non-insulin-dependent (NIDDM, type II)	Fasting PG > 140 mg/dl with 2 hour + intervening value >200 mg/dl on OGTT[†] more than once and in the absence of precipitating factors.
3. Other types	Type I or II criteria with genetic syndrome, drug therapy; pancreatic disease or other known causes or associations.
Impaired Glucose Tolerance (IGT)	FPG <140 mg/dl with 2 hour >140 mg/dl on OGTT[†].
Gestational Diabetes (GDM)	Two or more abnormal fasting of: FPG >105 mg/dl, 1 hour >190 mg/dl, 2 hour >165 mg/dl, 3 hour >145 mg/dl on OGTT.
Statistical Risk Classes	
1. Previous abnormality of glucose tolerance (Prev AGT)	Normal OGTT with previous abnormal OGTT, spontaneous hyperglycemia, or GDM.
2. Potential abnormality of glucose tolerance (Pot AGT)	Genetic propensity (e.g., identical twin with DM); islet cell antibodies.

* Details of this classification and its rationale can be found in National Diabetes Data Group: Classification and diagnosis of diabetes mellitus and other categories of glucose intolerance. Diabetes 28:1039, 1979.
[†]Oral glucose tolerance testing—1.75 mg/kg body weight, to a maximum of 75 gm.

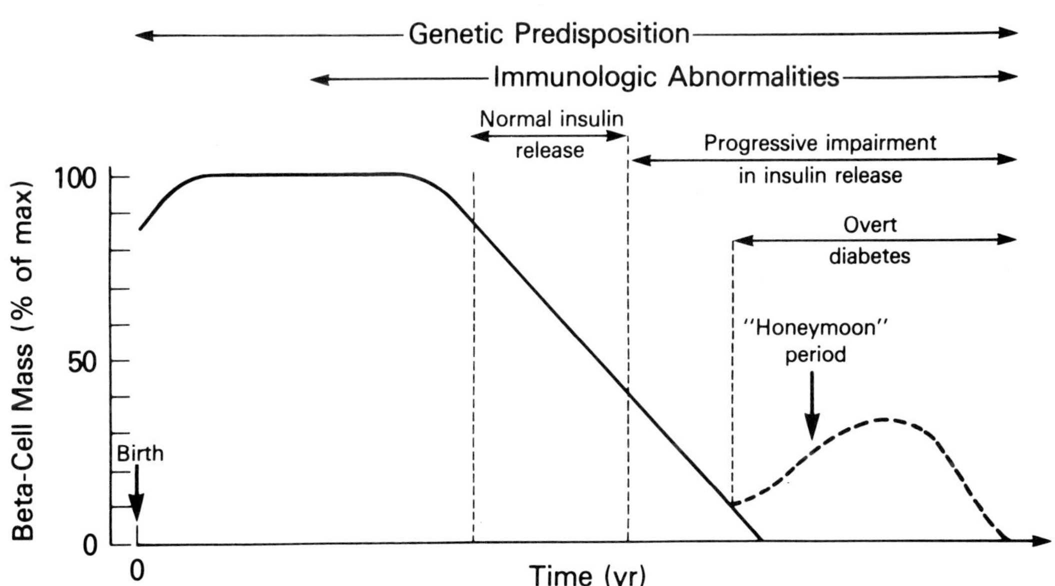

FIGURE 4–2. Proposed scheme of natural history of β cell defect. Timing of trigger in relation to immunologic abnormalities is unknown. Note that overt diabetes is not apparent until insulin secretory reserves are less than 10 to 20 per cent of normal. (From Sperling MA (ed): Physician's Guide to Insulin-Dependent (Type I) Diabetes. Diagnosis and Treatment. Arlington, VA, American Diabetes Association, 1988.)

been largely abandoned in favor of type I or IDDM. Type I diabetes is a distinct entity associated with certain human leukocyte antigens (HLAs), autoimmunity, and the presence of circulating antibodies to cytoplasmic and cell surface components of islet cells.[22,23] With few exceptions, diabetes in children is of the type I insulin-dependent variety.[24]

Type II Diabetes

Persons whose disease is in this subclass are not insulin dependent or ketosis prone, although they may use insulin for correction of symptomatic hyperglycemia and they may develop ketosis under special circumstances such as episodes of infection or stress. Because they are not insulin dependent, this condition is called non-insulin-dependent diabetes mellitus (NIDDM).

Serum insulin levels may be normal or occasionally low, but often are increased. In the majority of cases onset is after age 40, but NIDDM is known to occur in all ages, including childhood. Some 60 to 90 per cent of the subjects are obese. The condition was formerly called adult-onset diabetes, maturity-onset diabetes (MOD), or stable diabetes. This form of diabetes, manifests as abnormal carbohydrate tolerance, usually in obese individuals who secrete considerable amounts of insulin, and the problem is therefore one of insulin resistance.[25] Newer insights suggest there is also a relative insulinopenia in type II diabetes caused in part by the deposition in the pancreatic islets of an amyloid-like substance formed from a "diabetes-associated peptide."[25,26] Abnormal carbohydrate tolerance may also occur in children with a strong family history of type II diabetes that affects multiple family members in a pattern suggestive of dominant inheritance; the disease in these patients has been termed maturity-onset diabetes of the young (MODY) and may require insulin treatment. It is important to realize there are no statistically significant associations between this type of diabetes and specific HLAs, autoimmunity, or islet-cell antibodies. A variant of type II diabetes with clinical features intermediate between classical types I and II occurs predominantly in black adolescents.[24]

Secondary Diabetes

This subclass contains a variety of types of diabetes in some of which the etiologic relationship is known. Examples include diabetes secondary to pancreatic diseases such as cystic fibrosis or pancreatectomy for infantile hypoglycemia, diabetes secondary to endocrine disease such as Cushing syndrome, and diabetes secondary to the administration of drugs or poisons such as the rodenticide Vacor.[20,27] Certain genetic syndromes and abnormalities of the insulin receptor also are included in this category.[16,20,21] Again, there are no associations with specific HLAs, autoimmunity, or islet cell antibodies.

Impaired Glucose Tolerance

This condition was formerly known as asymptomatic diabetes, chemical diabetes, subclinical diabetes, borderline diabetes, or latent diabetes. It may represent a stage in the development of IDDM or NIDDM, but very few of these individuals go on to develop actual diabetes. Criteria for the diagnosis of impaired glucose tolerance are provided in Table 4–1.

Statistical Risk Classes

In addition to the above clinical classifications, individuals who do not have demonstrable impairment of glucose tolerance have been designated as having a greater statistical risk of future development of diabetes if they fall into one of two categories:

1. Previous abnormality of glucose tolerance. This was formerly called latent chemical diabetes or prediabetes and designated those individuals who previously had an abnormal glucose tolerance test or spontaneous hyperglycemia but at the time of classification had normal glucose tolerance.

2. Potential abnormality of glucose tolerance. This condition was known as prediabetes or potential diabetes and includes individuals presumed to be at increased risk for diabetes on genetic grounds and those with circulating islet cell antibodies.

This classification is summarized in Table 4–1.

PREVALENCE AND INCIDENCE

Surveys in the United States and elsewhere report an overall prevalence rate of 1 to 2:1000 school-age children.[28–30] This prevalence is highly correlated with age, ranging from 1:1430 children at 5 years to a peak of 1:360 children by age 16. Data on prevalence rates by racial or ethnic background are incomplete, but prevalence throughout the world varies widely, being highest in northern Scandinavia and lowest in Japan.[31] Among the American black population the prevalence of insulin-dependent diabetes is said to be 20 to 30 per cent of that in American Caucasians, a finding that has considerable implications regarding the genetic transmission of this disease.[32] However, some surveys report that the population-adjusted rate in American blacks is as high as two thirds that in the Caucasian population.[33] Analysis of the incidence rates shows a frequency of 12 to 16 new cases per 100,000 children per year.[28–33] Moreover, both prevalence and incidence of insulin-dependent diabetes in childhood in the United States are similar to those reported in Great Britain, parts of Sweden, and Australia.[28–33] Males and females appear to be equally affected, although there are reports of a preponderance of young males. A relative increased incidence in females at the time of puberty has also been suggested. There is no correlation with socioeconomic status. Peaks of presentation occur in two age groups: among 5- to 7-year-olds and at the time of puberty in both girls and boys. These age-related peaks correspond in the former to the increased exposure to infectious agents accompanying the beginning of school, and in the latter to the pubertal growth spurt induced by gonadal steroids together with increased pubertal growth hormone secretion, which may antagonize insulin action, thereby unmasking evolving diabetes.[34,35] This temporal pattern only infers a cause-and-effect relationship that remains to be proven.

The incidence of IDDM in childhood shows a cyclic variation that is both seasonal and long term. Independent studies confirm that newly recognized cases occur with greater frequency in the autumn and winter months both in the northern and southern hemispheres.[36] Children ages less than 6 years appear to have exaggerated seasonal variation in incidence of the disorder. In one study, peaks in the occurrence of mumps or mumps encephalitis were followed by peaks in the incidence of diabetes, with a mean time lag of 3.8 years,[37] but other studies have failed to demonstrate an increased

frequency of higher mumps or Coxsackie B antibody titers in recent-onset diabetes.[38] The incidence of diabetes is also increased in children with congenital rubella.[39] These associations with viral infections suggest a potential role for viruses as direct or indirect triggering mechanisms in the etiology of the disease.[40–43]

TYPE I DIABETES IN CHILDHOOD

Etiology, Genetics, and Pathogenesis

The ultimate cause of the initial clinical findings in this predominant form of diabetes in childhood is markedly diminished insulin secretion. Although basal insulin levels may be normal in newly diagnosed cases, insulin production in response to a variety of potent secretagogues is blunted, and usually completely disappears over a period of months to years. Some limited capacity for insulin secretion remains, however, and may persist for a variable period usually not exceeding 5 years. The greater the residual insulin-secreting capacity, as assessed by measurements of C peptide, the easier it is to maintain metabolic control with a minimum of exogenous insulin.[1,3]

The mechanisms leading to pancreatic beta cell failure are incompletely understood, but appear to be related to an autoimmune destruction of pancreatic islets in predisposed individuals. Type I diabetes has long been known to be associated with an increased prevalence of disorders such as Addison disease, Hashimoto thyroiditis, and pernicious anemia, in which autoimmune mechanisms are known to be pathogenic.[44,45] These conditions, including IDDM, are now known to be associated with an increased frequency of certain histocompatibility antigens, in particular HLA-DR3, and HLA-DR4.[41,46–57] The HLA system is the major histocompatibility complex, located on chromosome number 6, consisting of a cluster of genes that code for transplantation antigens and play a central role in the immune response.[51,56] Numerous disease associations and disease susceptibilities have been related to an increased frequency of one or several HLAs.[51,56] In type I diabetes, the inheritance of HLA-DR3 or -DR4 appears to confer a two- to threefold greater relative risk for developing the disease.[46–57] When both DR3 and DR4 are inherited together, however, the relative risk for developing diabetes is seven- to 10-fold greater, suggesting that DR3 and DR4 are additive in their effect of conferring relative risk.[52,56] Over 90 per cent of Caucasian patients with IDDM possess DR3 and/or DR4. A rare genetic type of properdin factor B (Bf[F1]) known to be closely linked to the HLA system on chromosome 6 was found in over 20 per cent of type I diabetics but in only 2 per cent of healthy subjects, yielding a relative risk of 15 for those who inherit this genetic marker.[54] Thus, D region specificities appear to be the more primary associations with type I diabetes.[55–57]

The molecular basis for autoimmune disease susceptibility conferred by the HLA-D complex [class II major histocompatibility molecules (MHC)] is an area of intense study. It is now known that the HLA-D region contains three subregions termed DP, DQ, and DR. Each class II antigen consists of one alpha and one beta chain, encoded by specific genes that are highly polymorphic, each gene having several alleles. Certain class II polymorphisms, especially on the HLA-DQβ chain, are either strongly associated with susceptibility to IDDM, or confer protection from diabetes when aspartic acid, rather than a nonaspartic amino acid, is at position 57 of the DQβ chain.[56,57] These findings provide a rational framework for the genetic factors associated with type I diabetes as suggested by the increased incidence in some families, the concordance rates in monozygotic twins, and the ethnic and racial differences in incidence.[52,58]

Finally, these findings have been used to provide models of the mode of genetic transmission for this disease and to provide predictions of recurrence risks to siblings and offspring.[56–61] Type I diabetes in the American black population is only about 20 to 30 per cent of that in American Caucasians, and this form of diabetes in blacks is associated with the same HLA genes as in Caucasians.[32] Because these genes are also about 20 to 30 per cent as common in American blacks as in Caucasians, so that the ratio of type I diabetes in American blacks to that in Caucasians is roughly equal to the fraction of Caucasian genes in the American black gene pool, it has been argued that the data are consistent with autosomal-dominant inheritance of type I diabetes.[32] On the other hand, on the basis of their studies by HLA typing in multiple affected family members, Rubinstein et al. suggested that the inheritance of diabetes was due to a re-

cessive gene closely linked to HLA D and with 50 per cent penetrance.[55] However, a more complex three-allele genetic model also fits the data, and this model exhibits the features of both dominant and recessive inheritance.[53,61] This model, based on the increased relative risk for individuals who have two different HLA alleles (e.g., DR3 and DR4) as compared to those with only one allele, and the differential immunologic associations with these different HLA alleles (e.g., persistent islet cell antibodies associated with HLA DR3), makes the following assumptions. First, there is a susceptibility locus "S," tightly linked to the HLA locus. Second, this S locus has two diabetogenic alleles, S_1 and S_2, that are in linkage disequilibrium and therefore in association respectively with DR3 and DR4. Third, different allelic combinations at the S locus are at risk for different forms of type I diabetes. When fitted to observations regarding prevalence, concordance rates in identical twins, and HLA identity in multiple affected siblings, the gene frequencies and penetrance rates can be calculated.[53,61] Evidence for at least two cooperating genes each linked to HLA alleles has been provided in other separate studies.[60] The model also predicts that there will be lower recurrence risks to relatives of blacks as compared to relatives of Caucasian diabetics. Multiple family pedigrees and HLA typing studies, suggest that in Caucasians, the recurrence risk to siblings is of the order of 2 to 5 per cent; the risk to offspring is also 2 to 5 per cent. In American blacks, these risks are only one half to two thirds of those in Caucasians.[53]

Although these recent genetic findings suggest that different genes on chromosome number 6 confer susceptibility to diabetes, factors other than pure inheritance are involved in producing clinical disease. Thus, the concordance rate among identical twins one of whom has insulin-dependent diabetes is at most only 50 per cent, suggesting the participation of an environmental triggering factor or factors.[48,58] Such a triggering factor may be a viral infection. In animals, a number of viruses can cause a diabetic syndrome, the appearance and severity of which depend on the genetic strain and immune competence of the species tested.[40–42] In man, epidemics of mumps, rubella, and the Coxsackie virus have been associated with subsequent increases in the frequency of type I diabetes, and the occurrence of acute diabetes mellitus induced by a Coxsackie B_4 virus has been documented.[43] The virus itself may be pancreatropic, initiating an inflammatory response in the islets (insulinitis); in those who have died early in the course of type I diabetes mellitus, the histology of the pancreas is indeed characterized by lymphocytic infiltration around the islets of Langerhans. Later, the islets become progressively hyalinized and scarred, a process suggesting an ongoing inflammatory response, possibly autoimmune in nature. In support of an autoimmune basis for type I diabetes, investigations show a high prevalence of circulating antibodies directed against the cytoplasmic components of islet cells and against the cell surface components of insulin-producing beta cells.[45,47,62–64] These antibodies, which are present in over 75 per cent of cases at the clinical onset of disease prior to insulin treatment, are therefore not insulin antibodies of the kind found universally in insulin-treated diabetics. The islet cell surface antibodies, in the presence of complement, are cytotoxic for beta cells in in vitro systems.[62,64] Similarly, T lymphocytes from diabetics have been shown to be cytotoxic to human insulinoma cells in culture.[64] These findings suggest that type I diabetes, akin to other autoimmune diseases such as Hashimoto thyroiditis, is a disease of "autoaggression," in which autoantibodies, in cooperation with complement, T cells, or other factors, are cytotoxic to their target cell, the insulin-producing islet cell.[44,45,47,62–64] Thus, the inheritance of certain genes intimately associated with the HLA system on chromosome 6 confers a predisposition for autoimmune disease, including diabetes, when triggered by an appropriate stimulus such as a virus. These findings offer an attractive hypothesis to explain the etiology and genetics of type I diabetes in which various subtypes with separate, distinct associations may exist.[52,57]

While these aspects are still the subject of research, it must be emphasized that not all insulin-dependent diabetic patients have one of the HLA types that are more frequently associated with this disease. However, HLA typing and detection of islet cell antibodies may permit more accurate information regarding the prediction and identification of those persons destined to develop type I diabetes.[23,65–69] Indeed, the existence of islet cell antibodies with progressive impairment of the "first phase" insulin response to intravenous glucose may precede by months to years the appearance of clinical diabetes. Similarly, anti-insulin antibodies can be detected in the "prediabetic phase" and at clinical presentation, before any exogenous insulin injection, suggesting an immune response to a modified endogenous insulin rendered immunogenic. Although the presence of islet cell antibodies (ICAs) in serum of unaffected individuals may vary with time, persistence of ICAs appears to be a strong predictive factor for developing IDDM in nonaffected siblings, especially when both HLA haplotypes are shared with the proband. The nature of the islet cell antigen evoking ICAs is unknown, but evidence suggests it is a 64,000 molecular weight component of islets.[68] This information, linking genetics, autoimmunity, and environmental triggers, is the basis for attempts to predict those persons destined to develop IDDM, and to prevent pancreatic endocrine destruction by immune intervention therapy such as cyclosporin, as early as possible.[23,65–69] These concepts are summarized in Figure 4–2.

Pathophysiology

The increasing destruction of beta cells leads progressively to more severe insulin deficiency. Insulin is the major anabolic hormone of the body. As indicated, normal insulin secretion in response to feeding is exquisitely modulated by neural, hormonal, and substrate-related mechanisms to permit precise disposition of ingested foodstuffs as energy to be utilized immediately or stored for future use; energy mobilization during the fasted state depends on low levels of insulin. Thus, in normal metabolism, there are regular swings between the fed, high-insulin, anabolic state and the fasted, low-insulin, catabolic state affecting three major tissues (Table 4–2). Type I diabetes mellitus, as it evolves, becomes a permanent low-insulin, catabolic state in which feeding will not reverse but rather exaggerate the catabolic processes listed in Table 4–2.

Although insulin deficiency is the primary defect, several secondary hormonal changes involving the classical stress hormones epinephrine, cortisol, growth hormone, and glucagon accelerate and exaggerate the rate and magnitude of the metabolic decompensation.[70–73] Increased plasma concentrations of these counterregulatory hormones are found in decompen-

TABLE 4–2.   MAJOR METABOLIC EVENTS DURING THE FED AND FASTED STATES

	High-Insulin (Fed) State	Low-Insulin (Fasted) State
Liver	Glucose uptake Glycogen synthesis Absent glyconeogenesis Lipogenesis Absent ketogenesis	Glucose production Glycogenolysis Gluconeogenesis Absent lipogenesis Ketogenesis
Muscle	Glucose uptake Glucose oxidation Glycogen synthesis Protein synthesis	Absent glucose uptake Fatty acid α-ketone oxidation Glycogenolysis Proteolysis and amino acid release
Adipose Tissue	Glucose uptake Lipid synthesis Triglyceride uptake	Absent glucose uptake Lipolysis and fatty acid release Absent triglyceride uptake

sated diabetes; they magnify the metabolic derangements through further impairing insulin secretion (epinephrine), antagonizing its action (epinephrine, cortisol, growth hormone), and promoting glycogenolysis, gluconeogeneis, lipolysis, and ketogenesis while decreasing glucose utilization and clearance. All of these secondary hormonal changes are restored to normal with adequate insulin therapy, and this indicates that the primary cause of the metabolic derangement is deficiency of insulin secretion and action.[13,70–73] Nevertheless, selective suppression of some of the counterregulatory hormones, (e.g., the suppression of glucagon and growth hormone secretion and splanchnic blood flow by the administration of somatostatin) ameliorates the hyperglycemia of diabetes, slows the rate of progression to ketoacidosis, and facilitates metabolic control.[13,14,72,73]

Insulin deficiency, acting in concert with excessive concentrations of epinephrine, cortisol, growth hormone, and glucagon, results in unrestrained glucose production while glucose utilization is impaired so that hyperglycemia develops (Table 4–2). Glucosuria results when the renal threshhold of approximately 160 mg/dl is exceeded; the resultant osmotic diuresis produces polyuria, dehydration, an increase in serum osmolality, and compensatory polydipsia. The plasma osmolality can be rapidly estimated from the formula:

$$\text{Serum osmolality (mOsm/kg)} = (\text{serum Na}^+ + \text{serum K}^+) \times 2 + \frac{\text{glucose}}{18}$$
$$(\text{mEq/L}) \quad (\text{mEq/L}) \quad (\text{mg/dl})$$

Since serum glucose is commonly elevated to levels of 600 mg/dl or higher at initial presentation, it is readily apparent that hyperosmolality is almost universally present during episodes of ketoacidosis.[74] This hyperosmolality contributes to the symptomatology, in particular cerebral obtundation during ketoacidosis, and has important implications for therapy.

In addition, in the presence of insulin deficiency and the elevated concentrations of counterregulatory hormones, there is brisk lipolysis and impaired lipid synthesis, leading to marked elevation in the plasma concentrations of total lipids, cholesterol, triglycerides, and free fatty acids. The hormonal interplay of insulin deficiency and glucagon excess shunts the free fatty acids to ketone body formation[74–76]; the rate of formation of these ketone bodies, principally β-hydroxybutyrate and acetoacetate, exceeds the capacity for peripheral utilization.[75] Glucagon, present in high concentrations in the plasma during episodes of ketoacidosis, plays a major role in the pathogenesis of the biochemical derangements associated with this complication.[76] First, it enhances the breakdown of glycogen by activating phosphorylase b through a cAMP-dependent mechanism. Second, again through a cAMP-dependent mechanism, it stimulates gluconeogenesis by enhancing the activity of the bifunctional enzyme 6-phosphofructose-2-kinase/fructose-2, 6-biphosphatase, and this leads to a decrease in the amount of fructose 2,6-biphosphate formed during glycolysis from fructose 6-phosphate. Fructose 2,6-biphosphate is a key regulator of carbohydrate metabolism and when its production rate falls, gluconeogenesis is enhanced and glycolysis is inhibited. Third, glucagon enhances ketogenesis as a result of the reduction in substrate flow from glucose and direct inhibition of acetyl-coenzyme A carboxylase. This stimulates the enzyme carnitine palmitoyl transferase I to convert fatty acyl esters to fatty acyl carnitine compounds, which are then able to traverse the mitochondrial membrane where they are converted to acetoacetate and β-hydroxybutyrate. Accumulation of these ketoacids results in metabolic acidosis and compensatory rapid deep breathing in an attempt to excrete excess carbon dioxide (Kussmaul respiration). Acetone, formed by nonenzymatic conversion of acetoacetate, is responsible for the characteristic fruity odor of the breath. Ketones are readily excreted in the urine in association with cations, further compounding losses of water and electrolytes. Typical losses of water and of the principal ions during development of diabetic ketoacidosis in children are depicted in Table 4–3. With progressive dehydration, acidosis, hyperosmolality, and diminished cerebral oxygen utilization, consciousness gradually becomes impaired and ultimately coma develops. Thus, insulin deficiency produces a profound catabolic state—an exaggerated starvation—in which all of the initial clinical features can be explained on the basis of known alterations in intermediary metabolism. The severity and duration of the symptoms are a reflection of the degree of insulinopenia.

Clinical Presentation

Most children present with a history of polyuria, polydipsia, polyphagia, and weight loss. These symptoms may be present for days to weeks, but in approximately half the children the duration of symptoms is less than 1 month. A subtle clue to the existence of polyuria may be the onset of enuresis in a previously toilet-trained child. An insidious onset with lethargy, weakness, and weight loss is quite common. The loss of weight is readily explicable on the basis of the catabolic state and the urinary losses of calories by considering a typical example.

A 10-year-old child normally has a caloric intake of some 2000 kcal, of which approximately 50 per cent is derived from carbohydrate. With the development of diabetes, polyuria of 5 L/day containing an average concentration of 5 per cent glucose commonly results. This represents a loss of 250 g of glucose, or 1000 kcal. The net effective caloric balance is only 1000 kcal, leading to hunger and polyphagia. Despite the increased food intake, however, calories cannot be utilized, further exacerbating catabolism and resulting in weight loss.

Pyogenic skin infections are uncommon as presenting complaints, but monilial vaginitis in teenage girls may occasionally be the presenting feature. Routine oral glucose tolerance tests have no place as a screening procedure for asymptomatic individuals, although other screening tests are being investigated.[23,65–67] It is also not necessary to perform a glucose tolerance test in children whose classic symptoms are associated with a random blood glucose of greater than 200 mg/dl.[20,21]

Diabetic Ketoacidosis

Only a minority of children (30 per cent or less) initially present with frank diabetic ketoacidosis (DKA), air hunger, Kussmaul respiration, acetone on the breath, obtundation of consciousness or coma, vomiting, dehydration, ketonemia, hyperglycemia, glucosuria, and ketonuria. Diabetic ketoacidosis is more likely to be present in children age 5 or less at the time of initial pre-

---

TABLE 4–3.   FLUID AND ELECTROLYTE MAINTENANCE AND LOSSES IN DIABETIC KETOACIDOSIS

Element	Maintenance Requirements*	Losses†
Water	1500 ml/m^2	100 ml/kg (range 60–100)
Sodium	45 mEq/m^2	6 mEq/kg (range 5–13)
Potassium	35 mEq/m^2	5 mEq/kg (range 4–6)
Chloride	30 mEq/m^2	4 mEq/kg (range 3–9)
Phosphate	10 mEq/m^2	3 mEq/kg (range 2–5)

* Maintenance is expressed in surface area to permit uniformity because fluid requirements change as weight increases.
† Losses are expressed per unit of body weight since the losses remain relatively constant as a function of total body weight.

sentation. Leukocytosis and abdominal pain that mimics appendicitis is extremely common in children and may be associated with an elevated serum amylase level that does not usually indicate the existence of pancreatitis.[74,75] The importance of this observation is not to assume the existence of a surgical emergency before a period of rehydration, electrolyte therapy, and insulin replacement; the abdominal pain frequently resolves after several hours of this treatment. It is also important to emphasize that hyperglycemia with blood glucose exceeding 200 mg/dl must be documented. Renal glucosuria, either as an isolated finding or as part of the Fanconi syndrome, in a child with vomiting and starvation ketosis may mimic the urinary findings of ketoacidosis (i.e., glucosuria and ketonuria). Blood glucose levels are normal, however, providing the clue that insulin therapy is not indicated.

The discovery of glucosuria during a hospital admission for trauma or infection rarely heralds the presence of diabetes; in most of these cases, the glucosuria remits during recovery. Inasmuch as this circumstance may indicate a limited capacity for insulin secretion, unmasked by the elevation in the plasma concentrations of the stress hormones, some authorities have recommended that these patients be periodically rechecked for the possibility of hyperglycemia and/or clinical features of diabetes mellitus.

The child differs little from adults in the basic pathophysiologic disturbances, clinical features, and trends in the treatment of DKA.[74,75] What distinguishes the child from the adult is the greater need for precision in the quantity, composition, and rate of fluid and electrolyte therapy, as well as in insulin dosage, and in providing close monitoring with individualization of therapy.

Diabetic ketoacidosis can be said to exist when there is hyperglycemia (blood glucose level 300 mg/dl or more) ketonemia (ketones strongly positive at greater than 1:2 dilution of serum), acidosis (pH 7.30 or less and bicarbonate less than 15 mEq/L), glucosuria, and ketonuria in addition to the clinical features described above. Serum sodium concentration may be normal or slightly low even though large deficits exist. Also, despite large deficits of potassium and phosphate, serum concentrations of these ions are not uniformly reduced prior to initiation of therapy.

Precipitating factors, even for the initial presentation, include stress such as trauma, infections, vomiting, and psychological disturbances. Recurrent episodes of ketoacidosis in established diabetics usually imply deliberate errors in recommended insulin dosage or unusual stress responses and indicate psychological disturbances or pleas to be removed from a home environment perceived to be stressful or intolerable. Diabetic ketoacidosis in children must be distinguished from the following:

1. Nonketotic hyperosmolar coma. Glucose is greater than 500 mg/dl and serum osmolality exceeds 300 mOsm/kg but ketones are absent in serum and urine. Although this syndrome is rare in children, it does occur.[74] The principles of fluid and electrolyte therapy are as outlined below, but insulin should be given with extreme caution to prevent a rapid fall in glucose and osmolality, and thereby induce cerebral edema.[77,78]

2. Lactic acidosis is extremely rare in childhood. Its presence usually indicates an inborn error of metabolism. Similarly, ketoacidosis in the absence of hyperglycemia also usually indicates an inborn error of metabolism.

3. The acidosis of salicylate intoxication generally occurs without hyperglycemia.

Treatment

Prevention through education of the family, patient, and responsible physician to recognize and treat diabetes prior to development of ketoacidosis is the best form of therapy. However, when the patient presents with established DKA the following principles should be employed.

The initial metabolic stabilization of a child with DKA is achieved by a combination of fluid and electrolyte therapy and insulin administration. The extent of metabolic decompensation (i.e., the presence of DKA) must be assessed clinically by estimating the degree of dehydration, observing for the presence of Kussmaul respiration, and noting whether there is an alteration in the conscious state. A biochemical confirmation of the presence of DKA must be sought by measurement of blood glucose and acid-base status, serum electrolyte concentrations (including calcium and phosphorus), and urinary ketones, and by an estimate of renal function through measurement of blood urea nitrogen (BUN) and/or creatinine. In addition, investigations such as bacterial cultures and a chest radiograph may be indicated.

In managing DKA, there are broad guidelines and principles that can be followed, but the precise treatment plan must be individualized. Children less than 2 years of age presenting with DKA or children with an arterial pH less than 7.0, blood glucose 1000 mg/dl or greater, or with an altered conscious state should be treated initially in an intensive care unit or equivalent setting where close monitoring of metabolic changes and meticulous supervision of therapy can be provided by experienced staff. A flow sheet detailing the composition of administered fluid, oral fluid intake, fluid output, timing and dose of insulin administered, electrolyte and acid-base status, and clinical parameters should be maintained; such a flow sheet is helpful in monitoring the patient's progress. Bladder catheterization is not needed routinely; urine bag collection or condom drainage provide an adequately accurate estimate of urine output in children. Repeated measurements of blood glucose, acid-base status, and serum electrolytes are obtained generally at 2-hour intervals for the initial 8 hours, 4-hour intervals for the next 16 hours, and then at 4- to 6-hour intervals until acidosis is completely resolved and the patient is fully conscious and able to take an adequate oral fluid intake without vomiting.

Fluid and Electrolytes. The fluid and electrolyte requirements of a child with DKA must be calculated more carefully than those of an adult because there is less margin for error. The maintenance fluid requirement of a child changes as the child grows, but is constant when expressed per unit of surface area; it is not constant when expressed per unit of body weight. In general, 1500 ml/m²/day is accepted as maintenance fluid requirement. By contrast, dehydration is expressed as a percentage of body weight; that is, 10 per cent dehydration implies a loss of 10 per cent of the body weight as water (Table 4–3). At presentation, clinical assessment usually underestimates the degree of dehydration in children. Children with DKA may be assumed to have lost 10 per cent of body weight as a rough estimate. The total fluid to be administered is the sum of maintenance and estimated dehydration plus ongoing losses. A schema for managing a child of 1 m² and weight of 30 kg is given in Table 4–4. Fluid replacement is extended over 36 hours to reduce the likelihood of a too-rapid drop in plasma osmolality, a factor that may predispose to cerebral edema. To reduce further the potential for developing cerebral edema, the initial replacement fluid consists of normal saline (0.9 per cent) so that a gradual decrease in plasma osmolality is achieved. Note that potassium therapy is initiated in the second hour and that some of the potassium is given as phosphate to provide phosphate repletion and reduce the provision of excess chloride. Initiation of insulin therapy and correction of acidosis may be followed by sharp reductions in the concentrations of potassium in the serum because of shifts of this ion to the intracellular compartment.

Provision of excess chloride is almost inevitable (see Table 4–5) and may aggravate acidosis.[79] The extent of excess chloride can be reduced through the use of phosphate, which is significantly depleted in diabetic ketoacidosis.[80] Moreover, phosphate together with glycolysis is essential for, and related to, the formation of 2,3-diphospho-

TABLE 4–4.   FLUID AND ELECTROLYTE LOSSES BASED ON ASSUMED 10 PER CENT DEHYDRATION IN A CHILD WITH DIABETIC KETOACIDOSIS (WEIGHT 30 KG; SURFACE AREA 1 M²)*

Fluid and Electrolyte	Approximate Accumulated Losses with 10 Per Cent Dehydration	Approximate Requirements for Maintenance (36 Hour)	Working Total (36 Hour)
Water (ml)	3000	2250	5500
Sodium (mEq)	180	65	250
Potassium (mEq)	150	50	200
Chloride (mEq)	120	45	165
Phosphate (mEq)	90	15	100

TABLE 4–5. REPLACEMENT PROCEDURE FOR CHILD (30 KG, 1 M^2) WITH DIABETIC KETOACIDOSIS (10 PER CENT DEHYDRATION)*†

Approximate Duration	Fluid (Composition)	Sodium	Potassium	Chloride	Phosphate (mEq)
Hour 1	500 ml of 0.9 per cent NaCl (normal saline)	75	—	75	—
Hour 2	500 ml of 0.45 per cent NaCl (0.5 normal saline) plus 20 mEq of KCl	35	20	55	—
Hour 3 to 12 (200 ml/hour for 10 hours)	2000 ml of 0.45 per cent saline with 30 mEq/L of potassium phosphate	150	60	150	40
Subtotal (initial 12 hours)	3000 ml	260	80	280	40
Next 24 hours (100 ml/hour)	0.2 normal saline in 5 per cent glucose with 40 mEq/L of potassium as the phosphate	75	100	75	60
Total over 36 hours	5400 ml	335	180	355	100

Bicarbonate therapy
For pH >7.20, no therapy necessary.
For pH between 7.10 and 7.20, 40 mEq/m^2 of bicarbonate over 2 hours, then reevaluate.
For pH <7.10, 80 mEq/m^2 of bicarbonate over 2 hours, then reevaluate.
New diabetics <2 years of age with DKA and 10 per cent dehydration or any diabetic with pH <7.00 should be managed in an intensive care unit or equivalent setting.

* All replacement values should be halved if dehydration is estimated to be 5 per cent. Maintenance requirements remain the same.

glycerate, (2,3-DPG), which affects the oxygen dissociation curve. With deficiency of 2,3-DPG, the oxygen dissociation curve is shifted to the left; that is, more oxygen is retained by hemoglobin and less is available to tissues, thereby predisposing to lactic acidosis.[81] Acidosis per se tends to shift the oxygen dissociation curve back to the right (Bohr effect), thereby "compensating" in part for 2,3-DPG deficiency. As acidosis due to the accumulation of ketoacids is corrected through the provision of insulin with or without provision of bicarbonate, the effects of 2,3-DPG deficiency may no longer be "compensated" and the release of oxygen to tissues may be impaired. Provision of phosphate promotes the formation of 2,3-DPG, permits the oxygen dissociation curve to shift to the right, and thus facilitates the release of oxygen to tissues and the correction of acidosis.[80] Hypophosphatemia is also associated with resistance to insulin action.

Although the restoration of 2,3-DPG concentrations by phosphate therapy is beneficial, it is important to be aware of the potential for precipitating hypocalcemia through excessive use of phosphate solutions. Hence, the use of potassium chloride alternating with a balanced solution of potassium phosphate as outlined in Table 4–4 is recommended. Administration of excessive quantities of phosphate may lead to hypocalcemia; therefore serum calcium should be measured periodically. Hypocalcemia requires appropriate treatment with calcium gluconate.

It should be noted that the nitroprusside reaction that is routinely used to measure "ketones" occurs primarily with acetone, less intensively with acetoacetate, but not with β-hydroxybutyrate. The normal ratio of β-hydroxybutyrate to acetoacetate is approximately 3:1, but it is commonly 8:1 and occasionally higher in DKA. Since with correction of acidosis, β-hydroxybutyrate is converted to acetoacetate, there is often an impression of persistence of ketonemia and ketonuria despite clinical improvement in the patient. For this reason, ketone bodies, as routinely measured, are not always a reliable index of therapeutic response.

Insulin.   These principles of fluid and electrolyte therapy and correction of acidosis form the cornerstone of treatment of

TABLE 4–6. CONTINUOUS LOW-DOSE INTRAVENOUS INSULIN THERAPY FOR DIABETIC KETOACIDOSIS

Priming dose: 0.1 U/kg regular insulin, intravenously
Continuous intravenous infusion: 0.1 U/kg/hour
  regular insulin beginning with second hour
Directions for making insulin infusion: Add 50 U
  regular insulin to 500 ml of physiologic saline
Flush 50 ml through the tubing to saturate insulin
  binding sites. For 30-kg patient, infuse at a rate of
  30 ml/hour
When the blood glucose concentration approaches
  300 mgg/dl and acidosis is resolved, discontinue
  the insulin infusion and start insulin therapy by
  subcutaneous injections of 0.2 to 0.4 U/kg at 6-hour
  intervals

ketoacidosis, and often result in clinical and biochemical improvement, even before the initiation of insulin therapy.[82] However, the provision of insulin is essential to restore normal intermediary metabolism and to hasten the correction of acidosis, which commonly persists longer than the hyperglycemia. The preferred method of insulin delivery is the continuous low-dose infusion method using a priming dose of 0.1 units/kg followed by 0.1 unit/kg/hour, as described in Table 4–6. This method is a very effective, simple, and physiologically sound form of therapy that has gained wide acceptance as the preferred method for administering insulin during diabetic ketoacidosis.[75,83]

Glucose concentrations often will reach levels of 200 to 300 mg/dl before acidosis is resolved completely. However, it is important to continue insulin administration at the standard rate of 0.1 U/kg/hour or, occasionally, 0.05 U/kg/hour, while adding 5 per cent or even 10 per cent glucose to the infusate in order to maintain glucose concentrations between 200 and 300 mg/dl. The reason for maintaining glucose concentration in the range of 200 to 300 mg/dl is to avoid hypoglycemia and prevent too rapid a fall in

plasma osmolality, because glucose contributes substantially to plasma osmolality. Administration of insulin by methods other than constant intravenous infusion is not recommended. Prior to introduction of this method of treatment insulin was administered by bolus injection (Table 4–7).

When blood glucose concentration approaches 300 mg/dl, the electrolyte solution is made up in 5 per cent glucose, and the rate of insulin infusion is maintained or halved to 0.05 units/kg/hour until acidosis is resolved. When acidosis is resolved, the insulin infusion may be discontinued 30 min after regular (short-acting) insulin is given subcutaneously at a dose of 0.2 to 0.4 units/ kg; these doses are repeated at 4- to 6-hour intervals while maintaining the glucose and electrolyte infusion, until the child can fully tolerate food. The dose of insulin is adjusted depending on the blood glucose concentration. Only regular (short-acting) insulin is used during this phase of treatment. One or 2 days of this insulin schedule permits assessment of approximate total daily insulin requirement (i.e., the sum of the doses used in a 24-hour day). This total is then provided as a "split, mixed insulin regimen" consisting of two parts of intermediate-acting (NPH or Lente) and one part regular insulin, with approximately two thirds of the total given in the morning before breakfast and the remainder before the evening meal. For newly diagnosed patients about 3 to 5 days are required to stabilize the insulin dose, whereas in established cases the dose used before the episode of ketoacidosis can be reintroduced sooner.

Use of Bicarbonate. With provision of fluid and electrolytes, as well as insulin, metabolic acidosis is corrected via the interruption of ketogenesis, the metabolism of ketones to bicarbonate, and the generation of bicarbonate by the distal renal tubule. Concerns over the use of bicarbonate center around four issues.[84] First, alkalosis shifts

TABLE 4–7. "TRADITIONAL" INSULIN REGIMEN FOR DIABETIC KETOACIDOSIS

Blood Glucose	Total Insulin Dose*	Intravenous Dose	I.M. or S.C. Dose	Frequency
>900 mg/dl	2 units/kg	1 unit/kg	1 unit/kg	Every 2 to 4 hours
600–900 mg/dl	1 unit/kg	0.5 unit/kg	0.5 unit/kg	Every 2 to 4 hours
300–600 mg/dl†	0.5 unit/kg	0.25 unit/kg	0.25 unit/kg	Every 2 to 4 hours

* These doses may be halved if serum ketones are only modestly elevated.
† When blood glucose approaches 300 mg/dl, start 5 per cent dextrose; cover with insulin, 0.25 unit/kg every 6 to 8 hours on a sliding scale.

the oxygen dissociation curve to the left, thereby diminishing the release of oxygen to tissues and potentially providing a mechanism for developing lactic acidosis. Second, alkalosis accelerates the entry of potassium into the intracellular space, and hence may produce hypokalemia. Third, provision of bicarbonate according to the calculated base deficit overcorrects and may result in alkalosis. Fourth, and perhaps most important, bicarbonate may lead to worsening in cerebral acidosis, while the plasma pH is being restored to normal. This is because HCO_3^- combines with H^+ and dissociates to CO_2 and H_2O. Whereas bicarbonate passes the blood-brain barrier slowly, carbon dioxide diffuses freely, thereby exacerbating cerebral acidosis and possibly cerebral depression. On the other hand, severe acidosis, with a pH of 7.1 or less, diminishes respiratory minute volume, may produce hypotension with peripheral vasodilation, impairs myocardial function, and may be a factor in insulin resistance.[84] For these reasons, administration of bicarbonate is recommended in certain cases. When the blood pH is 7.1 or less, some authorities recommend that 40 mEq/m^2 of bicarbonate be infused over 2 hours, and when the pH is 7.0 or less, 80 mEq/m^2 be infused over 2 hours, followed by reassessment of the patient. Bicarbonate never should be given as a bolus except during cardiopulmonary resuscitation.

Complications

With appropriate therapy, complications of DKA are uncommon in children. Iatrogenic complications include hypoglycemia, hypocalcemia from too vigorous use of phosphate, and hypokalemia from inadequate potassium replacement. The major complication of concern in children treated for DKA is cerebral edema, the etiology of which remains poorly understood. Clinically, cerebral edema develops in patients several hours after the institution of therapy, when clinical and biochemical indices suggest improvement. Inexplicably, there are manifestations of raised intracranial pressure, such as headache, deterioration in conscious state, development of fixed dilated pupils, and, occasionally, polyuria (secondary to diabetes insipidus), which may be misdiagnosed as osmotic diuresis caused by hyperglycemia. Once clinically obvious, this complication has a high morbidity and mortality. The traditional belief that the cause of the syndrome is raised intracranial pressure has led physicians to use agents such as mannitol (10 to 20 g/m^2 intravenously) as a means of reducing cerebral edema. More recently, the use of magnetic resonance imaging and computed tomography indicates that at least some of these children have cerebral thrombosis and infarction in addition to cerebral edema. The incidence of cerebral edema can be reduced by the prevention of DKA through the early diagnosis of diabetes mellitus and avoidance of recurrent episodes of DKA by effective patient-family education and support.

Comments

The schema outlined in Table 4–4 can be applied to children of all sizes by making the appropriate adjustment for the calculated surface area (obtained from standard nomograms) and for the child's weight. Adjustments also can be made if the estimated dehydration is more or less than the listed 10 per cent outlined in Tables 4–3 and 4–4. If the estimated dehydration is only 5 per cent, for example, maintenance fluid requirements remain the same but the estimated deficit requirement is halved. A detailed consideration of the pathophysiology of DKA and its treatment in children is presented elsewhere.[74]

As soon as possible, a recognizable precipitating cause, such as infection, should be appropriately treated. (Precipitating events for DKA such as myocardial infarction or cerebral thrombosis are not a consideration in childhood.) In addition, for both new patients and those with recurrent episodes of ketoacidosis, the time required for stabilization should be utilized to educate the parents and patients in the principles of management of the child with diabetes mellitus, including appropriate insulin dose, technique of injection, nutritional requirements, exercise, and monitoring of urine or blood. This education should be carried out by a team consisting of a physician, a dietitian, and a nurse with special training in diabetes.

Management of the Child with Type I Diabetes

The immediate goals of managing children with type I diabetes are the provision of adequate nutrition and insulin in a manner that prevents symptomatic hyperglycemia (i.e., polydipsia, polyuria, and nocturia) while avoiding hypoglycemia and permitting normal growth and development, both physical and emotional. Education of the parents and patient in the principles of management facilitates the achievement of these goals. Long-term goals include the minimization of risk for developing micro- or macrovascular complications by maintaining good metabolic (glycemic) control, although such control is not always achievable.

Insulin Regimens

The pattern of insulin concentration in the serum of normal humans during the course of one day consists of a basal level superimposed upon which are several secretory episodes coinciding with food intake. The rise in insulin levels is synchronous with and proportional to the rise in blood glucose. Moreover, insulin is secreted into the portal circulation and its first target organ is the liver, the key organ governing the initial disposal of a glucose load. It is naive, therefore, to expect that a single injection of intermediate-acting insulin given subcutaneously can mimic the normal pattern of insulin secretion; periods of excessive insulin action resulting in a tendency to hypoglycemia, and/or periods of inadequate insulin action resulting in hyperglycemia, are inevitable. Even with injections of regular, fast-acting insulin prior to each meal, normalization of blood glucose is not entirely achieved, although the degree of control may be improved and the wide fluctuations of blood glucose diminished. It is unrealistic, however, to expect children to permit multiple daily injections of insulin; as indicated, all regimens of insulin administration represent compromises. The intent of each regimen is the same; to achieve as near normal intermediary metabolism as will permit normal growth and development.

Table 4–8 lists the presently available insulins. They can be classified as short-acting, intermediate-acting and long-acting types; all are routinely available in a concentration of 100 U/ml (U-100) although higher concentrations are available for rare patients who exhibit profound insulin resistance, and diluted insulins (U-10) can be prepared for use in infants and toddlers. Refinements in manufacture have resulted in highly purified insulins with significantly less contamination by other pancreatic hormones such as proinsulin, glucagon, pancreatic polypeptide, and somatostatin. Antibodies to these and other contaminants had been previously demonstrated in the sera of insulin-treated diabetics.[85] These more highly purified insulins facilitate metabolic control, and result in fewer local or systemic allergic reactions, including lipoatrophy and lipohypertrophy. These insulins are extracted from beef and pork pancreas and are available as beef-pork mixtures, pure pork, or pure beef insulins. Human insulin prepared by recombinant DNA techniques or chemical modification of animal insulin is currently available for general use. It is probably less antigenic than other preparations, although antibodies to insulin are found in the serum of individuals who have received only human insulin. It is necessary to be aware of the fact that the onset and peak of action of human insulin are faster than those of other insulins and its duration of action is shorter. It is likely that in the future most if not all patients will be receiving human insulin if the cost is not higher than that of other insulins. In general, patients who were making satisfactory progress while receiving animal insulins were not advised to change to human insulin when the latter became available.[86]

At the onset of diabetes, or following recovery from ketoacidosis, the total daily dose of insulin is of the order of 0.5 to 1.0 U/kg. Long-acting insulins are not routinely used in children. In view of its gradual onset of action, intermediate-acting insulin is seldom used alone, and fast-acting regular insulin is given in addition. In most single-daily-dose regimens, approximately two thirds of the total dose is intermediate-acting insulin (NPH, Lente, etc.) and the remainder is the quick-acting form. The mixture is generally injected 30 min before breakfast.[87,88] The two insulins should be drawn up in the same syringe and always in the same sequence, so that the amount of residual insulin in the "dead space" remains constant. This ensures greater stability of control once a therapeutic dose is established. Disposable syringes with fine needles, minimal dead space, and easy-to-read calibration for use with U-100 insulin have become standard. For smaller children, syringes calibrated to a maximum of 50 units are available or dilute insulin solutions may be prepared with an appropriate

TABLE 4–8.   INSULINS CURRENTLY AVAILABLE IN THE UNITED STATES*

Product	Manufacturer	Strength
Short-acting (usual onset 0.5–2.0 h; usual duration 3–6 h)		
Human		
Humulin regular	Lilly	U-100
Humulin BR (only external insulin pumps)	Lilly	U-100
Novolin R (regular, formerly Actrapid human)	Squibb-Novo	U-100
Velosulin human (regular)	Nordisk-USA	U-100
Novolin R Penfill (regular)	Squibb-Novo	U-100
Beef		
Iletin II regular	Lilly	U-100
Semilente	Squibb-Novo	U-100
Pork		
Iletin II regular	Lilly	U-100, U-500
Purified pork R (regular, formerly Actrapid)	Squibb-Novo	U-100
Velosulin (regular	Nordisk-USA	U-100
Purified pork S (semilente, formerly Semitard)	Squibb-Novo	U-100
Regular	Squibb-Novo	U-100
Beef pork		
Iletin I (regular)	Lilly	U-40, U-100
Iletin I (Semilente)	Lilly	U-40, U-100
Intermediate acting (usual onset 3–6 h; usual duration 12–20 h)		
Human		
Humulin L	Lilly	U-100
Humulin NPH	Lilly	U-100
Insulatard human NPH	Nordisk-USA	U-100
Novolin L (lente, formerly Monotard human)	Squibb-Novo	U-100
Novolin N (NPH))	Squibb-Novo	U-100
Beef		
Iletin II Lente	Lilly	U-100
Iletin II NPH	Lilly	U-100
NPH	Squibb-Novo	U-100
Pork		
Iletin II Lente	Lilly	U-100
Iletin II NPH	Lilly	U-100
Insulatard NPH	Nordisk-USA	U-100
Purified pork lente (formerly Monotard)	Squibb-Novo	U-100
Purified pork N (NPH, formerly Protaphane)	Squibb-Novo	U-100
Beef pork		
Iletin I Lente	Lilly	U-40, U-100
Iletin I NPH	Lilly	U-40, U-100
Long acting (usual onset 6–12 h; usual duration 18–36 h)		
Human		
Humulin U (Ultralente)	Lilly	U-100
Beef		
Iletin II PZI	Lilly	U-100
Purified beef U (ultralente, formerly Ultratard)	Squibb-Novo	U-100
Ultralente	Squibb-Novo	U-100
Beef pork		
Iletin I PZI	Lilly	U-40, U-100
Iletin I Ultralente	Lilly	U-40, U-100
Premixed combinations		
Human		
Novolin 70/30	Squibb-Novo	U-100
Pork		
Mixtard (30% regular, 70% NPH)	Nordisk-USA	U-100

* From Sperling MA (ed): Physician's Guide to Insulin-Dependent (Type I) Diabetes. Diagnosis and Treatment. Arlington, VA, American Diabetes Association, 1988.

diluent fluid, which should not be saline or water, either of which may alter the behavior of the insulin. Diluent fluids are usually available from the manufacturer of the insulin. Adjustments in the dose of insulin can be made, depending on the pattern of blood glucose. For example, if the blood glucose is high in the self–blood glucose monitoring (SBGM) specimen obtained before noon, the dose of the quick-acting form of insulin is increased; if the level of blood glucose in the late afternoon or evening, is high, then the longer-acting insulin is increased. Each increase should be approximately 10 per cent, and except for the stabilization period following initial diagnosis, when changes may be made daily, subsequent changes should be made at 2- to 3-day intervals depending on response.

In the belief that a closer approximation of physiologic events that result in smoother control is achieved, twice-daily injections are now routinely recommended.[87,88] Of the daily total of insulin, two thirds is generally given before breakfast and one third before the evening meal; each injection consists of intermediate- and short-acting insulin usually in the proportion of 2:1 or 3:1. For example, for a 30-kg child, a typical regimen at a dose of 1 U/kg would consist of 14 units of NPH and 6 units of regular before breakfast, and 6 units of NPH plus 4 units of regular before the evening meal. Individual adjustment can and should be made according to response. It should be emphasized that this regimen is designed for eating schedules wherein the major meal is the evening dinner. Two daily injections offer greater flexibility in adjusting to variation in food intake, especially in young children, and reduce the number of episodes of hypoglycemia. This recommendation, however, is not intended to convey an attitude of rigidity, and in selected cases a single daily injection may be preferable. Advocating a regimen that cannot and will not be followed by the patient and the family support group may be worse for the child's welfare than an attitude on the part of the health management team that permits flexibility even though optimal control is not achieved.

The technique of insulin injection should be taught to the parents and patient. Injections are given at 90° to the plane of the skin and the sites are rotated between the arms, thighs, buttocks, and abdomen. With this rotation and the availability of the pure insulins, lipodystrophic changes, either atrophy or hypertrophy, have become quite rare. The rotation also helps to ensure absorption and prevent fibrosis. Some children find the abdominal wall to be a painful site for injection; in these children this site may be omitted. Depending on the physical and psychological maturity of the individual, children over the age of 10 to 12 years should be encouraged to administer their own insulin injections, and to monitor their own responses. The assumption of responsibility for self-monitoring may be a gradual process requiring a transitional period during which the parents and child participate. Once the child has assumed total responsibility, the parents must resist a tendency to overprotection. Further guidelines on adjusting the insulin dose are provided in the following sections. However, it should be stressed that the adolescent growth spurt is regularly associated with an increase in insulin requirements that may be reduced when puberty is completed.

Development of portable insulin delivery systems that may be computer controlled and that could provide insulin in a more physiologic manner is still an area of active research. The devices that depend on continuous glucose monitoring with computer controlled insulin delivery (closed loop) are too cumbersome for long-term use and still await the development of an implantable glucose sensor. The portable devices that provide preprogrammed continuous subcutaneous insulin delivery at two rates, constant basal and meal-related increments (open loop), can be adjusted for individual needs and have been used by some highly motivated patients for long periods; blood glucose, serum lipids, hormonal profiles, and glycosylated hemoglobin can be restored and maintained at normal levels.[89–94] Widespread use of these devices in children has not been uniformly successful because of difficulty in adhering to the demands of frequent self-monitoring of blood glucose and because of potential problems, including interruption of insulin delivery in patients who have no depots of intermediate-acting insulin.[94] The promise of near-normalization of blood glucose and other indices of metabolic control has not been fulfilled through the use of insulin delivery pumps, especially in children.[94]

Hypersensitivity to insulin is uncommon in children, but local skin reactions characterized by burning, itching, tenderness, erythema, or urticaria within hours of an injection sometimes occur. These reactions usually resolve spontaneously over a period of days, but a change in the insulin, especially avoiding a mixed beef-pork preparation or switching from NPH to Lente to omit the fish protein protamine, often is helpful. Desensitization may also be necessary, as may a short course of steroids.[95] Rarely, insulin resistance develops as a result of a local tissue enzyme that destroys injected insulin; these patients require expert care in specialized hospital units. After several months of insulin therapy, nearly all patients can be demonstrated to have antibodies to insulin. In the majority, these antibodies do not interfere with metabolic response, although they may promote instability by acting as a reservoir of insulin that may be released at unpredictable times.[95] Rarely, children with insulin antibodies develop true resistance characterized by an insulin requirement in excess of 2 U/kg/day. Antibodies causing allergy are usually of the immunoglobulin (Ig) E class; IgA and IgM antibodies may be responsible for resistance.[96]

Nutrition

The word "diet" connotes restriction and denial, and may therefore induce anxiety and often rebellion on the part of parents and patient. Avoidance of the word "diet" and discussion with patients and parents about "nutritional requirements" and "meal plans" is preferable. In this context, there is no special diet for the diabetic child; rather, there are nutritional requirements that must be met for optimal growth and development.[97] In addition, since the capacity to secrete insulin in response to a meal is negligible, and since the dose of insulin is predicated on caloric intake, regularity of the eating pattern for the chosen regimen of insulin dosage is essential. In general, the nutritional requirements of diabetic children are similar to those of healthy nondiabetic children of similar age, sex, weight, and activity, eating the foods of their own cultural, social, and ethnic background.[97] The guidelines listed below are generally applicable, but the needs of each child must be separately and individually planned and adjusted.

Total caloric intake is based on size or surface area and can be obtained from standard tables. The distribution of these calories should comprise approximately 55 per cent carbohydrate, 30 per cent fat, and 15 per cent protein. Approximately 70 per cent of the carbohydrate content should be derived from complex carbohydrates such as starch, while intake of sucrose or other highly refined sugars should be avoided. Complex carbohydrates require digestion and absorption so that the plasma glucose rises slowly, whereas freely available glucose as obtained from refined sugars, including carbonated beverages, is rapidly absorbed, causing marked hyperglycemia with wide swings in the degree of metabolic control. Carbonated beverages should therefore be of the sugar-free variety. Although concern in children is centered around the potential effect of a cumulative dose, recent studies provide no evidence of an association between saccharin in the moderate doses likely to be used and bladder cancer.[98] Sorbitol and xylitol are of little value as artificial sweeteners because they are metabolized and provide additional calories. Also, they are products of the polyol pathway, which is implicated in some of the complications of diabetes.[99] Fructose has antiketogenic effects and thus might theoretically serve as a useful substitute for glucose in diabetics. However, the caloric content of fructose is equal to that of glucose.

The fat intake is adjusted so that the polyunsaturated/saturated (P/S) ratio is increased to 1.2:1.0 from the usual American average of 0.3:1.0. To achieve this desirable ratio, fats derived from animal sources are reduced and substituted by polyunsaturated fats derived from vegetable sources. This can be achieved by substituting margarine for butter, vegetable oil for animal oils in cooking, and lean cuts of beef and increased amounts of veal, skinned chicken, turkey, and fish for fatty meats such as ham, bacon, and fatty ground beef. Cholesterol intake is reduced by these measures and by limiting the number of egg yolks consumed. There is ample evidence that these simple measures reduce serum low-density lipoprotein (LDL) cholesterol, a predisposing factor to atherosclerotic disease.

The total daily caloric intake may be divided so as to provide 20 per cent at breakfast, 20 per cent at lunch, and 30 per cent at dinner, leaving 10 per cent each for a midmorning, midafternoon, and evening snack; in older children the midmorning snack may be omitted and the extra 10 per cent of balanced calories taken with lunch. Various organizations, including the American Diabetes Association (ADA) and the American Heart Association (AHA) have prepared simplified methods of providing balanced meals based on the principles outlined above.[97] The ADA's meal plans are based on the principle of food exchanges; within each exchange group of carbohydrate, protein, and fat there are a wide variety of foods that can be substituted or exchanged. Thus, for practical purposes there are few if any restrictions, and each individual may select a diet based on personal taste or preference that may be translated into the exchanges or modified with the help of a physician and/or dietitian. Emphasis should be placed on regularity of food intake and on the constancy of carbohydrate intake; substitution within the carbohydrate exchanges is permissible so long as total carbohydrate intake is constant. Occasional excesses on special occasions such as birthdays, parties, and holidays are not only permissible, but encouraged so as not to foster rebellion and stealth in obtaining desired food. Similarly, cakes, doughnuts, and candies are permissible on occasions as long as the food exchange value and carbohydrate content are considered in that day's meal plan. Special adjustments in meal planning (and insulin) must be made during the adolescent growth spurt, and with vigorous exercise. Above all, adjustments must be constantly made to meet the needs of each individual, and flexibility rather than rigidity is of the essence in children. Special brochures and pamphlets describing the exchanges and sample meal plans for children are usually available from regional diabetes groups; their use should be encouraged as part of the educational process.[97]

In recent years it has become evident that diets with high fiber content are useful in improving control of blood glucose in diabetic subjects.[100] Inclusion of about 50 gm/day of selected forms of fiber from foods such as vegetables, wholemeal bread, bran cereals, and fruits in the diets of adult diabetics has led to significant reductions in concentration not only of blood glucose but also of total and LDL cholesterol. It appears likely that diets high in fiber content will be useful in enhancing control of glucose and atherogenic serum lipids in children with diabetes.

Exercise

Exercise is an integral component of growth and development. No form of exercise, including competitive sports of any kind, should be forbidden to the diabetic child, who should not be made to feel different or restricted. Instances in which diabetics have excelled in national or international sports are not rare. Although the physiologic adaptation in energy homeostasis associated with exercise in normal and insulin-dependent diabetic adults has been extensively investigated, direct information in children is lacking.[101–103] Nevertheless, the principles are likely to be the same as in older individuals. A major complication of exercise in diabetes is the occurrence of hypoglycemic reactions during or shortly after vigorous exercise. In diabetes, the major contributing factor to hypoglycemia with exercise is an increased rate of insulin absorption from its injection site consequent upon increased blood flow in the exercising limbs.[101,102] Thus, one approach to minimize hypoglycemia is to choose an injection site least likely to be exercised. For example, if the exercise involves primarily leg muscles the upper arms are used as the injection site, and vice versa. The abdomen may be the more suitable site when both arms and legs will be used. However, from the practical point of view, exercise usually involves all limbs, with an increased blood flow throughout the body. One additional carbohydrate exchange may be taken prior to the exercise, and readily available glucose in the form of orange juice, carbonated beverage, or candy should be available during and after exercise. With experience, and trial and error, each child and parent guided by the physician learns the optimal approach. Occasionally, when exercise is programmed at regular times and is frequently associated with hypoglycemia, the daily dose of insulin may need to be reduced by 10 per cent. Exercise training also improves glucoregulation by increasing insulin receptors, and lipid metabolism by raising high-density lipoprotein (HDL) cholesterol.[101,103]

Monitoring

A major change in the management of diabetes in the past few years has been the introduction of self–blood glucose monitoring (SBGM).[104,105] It is evident that older methods of treatment of diabetes have not resulted in a satisfactory diminution of morbidity and early mortality. As is pointed out elsewhere in this chapter it is likely that lack of adequate control of the level of glucose in the blood is correlated with the high incidence of complications. Measurement of urinary glucose does not permit an accurate assessment of blood glucose concentration for the following reasons. Glucosuria does not occur until the renal threshold is exceeded, and this may vary from 150 to 250 mg/dl in different individuals and may even vary in a single person from day to day. It has been suggested that the goal of "intensive therapy" to prevent or diminish the incidence of complications is the maintenance of the blood glucose concentration between 70 and 120 mg/ml before meals and less than 180 mg/dl after meals.[86] This goal may not be achievable in some patients, and less stringent published criteria for control ("average therapy") permit the blood glucose concentration to be between 160 and 200 mg/dl before meals.[86] It is evident that urine testing is an unsatisfactory method for monitoring patients in whom these goals have been set. Urine testing also provides no information on whether the blood glucose is approaching the hypoglycemic range. Thus, although urine testing is relatively easy to perform in many clinics, it is only recommended for home use if there is a concern that ketoacidosis may be developing, and then only ketones are measured. Despite concerns that SBGM may not be practical for the care of children, when the responsible physician has explained the advantages, SBGM has been accepted in a large of number of children affected by diabetes.[106] In setting stricter standards for control and the achievement of lower concentrations of blood glucose one runs the risk of increasing the incidence of hypoglycemia. This is a distressing complication at all ages but particularly in young children, in whom the developing brain is more vulnerable to damage than in older persons. Accordingly, in young children, particularly under the age of 6 years, it may be permissible to relax the more rigid standards of control and permit somewhat higher concentrations of blood glucose.

SBGM is performed by obtaining a drop of blood from a finger, toe, heel, or earlobe and placing it on strip of paper that has been chemically impregnated to change color according to the concentration of glucose in the blood. The color is then read off on a comparison chart or quantitated in a meter. Provided that adequate precautions have been taken to follow instructions to ensure that the specimen has been handled appropriately, results of this method of testing are quite satisfactory. A variety of automatic spring-loaded devices are available to reduce the pain and discomfort that is inevitable. A list of the commercially available finger-prick devices, test strips for visual reading, and blood glucose meters is provided on page 42 of reference 86.

The number of times that SBGM is performed over the day varies. Ideally, the blood glucose concentration before each meal and before bedtime should be known. Generally such a schedule of blood testing is not possible. Properly educated and motivated patients will perform SBGM two or three times daily for extended periods of time.[86] SBGM is also invaluable to determine the presence of nocturnal hypoglycemia, the Somogyi phenomenon, and the dawn phenomenon, as are discussed elsewhere in this chapter. The use of paper strips for SBGM has the additional advantage of providing an authentic record of the patient's self-monitoring. They should be brought to the physician at each visit as part of the records maintained by the patient.

Measurement of glycosylated hemoglobin (GHb) in blood provides a most useful index of control.[107,108] Hemoglobin A_{1c} is usually measured and taken to quantitate the hemoglobin to which glucose has been nonenzymatically attached. Because the reaction between glucose and amino groups of hemoglobin is slow, proportional to the prevailing blood glucose concentration, and continues as an irreversible reaction throughout the 120-day life span of the red blood cell, the level of GHb is a reflection of the integrated "time-averaged" blood glucose concentration over the preceding 2 to 3 months.[107,108] The test procedure, when properly performed in the laboratory, is not invalidated by an isolated episode of hyperglycemia nor is it subject to manipulation as are reported blood test results. In this regard, measurement of GHb is superior to random or fasting blood glucose measurements, which reflect an isolated instance in the continuum of metabolic change. Moreover, the stress of obtaining blood may be sufficient to raise blood glucose concentration, upon which is based the assessment of control or the recommended changes in insulin dosage. Consequently, GHb measurement provides an objective index of compliance and long-term control. Periodic evaluation by GHb measurement may also help resolve questions relating the degree of control to the subsequent development of complications. Care should be taken to ensure that the method used to measure HbA_{1c} removes the unstable fraction that rapidly forms during hyperglycemia and that can spuriously elevate HbA_{1c} levels.[108] Also, fetal hemoglobin elutes with glycohemoglobin in some assays, giving spuriously high values for HbA$_1$ in patients with thalassemia major and in infants. Conversely, patients with sickle cell trait (HbS) may have spuriously low levels of HbA$_1$ in certain assays. Thus, knowledge of potential hemoglobinopathy is important for correct interpretation of reported HbA$_1$ values, particularly when clinical impression is not congruent with test results.[108] These discrepancies occur because HbA$_{1c}$ and HbA$_1$ do not specifically represent GHb but rather fractions of hemoglobin that have different mobilities in electrophoretic analyses than the major fraction HbA. While interaction of glucose with hemoglobin changes its electrophoretic mobility, the fractions found in the HbA$_{1c}$ and HbA$_1$ bands contain moieties that are not glycosylated. Moreover, hemoglobin glycosylated at sites other than the NH$_2$-terminus of the beta chain is not found in the HbA$_{1c}$ and the HbA$_1$ fractions.[109]

Other measurements that should made at least once yearly include thyroxine and thyroid-stimulating hormone. After the disease has been present for 4 or 5 years, specimens of urine collected over 24 hours should be checked for microalbuminaria (an early indication of the presence of nephropathy). The patient should also be examined by an ophthalmologist, preferably one skilled in the early detection of the ocular complications of diabetes.

Natural History

The "Honeymoon" Period

After the initial presentation and stabilization, some 75 per cent of children require a progressive reduction in their insulin dose from approximately 1 U/kg to daily doses of 0.5 U/kg or less. Often recurrent hypoglycemia is the manifestation that prompts a reduction in recommended insulin dose. A minority of children actually can maintain normoglycemia in the absence of any administered insulin; this complete remission occurs in only 2 per cent or less of diabetics, but even in these patients glucose tolerance tests still demonstrate abnormal carbohydrate metabolism. The duration of the honeymoon phase is variable; it commonly lasts several weeks to months, but may last as long as 1 to 2 years. Recent investigations clearly demonstrate that residual insulin secretion, measured as C peptide, is present during this remission period and to a lesser extent for a variable period of several

years.[1,3] Virtually all diabetics have substantial C peptide secretion in the initial 2 years of disease, and approximately 20 per cent will have some C peptide response even after 5 years of clinical disease.[3] Stable, well-controlled diabetic subjects have higher C peptide secretion than nonstable subjects, and the required dose of insulin is inversely correlated to basal or stimulated C peptide response.

The reasons why this residual insulin secretion is inadequate to prevent the evolution of diabetes, including ketoacidosis, are not totally clear but presumably relate to stress-provoked secretion of catecholamines and other hormones that inhibit still further the insulin secretory capacity of the pancreatic beta cells as well as antagonizing insulin action at the periphery. In any event, the clinical remission phase is limited and, with isolated exceptions, clinical insulin-dependent diabetes inevitably recurs as a result of progressive destruction of β cells (Fig. 4–2). Although expert opinion varies, it is advisable to maintain insulin treatment unless a daily dose of 0.1 U/kg still causes hypoglycemia. If this occurs, insulin treatment may be discounted and the patient tested periodically for the reemergence of glucosuria. The physician may decide to completely discontinue insulin treatment if this appears to be in the patient's best interests. However, the patient and family should not be led to believe that the disease is "cured."

Hypoglycemic Reactions

All diabetic children experience a hypoglycemic reaction at sometime during the course of their disease. Hypoglycemia occurs suddenly or over minutes, in contrast to DKA, which develops over hours or days. The symptoms and signs are those due to an outpouring of catecholamines, including trembling, shaking, sweating, apprehension, and tachycardia, and those due to cerebral glucopenia, including hunger, drowsiness, mood or personality changes, mental confusion, seizures, and coma. There is now some evidence that these symptoms may occur with a sudden drop in blood glucose to levels that would not meet the criteria for hypoglycemia (less than 60 mg/dl) in healthy subjects.[110] The avoidance of severe hypoglycemic episodes should be a major objective of treatment; they have been implicated in ultimately provoking epileptic seizures and there is an increased frequency of abnormal electroencephalographic findings in diabetics.

The occurrence of hypoglycemia in a diabetic child indicates an inappropriate level of insulin effect for that individual's energy intake and expenditure. Common causes include the evolution of the honeymoon phase after initial diagnosis, deliberate or accidental errors in insulin dosage, inadequate caloric intake through missing meals, and exercise in the absence of increasing caloric intake. The most important factor in the treatment of hypoglycemia is education for patient and family to be familiar with the symptoms and signs and to avoid known precipitating factors outlined above. Acutely, a carbohydrate-containing snack, or a drink such as orange juice or sugar-containing carbonated beverage, or candy (each equivalent to 5 to 10 gm of glucose) should be taken. Patients, parents, and teachers should also be instructed in the use of glucagon; 0.5 mg given intramuscularly is particularly useful when the patient is losing consciousness or is vomiting. If exercise has been the precipitating factor, the patient should be instructed to take additional calories prior to exercise and, if hypoglycemia persists, to reduce the morning dose of insulin by 10 to 20 per cent.

The Somogyi and Dawn Phenomena

Hypoglycemic episodes that may be mild, that manifest as late nocturnal or early morning sweating, night terrors, headaches, and that alternate rapidly within 4 to 6 hours with ketosis, hyperglycemia, ketonuria, and severe glucosuria should arouse the suspicion of the Somogyi phenomenon. This syndrome has been aptly described as "hypoglycemia begetting hyperglycemia" and is believed to be due to an outpouring of counterregulatory hormones in response to insulin-induced hypoglycemia.[111,112,113] Occurrence of brittle diabetes in patients receiving daily insulin doses of more than 2 U/kg suggests that the phenomenon is present. Brittle diabetes implies that blood glucose concentrations fluctuate widely and rapidly, despite frequent upward adjustment of the insulin dose. Seventy per cent of patients in one series of 100 diabetic children were considered to be receiving insulin in excessive dosage; of those whose diabetes was considered unstable 90 per cent were being overdosed, and the dose

could be reduced by an average of 38 per cent in the whole group.[111] Thus, the Somogyi phenomenon may be a common cause of the instability or brittleness of diabetes in children. Appropriate treatment consists of reducing the dose of insulin to eliminate hypoglycemia. The early morning rise in blood glucose following recognized or unrecognized nocturnal hypoglycemia may also be the result of waning of activity of biologically available insulin unrelated to the action of counterregulatory hormones.[112,113]

The Somogyi phenomenon should be distinguished from the dawn phenomenon, defined as significant early morning hyperglycemia in the absence of antecedent hypoglycemia.[113,114] Normal persons are able to increase their insulin secretion to compensate for the nocturnal surges in growth hormone that antagonize insulin action. Because the early morning increase in insulin secretion does not occur in the diabetic, there is a rapid rise in the blood glucose concentration between 2 AM and 6 AM in the absence of antecedent hypoglycemia. Recognition of this condition may require measurement of blood glucose between 2 AM and 6 AM. Hypoglycemia is absent but a rapid increase from relatively normoglycemic levels to high blood glucose levels begins between 4 and 6 AM and may extend into the later morning, complicating the management of the diabetes.[113,114] Dealing with the dawn phenomenon requires measures such as a delay in the timing of the injection of intermediate-acting insulin or reduction in the size of the prebedtime snack.[114]

It may be difficult to distinguish between the Somogyi and dawn phenomena without home blood glucose monitoring, and parents or the patient are required on two or three occasions to monitor blood glucose concentrations between 2 AM and 6 AM. With the Somogyi phenomenon, the evening intermediate-acting insulin dose may need to be decreased. With the dawn phenomenon, the intermediate-acting insulin in the evening should be delayed. In the case of a highly motivated patient or family, three injections are prescribed, the usual combined short- and intermediate-acting insulin dose in the morning, a short-acting preparation dose at supper time, and an intermediate-acting insulin dose, delayed until approximately 9 PM.[88,113,114] This regimen may also be helpful in treatment of the Somogyi phenomenon by delaying the peak effect of the intermediate-acting insulin until approximately just before breakfast. Clearly, the appropriate at-home management would not be possible without determination of blood glucose profiles, now achieved by home blood glucose monitoring.[88,113,114]

Psychological Aspects

Diabetes in a child affects the life-style and interpersonal relationship of the entire family unit.[115,116] Feelings of anxiety and guilt are common in parents. Similar feelings coupled with denial and rejection are equally common in children, particularly during the normally rebellious teenage years. No specific personality disorder or psychopathology is characteristic of diabetes; similar feelings are observed in families with other chronic disorders.

In diabetics, these feelings find expression in nonadherence to instructions regarding nutrition and insulin therapy, or noncompliance with self-monitoring. Deliberate overdosing with insulin resulting in hypoglycemia, and omission of insulin or excesses in nutrition resulting in ketoacidosis, may be disguised pleas for psychological help or stratagems to escape family surroundings perceived as undesirable or intolerable, but occasionally are portents of suicidal intent. Overprotection on the part of parents is frequent, and often not in the best interests of the patient. Feelings of being different or of being alone are common, and not unjustified in view of the restrictions imposed by schedules requiring blood testing, insulin administration, and nutritional limitations. Perception of the likelihood of developing complications and of decreased life span in type I diabetes fosters anxiety. In addition, misinformation abounds regarding the risk of developing diabetes in siblings or offspring, or the risk of becoming severely ill during pregnancy.

Many, but not all, of these problems can be avoided by understanding, patience, counseling based on correct information, and the fostering of attitudes that permit perception of the patient not as a cripple but rather as a productive and potentially reproductive member of society. Recognizing the impact of these real and potential problems, various local and regional associations have organized peer discussion groups; feelings of isolation and frustration may be mitigated by the realization that others are also affected and share common problems. Summer camps for children, organized by various organizations, afford an excellent opportunity for learning and sharing under expert supervision. Reinforcement of education regarding diabetes, insulin dosage and technique of administration, nutrition, exercise, and hypoglycemic reactions can be performed via medical and paramedical personnel. The company of many peers with similar problems permits the development of newer insights for the diabetic child.

Infections and Trauma

In the child with diabetes, systemic or local infections are no more common than in nondiabetic children. During episodes of infection or trauma, diabetic children should take additional insulin: 10 to 20 per cent of the total daily insulin dose should be administered as the regular (short-acting) form before each meal if blood glucose monitoring shows that hyperglycemia is occurring.

Patients who are vomiting should be advised not to discontinue insulin injections, although the dose may be reduced by 50 per cent. If vomiting continues and the patient cannot tolerate clear liquids, admission to the hospital, and consideration of intravenous therapy with glucose and electrolytes, is warranted.

Surgery in the Diabetic Child

If surgery is elective, the patient should be admitted 24 hours prior to surgery, and the usual nutritional requirements and insulin provided. Supplemental regular insulin may also be given to achieve more optimal control of blood glucose. On the morning of surgery an infusion of 5 per cent glucose in 0.45 per cent saline plus 20 mEq of potassium chloride per liter is begun, and regular insulin is added to the infusate bottle so that 1 U of insulin is provided for each 2 to 4 gm of administered glucose. The blood glucose concentration should be monitored at periodic intervals before, during, and after surgery so that glucose levels remain at approximately 120 to 150 mg/dl through appropriate changes in the dose of insulin and/or glucose delivered. This regimen may be continued during the operative and postoperative period and discontinued when the patient is awake and capable of ingesting food and fluid. The rate of infusion should provide maintenance fluid requirements plus estimated losses during surgery. During the time when liquid foods are ingested, prior to intake of solid foods, regular insulin should be administered in a dosage of 0.2 U/kg at 6-hour intervals, with appropriate adjustments based on blood glucose profiles. When solid food is tolerated the insulin regimen used prior to surgery can be reinstituted. The care of the patient should be under the guidance of a physician experienced in diabetes, working in conjunction with the responsible surgeon.

An alternative and equally effective approach is to begin the electrolyte and glucose infusion on the morning of surgery, omit the intravenous insulin, and administer one half of the usual morning dose of insulin. Following recovery from anesthesia, subcutaneous regular insulin is given, 0.2 U/kg, and the dose repeated, increased, or decreased at 6-hour intervals, depending on the level of blood glucose, until the patient can fully tolerate the appropriate nutritional requirement, when the insulin regimen used prior to surgery can be reinstituted. This approach is particularly useful for surgery of short duration.

If emergency surgery needs to be undertaken, an intravenous line that provides 5 to 10 per cent glucose in 0.45 per cent saline plus 20 mEq of potassium chloride per liter is begun and insulin is added to the infusate so as to provide 1 U for each 2 to 4 gm of glucose infused. Again blood glucose concentration should be maintained at approximately 120 to 150 mg/dl. Where possible, rehydration and metabolic balance should be achieved before surgery is begun. Following surgery, the regimen described above can be instituted. Patients undergoing minor surgery under local anesthesia can have their usual insulin and food intake; losses through vomiting should be replaced by intravenous fluids.

The desirable objectives in managing a diabetic child who has surgery are to prevent hypoglycemia during anesthesia, severe fluid loss, or diabetic acidosis. The regimens described above are generally applicable, but vigilance and individual adjustment for each patient are necessary to achieve these desirable goals.

Neurovascular and Other Complications: Relation to Control

It has become apparent that the increasing survival of the diabetic child as a result of the availability of insulin, fluid and electrolyte therapy, antibiotics, and modern anesthesia is associated with an increasing incidence of complications that affect the microcirculation of the eye (retinopathy) and kidney (nephropathy) and the nerves (neuropathy) as well as large vessels and optic lens (cataracts). Statistics compiled by the National Diabetes Data Group indicate that retinopathy is present in 45 to 60 per cent of insulin-dependent diabetics after 20 years of disease and in 20 per cent after 10 years.[117] The incidence of proliferative retinopathy increases progressively with increasing duration of disease. Lens opacities are present in some 5 per cent of diabetics aged less than 19 years.[117] Diabetic nephropathy is also common (up to an incidence of 40 per cent after 25 years of diabetes in children), and renal disease may account for about half of the deaths in long-term insulin-dependent diabetics.[118] The arguments for and against a relationship between the degree of control and subsequent development of these complications has been summarized and reviewed in detail.[118–120] The bulk of clinical, experimental, and biochemical studies strongly suggest an association between control and later development of complications, although genetic predisposition or resistance to development of these complications also play a role.[120] In addition, these studies implicate some possible biochemical pathways that may be responsible for these complications. For example, the degree of glycosylation of proteins, which is proportional to the blood glucose concentration, is not restricted to hemoglobin but also affects other serum as well as tissue proteins and enzymes, a mechanism that has been implicated in some complications such as basement membrane thickening.[121] There is evidence that activation of the polyol pathway and disturbances in myoinositol metabolism are related to cataracts and neuropathy.[99,119] Typical lesions of diabetic nephropathy develop in normal kidneys within several years of their being transplanted to diabetics with chronic renal failure, and reversal of early changes has been reported in diabetic kidneys transplanted to nondiabetic recipients, implying that it is the diabetic environment and not genetic background that predisposes to these renal changes.[122,123] There has been a consistent failure to demonstrate any diabetic complications in the nonaffected identical twin of an insulin-dependent diabetic even after 20 years of recognized disease,[124] although genetic predisposition plays a role, as, for example, with hypertension and the risk of renal disease.[125,126]

Debate continues, however, because available modes of treatment have, until now, resulted in varying degrees of imperfect metabolic control without restoration of the fine moment-to-moment regulation of normal physiologic events. The potential relationship between degree of control and complications is currently under investigation in a multicenter trial, the Diabetes Control and Complications Trial (DCCT).[126] As long as reduction in incidence of these late complications remains a possibility, physicians treating children with diabetes have an enormous responsibility of maintaining as near normal metabolism as is compatible with the physical and psychological well-being of each child. Despite the potential for developing complications, survival for 40 years or more is feasible.[127]

Limited joint mobility due to thickening of the periarticular connective tissue of the fingers is a frequent complication of diabetes.[128,129] Aside from the difficulties resulting from the restriction of movement of the fingers, the complication is of importance because its incidence appears to correlate well with the development of microvascular disease.

Some complications, such as diabetic dwarfism associated with a glycogen-laden enlarged liver, are clearly related to under-insulinization, but this syndrome is only rarely encountered since the introduction of the longer acting insulins. The osteopenia that has been reported in diabetic children may be related to glycemic control, but this defect has no clinical relevance in the pediatric population.[129]

Long-Term Outcome

This outline of the long-term complications of insulin-dependent diabetes in children indicates that type I diabetes mellitus is not a benign disease. In 45 children less than 12 years of age at the time of diagnosis, there were 7 deaths within 10 to 25 years of diagnosis; 3 were directly attributable to diabetes and 2 more were due to suicide, with an additional 3 patients having attempted suicide.[130] Visual, renal, neuropathic, and other complications were frequent. Although diabetic children eventually attain

an adult height within the normal range, their final height is less than their genetic potential, and puberty may be considerably delayed.[131] Thus, compared to their unaffected identical twins, diabetics despite apparently satisfactory control experience delayed puberty and a substantial reduction in height with a mean difference of 5 cm when onset of disease is before puberty. When both twins were affected before puberty or when onset in one twin was after puberty, these differences in height and age at puberty were no longer present.[131] These findings indicate that conventional criteria for judging control had been inadequate, that control of insulin-dependent diabetes is almost never achieved by conventional means unless home monitoring of glucose and frequent insulin injections are used, and that the resolution of these problems remains a matter of urgency. In pilot studies, meticulous control was found to restore growth velocity including catch-up growth, correct hormonal derangements, and partially reverse or correct some objective derangements such as microalbuminuria or impaired nerve conduction velocity.[118–120,127] Nowhere is the impact of metabolic control more apparent than in pregnancy in a patient with type I diabetes and in fetal outcome.

Diabetes in Pregnancy

Type I diabetes mellitus complicates about 1:400 (0.25 per cent) pregnancies. Experience indicates that successful outcome for mother and baby is more likely when optimal metabolic control is maintained throughout and even preceding pregnancy.[132–134] When care is supervised by a team that includes physicians knowledgeable in the management of the pregnant diabetic and her newborn, perinatal mortality is similar to that of the general population. The risk of fetal morbidity and mortality is increased severalfold in poorly controlled diabetic pregnancy and also declines to near normal frequency with meticulous metabolic control.[132–134] Thus, there is strong impetus to attain metabolism as near normal as possible before conception and to maintain it throughout gestation. While there is general agreement on this objective, it is not always achieved and morbidity in mother and baby remain significant.[135–137] Many of the problems in both mother and fetus stem from the impact of diabetes on the normal metabolic adaptations of pregnancy.

Metabolism during Pregnancy

Normal pregnancy is characterized by insulin resistance, mediated largely by human placental lactogen (hPL), a hormone similar to growth hormone in both structure and function. Human placental lactogen is produced by the syncytiotrophoblast in increasing amounts as placental mass grows. The insulin resistance and increased lipolysis induced by this hormone are normally compensated by increased insulin secretion, which facilitates anabolic processes in the fed state. During fasting, when hPL levels remain high while insulin secretion is reduced, lipolysis with release of free fatty acids and formation of ketones as well as enhanced gluconeogenesis are the rule. The free fatty acids are utilized for maternal energy, while glucose is spared for fetal use. Ketosis appears sooner during fasting in pregnancy than in the nonpregnant state. Thus, accelerated catabolism, manifest as ketosis, appears during maternal fasting of relatively short duration (e.g. after missing breakfast).

In the early stages of pregnancy, there is a propensity for hypoglycemia in IDDM. This is due in part to the consumption of glucose by the developing conceptus before sufficient hPL is synthesized to antagonize exogenously administered insulin. In contrast, the second and third trimesters of pregnancy are characterized by an increasing insulin requirement of from 30 to 100 per cent to offset the anti-insulin effects of increasing hPL production. Thus, inadequate monitoring and inadequate upward adjustment of insulin may rapidly lead to diabetic ketoacidosis, a poor prognostic factor for fetal survival. On the other hand, a hypoglycemic episode late in the third trimester, in the absence of an obvious cause such as an error in insulin or omitted meal, implies a "failing placenta" that may require immediate action to deliver the infant. Adolescents with type I diabetes are most likely to fit in classes B and C of the modified White classification of pregnant diabetic women; adolescents are not likely to have vascular disease complicating diabetes.

The Infant of the Diabetic Mother

The infant of the diabetic mother has traditionally been viewed as a fat, plethoric, "giant" baby characterized by certain stigmata and complications in utero and in the immediate newborn period.[135,136] In utero, the complications are fetal death and stillbirth, congenital malformations, and macrosomia sometimes leading to traumatic delivery because of cephalopelvic disproportion.[132–134]

Fetal death and stillbirth are now uncommon but still occur, particularly with poor glycemic control, ketoacidosis, hydramnios, and preeclampsia. Expert management can reduce the risk of death and stillbirth while avoiding premature delivery and its complications through appropriate timing of the delivery. Fetal lung maturity is determined by measuring standard lecithin-sphingomyelin ratios and phosphatidylglycerol in amniotic fluid. Fetal hyperinsulinemia has been implicated as a factor responsible for fetal hypoxia that may contribute to death in utero.

Occurrence of major congenital malformations of the heart and brain and the caudal regression syndrome, including sacral agenesis, remains a major problem in pregnancy complicated by IDDM. Evidence in experimental animals and in women indicates that poor control is a major risk factor for congenital malformations.[132,133] The rate at which congenital malformations occur is reduced toward rates found in nondiabetic pregnancy by intensive treatment to attain near-normal glycemia before conception and maintain it throughout gestation.[132] Nevertheless, the rate of congenital malformations generally remains higher in diabetic pregnancy, about two- to fourfold the 2 per cent rate in nondiabetic pregnancy, and this accounts for one third to one half of all perinatal deaths in diabetic pregnancy.[132–134]

Macrosomia and several other complications, such as neonatal hypoglycemia (see Chapter 5) hypocalcemia, respiratory distress syndrome, and hyperbilirubinemia with polycythemia, including their sequelae, all are believed to have their genesis in the Pedersen hypothesis as outlined in Figure 4–3. Briefly, the inadequacy of maternal insulin results in an excess of circulating substrates such as glucose and amino acids that cross the placenta to the fetus. In addition, the polyuria consequent to maternal hyperglycemia may deplete maternal and hence fetal magnesium stores. The surfeit of circulating nutrients in the fetus promotes earlier maturation of insulin secretion, beta

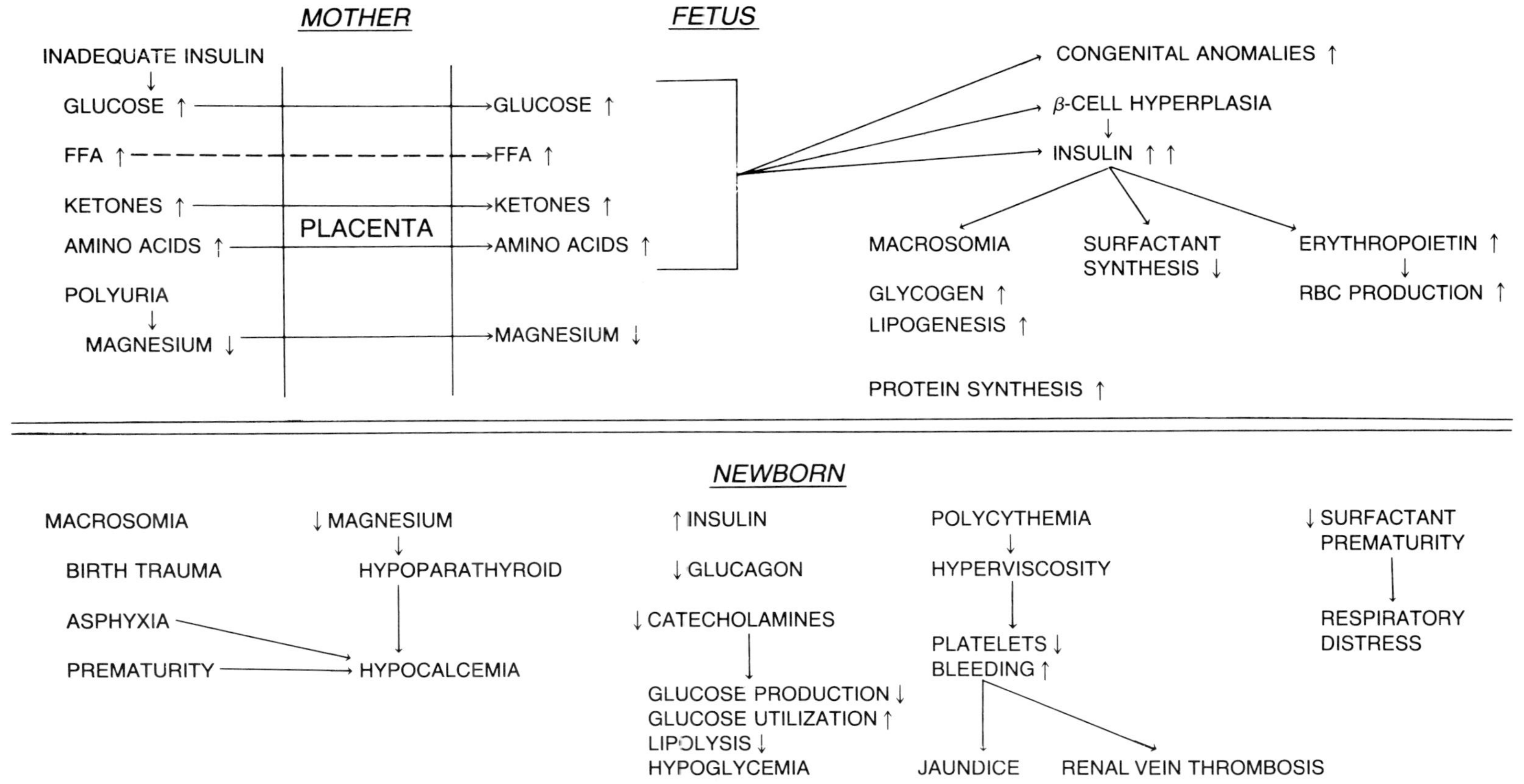

FIGURE 4–3. Proposed pathophysiology of development of abnormalities in the infant of the diabetic mother. Note that all the fetal and neonatal complications are attributed to the consequences of metabolic disturbances in the mother following inadequate insulin. This scheme is an adaptation of the Pedersen hypothesis as detailed in the text and refs 132–134.

cell hyperplasia, and fetal hyperinsulinemia. Hyperinsulinemia promotes macrosomia, impairs surfactant synthesis, and directly stimulates erythropoietin formation. It also is responsible for localized (ventricular septum) or generalized cardiac hypertrophy.[138] These factors combine to produce the well-known complications of the newborn infant born to a mother with insulin-dependent diabetes. There is considerable evidence for each of the proposed mechanisms and steps outlined in Figure 4–3, although knowledge regarding these aspects is far from complete.[132–137] Increasingly, however, evidence indicates that meticulous metabolic control during the third trimester of pregnancy reduces the rate and extent of these complications, just as meticulous metabolic control periconceptually during the critical 6- to 8-week period of organogenesis reduces the rate of congenital malformations.[132–137]

These concepts imply that care of an adolescent female with IDDM must include frank discussion concerning possible pregnancy, its impact on the patient, and the impact of diabetes on the offspring. Contraception should be available to those who do not wish to become pregnant. Young women who do not have vascular complications may be advised to use low-dose combined estrogen and progesterone birth control pills. If vascular complications or hypertension are present a progestin-only pill, or some other form of contraception, should be used.[86] For those who actively seek pregnancy, the importance of metabolic control before conception and during gestation must be emphasized. Adherence to the more stringent programs of self-monitoring and insulin administration is usually excellent, given the exceptionally high motivation for successful outcome in a wanted pregnancy. Monitoring of maternal and fetal well-being during pregnancy, optimal timing of delivery, its site, and management, and expert postnatal care to the newborn must be planned and integrated to involve appropriate specialists. Details of these aspects can be found in relevant reviews concerning diabetes and pregnancy, and the management of the newborn.[132–137]

TYPE II NON-INSULIN-DEPENDENT DIABETES AND IMPAIRED GLUCOSE TOLERANCE IN CHILDHOOD

In the general pediatric population, mass screening for abnormalities in carbohydrate intolerance via the oral glucose tolerance test has not been successful in identifying significant numbers of children with abnormalities[139]; mass screening methods for detection of diabetes by measuring urinary glucose are of little value in children. Attempts at early recognition of children considered at greater risk for the development of diabetes have identified a number of individuals with abnormalities in glucose tolerance, but of these only some 10 per cent or less progress to develop overt diabetes mellitus.[139,140] Precise indices of risk are not known, but children who may be considered at greater than normal risk include close relatives (including identical twins) of known diabetics, children who have stress glucosuria, or children who have symptoms suggestive of reactive postprandial hypoglycemia.[20] These patients constitute a group with an increased statistical risk and may be considered to have a potential abnormality of glucose tolerance (see Table 4–1)[20]; they also are the subjects of efforts to identify IDDM before the onset of clinical symptoms.[23]

When a glucose tolerance test is performed, it should be standardized according to the currently accepted criteria.[20] These include at least 3 days of standard diet containing 50 per cent of calories from carbohydrate, fasting from midnight before the morning of the test procedure, and a dose of glucose at 1.75 gm/kg not to exceed a total of 75 gm. The definition of abnormality is determined from the blood glucose response over the next 2 hours as outlined in Table 4–1. It must be emphasized that an oral glucose tolerance test is not indicated in children who have typical symptoms of diabetes and a random blood glucose in excess of 200 mg/dl.[20] Determination of serum insulin concentration has proven a useful research tool since those children with substantially reduced insulin response are more likely to progress to overt diabetes.[20,140] However, more recently first-phase insulin response, the sum of insulin values measured 1 and 3 min after a bolus of intravenous glucose, coupled with islet cell antibody (ICA) measurement, is being used as a screening method to detect persons considered to have evolving type I diabetes.[23,65–67]

The glucose responses during oral glucose tolerance testing are very similar in normal children at all ages. Consequently, the criteria outlined in Table 4–1 are applicable at all ages. These criteria are based on recommendations of the National Diabetes Data Group.[20] In contrast to glucose values, insulin responses during glucose tolerance testing show a progressive increase with growth from the age of 3 years through a mean age of 15 years. Glucose values are therefore a more reliable index of abnormality than the corresponding insulin values, which require adjustment for age and puberty.[34,35]

The term *impaired glucose tolerance* has been used in preference to previous terms such as *chemical diabetes, subclinical diabetes,* or *latent diabetes.* These latter terms imply a definitive prelude to the disease diabetes, whereas in reality abnormal oral glucose tolerance on repeat testing may show spontaneous shifts in the direction of improvement or stability for many years.[20] Even patients with subnormal insulin responses to oral glucose may not show further deterioration, but it is in this category that progression to overt diabetes is most likely to develop.[23,140] First-phase insulin response to a pulse of intravenous glucose, coupled with ICA measurement, may prove to be more discriminating.[23,65-67] The intent of using the term *impaired glucose tolerance* is to avoid the stigma associated with the term *diabetes.* This stigma can influence the choice of vocation, availability of insurance, and self-image. The use of oral hypoglycemic agents for these children has been investigated in clinical trials with inconclusive results,[139] probably because they are most likely normal or evolving into type I diabetes. Oral hypoglycemic agents should therefore be restricted to investigations and not routinely used in children.

In those children who go on to develop fasting hyperglycemia, insulin may be necessary for correction of hyperglycemia but ketosis may not develop. Thus, these children, most of whom are adolescents, have the characteristics of insulin-requiring but not insulin-dependent diabetes (type II), previously called maturity-onset diabetes. The term *maturity-onset diabetes of the young* (MODY) has been applied to these subjects.[58,140] As a group, MODY may contain individuals who do not require insulin even after many years of follow-up. The striking distinguishing feature among this group is the strong family history of non-insulin-requiring diabetes in 85 per cent of cases. In approximately one half of the affected families, there is direct vertical trans-

mission of this form of diabetes through three generations, and 50 per cent of tested siblings have impaired glucose tolerance. Chlorpropramide-induced alcohol flushing has been demonstrated in many of these patients.[58] The chlorpropramide alcohol flush was considered to represent sensitivity to the endogenous opiate enkephalin. Thus, MODY may represent a separate genetic entity with a better prognosis for longevity and possibly fewer vascular complications.[58]

DISEASES ASSOCIATED WITH CHILDHOOD DIABETES

Cystic Fibrosis and Diabetes Mellitus

Because of improvement in medical care, many children with cystic fibrosis now survive to the late teens and early adult years. In addition to the primary insufficiency of pancreatic exocrine function, there is a high incidence of pancreatic endocrine dysfunction, manifesting as glucose intolerance and progressing occasionally to overt diabetes mellitus.[141] When hyperglycemia develops, the accompanying metabolic derangements are usually mild and, when insulin therapy becomes necessary, relatively low doses suffice for adequate management. Ketoacidosis is uncommon in this group but can occur as pancreatic endocrine function progressively deteriorates. Treatment with insulin is as outlined for type I diabetes, but dietary management may be limited by the constraints of the primary malabsorption.

Autoimmune Diseases

Chronic lymphocytic thyroiditis (Hashimoto thyroiditis) is frequently associated with type I diabetes in children (Chapter 3). The prevalence of thyroid cytoplasmic antibodies in the sera of patients with type I diabetes is 2 to 20 times the rate found in control populations, and as many as 1:5 insulin-dependent diabetics may have thyroid antibodies in their serum.[44,45] However, only a small proportion go on to develop clinical hypothyroidism and in these the interval between diagnosis of diabetes and thyroid disease is, on the average, 5 years. Therefore, routine palpation of the thyroid gland in all children with insulin-dependent diabetes is recommended. If the gland feels firm and/or enlarged, thyroid antibodies and serum thyroid-stimulating hormone

(TSH) concentrations should be measured. A TSH level of greater than 10 μU/ml indicates existing or incipient failure of thyroid function, which warrants replacement with thyroid hormone. A slowing in the rate of growth may also indicate thyroid failure and suggests the need for measurements of serum thyroxine and TSH concentration. Because thyroid disease may not become evident for a long time some pediatric endocrinologists measure serum thyroxine and TSH at least once yearly. When two features such as diabetes and thyroid disease coexist, the possibility of adrenal insufficiency should be borne in mind (Chapter 3). This may be heralded by decreasing insulin requirements (due to an increasing frequency of hypoglycemia), increasing pigmentation of the skin and buccal mucosa, salt craving, weakness, asthenia, postural hypotension, or frank addisonian crisis indicating primary adrenal failure. This syndrome is most unusual in the first decade of life but may become apparent in the second decade of life or later.[26,27] Those with autoimmune disturbances involving multiple endocrine glands are more likely to have association with the HLA-DR3 antigen and to have persistence of islet cell antibodies for many years.[45,52]

In addition to thyroid and adrenal disease, circulating antibodies to gastric parietal cells, or to intrinsic factor, are two to three times more common in patients with type I diabetes than in normal subjects. There is a good correlation between the existence of gastric parietal cell antibodies and the presence of atrophic gastritis, and between circulating antibodies to intrinsic factor and malabsorption of vitamin B_{12}. Thus, the possibility of megaloblastic anemia should be considered in type I diabetes, although its occurrence in children is rare.[44]

A variant of the multiple endocrine deficiency syndrome is characterized by type I diabetes, idiopathic intestinal mucosal atrophy with inflammation and severe malabsorption, IgA deficiency, and circulating antibodies to multiple endocrine organs, including thyroid, adrenal, pancreas, parathyroid, and gonads. In addition, nonaffected family members have an increased frequency of vitiligo, Graves disease, low complement levels, and multiple sclerosis, and a high frequency of antibodies to endocrine tissue.

Rare Genetic Syndromes

A number of rare genetic syndromes associated with insulin-dependent diabetes mellitus or with carbohydrate intolerance have been described.[20] These syndromes represent a broad spectrum of diseases from premature cellular aging, as in the Werner or Cockayne syndromes, to marked obesity associated with hyperinsulinism, resistance to insulin action, and carbohydrate intolerance, as in the Prader-Willi syndrome. Some of these syndromes are characterized by primary disturbances in the insulin receptor or in antibodies to the insulin receptor without any impairment in insulin secretion.[16–20] Although rare, these syndromes provide unique models to study the multiple etiologies of disturbed carbohydrate metabolism from defective insulin secretion, or from defective insulin action at the cell receptor or postreceptor step.[16–20] These syndromes are briefly summarized in Table 4–9.

TRANSIENT DIABETES OF THE NEWBORN

Onset of persistent, insulin-dependent diabetes before the age of 6 months is most unusual. The syndrome of transient diabetes mellitus in the newborn has its onset in the first week of life and is self-limited in duration, lasting only several weeks to months before spontaneous resolution.[142,143] It occurs almost invariably in infants who are small for gestational age and is characterized by hyperglycemia and pronounced glucosuria resulting in severe dehydration, but with only minimal or no ketonemia or ketonuria. An insulin secretory response to glucose or tolbutamide is low or absent; basal insulin concentration is normal. Following spontaneous recovery, the insulin responses to these same stimuli are brisk and normal. The syndrome may be due to immaturity of cAMP generation within islets.[143] Occurrence of the syndrome in consecutive siblings has been reported. Permanent diabetes has not recurred in any affected infant who has recovered. The syndrome of transient diabetes of the newborn should be distinguished from severe hyperglycemia occurring in diseases associated with abnormalities of the central nervous system and disturbances of electrolytes. These patients are usually older infants rather than newborns, and they respond

TABLE 4–9. CONDITIONS AND SYNDROMES ASSOCIATED WITH DIABETES MELLITUS AND IMPAIRED GLUCOSE TOLERANCE*

Pancreatic Disease	Hormonal	Insulin Receptor Abnormalities	Genetic Syndromes

Neonatal
  Congenital absence of
    the pancreatic islets
  Transient diabetes of
    the newborn
  Functional immaturity
    of insulin secretion
Postinfancy
  Acquired—trauma,
    infections, etc.
  Inherited cystic
    fibrosis, hereditary
    relapsing
    pancreatitis,
    hemochromatosis
	Hypoinsulinemic—
	  Endocrine overactivity
	    Catecholamines, e.g.,
	      pheochromocytoma
	    Somatostatinoma
	    Mineralocorticoids, e.g.,
	      aldosteronoma
	  Underactivity
	    Hypoparthyroidism-hypocalcemia
	    Type I isolated growth hormone
	      deficiency
	    Multitropic pituitary deficiency
	    Laron dwarfism
	    Hypothalamic lesions—"Piqure"
	      diabetes (of Claude Bernard)
	Hyperinsulinemic—states of insulin
	    resistance
	  Overactivity
	    Glucocorticoids
	    Progestins and estrogens
	    Growth hormone—acromegaly
	    Glucagon
	  Underactivity
	    Type II isolated growth hormone
	      deficiency
		a. Defect in insulin receptor
		    Congenital lipodystrophy
		    Associated with virilization,
		    acanthosis nigricans
		b. Antibody to insulin
		    receptor–associated
		    immune disorders
			a. Inborn errors of metabolism
			b. Insulin-resistant syndromes
			c. Hereditary neuromuscular
			    disorders
			d. Progeroid syndrome
			e. Cytogenetic disorders,
			    Downs' syndrome,
			    Turners' syndrome,
			    Klinefelters' syndrome
			f. IGT with obesity[†]
			    Prader-Willi syndrome

* Detailed in National Diabetes Data Group: Classification and diagnosis of diabetes mellitus and other categories of glucose intolerance. Diabetes 28:1039, 1979.
[†]IGT = impaired glucose intolerance.

promptly to rehydration with a minimal requirement for insulin.[142]

Once the disease is recognized, therapy with insulin is mandatory. One to two units per kilogram of an intermediate-acting insulin in divided doses results in dramatic improvement and accelerated growth and weight gain. Attempts at gradually withdrawing the insulin therapy may be made as soon as recurrent hypoglycemia becomes manifest or after 2 months of age. The parents should be assured regarding the transient nature of the disease and the excellent prognosis, although there have been a few case reports of development of permanent diabetes.[144]

INSULIN RESISTANCE SYNDROMES

Insulin resistance is found in many conditions such as type II diabetes, obesity, chronic renal failure, and various forms of muscular dystrophy. It also occurs in states of excess of counterregulatory hormones, such as acromegaly and Cushing syndrome. It is a constant feature of leprechaunism (Donahue syndrome), a rare disorder characterized by intrauterine and postnatal growth impairment, diminished fat and muscle mass, characteristic facies, abnormal gonadal function, hyperinsulinemia, and early death.[145] Abnormalities of the insulin receptor are associated with the disturbance of carbohydrate metabolism and could possibly be implicated in the pathogenesis of the syndrome.

Other forms of insulin resistance associated with abnormalities of the insulin receptor are classified as types A, B, and C syndromes of insulin resistance.[146] Type A occurs in females generally between the ages of 8 and 16 years and is characterized by the presence of acanthosis nigricans, virilization and amenorrhea (often associated with polycystic ovaries), hyperglycemia, and high circulating levels of insulin. The concentration of insulin receptors on circulating monocytes is reduced and antibodies to the insulin receptor are not found in the serum. The type B syndrome is found predominantly in females and may occur in children as well as adults. The insulin resistance is mediated by autoimmune mechanisms, and high titers of antibodies to the insulin receptor are found in the plasma, as are high levels of insulin and glucose. Other evidence of autoimmune disorders may be present, such as systemic lupus erythematosus, ataxia telangiectasia, arthralgias, and alopecia. Patients have been described who have the features of the type A syndrome with the exception that the insulin receptors on their circulating monocytes are normal in number and affinity and antibodies to the receptor are not present in significant titers. These patients are designated as having the type C syndrome of insulin resistance. Congenital and acquired lipodystrophy may be associated with insulin resistance. In some cases receptor abnormalities have been found, as in the type A syndrome, but in many insulin receptor binding is normal or even increased. Lipoatrophy may be complete or partial, and other features that may be present include acanthosis nigricans, excessive growth, and hypertrophied external genitalia. Other abnormalities may also be present.[147]

FUTURE DIRECTIONS

Several avenues of research are being followed to elucidate the etiology of type I diabetes,[23] "cure" existing disease by pancreas or islet transplantation,[148,149] arrest the ongoing destruction of islets through immunologic suppression with agents such as cyclosporin,[23,69] improve methods of insulin delivery,[89–94] and reduce long-term complications.[150–152] The association of certain HLA subtypes with diabetes and their relation to autoimmune diseases offer the promise for unmasking the primary cause of insulin-dependent diabetes mellitus.[23,57] These associations, and the possible protracted course of islet destruction with progressively impaired first-phase insulin secretion, point the direction for attempts to prevent the clinical appearance of disease in genetically predisposed individuals, or arrest it to preserve residual insulin secretion.[23,69] Transplantation of whole pancreas has been successfully performed in a number of individuals, but the approach is generally limited by problems of rejection and by reactivation of immune-mediated destruction of β cells.[148] Transplantation of isolated fetal pancreatic islets to enhance growth potential, and their culture prior to transplantation, may overcome the problems of rejection and of adequate islet tissue.[149] Also, inhibitors of certain enzymes such as aldose reductase or processes believed to participate in the development of diabetic complications are undergoing clinical trials.[150–152]

Because type I diabetes is mediated by autoimmune processes, much attention has been paid recently to the possibility that intervention early in the course of the disease with immunosuppressive agents such as cyclosporine will reverse the progress of islet destruction and induce a remission. Some of the evidence gathered thus far suggests that this may be possible,[69] but the remissions do not appear to be permanent and it may be necessary to continue administration of the immunosuppressive agent indefinitely. Enthusiasm for prolonged regimens of therapy has to be tempered with the knowledge that cyclosporine administered over prolonged periods of time may lead to serious toxic effects, especially in the kidneys. Whether other immunosuppressive agents will be effective is not yet known.

REFERENCES

1. Sperling MA: Insulin biosynthesis and C-peptide. Am J Dis Child 134:1119, 1980.
2. Steiner DF: Insulin today. Diabetes 26:322, 1977.
3. Binder C, Rubenstein AR: Proceedings of an International C-Peptide Research Symposium. Diabetes 27(Suppl 1):145, 1978.
4. Gabbay KH: The insulinopathies. N Engl J Med 302:165, 1980.
5. Given BD, Mako ME, Tager HS, et al: Diabetes due to secretion of an abnormal insulin. N Engl J Med 302:129, 1980.
6. Gruppuso PA, Gorden P, Kahn CR, et al: Familial hyperproinsulinemia due to a proposed defect in conversion of proinsulin to insulin. N Engl J Med 311:629, 1984.
7. Haneda M, Polonsky KS, Bergenstal RM, et al: Familial hyperinsulinemia due to a structurally abnormal insulin. Definition of an emerging new clinical syndrome. N Engl J Med 310:1288, 1984.
8. Permutt MA, Chirgwin J, Rotwein P, et al: Insulin gene structure and function: A review of studies using recombinant DNA methodology. Diabetes Care 7:386, 1984.
9. Tager HS: Abnormal products of the human insulin gene. Diabetes 33:693, 1984.
10. Polonsky KS, Licinio-Paixae J, Given BD, et al: Use of biosynthetic human C-peptide in the measurement of insulin secretion rates in normal volunteers and type I diabetic patients. J Clin Invest 77:98, 1986.
11. Tillil H, Shapiro ET, Given BD, et al: Reevaluation of urine C-peptide as measure of insulin secretion. Diabetes 37:1195, 1988.
12. Sperling MA: Control of insulin secretion. Calif Med 119:17, 1973.
13. Felig P, Wahren J, Sherwin R, et al: Insulin, glucagon, and somatostatin in normal physiology and diabetes mellitus. Diabetes 25:1091, 1976.
14. Unger RJ, Orci L: Glucagon and the A cell. Physiology and pathophysiology. N Engl J Med 304:1518, 1575, 1981.
15. Woods SC, Porte D Jr: Neural control of the endocrine pancreas. Physiol Rev 54:596, 1974.
16. Flier JS, Kahn CR, Roth J: Receptors, antireceptor antibodies and mechanisms of insulin resistance. N Engl J Med 300:413, 1979.
17. Pollet RJ, Levey GS: Principles of membrane receptor physiology and their application to clinical medicine. Ann Intern Med 92:663, 1980.
18. Kaplan SA: The insulin receptor. J Pediatr 104:327, 1984.
19. Rosen OM: After insulin binds. Science 237:1452, 1987.
20. National Diabetes Data Group: Classification and diagnosis of diabetes mellitus and other categories of glucose intolerance. Diabetes 28:1039, 1979.
21. Rosenbloom AL, Korhman A, Sperling M: Classification and diagnosis of diabetes mellitus in children and adolescents. J Pediatr 98:320, 1981.
22. Nerup J, Mandrup-Poulsen T, Molvig J: The HLA-IDDM association: Implications for etiology and pathogenesis of IDDM. Diabetes Metab Rev 3:779, 1987.
23. Riley WJ, Winter WE, Mclaren NK: Identification of insulin-dependent diabetes mellitus before onset of clinical symptoms. J Pediatr 112:314, 1988.
24. Winter WE, Maclaren NK, Riley WJ, et al: Maturity-onset diabetes of youth in Black Americans. N Engl J Med 316:285, 1987.
25. Cahill GF Jr: Beta-cell deficiency, insulin resistance, or both? N Engl J Med 318:1268, 1988.
26. Clark A, Cooper GTS, Lewis CE, et al: Islet amyloid formed from diabetes-associated peptide may be pathogenic in type II diabetes. Lancet 1:231, 1987.
27. Karam JH, Lewitt PE, Young CW, et al: Insulinopenic diabetes after rodenticide (Vacor) ingestion: A unique model of acquired diabetes in man. Diabetes 29:971, 1980.
28. Calnan M, Peckham CS: Incidence of insulin dependent diabetes in the first 16 years of life. Lancet 1:589, 1977.
29. Holmgren G, Samuelson G, Hermansson B: The prevalence of diabetes mellitus: A study of children and their relatives in a northern Swedish county. Clin Genet 5:465, 1974.
30. Kyllo CJ, Nuttall FQ: Prevalence of diabetes mellitus in school-age children in Minnesota. Diabetes 27:57, 1978.
31. LaPorte RE, Dorman JS, Orchard TJ: Preventing insulin dependent diabetes mellitus: The environmental challenge. Br Med J 295:479, 1987.
32. Macdonald MJ: The frequencies of juvenile diabetes in American blacks and Caucasians are consistent with dominant inheritance. Diabetes 29:110, 1980.
33. LaPorte RE, Fishbein HA, Drash AL, et al: The incidence of insulin dependent diabetes mellitus in Allegheny County, Pennsylvania (1965–1976). Diabetes 30:279, 1981.
34. Bloch CA, Clemons P, Sperling MA: Puberty decreases insulin sensitivity. J Pediatr 110:481, 1987.
35. Amiel SA, Sherwin RS, Simonson DC, et al: Impaired insulin action in puberty. A contributing factor to poor glycemic control in adolescents with diabetes. N Engl J Med 315:215, 1986.

36. Fleegler FM, Rogers KD, Drash AL, et al: Age, sex and season of onset of juvenile diabetes in different geographic areas. Pediatrics 63:374, 1979.

37. Sultz HA, Hart BA, Zielezny M, et al: Is mumps virus an etiologic factor in juvenile diabetes mellitus? J Pediatr 86:654, 1975.

38. Samantray SK, Christopher S, Mukundan P, Johnson SC: Lack of relationship between viruses and human diabetes mellitus. Aust NZ J Med 7:139, 1977.

39. Menser MA, Forrest JM, Bransby RD: Rubella infection and diabetes mellitus. Lancet 1:57, 1978.

40. Craighead JE: Current views on the etiology of insulin-dependent diabetes mellitus. N Engl J Med 299:1439, 1978.

41. Drash AL: The etilogy of diabetes mellitus. N Engl J Med 300:1211, 1978.

42. Rayfield EJ, Seto Y: Viruses and the pathogenesis of diabetes mellitus. Diabetes 27:1126, 1978.

43. Yoon JW, Austin M, Onodera T, Notkins AL: Virus-induced diabetes mellitus: Isolation of a virus from the pancreas of a child with diabetic ketoacidosis. N Engl J Med 300:1173, 1979.

44. MacCuish AC, Irvine WJ: Autoimmunological aspects of diabetes mellitus. Clin Endocrinol Metab 4:435, 1975.

45. Neufeld M, MacLaren NK, Riley NJ, et al: Islet cell and other organ-specific antibodies in U.S. Caucasians and blacks with insulin-dependent diabetes mellitus. Diabetes 29:589, 1980.

46. Cudworth AG, Gorsuch AN, Wolf E, Festeinstein H: A new look at HLA genetics with particular reference to type-1 diabetes. Lancet 2:389, 1979.

47. Irvine WF, McCallum CF, Gray RS, et al: Pancreatic islet-cell antibodies in diabetes mellitus correlated with the duration and type of diabetes, coexistent autoimmune disease and HLA type. Diabetes 26:138, 1977.

48. Nelson PG, Pyke DA, Cudworth AG, et al: Histocompatibility antigens in diabetic identical twins. Lancet 2:193, 1975.

49. Nerup F, Platz P, Ortved-Anderson O, et al: HLA antigens and diabetes mellitus. Lancet 2:864, 1974.

50. Rodey GE, White N, Frazer TE, et al: HLA-DR specificities among Black Americans with juvenile-onset diabetes. N Engl J Med 301:810, 1979.

51. Rosenberg LE, Kidd KK: HLA and disease susceptibility: A primer. N Engl J Med 297:1060, 1977.

52. Rotter JI, Rimoin DL: Heterogeneity in diabetes mellitus—update 1978. Diabetes 27:599, 1978.

53. Rotter JI, Hodge SE: Racial differences in juvenile-type diabetes are consistent with more than one mode of inheritance. Diabetes 29:115, 1980.

54. Raum D, Stein R, Alper CA, Gabbay KH: Genetic marker for insulin-dependent diabetes mellitus. Lancet 1:1208, 1979.

55. Rubinstein P, Suciu-Foca N, Nicholson JF: Genetics of juvenile diabetes mellitus. N Engl J Med 297:1036, 1977.

56. Todd JA, Acjha-Orbea H, Bell JI, et al: A molecular basis for MHC class II-associated autoimmunity. Science 240:1003, 1988.

57. Morel PA, Dorman JS, Todd JA, et al: Aspartic acid at position 57 of the HLA-DQβ chain protects against type I diabetes: A family study. Proc Natl Acad Sci (USA) 85:8111, 1988.

58. Pyke DA: Diabetes: The genetic connections. Diabetologia 17:333, 1979.

59. Gamble DR: An epidemiological study of childhood diabetes affecting two or more siblings. Diabetologia 19:341, 1980.

60. Deschamps I, Lestradet H, Bonati C, et al: HLA genotype studies in juvenile insulin-dependent diabetes. Diabetologia 19:189, 1980.

61. Hodge SE, Rotter JI, Lange KL: A three-allele model for heterogeneity of juvenile onset insulin-dependent diabetes. Ann Hum Genet 43:399, 1980.

62. Dobersen MJ, Scharff JE, Ginsberg-Fellner F, Notkins AL: Cytotoxic autoantibodies to beta cells in the serum of patients with insulin-dependent diabetes mellitus. N Engl J Med 303:1493, 1980.

63. MacLaren NK, Huang SW, Fogh J: Antibody to cultured human insulinoma cells in insulin-dependent diabetes. Lancet 1:997, 1975.

64. Huange SW, MacLaren N: Insulin-dependent diabetes: A disease of autoaggression. Science 192:64, 1976.

65. Tarn AC, Dean BM, Schwarz G, et al: Predicting insulin-dependent diabetes. Lancet 1:845, 1988.

66. Eisenbarth GS: Genes, generator of diversity, glycoconjugates, and autoimmune β-cell insufficiency in type I diabetes. Diabetes 36:355, 1987.

67. Winter WE, Maclaren NK: Type I insulin dependent diabetes: An autoimmune disease that can be arrested or prevented with immunotherapy? Adv Pediatr 32:159, 1985.

68. Colman PG, Campbell IL, Kay TWH, et al: 64,000-M_r autoantigen in type I diabetes. Evidence against its surface location on human islets. Diabetes 36:1432, 1987.

69. Bougneres PF, Carel JC, Castano L, et al: Factors associated with early remission of type I diabetes in children treated with cyclosporine. N Engl J Med 318:663, 1988.

70. Sperling, MA: The contribution of hyperglycemic hormones to the pathogenesis of diabetes mellitus. Am J Dis Child 131:1145, 1977.

71. Schade DS, Eaton RP: The temporal relationship between endogenously secreted stress hormones and metabolic decompensation in diabetic man. J Clin Endocrinol Metab 50:131, 1980.

72. Cryer PE, Gerich JE: Glucose counterregulation, hypoglycemia, and intensive therapy in diabetes mellitus. N Engl J Med 313:232, 1985.

73. Raskin P, Unger RH: Hyperglucagonemia and its suppression: Importance in the metabolic control of diabetes. N Engl J Med 299:433, 1978.

74. Sperling MA: Diabetic ketoacidosis. Pediatr Clin North Am 31:591, 1984.

75. Kreisberg RA: Diabetic ketoacidosis: New concepts and trends in pathogenesis and treatment. Ann Intern Med 88:681, 1978.

76. Foster DW, McGarry JD: The metabolic derangements and treatment of diabetic ketoacidosis. N Engl J Med 309:159, 1983.

77. Duck SC, Wyatt DR: Factors associated with brain herniation in the treatment of diabetic ketoacidosis. J Pediatr 113:10, 1988.

78. Harris GD, Fiordalisi I, Finberg L: Safe man-

agement of diabetic ketoacidemia. J Pediatr 113:65, 1988.

79. Hammeke M, Bear R, Lee R, et al: Hyperchloremic metabolic acidosis in diabetes mellitus. Diabetes 27:16, 1978.

80. Keller U, Berger W: Prevention of hypophosphatemia by phosphate infusion during treatment of diabetic ketoacidosis and hyperosmolar coma. Diabetes 29:87, 1980.

81. Kanter Y, Gerson JR, Bessman AN: 2,3-Diphosphoglycerate, nucleotide phosphate, and organic and inorganic phosphate levels during the early phases of diabetic ketoacidosis. Diabetes 26:429, 1977.

82. Waldhausl W, Kleinberger G, Korn A, et al: Severe hyperglycemia: Effects of rehydration on endocrine derangements and blood glucose concentration. Diabetes 28:577, 1979.

83. Heber D, Molitch ME, Sperling MA: Low-dose continuous insulin therapy for diabetic ketoacidosis: Prospective comparison with "conventional" insulin therapy. Arch Intern Med 137:1377, 1977.

84. Kaye R: Diabetic ketoacidosis—the bicarbonate controversy. J Pediatr 87:156, 1973.

85. Bloom SR, Adrian TE, Barnes AJ, et al: Autoimmunity in diabetics induced by hormonal contaminants of insulin. Lancet 1:14, 1979.

86. Sperling MA (ed): Physician's Guide to Insulin-Dependent (Type I) Diabetes. Diagnosis and Treatment. Alexandria, VA, American Diabetes Association, 1988.

87. Werther GA, Jenkins PA, Turner RC, Baum JD: Twenty-four-hour metabolic profiles in diabetic children receiving insulin injections once or twice daily. Br Med J 281:414, 1980.

88. Sperling MA: Outpatient management of diabetes mellitus. Pediatr Clin North Am 34:917, 1987.

89. Tamborlane WV, Press CM: Insulin infusion pump treatment of type I diabetes. Pediatr Clin North Am 31:721, 1984.

90. Mecklenburg RS, Benson EA, Benson JW Jr, et al: Long-term metabolic control with insulin pump therapy. Report of experience with 127 patients. N Engl J Med 313:465, 1985.

91. Brownlee M, Cerami A, Li JJ, et al: Association of insulin pump therapy with raised serum amyloid A in type I diabetes mellitus. Lancet 1:411, 1985.

92. Micossi P, Cristallo M, Galimberti G, et al: One-year trial of a remote-controlled implantable insulin infusion system in type I diabetic patients. Lancet 2:866, 1988.

93. Bougneres PF, Landier F, Lemmell C, et al: Insulin pump therapy in young children with type I diabetes. J Pediatr 105:212, 1984.

94. Brink SJ, Stewart C: Insulin pump treatment in insulin-dependent diabetes mellitus. Children, adolescents, and young adults. JAMA 255:617, 1986.

95. Witters LA, Ohman JL, Weir GC, et al: Insulin antibodies in the pathogenesis of insulin allergy and resistance. Am J Med 63:703, 1977.

96. Kumar D: Anti-insulin IgE in Diabetics. J Clin Endocrinol Metab 45:1159, 1977.

97. Bantle JP: The dietary treatment of diabetes mellitus. Med Clin North Am 72:1285, 1988.

98. Saccharin and bladder cancer. Lancet 1:855, 1980.

99. Gabbay KH: The sorbitol pathway and the complications of diabetes. N Engl J Med 288:831, 1973.

100. Rivellese A, Riccardi G, Giacco A, et al: Effect of dietary fiber on glucose control and serum lipoproteins in diabetic patients. Lancet 2:447, 1980.

101. Horton ES: Exercise and diabetes mellitus. Med Clin North Am 72:1301, 1988.

102. Zinman G, Murray FT, Vranic M, et al: Glucoregulation during moderate exercise in insulin treated diabetics. J Clin Endocrinol Metab 45:641, 1977.

103. Landt KW, Campaigne BN, James FW, et al: Effects of exercise training on insulin sensitivity in adolescents with type I diabetes. Diabetes Care 5:461–465, 1985.

104. Sonksen PH, Judd SL, Lowy D: Home monitoring of blood-glucose: Method for improving diabetic control. Lancet 1:729, 1978.

105. Walford S, Gale EAM, Allison SP, et al: Self-monitoring of blood glucose: Improvement of diabetic control. Lancet 1:732, 1978.

106. Geffner ME, Kaplan SA, Lippe BM, Scott ML: Self blood glucose monitoring and intensive insulin therapy: Acceptability and efficacy in childhood diabetes. JAMA 249:2913, 1983.

107. Goldstein DE, Walker B, Rawlings SS, Hess RL, England JE, Peth SB, Hewett JE: Hemoglobin A_{1c} levels in children and adolescents with diabetes mellitus. Diabetes Care 3:503, 1980.

108. Goldstein DE: Clinical impression versus laboratory result. J Pediatr 109:649, 1986.

109. Abraham EC, Perry RE, Stallings M: Application of affinity chromatography for separation of glycosylated hemoglobins. J Lab Clin Med 102:187, 1983.

110. Santiago JV, Clarke WL, Shah SD, Cryer PE: Epinephrine, norepinephrine, glucagon, and growth hormone release in association with physiological decrements in the plasma glucose concentration in normal and diabetic man. J Clin Endocrinol Metab 51:877, 1980.

111. Rosenbloom AL, Giordano BP: Chronic overtreatment with insulin in children and adolescents. Am J Dis Child 131:881, 1977.

112. Gale EAM, Kurtz AB, Tattersall RB: In search of the Somogyi effect. Lancet 2:279, 1980.

113. Bolli G, Gottesman I, Campbell P, et al: Glucose counterregulation and waning of insulin in the Somogyi phenomenon. N Engl J Med 311:1214, 1984.

114. Campbell P, Bolli G, Cryer P, et al: Pathogenesis of a dawn phenomenon in patients with insulin-dependent diabetes mellitus. N Engl J Med 312:1473, 1985.

115. Cerreto MC, Travis LB: Implications of psychological and family factors in the treatment of diabetes. Pediatr Clin North Am 31:689, 1984.

116. Jacobson AM, Leibovich JB: Psychological issues in diabetes mellitus. Psychosomatics 25:7, 1984.

117. Diabetes in America: Diabetes Data Compiled 1984. US Department of Health and Human Services Publication No. 85-1468 (NIH). Washington, DC, US Government Printing Office, 1985.

118. Skyler JS: Complications of diabetes mellitus: Relationship to metabolic dysfunction. Diabetes Care 2:499, 1979.

119. Greene DA, Lattimer SA, Sima AAF: Sorbitol

phosphoinositides and Na-K ATPase in pathogenesis of diabetic complications. N Engl J Med 316:599, 1987.

120. Leslie ND, Sperling MA: Relation of metabolic control to complications in diabetes mellitus. J Pediatr 108:491, 1986.

121. Kirschenbaum DM: Glycosylation of proteins: Its implications in diabetic control and complications. Pediatr Clin North Am 31:611, 1984.

122. Mauer SM, Barbosa J, Vernier R, et al: Development of diabetic vascular lesions in normal kidneys transplanted into patients with diabetes mellitus. N Engl J Med 295:916, 1976.

123. Abouna GM, Kremer GD, Daddah SD, et al: Reversal of diabetic nephropathy in human cadaveric kidneys after transplantation to non-diabetic recipients. Lancet 2:1274, 1983.

124. Karam JH, Rosenthal M, O'Donnell JJ, et al: Discordance of diabetic microangiopathy in identical twins. Diabetes 25:24, 1976.

125. Krolewski AS, Canessa M, Warram JH, et al: Predisposition to hypertension and susceptibility to renal disease in insulin-dependent diabetes mellitus. N Engl J Med 318:140, 1988.

126. Mogensen CW: Mangement of diabetic renal involvement and disease. Lancet 1:867, 1988.

127. Pax-Guevara AT, Hsu TH, White P: Juvenile diabetes mellitus after forty years. Diabetes 24:559, 1976.

128. Rosenbloom AL, Silverstein JH, Lezotte DC, Richardson K, McCallum M: Limited joint mobility in childhood diabetes mellitus indicates increased risk for microvascular disease. N Engl J Med 305:191, 1981.

129. Rosenbloom AL: Skeletal and joint manifestations of childhood diabetes. Pediatr Clin North Am 31:569, 1984.

130. MacGregor M: Juvenile diabetics growing up. Lancet 1:944, 1977.

131. Tattersal RB, Pyke DA: Growth in diabetic children: Studies in identical twins. Lancet 2:1105, 1973.

132. Landon MB, Gabbe SG: Diabetes and pregnancy. Med Clin North Am 72:1493, 1988.

133. Freinkel N: Of pregnancy and progeny. Diabetes 29:1023, 1980.

134. Freinkel N, Dooley SL, Metzger BE: Care of the pregnant woman with insulin dependent diabetes mellitus. N Engl J Med 313:96, 1985.

135. Menon RM, Sperling MA: Carbohydrate metabolism. Semin Perinatol 12:157, 1988.

136. Pildes RS: Infants of diabetic mothers. N Engl J Med 289:902, 1973.

137. McMahan MJ, Mimouni F, Miodovnik M, et al: Surfactant associated protein (SAP-35) in amniotic fluid from diabetic and nondiabetic pregnancies. Obstet Gynecol 70:94, 1987.

138. Mace S, Hirshfield SS, Riggs T, Faranoff AA, Merkatz IR: Echocardiographic abnormalities in infants of diabetic mothers. J Pediatr 95:1013, 1979.

139. Rosenbloom AL, Drash A, Guthrie R: Chemical diabetes in childhood: Conference summary. Metabolism 22:413, 1973.

140. Fajans SS, Cloutier MC, Crowther RL: Clinical and etiologic heterogeneity of idiopathic diabetes mellitus. Diabetes 27:1112, 1978.

141. Lippe BM, Sperling MA, Dooley RR: Pancreatic alpha and beta cell functions in cystic fibrosis. J Pediatr 90:751, 1977.

142. Schiff D, Colle E, Stern L: Metabolic and growth patterns in transient neonatal diabetes. N Engl J Med 287:119, 1972.

143. Pagliara AS, Karl IE, Kipnis DB: Transient neonatal diabetes: Delayed maturation of the pancreatic beta cell. J Pediatr 82:97, 1973.

144. Daugberg PS: A case of permanent diabetes in a neonate. Dan Med Bull 28:216, 1981.

145. Geffner ME, Kaplan SA, Bersch N, et al: Leprechaunism: In vitro insulin action despite genetic resistance. Pediatr Res 22:286, 1987.

146. Flier JS, Kahn CR, Roth J: Receptors, antireceptor antibodies and mechanisms of insulin resistance. N Engl J Med 300:413, 1979.

147. Wachslicht-Rodbard H, Muggeo M, Kahn CR, et al: Heterogeneity of the insulin-receptor interaction in lipoatrophic diabetes. J Clin Endocrinol Metab 52:416, 1981.

148. Sutherland, DER, Goetz FC, Chin PL, et al: Pancreas transplantation. Pediatr Clin North Am 31:735, 1984.

149. Lacy PE, Davie JM: Transplantation of pancreatic islets. Annu Rev Immunol 2:183, 1984.

150. Editorial: Current status of aldose reductase inhibitors. Diabetes Care 10:123, 1987.

151. Brownlee M, Vlassara H, Kooney A, et al: Aminoguanidine prevents diabetes-induced arterial wall protein cross-linking. Science 232:1629, 1986.

152. Winegrad AI: Does a common mechanism induce the diverse complications of diabetes? Diabetes 36:396, 1987.

5

HYPOGLYCEMIA

Mitchell E. Geffner

One approach to the determination of the cause of hypoglycemia in children is based on the ages at which different types of hypoglycemia are most likely to occur.[1] While this schema is useful for the most common causes, the recent recognition of many new etiologies for the disorder limits the value of age-related stratification. An alternative approach to the diagnosis and management of pediatric hypoglycemia is based on an understanding of the metabolic control mechanisms of glucose homeostasis. Most causes of hypoglycemia can be divided into two general categories: (1) *overutilization*, which results from excessive tissue uptake of glucose (invariably the result of exaggerated or dysregulated insulin secretion), and (2) *underproduction*, which results from deficient precursor conversion to glucose (glycogenolysis and/or gluconeogenesis). This alternative schematization is in line with the fact that hypoglycemia is a manifestation of the failure of these controls for maintenance of normoglycemia.[2] With such a mechanistic approach, a simplified pathophysiologic algorithm can be developed that, in turn, permits a logical diagnostic approach to the child with hypoglycemia.

GLUCOSE MEASUREMENTS AND DEFINITIONS OF HYPOGLYCEMIA

To be certain of the diagnosis of hypoglycemia, one must be cognizant of the circumstances surrounding the glucose measurement itself. First, the concentration of the glucose in serum or plasma (as measured in the clinical laboratory) is 12 to 15 per cent higher than a simultaneous measurement in whole blood (as measured at the bedside or at home by fingerprick collection). This difference could have a significant impact on the glucose level chosen for the diagnostic evaluation of hypoglycemia. This discordance in the measurement occurs because the plasma and serum concentrations are determined using only the liquid phase of the blood sample, whereas, with whole blood, a significant part of the volume used for measurement is comprised of a solid phase, including hemoglobin. The glycolytic enzymes of erythrocytes can lower the concentration of glucose by as much as 18 mg/dl/hour when the blood is kept at room temperature.[3] It is necessary, therefore, that the plasma or serum be separated from the erythrocytes immediately after the blood is drawn and refrigerated until the glucose measurement is performed. Alternatively, sodium fluoride, an inhibitor of glycolysis, is added to the tube in which the blood is collected, conventionally known as a "gray-top tube."

The criteria for the diagnosis of hypoglycemia in infancy remain controversial. Originally, hypoglycemia in the first 72 hours of life was defined as a blood glucose of less than 30 mg/dl (serum/plasma less than 35 mg/dl) in term infants and less than 20 mg/dl (serum/plasma less than 25 mg/dl) in premature infants.[1] More recent studies have suggested that hypoglycemia in term infants be defined as less than 40 to 45 mg/dl after the first 24 hours of life.[4,5] Incidence figures for neonatal hypoglycemia will depend on operational definitions.[6] The frequency of observed glucose values below a certain level may vary in populations of newborns depending on differences in gestational age, birth weight, exact age at time of measurement, method and quantify of recent feedings, and sampling time related to feeding. Beyond 48 hours of age, normal blood glucose concentrations are greater than 40 mg/dl (plasma/serum greater than 45 mg/dl), with mean whole blood values in the first month of life generally between 60 and 70 mg/dl (plasma/serum 70 to 80 mg/dl).[1]

MECHANISMS OF NORMAL GLUCOSE HOMEOSTASIS

The maintenance of normoglycemia is the result of a complex interaction between the glucose-lowering action of insulin on the one hand and the glucose-raising action of the anti-insulin or counterregulatory hormones (glucagon, epinephrine, norepinephrine, cortisol, and growth hormone) on the other hand (Fig. 5–1). These hormones, separately or collectively, regulate multiple steps in the mobilization of preformed glucose from hepatic glycogen stores (via glycogenolysis) in the liver and formation of new glucose from nonglucose substrates (via gluconeogenesis). Glucagon, through breakdown of hepatic glycogen, has a critical role in short-term protection against hypoglycemia. Epinephrine may also activate glycogenolysis, particularly in states of glucagon deficiency.

When hepatic glycogen is depleted (usually in less than 24 hours, depending on age), gluconeogenesis becomes the sole source of glucose production[7] (Fig. 5–1). The available substrates from peripheral tissues include amino acids (alanine, threonine, serine, and glycine) from muscle, lactate and pyruvate mostly from muscle, and

glycerol from fat. Counterregulatory hormonal control of gluconeogenesis involves regulation of substrate supply, hepatic uptake of precursors, and their conversion to glucose. Epinephrine stimulates gluconeogenesis by increasing availability of lactate and pyruvate from muscle and of glycerol from fat, with norepinephrine also a potent stimulus of lipolysis.[8] Cortisol, in a time-dependent fashion, provides additional substrate in the form of amino acid[9] and also facilitates epinephrine-induced lipolysis.[10] Growth hormone, in a delayed fashion, also mobilizes fat and provides gluconeogenic substrate in the form of glycerol.[11] Finally, multiple counterregulatory hormones regulate hepatic uptake of substrates, with glucagon playing an important role in hepatic amino acid uptake and conversion.[12]

The regulatory control varies depending on factors such as chronologic age (infancy versus later childhood) and recent food intake [fasting (postabsorptive) versus fed (absorptive) state]. The importance of age is evident by the increased susceptibility of the neonate to hypoglycemia and by the normally lower plasma glucose concentrations found in the early hours of life (compared to older children). The newborn infant, once separated from maternal glucose sources,

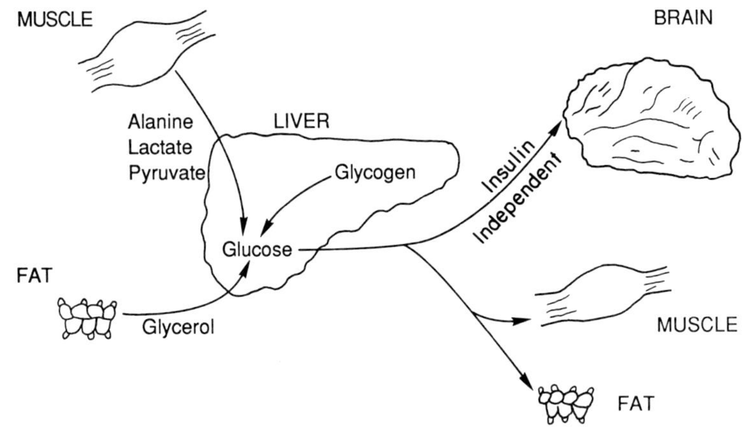

FIGURE 5–1. Hormones and substrates for glucose homeostasis.

enters a state with no food, at least initially, in the gastrointestinal tract. Importantly, at this time the infant has a large glucose requirement (as high as 8 mg/kg/min) compared to the adult, who requires approximately 2.3 mg/kg/min.[13] This large age-related requirement stems from the obligatory need for glucose as a fuel by the newborn brain, which occupies a larger percentage of total body mass than at any other age. Consumption by other glucose-requiring tissues, such as the retina, renal medulla, and leukocytes, is negligible.

Although the fetal liver contains large amounts of glycogen that have been mostly deposited during the last trimester, the neonatal glycogenolytic response to glucagon is slow but sustained.[1] The maturation of gluconeogenic enzymes responsible for conversion of amino acids and lactate into glucose is delayed, resulting in elevated serum concentrations of these precursors. Concomitantly, the ability of the liver to generate ketone bodies from available free fatty acids is restricted in the newborn period, which leads to a near-exclusive dependence of the central nervous system on glucose as its metabolic fuel[14] (Table 5–1).

For these reasons, the normal newborn can be expected to have lower plasma glucose concentrations compared to older children and, with even minor stresses, to develop significant hypoglycemia. Premature infants are at increased risk for hypoglycemia because their foreshortened intrauterine existence precludes sufficient hepatic glycogen storage. If an infant is undergrown (small for gestational age), glycogen and other metabolic fuels are often depleted, resulting in increased susceptibility to neonatal hypoglycemia.

Gluconeogenic enzyme activity can be detected in the fetal liver as early as the second month of gestation and increases to term.[15] Thus, the fetus is not completely reliant on maternal glucose provision. Simultaneous with a rapid fall in hepatic glycogen content over the first few days of life, the infant becomes dependent on gluconeogenic enzyme activities, which increase in response to postnatal surges in glucagon and catecholamine secretion.[16] Thus, hepatic glycogenolysis appears to be crucial for the immediate postnatal adaptation from the glucose-replete in utero state to the glucose-depleted fasted state characterizing the first few hours of extrauterine life. After depletion of glycogen stores, the infant becomes dependent on gluconeogenesis to maintain normoglycemia.

As the infant grows older, hepatic glycogen is usually sufficient to offset hypoglycemia for up to 12 hours of fasting and, by late childhood and adulthood, for 24 hours. As in infancy, with prolonged fasting glycogen stores become exhausted and gluconeogenesis becomes the exclusive source of glucose. Infants and young children have diminished muscle mass per unit of body weight compared to older children and adults and, therefore, have more limited stores of substrate for gluconeogenesis. Thus, the younger the child the greater the susceptibility to hypoglycemia.

SIGNS, SYMPTOMS, AND PROGNOSIS OF HYYPOGLYCEMIA

The clinical features of infants with hypoglycemia are relatively nonspecific and range from jitteriness, tremors, cyanosis, apnea, limpness, lethargy, and poor feeding to repeated convulsions during the early months of life. In the immediate newborn period, the clinical picture may resemble that of sepsis. The older child, in whom the prevalence of hypoglycemia is lower, first develops epinephrine-mediated signs and symptoms (e.g., sweating, shakiness, and hunger); if the condition is not corrected, the infant can progress to neuroglycopenic symptoms (e.g., mental clouding, loss of consciousness, and convulsions).

These symptoms should lead to a vigorous search for the diagnosis and etiology of hypoglycemia. In the process, aggressive treatment measures (see below) are indicated to avoid persistence and/or recurrence of prolonged hypoglycemia, which, if occurring in the first year of life, may lead to permanent neurologic sequelae. On the other hand, there is no evidence linking short-term hypoglycemia, even early in life, to permanent brain damage. Additonally, there are no data

---

TABLE 5–1. FACTORS CONTRIBUTING TO HYPOGLYCEMIA IN INFANCY

Large obligatory glucose requirement
Gastrointestinal tract initially devoid of nutrients
Limited glycogen stores
Diminished gluconeogenesis
    Delayed maturation of gluconeogenic enzymes
    Diminished hepatic ketogenesis

on the long-term neurologic outcomes of term neonates with blood sugars on the first 3 days of life between 30 and 40 mg/dl. If hypoglycemia is persistent and goes undiagnosed or is incompletely treated during the first months of life, microcephaly may occur[17] and developmental delay becomes obvious. The final prognosis of the hypoglycemic infant, however, must await full growth and development because significant improvement in neurologic function and brain growth may occur over the first few years of life.[18] Single episodes of hypoglycemia that occur in older children, usually in those with type 1 diabetes, while to be avoided, rarely result in any permanent neurologic sequelae.

ETIOLOGY AND TREATMENT OF HYPOGLYCEMIA

Overutilization of Glucose

Overutilization of glucose as a cause of hypoglycemia almost always results from hyperinsulinemic states, which occur most commonly in infancy but may occur in later childhood. In infancy, this form of hypoglycemia encompasses a spectrum of disorders characterized by diffuse islet cell hyperplasia, insulin-secreting tumors (microadenomas, adenomatosis, or both), and even completely normal pancreatic histology.[17,19–22] These disorders are best collectively designated as the islet cell dysmaturation syndrome[23] (Table 5–2), which should replace the term *nesidioblastosis*, a histologic description of endocrine tissue (islets) budding from exocrine tissue (acini). Once thought to be pathognomonic for infantile hyperinsulinemia, nesidioblastosis is now known to be a normal developmental finding in the first year of life based on pancreatic autopsy specimens from infants dying from trauma.[24] It has been suggested, at least in some studies, that dysregulated

TABLE 5–2. HISTOLOGIC FINDINGS IN ISLET CELL DYSMATURATION SYNDROME

Islet cell hyperplasia
Islet cell hypertrophy
(Micro)adenoma
Adenomatosis
Normal histology
?Delta cell deficiency

TABLE 5–3. ETIOLOGY OF HYPERINSULINEMIC HYPOGLYCEMIA IN CHILDHOOD

Islet cell dysmaturation syndrome
Infant of a diabetic mother
Beckwith-Wiedemann syndrome
Erythroblastosis fetalis
Trisomy 13
Total parenteral nutrition
Dumping syndrome
Type 1 diabetes mellitus
Drug-induced
    Maternal tocolytics
    Quinine for antimalarial treatment

insulin secretion in infancy may result from associated pancreatic (delta cell) somatostatin deficiency with resultant loss of paracrine inhibitory control over insulin secretion by adjacent β cells.[25,26] Several families have been described with more than one affected infant, suggesting a role for genetic factors in the pathogenesis of some cases of neonatal hyperinsulinemia.[27] Discrete or multiple insulinomas in older children are rare, but, if found, should prompt a search for coexisting endocrine tumors involving the pituitary and parathyroid glands (familial multiple endocrine neoplasia type 1 or Wermer syndrome)[28] (see Chapter 7).

Certain conditions in infancy may predispose to hyperinsulinemic hypoglycemia and should be suspected when certain specific physical findings are present (Table 5–3). The hypersomatotropic (overgrown) infant of a diabetic mother (IDM) is the most common of these conditions, with transient hypoglycemia developing within a few hours of birth because of the fetal-neonatal hyperinsulinemic response to maternal-fetal hyperglycemia. Failure of the IDM to down-regulate the number of insulin receptors on target tissues in response to prevailing hyperinsulinemia is also presumed to contribute to the postnatal hypoglycemia.[29] Fifty per cent of infants with the Beckwith-Wiedemann syndrome (macrosomia, macroglossia, and omphalocele) develop pancreatic β cell hyperplasia and hypoglycemia.[30] Hyperinsulinemic hypoglycemia also occurs in infants with severe erythroblastosis fetalis secondary to β cell hyperplasia.[31] Infants with Trisomy 13 may also be at increased risk for hyperinsulinemic hypoglycemia.[32]

Iatrogenic hyperinsulinemic hypoglycemia can occur in patients of all ages receiving hypertonic dextrose as part of total parenteral nutrition (TPN) regimens. With home programs limited to overnight administration of large amounts of glucose, significant compensatory hyperinsulinemia occurs,[33] predisposing such patients to severe hypoglycemia if the infusion is inadvertently interrupted or if the discontinuation (tapering) procedure is not gradual. Hyperinsulinemia may also contribute to the late hypoglycemia seen in children with the "dumping" syndrome.[34]

Children with type 1 diabetes are at risk for hyperinsulinemic hypoglycemia. With the current emphasis on tight glycemic control, modern insulin regimens induce hyperinsulinemia in the peripheral bloodstream in order to provide adequate levels of insulin to the liver via the portal circulation.[35] This, along with variations in eating and exercise patterns and acquired derangements in counterregulatory hormone secretion,[36] predisposes diabetic children to hypoglycemia.

Certain drugs may cause hyperinsulinemic hypoglycemia. Infants born to mothers receiving β-sympathomimetic tocolytic agents, such as terbutaline, are at risk for developing transient hyperinsulinemic hypoglycemia secondary to transplacental passage of the drug.[37] Severe hypoglycemia secondary to hyperinsulinemia has also been reported to occur in adolescents and adults with falciparum malaria, at least in part related to quinine-induced enhancement of insulin secretion.[38]

The inclusion of leucine sensitivity in the differential diagnosis of hyperinsulinemic hypoglycemia has been intentionally omitted. Leucine is one of several insulinotropic amino acids and is a normal dietary constituent. It would appear that all forms of hyperinsulinemic hypoglycemia are, indeed, leucine sensitive,[39] and therefore leucine sensitivity should not be construed as a distinct pathologic entity. If a child with hyperinsulinemia is able to maintain normoglycemia solely by dietary leucine restriction, this child probably has the mildest form of the islet cell dysmaturation syndrome.

The diagnosis of hyperinsulinemia is, at times, difficult to make. It should be suspected on the basis of the following (see section on "Diagnosis of Childhood Hypoglycemia" and Table 5–4): (1) rapid development of hypoglycemia after the onset of fasting; (2) high exogenous glucose requirements (12 mg/kg/min or more) to maintain

TABLE 5–4. DIAGNOSTIC CRITERIA FOR HYPERINSULINEMIC HYPOGLYCEMIA

Suggestive
  Rapid development of hypoglycemia with fasting
  High exogenous glucose requirement to maintain normoglycemia
  Absence of ketonemia, ketonuria, and acidosis at time of hypoglycemia
  Rise in plasma glucose concentration >30 mg/dl from hypoglycemic baseline level following glucagon administration
Diagnostic
  Serum insulin level >10 μU/ml at time of hypoglycemia
  Insulin-glucose ratio >0.3:1 at time of hypoglycemia
Supportive
  Restoration of normoglycemia with diazoxide and/or somatostatin
  Elevated serum C peptide and/or proinsulin levels at time of hypoglycemia

normoglycemia; (3) lack of ketonemia, ketonuria, and acidosis at the time of hypoglycemia; and (4) increase in the plasma glucose concentration of greater than 30 mg/dl following glucagon administration at the time of hypoglycemia.[40] The fifth and key criterion for the diagnosis of hyperinsulinemia is the finding of a high plasma or serum insulin concentration (usually greater than 10 μU/ml) or a high insulin-glucose ratio (greater than 0.3:1)[19] at the time of documented hypoglycemia. Because reports of insulin assays are often not immediately available, the first four criteria are important in guiding initial therapeutic strategies. Occasionally the use of pharmacologic agents [e.g., diazoxide or, on an experimental basis, somatostatin (see later in this chapter)] may facilitate confirmation of the diagnosis if their use restores normoglycemia.

It should be pointed out that failure to develop ketonemia at the time of hypoglycemia also occurs in patients with carnitine deficiency who are unable to transport fatty acids into mitochondria, where they are normally oxidized to ketone bodies.[41] However, patients with this rare disorder fail to manifest the other criteria of glucose overutilization and present, in the systemic variant, with episodes of lethargy and somnolence associated with hyperammonemia, increased levels of transaminase activity in the serum, hepatomegaly, and cardiomegaly. On the other hand, ketonuria may occur in the hyperinsulinemic infant despite very low serum ketone levels because of an age-related diminution in the renal threshhold for ketones.[42]

If each of the criteria for the diagnosis of hyperinsulinemic hypoglycemia is present except for the elevated insulin level or insulin-glucose ratio, alternative diagnostic possibilities suggesting overutilization need to be considered. First, several infants have been described with (transient) glucagon deficiency[43] who became hypoglycemic because of partially unopposed insulin action. Theoretically, this diagnosis can be made by measuring the plasma glucagon concentration at the time of hypoglycemia, since limited age-related normal data are available. Second, a single infant has been described who had hypoglycemia secondary to circulating, *stimulatory* anti-insulin–receptor antibodies that disappeared following treatment with prednisone for 3 months.[44] Third, a few children have been reported with the insulin autoimmune syndrome in which antibodies to insulin arise de novo[45] or perhaps secondary to a structurally abnormal insulin molecule.[46] These antibodies can sequester insulin and release it rapidly and unpredictably, resulting in hypoglycemia.[47] Finally, and perhaps most importantly, elimination of the diagnosis of hyperinsulinemia should not be based on a single "normal" insulin measurement. Because of the short biologic half-life of insulin (approximately 1.5 min), it is possible that some simultaneous insulin and glucose measurements may fail to provide evidence for either absolute or relative hyperinsulinemia.[48] Additionally, because of assay variations, the insulin radioimmunoassay may need to be repeated by a different technique before concluding that a "normal" value is, indeed, an accurate representation. Occasionally, simultaneous measurements of proinsulin and/or C peptide levels can be helpful, but usually only as confirmatory tests.[49]

While the evaluation for hyperinsulinemia is underway, it is imperative to maintain normoglycemia. Because of the high exogenous glucose requirement to offset the ongoing overutilization, placement of a central catheter may be necessary. Once the diagnosis has been established, or, occasionally, as part of a diagnostic trial, medical therapy with oral diazoxide should be initiated (Table 5–5). This medication acts predominantly by suppressing insulin secretion by the β cells and, when administered orally, does not cause any lowering of the blood

TABLE 5–5. THERAPEUTIC STRATEGIES FOR THE ISLET-CELL DYSMATURATION SYNDROME

Medical: mainstay
  Diazoxide
Medical: adjunctive
  Diphenylhydantoin
  Chlorothiazide
  Low-leucine diet
  Corticosteroids
  Growth hormone
  Long-acting epinephrine
  Glucagon (including continuous subcutaneous
    infusion and protamine-zinc* forms)
  Somatostatin (native* or long-acting*)
Surgical: mainstay
  Subtotal pancreatectomy (85–90%)
Surgical: alternative
  Lesionectomy
  Total pancreatectomy

* Experimental.

pressure. The starting dose is 10 mg/kg/day (maximum dose 30 mg/kg/day) given in three divided doses. Diazoxide is successful as sole therapy in about two thirds of cases, particularly if symptoms of hypoglycemia begin after 1 month of age.[19]

The most common acute side effect of diazoxide is salt and water retention, which, in its most severe form, can lead to congestive heart failure. Its most common chronic side effect, which occurs nearly universally after a few months of use, is hypertrichosis characterized by clumps of hair on the forehead, back, and limbs, which is unrelated to hyperandrogenism. Other less common side effects include hyperosmolar nonketotic coma, decreased neutrophil counts, and a decreased serum immunoglobulin (Ig) G level (with perhaps an increased risk of bacterial sepsis).[17] More recently, long-term use of diazoxide has been linked to coarsening of the facies with associated gingival hyperplasia, thickening of the lips, and widening of the spaces between teeth.[50] Some patients have been cured after over 10 years of diazoxide therapy,[51] following which the drug could be discontinued. However, because of the significant long-term toxicity of diazoxide, it is unclear whether this is an advisable practice when surgery may be curative.

Pharmacologic agents such as diphenylhydantoin, which inhibits insulin secretion, and chlorothiazide, which is structurally similar to diazoxide, have been employed as adjuncts to diazoxide, but are generally not recommended (Table 5–5).

Low-leucine diets are occasionally helpful.[52] In selected patients, short-term use of counterregulatory (anti-insulin) agents such as corticosteroids, growth hormone, long-acting forms of epinephrine, and glucagon (by infusion or complexed to protamine-zinc) has been efficacious. More recently, native and long-acting analogs of somatostatin have been used on an experimental basis in infants with hyperinsulinemic hypoglycemia, either alone or in conjunction with other agents in both short- and long-term regimens.[53–56] Long-term use of somatostatin in infancy and childhood must be considered with extreme caution because of simultaneous suppressive effects on the secretion of somatotropin and other hormones.

If medical therapy is deemed unsuccessful or unsafe (because of side effects), an 85 to 90 per cent subtotal pancreatectomy[57] (Table 5–5) should be performed by an experienced pediatric surgeon. If an adenoma can be found, subtotal pancreatectomy is probably still advisable because the remaining pancreatic islet tissue may still be dysfunctional. If an initial surgical procedure does not fully restore normoglycemia, reinstitution of diazoxide therapy may be effective or, on occasion, a second surgical procedure (further subtotal or, rarely, total pancreatectomy) is necessary. Surgical failure can occur if too little pancreatic tissue is removed, if tumorous tissue is inadvertently retained in vivo, or if significant pancreatic tissue regrowth occurs. If too much pancreatic tissue is excised, permanent insulin-requiring diabetes and malabsorption may develop. Transient postsurgical hyperglycemia (occasionally requiring exogenous insulin therapy) is a frequent concomitant of successful surgery, but it rarely lasts beyond 1 week unless excessive pancreatic tissue has been removed.

Underproduction of Glucose

As outlined in Figure 5–1, the major precursors that can be converted to glucose include glycogen, amino acids, lactate, pyruvate, and glycerol. In certain hypoglycemic disorders associated with underproduction of glucose, there can be an actual deficiency of substrate, or, more likely, a specific enzyme defect or missing counterregulatory hormone, preventing mobilization or transport of substrate. The enzyme deficiencies tend to be inherited in an autosomal-recessive fashion, whereas disturbances of coun-

terregulatory hormones are usually sporadic. These defects can be best appreciated in terms of the metabolic pathway(s) (glycogenolysis and/or gluconeogenesis) in which they occur (Fig. 5–2 and Table 5–6). This conceptual approach also helps predict the rapidity of onset of hypoglycemia, precipitating factors, associated abnormalities, and aims of therapy.

Defects in Glycogenolysis

Glycogen Storage Disease. Deficiency of the enzyme glucose-6-phosphatase results in a primary defect of *both* glycogenolysis and gluconeogenesis, leading to fairly rapid onset of profound hypoglycemia.[58] This occurs because this pivotal enzyme normally catalyzes the conversion of glucose 6-phosphate formed from *both* glycogen breakdown and gluconeogenic precursors to glucose (Fig. 5–2). Enhanced peripheral glucose utilization also occurs, adding further to the risk of hypoglycemia.[59] As a result of impaired glycogenolysis, glycogen is deposited in the liver. Hence, this disorder is a typical *glycogen storage disease* (GSD), the so-called GSD IA variety or von Gierke disease. The GSD IA enzyme deficiency is demonstrable in liver, kidney, and intestinal mucosa, and the diagnosis is confirmed directly by enzyme assay in liver tissue. A newly described GSD IB form appears to be due to a defective hepatic glucose 6-phosphate transport system rather than to an enzyme deficiency per se.[60]

Patients with either type are prone to hepatomegaly and may develop a protuberant abdomen, nephromegaly, cherubic facies, and growth failure. Common laboratory findings include, in addition to hypoglycemia, lactic acidosis, hyperlipidemia, ketosis, hyperuricemia, increased levels of transaminases in the serum, hyperalaninemia, and hyperglucagonemia. Many of the secondary metabolic derangements result from shunting of intermediates through the glycolytic pathway. These patients also have a propensity to develop hepatomas (usually after puberty) with malignant potential,[61] as well as bleeding diatheses associated with prolonged bleeding times and abnormal platelet function.[62] Additionally, patients with GSD IB develop neutropenia, neutrophil dysfunction, and increased risk of bacterial infection.[60,62] The aim of treatment is to correct hypoglycemia and lactic acidosis, achieve normal growth, and prevent ne-

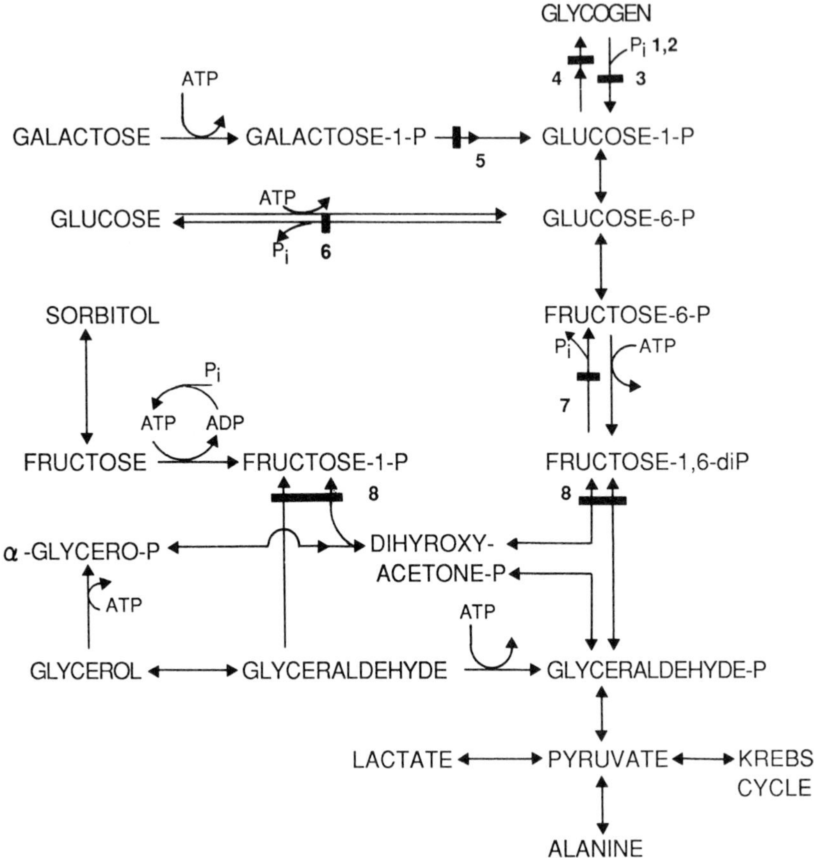

FIGURE 5–2. 1, phosphorylase kinase (GSD IX); 2, phosphorylase (GSD VI); 3, debranching enzyme (GSD III); 4, glycogen synthetase (GSD 0); 5, galactose 1-phosphate uridyl transferase (classical galactosemia); 6, glucose-6-phosphatase (Von Gierke disease or GSD IA); 7, fructose-1,6-diphosphatase; 8, fructose 1-phosphate aldolase (hereditary fructose intolerance); P = phosphate; diP = diphosphate; P_i = inorganic phosphate; ATP = adenosine triphosphate; ADP = adenosine diphosphate. Metabolic pathways for glucose homeostasis.

(Modified from Gitzelmann R, Steinmann B, van den Berghe G: Essential fructosuria, hereditary fructose intolerance, and fructose-1,6-diphosphatase deficiency. *In* Stanbury JB, Wyngaarden JB, Frederickson DS, Goldstein JL, Brown MS (eds): The Metabolic Basis of Inherited Disease. New York, McGraw-Hill, 1983, p 120.)

TABLE 5–6. MECHANISMS OF UNDERPRODUCTION OF GLUCOSE IN CHILDHOOD HYPOGLYCEMIA

	Defective Glycogenolysis		Defective Gluconeogenesis	
Etiology of Glucose Underproduction	*Primary*	*Secondary*	*Primary*	*Secondary*
Glucose-6-phosphatase deficiency (GSD IA or Von Gierke disease)	●		●	
Debranching enzyme deficiency (GSD III)	●			
Galactose 1-phosphate uridyl transferase deficiency (classic galactosemia)		●		
Fructose-1,6-diphosphatase deficiency		●	●	
Fructose 1-phosphate aldolase deficiency (hereditary fructose intolerance)		●		●

phropathy.[63] This usually requires continuous nocturnal enteral provision of glucose of glucose polymers,[64] combined with frequent daytime oral feedings supplemented with uncooked starch.[65] Longitudinal studies suggest that reestablishment of normoglycemia leads to significant improvement of the secondary metabolic defects, reduction in liver size, and normalization of growth.[66] In one case of GSD IA, liver transplantation was employed to treat a patient with associated multiple hepatic adenomas, resulting in complete metabolic normalization through 1 year of reported follow-up.[67]

Other classic forms of glycogen storage disease,[63] caused by deficiencies of debranching enzyme (GSD III), phosphorylase (GSD VI), and phosphorylase kinase (GSD IX), may also be associated with hypoglycemia, but less often than GSD I, presumably because the enzyme defects are incomplete and because gluconeogenesis remains intact. The rare glycogen storage disease designated GSD 0, in which a deficiency of the enzyme glycogen synthetase in liver and muscle has been described, may also be associated with fasting hypoglycemia.[68] In a strict sense, this condition is not a glycogen *storage* disease, but rather a disease in which there is an inability to store glycogen in the liver. Affected patients also develop postprandial *hyper*glycemia secondary to an inability to store glucose in the absorptive state.

Galactosemia. Galactosemia is most commonly due to a deficiency of the hepatic enzyme galactose 1-phosphate (Gal-1-P) uridyl transferase, the normal role of which is to convert galactose to glucose[69] (Fig. 5–2). In deficiency states, ingestion of lactose-containing formulas or breast milk results in an inability to process galactose, leading to an accumulation of Gal-1-P, the precursor immediately proximal to the enzyme block, which *secondarily* inhibits hepatic glycogenolysis. This results in hypoglycemia in the first few days of life and may be associated with gastrointestinal symptoms and failure to thrive. For unclear reasons, affected infants are predisposed to *Escherichia coli* sepsis,[70] the symptoms of which may mimic those due to the primary defect. Other characteristic findings in the infant with galactosemia include hepatosplenomegaly, jaundice, cataracts, and mental retardation. Although newborn screening programs are widespread in this country and early elimination of dietary lactose appears

to control most of the manifestations of the disease, many adolescent and adult women with galactosemia develop primary ovarian failure that is believed to be due to prenatal and early postnatal ovarian exposure to elevated levels of galactose metabolites.[71]

Defects in Gluconeogenesis

Frustose-1,6-Diphosphatase Deficiency. The most typical disorder in this category, fructose-1,6-diphosphatase deficiency leads to a blockade of the gluconeogenic pathway at the level of fructose 1,6-diphosphate (F-1,6-diP) (Fig. 5–2), preventing further channeling of gluconeogenic substrates to form new glucose.[72] Because affected individuals have an intact glycogenolytic pathway, hypoglycemia does not characteristically occur with short-term fasts.[73] On the other hand, administration of substrates such as glycerol and alanine or ingestion of large amounts sucrose, fructose, or sorbitol, all of which enter the gluconeogenic pathway proximal to F-1,6-diP, are shunted in the direction of glycolysis to form lactate. Hypoglycemia than ensues, perhaps because of a secondary inhibitory effect of accumulating phosphorylated intermediates upon glycogenolysis.[72] Affected patients usually present shortly after birth with hepatomegaly and recurrent episodes of hypoglycemia, ketosis, and acidosis along with many of the biochemical features seen in GSD 1. In older children, fasting and infection may trigger episodes of hypoglycemia. Treatment that is aimed at avoidance of the known dietary precipitants can prevent hypoglycemia, reduce hepatomegaly, and improve growth.

Hereditary Fructose Intolerance. Hereditary fructose intolerance is due to a deficiency in the enzyme fructose 1-phosphate (F-1-P) aldolase, which is normally found in the liver, kidney, and intestines. As a result of this deficiency, fructose cannot be shuttled into the gluconeogenic pathway for conversion to glucose, resulting in a specific accumulation of F-1-P, the precursor immediately proximal to the enzyme block[74] (Fig. 5–2). This same enzyme is normally involved in the glycolytic pathway and catalyzes conversion of F-1,6-diP to D-glyceraldehyde. Accumulation of F-1-P, following intake of fructose, impedes both glycogenolysis and gluconeogenesis,[75] leading to hypoglycemia, poor feeding, vomiting, hepatomegaly, jaundice, renal tubulopathy, growth retardation, and even death.[76] Patients develop a strong aversion for sweets and can remain healthy with avoidance of dietary sucrose and fructose.

Substrate Disturbances. Disordered gluconeogenesis is also associated with genetic disturbances of substrate mobilization involving amino acid (e.g., maple syrup urine disease) or lipid (e.g., systemic carnitine deficiency) pathways. The exact mechanisms responsible for the pathogenesis of hypoglycemia in these rare disorders is unknown. Roles for both decreased amounts of substrate and diversion of substrates have been implicated in the amino acid disorders, whereas liver damage in conjunction with simultaneous overutilization of glucose may be contributory in disorders of fatty acid oxidation. A rare disorder associated with presumed substrate-limited hypoglycemia is glycerol intolerance.[77] It is reported to cause intermittent hypoglycemia, and symptoms of low blood glucose follow administration of glycerol or medium-chain triglycerides. In this condition, unlike fructose-1,6-diphosphatase deficiency, fructose challenge does not lead to hypoglycemia. No specific glycolytic or gluconeogenic enzymatic defect has been identified.

The prototype disorder of gluconeogenesis related to substrate deficiency is so-called ketotic hypoglycemia, which appears to be the most common cause of childhood hypoglycemia outside the newborn period, with a peak incidence between 18 months and 3 years of age. Occasional cases may begin later, with spontaneous resolution before puberty in all cases. Although the pathogenesis of the hypoglycemia is frequently ascribed to a deficiency of gluconeogenic amino acids, particularly alanine,[78] it is equally likely that the hypoalaninemia is the result, rather than the cause, of the hypoglycemia.[79] Affected children usually present with neuroglycopenic symptoms in the late morning with a history of having omitted breakfast and possibly also the previous night's supper, because of anorexia from an intercurrent illness. At the time of hypoglycemia, ketonemia and ketonuria are present with suppression of insulin secretion and appropriately increased serum concentrations of counterregulatory hormones. Compared to age-matched nonhypoglycemic children, youngsters prone to this form of hypoglycemia are traditionally thin for age with less muscle mass, which may be responsible for depletion of gluconeogenic amino acids. No specific enzymatic

defect or counterregulatory hormonal abnormality has been found in this condition. Ketotic hypoglycemia is more than likely a normal developmental phenomenon related to age,[80] and hence its alternate name, fasting functional hypoglycemia, should be preferentially used. Treatment consists of close monitoring of oral intake, inclusion of a routine prebedtime snack consisting of both protein and carbohydrate, avoidance of late arising, and monitoring of ketones during intercurrent illness. The diagnosis of the condition is quite straightforward and the patient can easily be handled by the nonspecialist.

Counterregulatory Hormone Deficiency. Counterregulatory hormone deficiency states can also be associated with hypoglycemia. As described in detail in Chapter 1, the infant with congenital growth hormone deficiency is prone to hypoglycemia. Similarly, any cause of glucocorticoid deficiency [as part of conditions causing primary adrenocortical failure (e.g., Addison disease, congenital adrenal hyperplasia or hypoplasia) or associated with central corticotropin-releasing factor or adrenocorticotropic hormone deficiency] may predispose to the development of hypoglycemia. A more detailed discussion of these disorders is provided in Chapter 6. While it has been suggested that the major cause of unclassified hypoglycemia in childhood is epinephrine deficiency,[81] these findings require further verification.

Acquired defects of gluconeogenesis may also occur as a component of liver disease (e.g., Reye syndrome). An important form of drug-induced inhibition of hepatic gluconeogenesis is that associated with alcohol. This may occur as a result of direct alcohol intake, particularly by the diabetic adolescent or, indirectly, from mouthwash experimentation by younger, otherwise normal children. Another acquired form of hypoglycemia is that of Jamaican vomiting sickness, which is due to the action of "hypoglycins" present in the unripe akee fruit. These substances cause decreased transport and oxidation of long-chain fatty acids that limit production of critical intermediates and energy sources necessary for gluconeogenesis.[1]

DIAGNOSIS OF CHILDHOOD HYPOGLYCEMIA

While various and sometimes complex algorithms have been employed to facilitate

TABLE 5–7. THE CRITICAL SAMPLE IN THE EVALUATION OF CHILDHOOD HYPOGLYCEMIA

Substrates	Hormones
Original	
Glucose (pre- and postglucagon)	Insulin
Ketones	Growth hormone
Free fatty acids	Cortisol
Lactate	Glucagon
Alanine	Thyroxine, triiodothyronine, thyroid-stimulating hormone
Uric acid	
Current modifications	
Glucose (pre- and postglucagon)	Insulin
Ketones	
+ 5–10 ml serum/plasma (provisional)	

the diagnosis of childhood hypoglycemia,[82] the following simplified strategy, based on the division of potential etiologies into those associated with overutilization of glucose and those associated with underproduction of glucose, can be successfully applied to most cases. This pathophysiologic approach underlies the concept of the "critical blood sample"[83] for measurement of glucose, ketones, insulin, counterregulatory hormones, and relevant substrates at the time of hypoglycemia (Table 5–7). However, the complete critical sample, as usually described,[83] is costly and measurement of all its recommended components is frequently not necessary. Alternatively, the following further modifications of this approach should be considered.

At the time of spontaneous or induced (by a controlled, in-hospital fast) hypoglycemia (bedside reagent strip whole-blood glucose less than 35 mg/dl), a blood sample (by venipuncture) should be obtained for laboratory measurement of serum concentrations of glucose, ketones, and insulin. Five to 10 ml of blood should be drawn simultaneously, placed in appropriate tubes, and held for possible measurement of other related hormones and substrates (depending on the outcome of the initial laboratory results and clinical presentation). This should be followed immediately by the intravenous, intramuscular, or subcutaneous injection of glucagon (30 μg/kg, maximum dose 1 mg) with bedside and laboratory glucose mea-

surements 10, 20, and 30 min later. The *routine* use of free fatty acid, lactate, alanine, uric acid, glucagon, or thyroid function tests in all cases should be discouraged.

As mentioned earlier (Table 5–4), spontaneous or rapid development of hypoglycemia with fasting (usually less than 4 hours), lack of associated ketonemia (or ketonuria), a rise in plasma or serum glucose concentration over 30 mg/dl above hypoglycemic baseline, and subsequent glucose requirement of 12 mg/kg/min or more to maintain normoglycemia virtually ensure the diagnosis of hyperinsulinemia, the most common cause of persistent hypoglycemia in the first year of life. An elevated serum insulin level (or insulin-glucose ratio) at the time of hypoglycemia is diagnostic. The need for measurement of blood levels of other substrates and counterregulatory hormones is therefore unnecessary if these criteria are met.

The most likely cause of hypoglycemia in the older child (over 18 months of age) is the fasting functional form of ketotic hypoglycemia. However, any cause of hypoglycemia secondary to underproduction of glucose (except systemic carnitine deficiency) will be of the ketotic variety since insulin production will be inhibited and lipolysis activated. Additionally, in the underproduction states, the glycemic response to glucagon will be less than 30 mg/dl above hypoglycemic baseline (and sometimes zero) because (nearly) all glycogen will be depleted in the face of inhibition of insulin secretion.[40] In this setting it is conceivable that the other substrates and hormones of the critical sample would need to be measured. However, most of the time the history, physical examination, and other laboratory tests determined prior to hypoglycemia should clarify the need for analysis of additional components of the critical sample.

For example, the presence of significant hepatomegaly and a protuberant abdomen in the growth-delayed child with associated ketonemia, hyperlipidemia, hyperuricemia, acidosis, and blunted glycemic response to glucagon suggests the presence of GSD I. This constellation of findings necessitates performance of a specific diagnostic test (liver biopsy) and evaluation for associated metabolic, hematologic, and hepatic abnormalities.

Alternatively, hypopituitarism is suggested by the presence of short stature (although this may not be present in the first year of life), a relative excess of weight for height, microphallus in the male, ketonemia, and blunted glycemic response to glucagon. Here the critical sample should be processed for growth hormone (and cortisol) with attention given to other possible hypothalamic-pituitary–target organ hormone abnormalities. In the interpretation of the growth hormone response, it should be remembered that serum growth hormone levels in the first year of life are normally "high" in the basal state (compared to later childhood) and may hyperrespond to hypoglycemic stimuli.[84] In addition, growth hormone responses to hypoglycemia induced by prolonged fasting may be blunted in the non-growth-hormone–deficient child,[85] thereby making the *routine* performance of this test difficult to interpret.

The presence of hyperpigmentation in the child with hypoglycemia, ketonemia, and a blunted glycemic response to glucagon suggests the diagnosis of primary adrenal insufficiency and requires measurement of the serum cortisol level in the critical sample. Attention should be paid to the possibility of associated mineralcorticoid insufficiency, and possible involvement of other endocrine glands. The interpretation of the serum cortisol response to hypoglycemia must take into account the known "low morning levels that occur in infancy (as low as 2 μg/dl)[86] and possible associated hepatic disorders that could affect cortisol-binding globulin concentrations.

Other metabolic defects should be suspected based on specific feeding history, family history, and physical examination. Carefully performed challenge tests (e.g., glycerol, galactose, fructose) may help to delineate a presumed defect and measurement of enzyme activity may be necessary to make a specific diagnosis.

In still other situations in which older children and adolescents complain of symptoms suggestive of hypoglycemia (e.g., lightheadedness, shakiness, diaphoresis, weakness, and fatigue), before embarking on a complex evaluation, documentation of hypoglycemia at the time of alleged symptoms is mandatory. In this setting, the diagnosis of reactive hypoglycemia has historically been made based on the induction of hypoglycemia (not necessarily with associated symptoms) 3 to 5 hours after an oral glucose load. Because of the benign nature of this "problem," its simple dietary "therapy,"

and popularization by media and self-styled nutritionists, reactive hypoglycemia is frequently diagnosed to account for such symptomatology. Careful analysis, however, reveals that 10 per cent of normal subjects have glucose values of less than 47 mg/dl and 2.5 per cent have values of less than 39 mg/dl during an oral glucose tolerance test. Furthermore, psychological assessments of these patients, including children, reveal a high incidence of underlying neuroses and emotional disturbances (conversion V profile on the Minnesota Multiphasic Personality Inventory),[87] with parental belief systems frequently passed on to "symptomatic" children. These findings have led to the characterization of reactive hypoglycemia as a nondisease of epidemic proportions.[88] For the rare patient with true reactive, postprandial hypoglycemia, simultaneous hypoglycemia and symptoms are best diagnosed either spontaneously or following a standardized meal challenge test.[89] In any case, reactive hypoglycemia does not appear to be a forerunner of future diabetes.[90]

While new methods for the workup of the hypoglycemic child, such as the 2-deoxyglucose test,[91] have been proposed, the simplified version of the critical sample at the time of hypoglycemia remains the cornerstone for the diagnostic evaluation.

REFERENCES

1. Cornblath M, Schwartz R: Disorders of Carbohydrate Metabolism in Infancy. Philadelphia, WB Saunders Company, 1976.
2. Sauls JS Jr, Ulstrom RA: Hypoglycemia. *In* Kelley VC (ed): Brennenmann's Practice of Pediatrics. Hagerstown, MD, WF Prior Co, 1966, chap 40.
3. Klaus MH, Fanaroff AA: Care of the High-Risk Neonate. Philadelphia, WB Saunders Company, 1973, p 170.
4. Srinivasan G, Pildes RS, Cattamanchi G, Voora S, Lilien LD: Plasma glucose values in normal neonates: A new look. J Pediatr 109:114, 1986.
5. Heck LJ, Erenberg A: Serum glucose levels in term neonates during the first 48 hours of life. J Pediatr 110:119, 1987.
6. Sexson WR: Incidence of neonatal hypoglycemia: A matter of definition. J Pediatr 105:149, 1984.
7. Lecavalier L, Bolli G, Gerich J: Major role for gluconeogenesis during counter-regulation in man. Diabetes 36(Suppl):9A, 1987.
8. Frizzell RT, Campbell PJ, Cherrington AD: Gluconeogenesis and hypoglycemia. Diabetes Metab Rev 4:51, 1988.
9. Simmons PS, Miles JM, Gerich JE, Haymond MW: Increased proteolysis: An effect of increases in plasma cortisol within the physiologic range. J Clin Invest 73:412, 1984.

10. Exton JH, Friedmann N, Wong EHA, Brineaux JP, Corbin JD, Park CR: Interaction of glucocorticoids with glucagon and epinephrine in the control of gluconeogenesis and glycogenolysis in liver and of lipolysis in adipose tissue. J Biol Chem 11:3579, 1972.

11. Gerich JE, Lorenzi M, Bier DM, Tsalikian E, Schneider V, Karam JH, Forsham PH: Effects of physiologic levels of glucagon and growth hormone on human carbohydrate and lipid metabolism. J Clin Invest 57:875, 1976.

12. Davis MA, Williams PE, Cherrington AD: Effect of glucagon on hepatic lactate metabolism in the conscious dog. Am J Physiol 248 (Endocrinol Metab 11):E463, 1985.

13. Bier DM, Leake RD, Haymond MW, Arnold KJ, Gruenke LD, Sperling MA, Kipnis DM: Measurement of "true" glucose production rates in infancy and childhood with 6,6-dideuteroglucose. Diabetes 26:1016, 1977.

14. Stanley CA, Anday EK, Baker L, Delivoria-Papadopolous M: Metabolic fuel and hormone responses to fasting in newborn infants. Pediatrics 64:613, 1979.

15. Shelley HJ, Neligan GA: Neonatal hypoglycaemia. Br Med Bull 22:34, 1966.

16. Ogata ES: Carbohydrate metabolism in the fetus and neonate and altered neonatal glucoregulation. Pediatr Clin North Am 33:25, 1986.

17. Landau H, Perlman M, Meyer S, Isacsohn M, Krausz M, Mayan H, Lijovetsky G, Schiller M: Persistent neonatal hypoglycemia due to hyperinsulinism: Medical aspects. Pediatrics 70:440, 1982.

18. Aynsley-Green A, Polak JM, Bloom SR, Gough MH, Keeling J, Ashcroft SJH, Turner RC, Baum JD: Nesidioblastosis of the pancreas: Definition of the syndrome and the management of the severe neonatal hyperinsulinaemic hypoglycaemia. Arch Dis Child 56:496, 1981.

19. Stanley CA, Baker L: Hyperinsulinism in infants and children: Diagnosis and therapy. Adv Pediatr 23:315, 1976.

20. Witte DP, Greider MH, DeSchryver-Kecskemeti K, Kissane JM, White NH: The juvenile human endocrine pancreas: Normal v idiopathic hyperinsulinemic hypoglycemia. Semin Diagn Pathol 1:30, 1984.

21. AvRuskin TW, Crigler JF, Soeldner JS: Diazoxide treatment of neonatal and infant hypoglycemia: A review and reassessment. J Pediatr Endocrinol 1:49, 1985.

22. Schwartz JF, Zwiren GT: Islet cell adenomatosis and ademona in an infant. J Pediatr 79:232, 1971.

23. Case records of the Massachusetts General Hospital. N Engl J Med 299:241, 1978.

24. Jaffe R, Hashida Y, Yunis EJ: Pancreactic pathology in hyperinsulinemic hypoglycemia of infancy. Lab Invest 42:356, 1980.

25. Rahier J, Fält K, Müntefering H, Becker K, Gepts W, Falkmer S: The basic structural lesion of persistent neonatal hypoglycaemia with hyperinsulinism: Deficiency of pancreatic D cells or hyperactivity of B cells? Diabetologia 26:282, 1984.

26. Bishop AE, Polak JM, Garin Chesa P, Timson CM, Bryant MG, Bloom SR: Decrease of pancreatic somatostatin in neonatal nesidioblastosis. Diabetes 30:122, 1981.

27. Schwartz SS, Rich BH, Lucky AW, Straus FH, Gonen B, Wolfsdorf J, Thorp FW, Burrington JD, Madden JD, Rubenstein AH, Rosenfield RL: Familial nesidioblastosis: Severe neonatal hypoglycemia in two families. J Pediatr 95:44, 1979.

28. Brandi ML, Marx SJ, Aurbach GD, Fitzpatrick LA: Familial multiple endocrine neoplasia type I: A new look at pathophysiology. Endocr Rev 8:391, 1987.

29. Neufeld ND, Kaplan SA, Lippe BM, Scott M: Increased monocyte receptor binding of [^{126}I] insulin in infants of gestational diabetic mothers. J Clin Endocrinol Metab 47:590, 1978.

30. Schiff D, Colle E, Wells D, Stern L: Metabolic aspects of the Beckwith-Wiedemann syndrome. J Pediatr 82:258, 1973.

31. Falorni A, Fracassini F, Massi-Benedetti F, Amici A: Glucose metabolism, plasma insulin, and growth hormone secretion in newborn infants with erythroblastosis fetalis compared with normal newborns and those born to diabetic mothers. Pediatrics 49:682, 1972.

32. Smith VS, Giacoia GP: Hyperinsulinaemic hypoglycaemia in an infant with mosaic trisomy 13. J Med Genet 22:228, 1985.

33. Byrne WJ, Lippe BM, Strobel CT, Levin SR, Ament ME, Kaplan SA: Adaptation to increasing loads of total parenteral nutrition: Metabolic, endocrine, and insulin receptor responses. Gastroenterology 80:947, 1981.

34. Rivkees SA, Crawford JD: Hypoglycemia pathogenesis in children with dumping syndrome. Pediatrics 80:937, 1987.

35. Rizza RA: Use of artificial devices in intensive insulin therapy of diabetes mellitus. Clin Chem 32:B97, 1986.

36. Santiago JV, White NH, Skor DA, Levandoski LA, Bier DM, Cryer PE: Defective glucose counterregulation limits intensive therapy of diabetes mellitus. Am J Physiol 247 (Endocrinol Metab 10):E215, 1984.

37. Procianoy RS, Pinheiro CEA: Neonatal hyperinsulinism after short-term maternal beta sympathomimetic therapy. J Pediatr 101:612, 1982.

38. White NJ, Warrell DA, Chanthavanich P, Looareesuwan S, Warrell MJ, Krishna S, Williamson DH, Turner RC: Severe hypoglycemia and hyperinsulinemia in falciparum malaria. N Engl J Med 309:61, 1983.

39. Fajans SS: Leucine-induced hypoglycemia. N Engl J Med 272:1224, 1965.

40. Finegold DN, Standley CA, Baker L: Glycemic response to glucagon during fasting hypoglycemia: An aid in the diagnosis of hyperinsulinism. J Pediatr 96:257, 1980.

41. Chapoy PR, Angelini C, Brown WJ, Stiff JE, Shug AL, Cederbaum SD: Systemic carnitine deficiency—a treatable inherited lipid-storage disease presenting as Reye's syndrome. N Engl J Med 303:1389, 1980.

42. Wolfsdorf JI, Sadeghi-Nejad A, Senior B: Ketonuria does not exclude hyperinsulinemic hypoglycemia. Am J Dis Child 138:168, 1984.

43. Mehta A, Wootton R, Cheng KN, Penfold P, Halliday D, Stacey TE: Effect of diazoxide or glucagon on hepatic glucose production rate during extreme neonatal hypoglycaemia. Arch Dis Child 62:924, 1987.

44. Elias D, Cohen IR, Shechter Y, Spirer Z, Golander A: Antibodies to insulin receptor followed by anti-idiotype. Antibodies to insulin in child with hypoglycemia. Diabetes 36:348, 1987.

45. Nakagawa S, Suda N, Kudo M, Kawasaki M: A new type of hypoglycaemia in a newborn infant. Diabetologia 9:367, 1973.

46. Seino S, Fu ZZ, Marks W, Seino Y, Imura H, Vinik A: Characterization of circulating insulin in insulin autoimmune syndrome. J Clin Endocrinol Metab 62:64, 1986.

47. Ichikara K, Shima K, Saito Y, Nonaka K, Tarui S, Nishikawa M: Mechanism of hypoglycemia observed in a patient with insulin autoimmune syndrome. Diabetes 26:500, 1977.

48. Wolfsdorf JI, Senior B: The diagnosis of insulinoma in a child in the absence of fasting hyperinsulinemia. Pediatrics 64:496, 1979.

49. Aynsley-Green A, Jenkins P, Tronier B, Heding LG: Plasma proinsulin and c-peptide concentrations in children with hyperinsulinaemic hypoglycaemia. Acta Paediatr Scand 73:359, 1984.

50. Albers N, Conte FA, Rosenthal SM, Kaplan SL, Grumbach MM: Outcome and side-effects of long-term treatment with diazoxide in children with hyperinsulinemic hypoglycemia. Clin Res 36:213A, 1988.

51. Grant DB, Dunger DB, Burns EC: Long-term treatment with diazoxide in childhood hyperinsulinism. Acta Endocrinol 113(Suppl 279):340, 1986.

52. Zuniga O, Golden MP, Sargeant DT, Graham MJ, Bradvica C, Santiago J, White NH: Persistent leucine sensitivity following partial pancreatectomy and diazoxide treatment. Am J Dis Child 137:393, 1983.

53. Roti E, Ghinelli C, Bandini P, Del Rossi C, Emanuele R, Robuschi G, Gnudi A: Effects of somatostatin in a case of severe hypoglycemia due to nesidioblastosis. J Endocrinol Invest 4:209, 1981.

54. Bougnères PF, Landier F, Garnier P, Job JC, Chaussain JL: Treatment of insulin excess by continuous subcutaneous infusion of somatostatin and glucagon in an infant. J Pediatr 106:792, 1985.

55. Bruining GJ, Bosschaart AN, Aarsen RSR, Lamberts SWJ, Sauer PJJ, Del Pozo E: Normalization of glucose homeostasis by a long-acting somatostatin analog SMS 201-995 in a newborn with nesidioblastosis. Acta Endocrinol 113(Suppl 279):334, 1986.

56. Jackson JA, Hahn Jr HB, Oltorf CE, O'Dorisio TM, Vinik AI: Long-term treatment of refractory neonatal hypoglycemia with long-acting somatostatin analog. J Pediatr 111:548, 1987.

57. Fonkalsrud EW, Trout HH, Lippe B, LaFranchi S, Dakake C: Idiopathic hypoglycemia in infancy. Arch Surg 108:801, 1974.

58. Slonim AE: Recent advances in treatment of the glycogenoses. J Pediatr Endocrinol 1:21, 1985.

59. Tsalikian E, Simmons P, Howard C, Haymond MW: Near normal glucose production in type 1 GSD. Pediatr Res 16:265A, 1982.

60. Schaub J, Heyne K: Glycogen storage disease type Ib. Eur J Pediatr 140:283, 1983.

61. Zangeneh F, Limbeck GA, Brown BI, Emch JR, Arcasoy MM, Goldenberg VE, Kelley VC: Hepatorenal glycogenosis (type I glycogenosis) and carcinoma of the liver. J Pediatr 74:73, 1969.

62. Ambruso DR, McCabe ERB, Anderson D, Beaudet A, Ballas LM, Brandt IK, Brown B, Coleman R, Dunger DB, Falletta JM, Friedman HS, Haymond MW, Keating JP, Kinney TR, Leonard JV, Mahoney Jr DH, Matalon R, Roe TF, Simmons P, Slonim AE: Infectious and bleeding complications in patients with glycogenosis Ib. Am J Dis Child 139:691, 1985.

63. Fernandes J, Leonard JV, Moses SW, Odièvre M, di Rocco M, Schaub J Smit GPA, Ullrich K, Durand P: Glycogen storage disease: Recommendations for treatment. Eur J Pediatr 147:226, 1988.

64. Schwenk WF, Haymond MW: Optimal rate of enteral glucose administration in children with glycogen storage disease type I. N Engl J Med 314:682, 1986.

65. Sidbury JB, Chen YT, Roe CR: The role of raw starches in the treatment of type I glycogenosis. Arch Intern Med 146:370, 1986.

66. Michels VV, Beaudet AL, Potts VE, Montandon CM: Glycogen storage disease: Long-term follow-up of nocturnal intragastric feeding. Clin Genet 21:136, 1982.

67. Malatack JJ, Finegold DN, Iwatsuki S, Shaw Jr BW, Gartner JC, Zitelli BJ, Roe T, Starzl TE: Liver transplantation for type I glycogen storage disease. Lancet 1:1073, 1983.

68. Hug G: Glycogen storage disease. Birth Defects 12:145, 1976.

69. Kliegman RM, Sparks JW: Perinatal galactose metabolism. J Pediatr 107:831, 1985.

70. Dennehy PH, O'Shea PA, Abuelo DN: A newborn infant with bilious vomiting and jitteriness. J Pediatr 106:161, 1985.

71. Kaufman FR, Donnell GN, Roe TF, Kogut MD: Gonadal function in patients with galactosaemia. J Inherited Metab Dis 9:140, 1986.

72. Melancon SB, Khachadurian AK, Nadler HL, Brown BI: Metabolic and biochemical studies in fructose 1,6-diphosphatase deficiency. J Pediatr 82:650, 1973.

73. Baker L, Winegrad AI: Fasting hypoglycaemia and metabolic acidosis associated with deficiency of hepatic fructose-1,6-diphosphatase activity. Lancet 2:13, 1970.

74. Odièvre M, Gentil C, Gautier M, Alagille D: Hereditary fructose intolerance in childhood. Am J Dis Child 132:605, 1978.

75. Kaufmann U, Froesch ER: Inhibition of phosphorylase-a by fructose-1-phosphate, α-glycerophosphate and fructose-1,6-diphosphate: Explanation for fructose-induced hypoglycaemia in hereditary fructose intolerance and fructose-1,6-diphosphatase deficiency. Eur J Clin Invest 3:407, 1973.

76. Mock DM, Perman JA, Thaler MM, Morris Jr RC: Chronic fructose intoxication after infancy in children with hereditary fructose intolerance. N Engl J Med 309:764, 1983.

77. Maclaren NK, Cowles C, Ozand PT, Shuttee R, Cornblath M: Glycerol intolerance in a child with intermittent hypoglycemia. J Pediatr 86:43, 1975.

78. Haymond MW, Karl IE, Pagliara AS: Ketotic hypoglycemia: An amino acid substrate limited disorder. J Clin Endocrinol Metab 38:521, 1974.

79. Wolfsdorf JI, Sadeghi-Nejad A, Senior B: Hypoalaninemia and ketotic hypoglycemia: Cause or consequence? Eur J Pediatr 138:28, 1982.

80. Saudubray JM, Marsac C, Limal JM, Dumurgier E, Charpentier C, Ogier H, Coudè FX: Variation in plasma ketone bodies during a 24-hour fast in normal and in hypoglycemic children: Relationship to age. J Pediatr 98:904, 1981.

81. Hansen IL, Levy MM, Kerr DS: Differential diagnosis of hypoglycemia in children by responses

to fasting and 2-deoxyglucose. Metabolism 32:960, 1983.

82. Phillip M, Bashan N, Smith CPA, Moses SW: An algorithmic approach to diagnosis of hypoglycemia. J Pediatr 110:387, 1987.

83. Cornblath M: Hypoglycemia in infancy and childhood. Pediatr Ann 10:49, 1981.

84. Cornblath M, Parker ML, Reisner SH, Forbes AE, Daughaday WH: Secretion and metabolism of growth hormone in premature and full-term infants. J Clin Endocrinol 25:209, 1965.

85. Kerr DS, Hansen IL, Levy MM: Metabolic and hormonal responses of children and adolescents to fasting and 2-deoxyglucose. Metabolism 32:951, 1983.

86. Stark P, Beckerhoff R, Leumann EP, Vetter W, Siegenthaler W: Control of plasma aldosterone in infancy and childhood. Helv Paediatr Acta 30:349, 1975.

87. Johnson DD, Dorr KE, Swenson WM, Service J: Reactive hypoglycemia. JAMA 243:1151, 1980.

88. Yager J, Young RT: Non-hypoglycemia is an epidemic condition. N Engl J Med 291:907, 1974.

89. Hogan MJ, Service FJ, Sharbrough FW, Gerich JE: Oral glucose tolerance test compared with a mixed meal in the diagnosis of reactive hypoglycemia. Mayo Clin Proc 58:491, 1983.

90. Gastineau CF: Is reactive hypoglycemia a clinical entity? Mayo Clin Proc 58:545, 1983.

91. Hansen IL, Levy MM, Kerr DS: The 2-deoxyglucose test as a supplement to fasting for detection of childhood hypoglycemia. Pediatr Res 18:490, 1984.

6

THE ADRENAL CORTEX

Maria I. New, Patrizia del Balzo, Christopher Crawford, and Phyllis W. Speiser

THE ADRENAL CORTEX: STRUCTURE AND FUNCTIONS

Steroid hormones in plasma arise from the secretory activity of the adrenal cortex, the male and female gonads, and the placenta in pregnancy. Limited steroid synthesis has also been shown to occur in nonendocrine tissues such as brain,[1] the steroids produced in this case presumed to function in intracellular (autocrine) or paracrine roles. Pathologically, steroids may be generated in considerable amounts by adenomas and actively secreting carcinomas, or may be introduced by therapeutic administration.

Steroidogenesis

Regulation of Steroidogenesis

Adrenocorticotropin. The integrity of the adrenal gland and its ability to syntheisze steroid hormones are dependent upon pituitary secretion of the peptide adrenocorticotropin (ACTH).[2,3] Adrenocorticotropin is one of a group of trophic hormones that are cleavage products of a large molecular weight precursor, pro-opiomelanocortin (POMC), synthesized in the anterior and intermediate lobes of the pituitary. In the anterior lobe POMC is processed to three major biologically active peptides: ACTH, β-lipotropin, and a large NH_2-terminal fragment, N-POMC (pro-γ-melanotropin), that has been shown to potentiate the adrenal steroidogenic response to ACTH[4] (Fig. 6–1). Release of ACTH from the pituitary is in turn modulated by the neuronal peptide corticotropin-releasing factor (CRF)[5] originating in the hypothalamus[6–8]; the primary action of CRF[9] is augmented by (arginine) vasopressin (AVP)[10] (recently reviewed in ref. 11).

The hypothalamic-pituitary-adrenal axis forms a regulated system (Fig. 6–2). Corticotropin-releasing factor stimulates the secretion of ACTH by the pituitary; ACTH is released in pulsatile fashion into the circulation, where it has a relatively short plasma half-life, and the binding of ACTH to specific receptors in the adrenal cortex promotes cortisol synthesis. Negative feedback control is exerted by cortisol, directly inhibiting ACTH release from the pituitary, and modulating release of CRF from the hypothalamus relative to a set-point determined by the central nervous system for the expected plasma cortisol level. Net ACTH release has basal, diurnal, and stress-induced components. Plasma cortisol levels below the central (hypothalamic-pituitary) set-point will increase the rate and intensity of ACTH secretory pulses. Adrenal enzyme deficiencies causing impaired synthesis and decreased secretion of cortisol thus lead to chronic elevations of ACTH, with overstimulation and consequent hyperplasia of the adrenal cortex.

Angiotensin II/[K^+]. The zona glomerulosa, in which aldosterone synthesis occurs, is responsive to changes in plasma volume via the renin-angiotensin system,[12] and responsive to the state of serum electrolyte balance directly via the serum K^+ concentration, and the rate of aldosterone synthesis is primarily modulated by these two factors, angiotensin II and potassium. Angiotensin II is the main effector peptide in the regulation of blood pressure and salt and water homeostasis by the renin-angiotensin system. Binding to specific receptors on cells of the zona glomerulosa and stimulating early (cholesterol to pregnenolone) steroid synthesis, angiotensin II is also a potent pressor agent, acting directly and immediately on the vasculature to increase renal perfusion pressure.[13] There is a latency period of about 60 min before the effects of

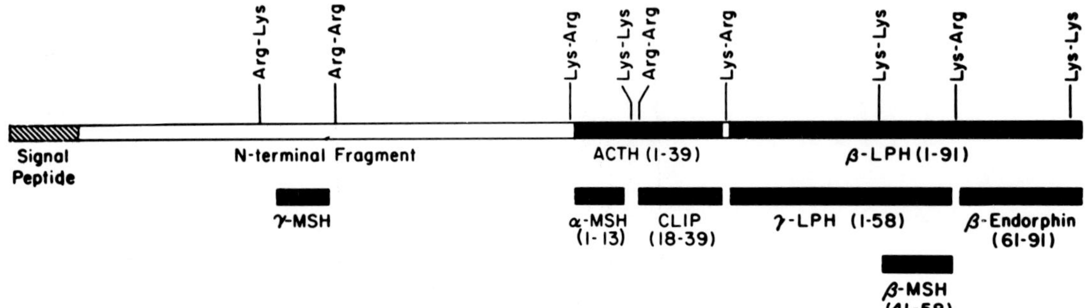

FIGURE 6–1. Schematic of the cleavage products of the bovine precursor peptide molecule pro-opiomelanocortin (POMC). The top bar shows (after the signal peptide) the three major anterior lobe peptides, (1) NH_2-terminal (16-kb) fragment, (2) ACTH, and (3) β-lipotropin. The two sites of proteolytic cleavage for these three components are arginine-lysine (RK) pairs. Further cleavage (at RR, RK, KK, and KR sites) generates these subfragments: (1) γ-melanotropin (γ-MSH) processed from a short precursor section in NH_2-terminal fragment, (2) α-melanocyte-stimulating hormone (α-MSH) and corticotropin-like intermediate lobe peptide (CLIP) from ACTH, and (3) γ-lipotropin (γ-LPH), β-melanocyte-stimulating hormone (β-MSH), and β-endorphin from β-lipoprotein (β-LPH). (From Krieger DT, Liotta AS, Brownstein MJ, Zimmerman EA: ACTH, β-lipotropin and related peptides in brain, pituitary, and blood (review). Recent Prog Horm Res 36:277, 1980.)

increased aldosterone synthesis are seen at the renal tubule.

The enzyme renin is secreted by specialized epithelioid cells of the juxtaglomerular afferent arterioles in the kidneys. Its secretion is controlled by (1) renal perfusion pressure, (2) renal adrenergic nerve activity, and (3) the distal tubular sodium load, communicated by the macula densa; renin secretion is subject as well to modification by numerous hormonal substances. Angiotensinogen is a glycoprotein of molecular weight 54,000 to 57,000 Da whose synthesis in the liver is significantly induced by glucocorticoids (and contraceptive steroids); because renin exhibits absolute specificity for binding of NH_2-terminal sequences of angiotensinogen, this peptide is also simply termed *renin substrate*. Angiotensin I results from the cleavage of angiotensinogen in plasma by renin. Angiotensin II is generated from the processing of the decapeptide angiotensin I by angiotensin I–converting enzyme (ACE), predominantly in the pulmonary vascular bed but also locally in other tissues, and is cleared nonspecifically with a half-life in the circulation of 15 to 30 min (see Fig. 6–3).

Aldosterone secretion is also stimulated directly by high serum K^+ concentration, less sensitively by low serum Na^+ concentration, and by ACTH.[14] Adrenocorticotro-

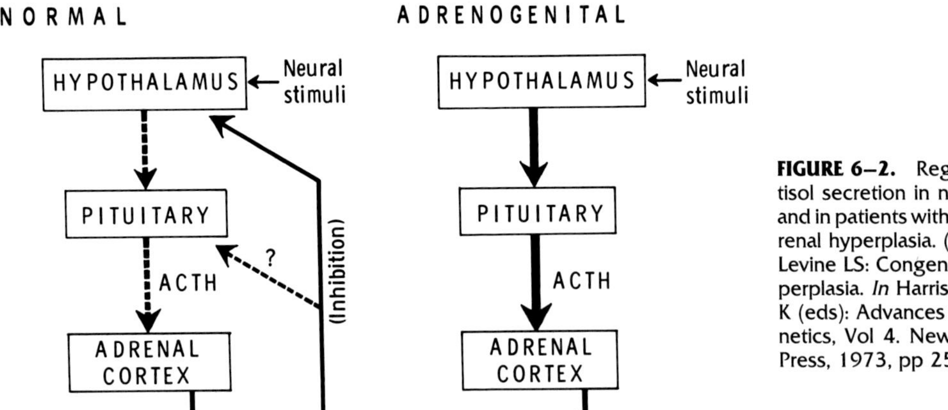

FIGURE 6–2. Regulation of cortisol secretion in normal subjects and in patients with congenital adrenal hyperplasia. (From New MI, Levine LS: Congenital adrenal hyperplasia. *In* Harris H, Hirschhorn K (eds): Advances in Human Genetics, Vol 4. New York, Plenum Press, 1973, pp 251–326.)

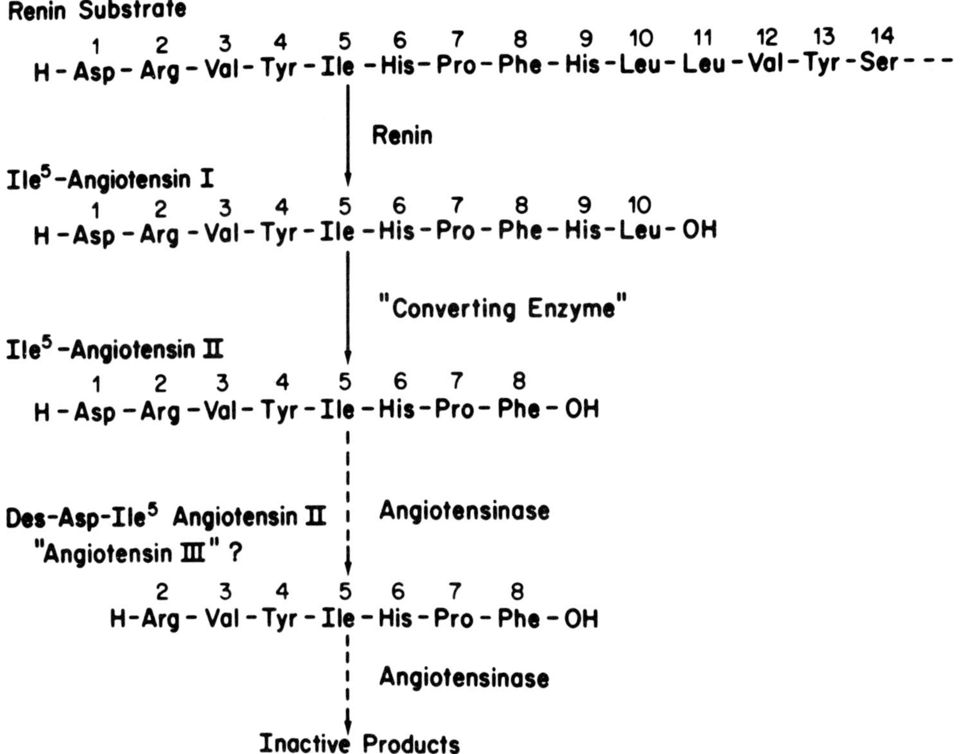

FIGURE 6–3. Factors regulating the synthesis/secretion of aldosterone by the adrenal cortex. (From New MI, Peterson RE: Disorders of aldosterone secretion in childhood. Pediatr Clin North Am 13:43, 1966.)

pin has a permissive role through its general effect on adrenocortical function, but in addition to this the zona glomerulosa is transiently very sensitive to ACTH, especially when the late aldosterone synthetic stages specific to this zone have been potentiated by chronic angiotensin II stimulation or electrolyte imbalance (K^+ loading/Na^+ restriction).[15,16] Other mediators have been named, but their physiologic significance remains unconfirmed. Thus the four major factors affecting aldosterone synthesis by the zona glomerulosa are angiotensin II, K^+, Na^+, and ACTH (Fig. 6–4).

Steroid Synthetic Pathways

Steroids secreted by the adrenal cortex are of three types: mineralocorticoids, glucocorticoids, and sex steroids. Corticosteroids (mineralocorticoids and glucocorticoids), produced uniquely in the adrenals, and the follicular/luteal and placental progestagens are C_{21} steroids. Sex steroids, which are synthesized in the gonads and adrenals, may be androgenic (C_{19} steroids) or estrogenic (C_{18} steroids); adrenal sex steroid production is essentially of androgens only.

The first and rate-limiting step in steroid synthesis is the conversion of the C_{27} sterol cholesterol to the C_{21} steroid pregnenolone by removal of a six-carbon fragment. This step, called side-chain cleavage, takes place at the mitochondrial inner membrane.[17]

Pregnenolone is the common precursor for all other steroids. After formation in the mitochondrion it is exported to the smooth endoplasmic reticulum (SER), where steroid intermediates are synthesized by the enzymes steroid 17α-hydroxylase/17,20-lyase and 3β-hydroxysteroid dehydrogenase (3β-ol dehydrogenase).

The action of the 3β-ol dehydrogenase enzyme, converting pregnenolone to progesterone and 17α-hydroxypregnenolone to 17α-hydroxyprogesterone, is NAD^+ dependent. In the C_{19} series, 3β-ol dehydrogenase acts to a lesser extent, converting the Δ^5 androgen precursor dehydroepiandrosterone (DHEA) to Δ^4-androstenedione.

Cytochrome P450c17 is a single SER-bound (i.e., microsomal) cytochrome P450 exhibiting dual activity.[18] In addition to its 17α-hydroxylase function, P450c17 cleaves the 17,20 carbon-carbon bond of 17α-hy-

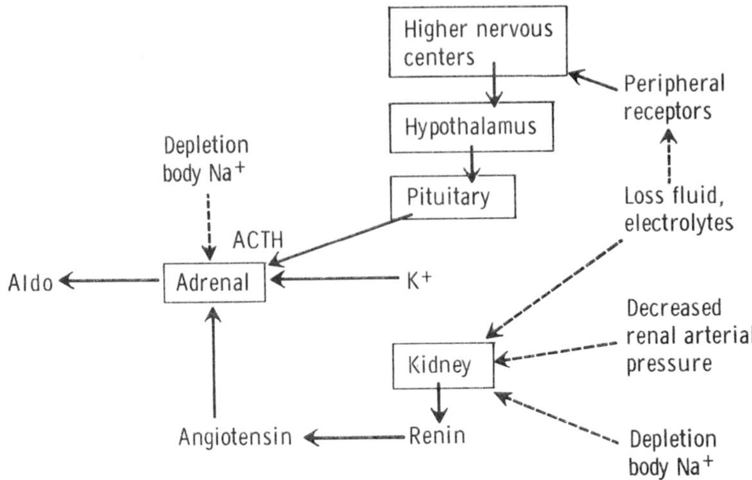

FIGURE 6–4. Biochemistry of the renin-angiotensin system. Ile[5]-angiotensin contains isoleucine in the 5 position and is the form of peptide that occurs in man. The existence of des-Asp[1]-angiotensin II as an intermediate in the pathway has not been definitely established. (From Oparil S, Haber E: N Engl J Med 291:389, 1974.)

droxylated steroids (17,20-lyase activity) to produce 17-ketosteroids. Thus, the Δ^5-17α-hydroxypregnenolone, instead of going to Δ^4-17α-hydroxyprogesterone, may be further converted by P450c17 to DHEA, and Δ^4-17α-hydroxyprogesterone may be further converted to Δ^4-androstenedione. Because C_{19} production requires the 17,20-lyase function, and C_{18} (estrogen) production requires C_{19} substrates, cytochrome P450c17 therefore determines all sex steroid production. Both pathways from C_{21} to C_{19} compounds are operative, for instance in testosterone synthesis in the testis,[19] whereas in the normal adrenal only the Δ^5 pathway (to DHEA) is active and the Δ^4 pathway is quantitatively minor. When concentrations of substrate are excessive, as occurs in several of the forms of congenital adrenal hyperplasia, the resulting production of adrenal androgens can be physiologically significant.

The 21-hydroxylase enzyme is also a microsomal cytochrome P450, P450c21; it accepts both 17α-hydroxyprogesterone and progesterone as substrates. 21-Hydroxylation of 17α-hydroxyprogesterone produces 11-deoxycortisol (compound S),[20] the immediate precursor of cortisol. 21-Hydroxylation of progesterone produces deoxycorticosterone (DOC) for aldosterone synthesis in the zona glomerulosa.

Transport of compound S and DOC to the mitochondrial inner membrane provides the substrates for a second mitochondrial cytochrome P450 enzyme, P450c11,[21] to convert to the final adrenal corticosteroid products.[22] 11β-Hydroxylation of compound S

yields cortisol in a single step. In the zona glomerulosa, P450c11 is responsible for three steps in sequence, completing aldosterone synthesis: in addition to 11β-hydroxylation of DOC to corticosterone (compound B), 18-hydroxylase and 18-oxidase activities of P450c11 convert compound B to 18-hydroxycorticosterone and then to aldosterone.[22,23] These steps are also called corticosterone methyloxidase (CMO) type I (18-hydroxylase) and type II (18-oxidase); the terminal 18-oxidase or CMO II function takes place only in the glomerulosa. In the zona fasciculata, there is some 18-hydroxylation of DOC and substance B.

Development and Physiology

Histology and Zonation

There are three histologically discernible zones in the adult cortex: the (outer) zona glomerulosa, the middle zona fasciculata, which is the widest zone, and the inner zona reticularis. The gland is extensively vascularized. Arterial branches supplying blood to the adrenals feed into a subcapsular plexus from which blood flow proceeds centripetally to a central (medullary) portal vein. This directional perfusion creates high blood concentration gradients of secreted steroids (hormones and intermediates) that in certain cases affect enzymatic activities and locally influence cellular development and thus the organization of the zones.

A functional division exists between the zona glomerulosa and the zona fasciculata.

(The lipid-rich zona fasciculata and denser zona reticularis are not enzymatically distinct, the moving boundary between them appearing to be a function of the degree and duration of ACTH stimulation and concomitant lipid depletion.) Clinical data on regulation and secretion support the concept of the zona glomerulosa and the zona fasciculata behaving as two separate glands: cortisol is produced in the zona fasciculata under the control of ACTH, and aldosterone originates from the zona glomerulosa, which while still tonically dependent on ACTH is principally governed by angiotensin II and serum [K$^+$].

Fetal Development

The adrenal cortex arises from mesodermal cells migrating from the celomic epithelium—as do the steroidogenic gonadal tissues—very early in the embryonic period. A distinct cortical mass is seen in the fourth week, becoming an active secretor of steroids by the sixth week; this cell population, organized into a provisional zone, comprises the functional cortex in the fetal period. The provisional cortex functions co-ordinately with the placenta and fetal liver in steroidogenesis in the fetal compartment. This will not be discussed here. The permanent (i.e., adult) cortex derives from a second migration of cells that forms around the fetal cortex, remaining as a thin peripheral rim until the end of gestation and becoming active only with the involution of the fetal cortex in the neonatal period. Throughout the intrauterine period the (fetal) cortex has grown significantly, reaching one third the size of the kidneys at term (10 times the relative size of the adult cortex). With its rapid regression soon after birth, the permanent cortex assumes the steroidogenic functions and develops the zonal organization of the adult gland.

Sexual Differentiation.   According to the model developed first by Jost,[24,25] normal male differentiation is dependent on two functions of the fetal testes: first, the secretion of sufficient quantities of testosterone to stabilize the mesonephric tubules as the wolffian ducts and to direct their formation into the male internal genital structures (the epididymides, vasa deferentia, seminal vesicles, and ejaculatory ducts); and second, the secretion of anti-müllerian hormone (AMH), a glycoprotein[26] factor synthesized by the Sertoli cells of the testis[27] to suppress development of the müllerian ducts into the female internal structures (the fallopian tubes, uterus, cervix, and upper vagina) (Fig. 6–5).

Normal differentiation of the testis itself takes place under the influence of a testis-determining gene (Tdf),[28] which is located on the short arm of the Y chromosome and is distinct from the gene for the earlier-known male-specific H-Y antigen.[29] Normal ovarian differentiation requires no specific chromosomal primer and occurs constitutively in the absence of a testis-determining gene. Anti-müllerian hormone secretion starts in the developing testis between 6 and 7 weeks of gestation with differentiation of the Sertoli cells.[30] Leydig cells begin to produce testosterone at approximately 8 weeks, autonomously at first,[31] but soon coming under gonadotropin control.

Testosterone is also required for suppression of the breast anlage and indirectly for normal formation of the male external genitalia. In order to act on the external genital primordium and other androgen-responsive cell types, testosterone must first undergo conversion at the tissue site to 5α-dihydrotestosterone (DHT).[32,33] The differentiation promoted by DHT includes formation of the scrotum from the genital swellings, midline closure and elongation of the genital folds, forming the body of the phallus, and extension of the urogenital sinus by fusion along the ventral groove to form a penile urethra.

Raised androgen levels from abnormal fetal adrenal androgen production (as in virilizing adrenal hyperplasia) or from a maternal androgen-producing tumor or exogenous androgen administration during pregnancy do not affect genital development in the male fetus because of the already high levels of androgens produced by the gonads, but are high enough to cause significant masculinization of the external genitalia in females.[34] In pregnancies at risk for a child affected with virilizing adrenal hyperplasia, suppression of fetal adrenal androgen production with decisive lessening of genital ambiguity in females has been achieved by administering dexamethasone to the mother.

BLOCKS IN ACTIVITY OF STEROIDOGENIC ENZYMES

Congenital Adrenal Hyperplasia

Congenital adrenal hyperplasia (CAH) refers to the histologic alterations in adrenal

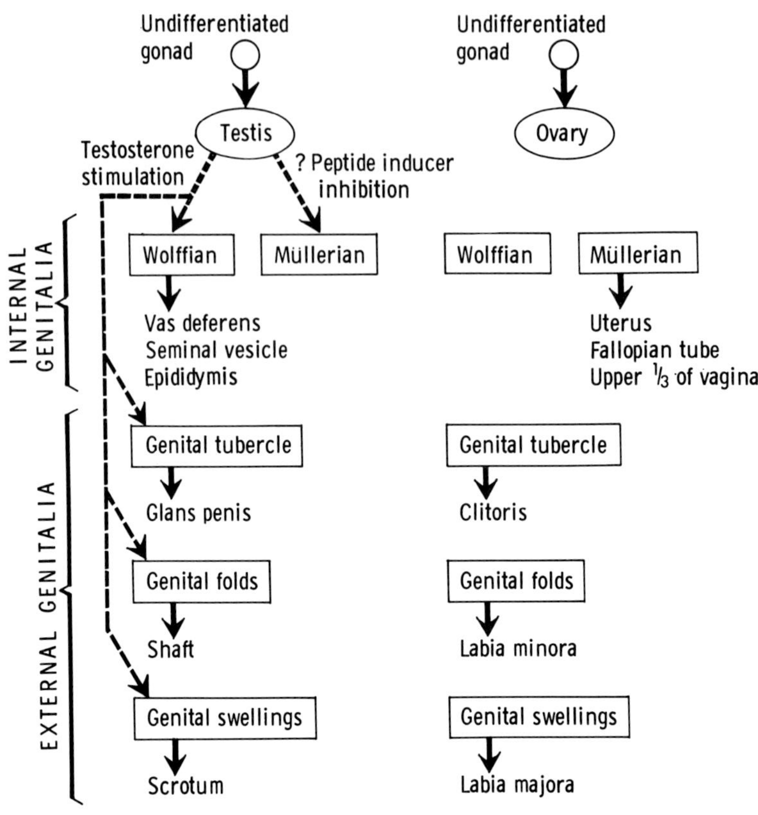

FIGURE 6–5. Fetal sex differentiation. (From New MI, Levine LS: Congenital adrenal hyperplasia. *In* Harris H, Hirschhorn K (eds): Advances in Human Genetics, Vol. 4, New York, Plenum Press, 1973, pp 25–326.)

cortical tissue that follow from chronically elevated plasma levels of ACTH; ACTH elevations are secondary to low plasma cortisol arising biochemically from reduced or absent activity of one of the five enzymes of cortisol synthesis from cholesterol in the adrenal cortex. Each enzyme deficiency produces characteristic alterations in synthesized and secreted levels of adrenal steroid hormones and their precursors. The particular imbalances resulting in each case cause abnormalities of fetal genital development and pseudohermaphroditism, and accompanying specific recognizable metabolic disturbances.

The following enzymatic defects of steroidogenesis and their associated clinical syndromes have been described[35,36] (see Table 6–1):

1. 21-Hydroxylase deficiency: classical (salt-wasting and simple virilizing) and nonclassical

2. 11β-Hydroxylase deficiency (hypertensive CAH) with CMO types I and II (salt-wasting)

3. 3β-ol Dehydrogenase deficiency (classical and nonclassical)

4. 17α-Hydroxylase deficiency with 17,20-lyase deficiency

5. Cholesterol desmolase deficiency (lipoid hyperplasia)

The 21-hydroxylase and 11β-hydroxylase deficiencies, occurring late in cortisol synthesis (see Fig. 6–6), cause channeling of accumulating common precursor steroids into androgen pathways, resulting in genital ambiguity in females and hyperandrogenic effects in both sexes. Accompanying the virilizing effects, imbalances in salt metabolism distinguish these two forms: in 21-hydroxylase deficiency, deficient aldosterone synthesis causes salt wasting and hypovolemia in 75 per cent of cases, whereas excess DOC in 11β-hydroxylase deficiency causes hypertension.

In the more proximal 17α-hydroxylase/17,20-lyase deficiency, blocked production of both 17α-hydroxy (glucocorticoid) and C_{19}/C_{18} steroids causes pseudohermaphroditism in males and sexual infantilism in females, in conjunction with low cortisol; channeling of steroids in the 17-deoxy pathway produces mineralocorticoid excess and hypertension. In the 3β-ol dehydrogenase defect, poor or absent conversion to Δ^4 ste-

TABLE 6–1. FORMS OF ADRENAL HYPERPLASIA

Deficiency	Syndrome	Ambiguous Genitalia	Postnatal Virilization	Salt Metabolism	Steroids Increased*	Steroids Decreased*	Enzyme	Chromosomal Location	Frequency	Gene Cloned
Cholesterol desmolase	Lipoid hyperplasia	Males	No	Salt wasting	None	All	P450scc	15	Rare	Yes
3β-OH-steroid dehydrogenase	Classic	Males	Yes	Salt wasting	DHEA, 17-OH-pregnenolone	Aldo, T, cortisol	3β-OH-steroid dehydrogenase	—	Rare	No
	Nonclassic	No	Yes	Normal	DHEA, 17-OH-pregnenolone	—	3β-OH-steroid dehydrogenase	—	?Frequent	—
17α-Hydroxylase	—	Males	No	Hypertension	DOC, corticosterone	Cortisol, T	P450c17	10	Rare	Yes
17, 20-Lyase	—	Males	No	Normal	—	DHEA, T, Δ^4-A	P450c17	10	Rare	Yes
21-Hydroxylase									1:12,000	Yes
	Salt wasting	Females	Yes	Salt wasting	17-OHP, Δ^4-A	Aldo, cortisol	P450c21	6p (HLA-B40; HLA-Bw47,DR7)	75%	—
	Simple virilizing	Females	Yes	Normal	17-OHP, Δ^4-A	Cortisol	p450c21	6p (HLA-B5)	25%	—
	Nonclassic	No	Yes	Normal	17-OHP, Δ^4-A	—	P450c21	6p (HLA-B14, DR1)	0.1–1% (3% in European Jews)	—
11-Hydroxylase	Classic	Females	Yes	Hypertension	DOC, 11-deoxycortisol (S)	Cortisol ± Aldo	P450c11	8q	1:100,000	Yes
	Nonclassic	No	Yes	Normal	11-deoxycortisol ± DOC	—	P450c11	8q	?Frequent	—
Corticosterone methyloxidase type II	Salt wasting	No	No	Salt wasting	18-OH-corticosterone	Aldo	P450c11	8q	Rare (except in Iranian Jews)	—

* Aldo, aldosterone; Δ^4-A, Δ^4-androstenedione; DHEA, dehydropeiandrosterone; DOC, 11-deoxycorticosterone; 17-OHP, 17α-hydroxyprogesterone; T, testosterone.

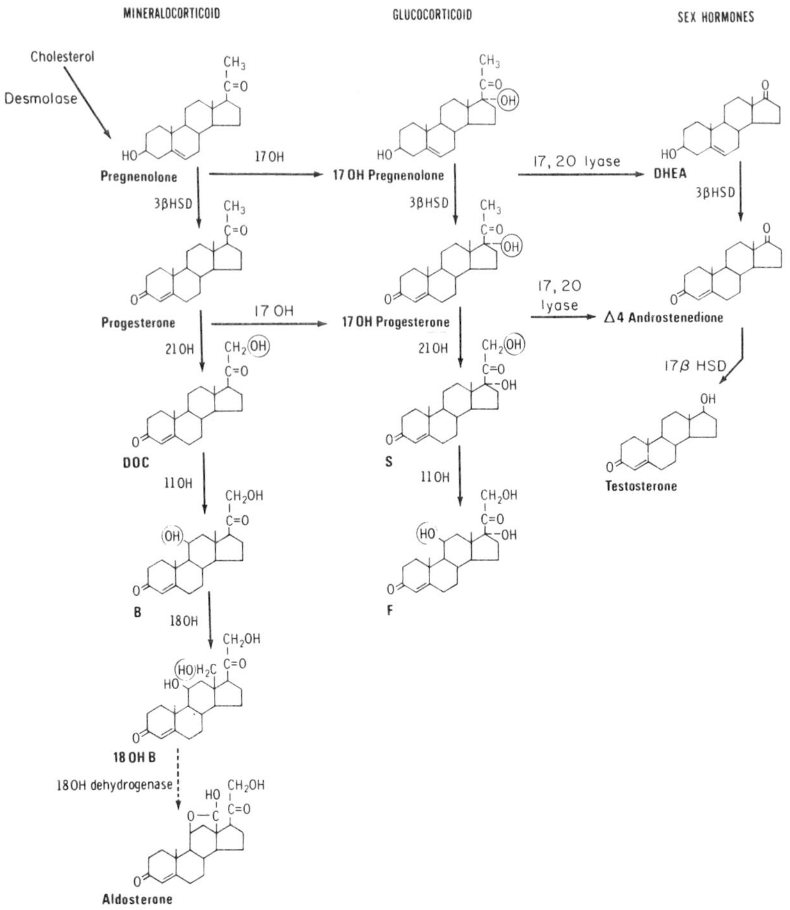

FIGURE 6–6. Simplified scheme for adrenal steroidogenesis. Each hydroxylation step is indicated and the newly added hydroxyl group is circled. (Adapted from New and Levine.[78])

roids allows production only of the Δ^5 steroid precursors, which are relatively inactive, causing salt wasting and cortisol insufficiency. While lack of potent Δ^4 androgens produces pseudovaginal hypospadias in the male, enormously high levels of the weak androgen, DHEA, may cause limited virilization (clitoral enlargement) in females. Cholesterol desmolase deficiency blocks all steroid production, with buildup of cholesterol substrate (lipoid adrenal hyperplasia), and accordingly, among its very serious effects, results in pseudohermaphroditism in genetic males.

The 17,20-lyase deficiency is a variant of 17α-hydroxylase deficiency, in which glucocorticoid and mineralocorticoid levels are relatively unaffected and a block in (adrenal and gonadal) C_{21} to C_{19} steroid conversion results in a specific clinical phenotype. Sexual ambiguity is not a feature of the 18-hydroxylase (CMO I) or 18-dehydrogenase (CMO II) deficiencies causing hypotension, since these distal blocks in aldosterone syn-

thesis have quantitatively small effects on the steroid economy and adrenal sex steroid secretion is thus unaffected.

21-Hydroxylase Deficiency (Virilizing CAH)

Virilization in 21-Hydroxylase Deficiency. The prominent feature of 21-hydroxylase deficiency is progressive virilism with advanced somatic development. The classic disorder most often exhibits salt wasting from deficient aldosterone synthesis, and is of the simple virilizing type in about one fourth of cases. Developmental genital anomalies are manifest in females as varying degrees of genital ambiguity, which should flag the diagnosis in the female (Fig. 6–7). Because genital formation in males is normal, the syndrome often goes unrecognized at birth until signs of androgen excess such as accelerated height and precocious sexual hair appear later in childhood.[37] Adrenocortical cell differentiation and the for-

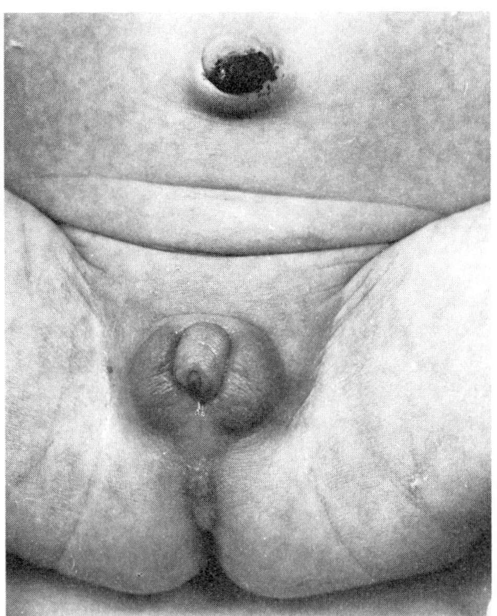

FIGURE 6–7. Ambiguous genitalia in a newborn female due to 21-hydroxylase deficiency. Note the enlarged clitoris, single orifice on the perineum, and scrotalization of the labia majora. (From New MI, Dupont B, Grumbach K, Levine LS: Congenital adrenal hyperplasia and related conditions. *In* Stanbury JB, et al. (eds): The Metabolic Basis of Inherited Disease. 5th ed. New York, McGraw-Hill, 1983.)

mation of the fetal zone occur early in embryogenesis, and although the biochemical schedule of steroid synthesis has not been completely elucidated, it is clear that genital development in the fetus takes place under the influence of active adrenal steroid synthesis. Thus, in the female, the extent of masculinization of the external genitalia ranges from mild clitoral enlargement, through varying degrees of fusion of the labioscrotal folds (posterior to anterior), to the profound morphologic anomaly of a penile urethra.

Genetic sex, gonadal differentiation, and internal genital morphogenesis are normal in 21-hydroxylase deficiency. Since there is no anomalous secretion of AMH, the müllerian ducts in the female develop normally into uterus and fallopian tubes. Wolffian duct stabilization and differentiation proceeds under the control of high intraluminal levels of gonadal androgens in the male; this process appears to be unaffected by elevated adrenal androgens and there is no observable wolffian development in females with 21-hydroxylase deficiency congenital adrenal hyperplasia.

21-Hydroxylase deficiency is the most common cause of ambiguous genitalia in the newborn female, and because affected females have the capacity for an entirely normal female sex role, including childbearing, it is very important to recognize this disorder in newborns born with ambiguous genitalia. Although the male is not jeopardized by inappropriate sex assignment, premature masculinization and accelerated physical development cause problems of adjustment. In addition, continued adrenal androgen excess may suppress the pituitary-gonadal axis, preventing maturation of the testes and resulting in infertility. In both sexes there is early fusion of the epiphyses with resulting short stature.

Salt Wasting in 21-Hydroxylase Deficiency. In three fourths of classical cases (i.e., those presenting at birth) of 21-hydroxylase deficiency there is renal salt wasting from deficient aldosterone synthesis[35]; this is defined by hyponatremia and hyperkalemia, inappropriately high urinary sodium, and low serum and urinary aldosterone with concomitantly high plasma renin activity (PRA). The increase in the proportion of salt-wasting cases in recent years can be attributed to better case identification and patient survival. In addition to inadequate secretion of aldosterone or other salt-retaining steroids, other precursors with natriuretic action produced in excess may counter the marginally competent sodium-conserving mechanism of the immature newborn renal tubule.[38–41] Salt losing in infancy from an aldosterone biosynthetic defect may improve with age,[42,43] and possible adjustments in sodium intake and mineralocorticoid replacement in patients labeled neonatally as salt wasters can be made on the basis of careful monitoring of PRA.

The degree of genital ambiguity in a female newborn does not indicate the form of 21-hydroxylase deficiency. Although correlation of the severity of salt wasting with the extent of virilization has been claimed,[44] in the case description of a genetic female with fully masculine phenotype, the patient described was no longer a salt waster by 4 years of age.[45] Thus even mildly virilized newborn females with 21-hydroxylase deficiency should be observed carefully for signs of adrenal insufficiency in the first weeks of life.

With few exceptions,[46] the literature has indicated that the presence or absence of salt wasting in 21-hydroxylase deficiency is seen consistently within a family, and subsequent affected offspring have thus been predicted to have the same form of the disease as the index case. A recent report, however, has identified discordance for salt wasting and aldosterone synthetic capacity in several families among siblings who in addition carried identical human leukocyte antigen (HLA)-B antigen markers (see next section) for the genetic defect.[43] Distinct zonal defects in the two classical forms of 21-hydroxylase deficiency have been clinically investigated.[47]

HLA and 21-Hydroxylase Deficiency. The human major histocompatibility complex (MHC), or HLA, located on the short arm of chromosome 6 (between subregions 6p21.1 and 6p21.3), is an assembly of genes coding for cell surface antigens that are the major barriers for allogenic transplantation (hence the name MHC). The class I antigens, and others, the class II antigens, are expressed on activated lymphocytes and provide a basis for control of the immune response; in addition there are class III genes coding for expressed factors with functions outside the histocompatibility and immune responses, including adrenal cytochrome P450 specific for steroid 21-hydroxylation (P450c21).

Classic genetic analysis showed the HLA complex to span a recombinative distance of approximately 3 cM (centimorgans).[48] During the period 1976 to 1982 the gene for 21-hydroxylase deficiency was mapped within HLA between HLA-B and HLA-DR (a distance of 0.8 cM), segregating more frequently with HLA-B (reviewed in ref. 49). Molecular genetic studies of the human MHC led to the isolation and characterization of essentially all active genes within this extended region,[50–52] which has recently been determined to be a DNA segment of approximately 3500 kb (kilobase pairs) in length. (See also section on "Molecular Genetics in CAH" later in this chapter.)

HLA Linkage. Linkage between HLA and 21-hydroxylase deficiency was first shown by Dupont et al.[53] Reports from the same group[54] and other groups soon after (reviewed in ref. 49) confirmed linkage with HLA. Compiled data on intra-HLA recombinations strongly indicated a gene locus for 21-hydroxylase between HLA-B and -DR.[55] The more recent molecular studies have confirmed this location in class III. Steroid 21-hydroxylase deficiency is a monogenic trait, and the close genetic linkage of the 21-hydroxylase gene to HLA is utilized for genotyping siblings in pedigrees with an affected index case; thus a sibling sharing both HLA haplotypes with the index case is predicted to be affected, one who shares a single haplotype is predicted to be a heterozygote, and one who shares no HLA haplotype is predicted to be unaffected (Fig. 6–8).

Linkage Disequilibrium. The study by Dupont et al.[53] first showing linkage between HLA and the gene for 21-hydroxylase deficiency obtained a total maximum locus of deficiency (lod) score of 3.394 (recombinant fraction θ = 0.00) with data from six families. The most recent calculated lod scores are in excess of 22 (θ = 0.00). In addition to linkage of the 21-hydroxylase locus with the neighboring HLA-B and -DR antigen loci, 21-hydroxylase deficiency alleles are found in linkage disequilibrium with HLA antigen genes or haplotypic combinations that may include specific alleles of C4 of serum complement.[56] The salt-wasting form of 21-hydroxylase deficiency shows increased association with HLA-Bw60(40) and with HLA-Bw47 within the extended haplotype HLA-A3,Bw47,DR7, which also carries a null allele at C4B.[57,58] Simple virilizing disease is associated with HLA-Bw51(5) in selected ethnic groups.[58] Nonclassical disease is associated with the haplotype HLA-B14,DR1, which has been shown to have a duplicated C4A isotype.[59–61] The nonclassical association with HLA-B14,DR1 has been observed in all ethnic groups examined[62] except the Yugoslav population.[63] Negative association with 21-hydroxylase deficiency has been noted for the haplotype HLA-A1,B8,DR3, which carries a null allele at C4A; this haplotype occurs with somewhat greater frequency in certain autoimmune disorders.

3β-Hydroxysteroid Dehydrogenase Deficiency

The enzyme 3β-hydroxysteroid dehydrogenase (3β-HSD), or 3β-ol dehydrogenase, is necessary for the synthesis of all adrenal and gonadal steroids beyond the relatively inactive 3β-ol Δ^5 precursors. First described by Bongiovanni in 1962,[64] 3β-HSD deficiency seemed most likely to have a monogenic autosomal recessive mode of transmission based on pedigree analysis.[64–66]

As gonadal 3β-ol dehydrogenase enzyme activity is reduced also (although not always equally with the adrenal defect), gonadal

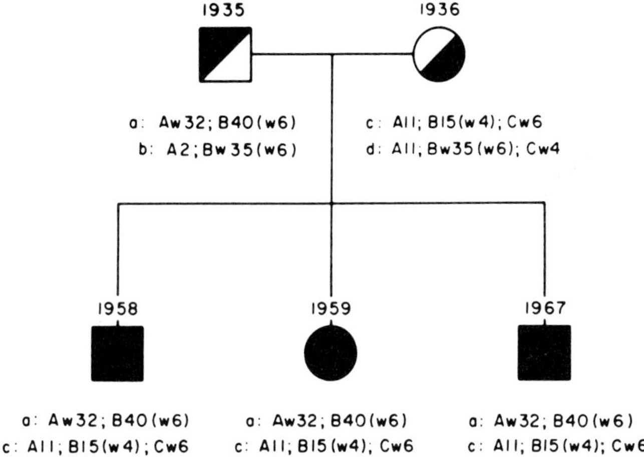

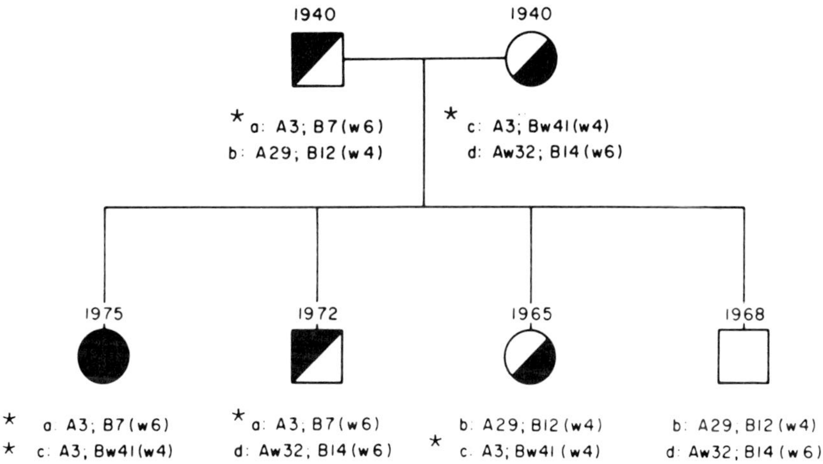

FIGURE 6–8. Pedigrees for two families with 21-hydroxylase deficiency. The HLA type and haplotypes for the HLA-A, HLA-B and HLA-C alleles are given in each family. The paternal haplotypes are labeled a and c and the maternal haplotypes c and d. The parents are obligate heterozygous carriers for the 21-hydroxylase deficiency gene, denoted by the half-black symbols. In *A*, three affected siblings are phenotypically, genotypically identical. In *B*, one affected child is HLA-genotypically different from the three unaffected siblings. One sibling, who carries the parental A and D haplotypes, is presumed to be a heterozygous carrier for 21-hydroxylase deficiency because he shares the haplotype with the patient. Another sibling has the parental b and c haplotypes and shares the c haplotype with the patient, and should be a carrier of the 21-hydroxylase deficiency gene. The child with the b and d haplotypes should be normal for the gene. (From Levine LS, Zachmann M, New MI, Prader A, Pollack MS, O'Neill GJ, Yang SY, Oberfield SE, Dupont B: Genetic mapping of the 21-hydroxylase deficiency gene within the HLA linkage group. N Engl J Med 299:911, 1978.)

androgen production is deficient. In genetic males, incomplete genital development results in recognizable ambiguity at birth. In affected females on the other hand, the very high levels of circulating DHEA—and perhaps some peripheral conversion of DHEA to more potent androgens—may produce a limited androgen effect (restricted to clitoral enlargement).

A high ratio of Δ^5 to Δ^4 steroids, characterized specifically by elevated serum levels of the Δ^5 steroids pregnenolone, 17-hydroxypregnenolone, and DHEA, and increased excretion of the Δ^5 metabolites pregnenetriol and 16-pregnenetriol in the urine, are diagnostic for this enzyme disorder.

Deficient aldosterone production in cases of a complete or near-complete 3β-ol dehydrogenase enzyme block results in salt wasting[64–74]; in other cases the ability to conserve sodium has been intact.[64,66,68,70,74] Thus, in 3β-ol dehydrogenase deficiency, as in 21-hydroxylase and 11β-hydroxylase deficiency (see following section), the other common forms of congenital adrenal hyperplasia, there is a phenotypic spectrum for each clinical feature, and salt wasting may be present to some degree.[66] As with the 21-hydroxylase and 11β-hydroxylase enzymes (see next section), it is not possible to judge the degree of severity of the 3β-ol dehydrogenase defect based on the appearance of the external genitalia at birth.

Hypertensive Forms of CAH

11β-Hydroxylase Deficiency. Abnormal adrenal steroid secretion attributable specifically to impeded 11β-hydroxylation was first reported by Eberlein and Bongiovanni in 1955.[75] The characteristic steroid profile of 11β-hydroxylase deficiency shows elevated compounds S and DOC in the serum, with marked urinary elevation of the corresponding tetrahydro metabolites, THS and THDOC, and complete absence of any 11-oxygenated C_{19} or C_{21} steroids in the blood or urine.[76]

Hypertension with hypokalemic alkalosis is the single clinical feature distinguishing 11β-hydroxylase from 21-hydroxylase deficiency, yet elevation of blood pressure correlates poorly with the serum abnormality[77] and either feature (or both) may be absent. Hypertension is attributable to elevated DOC.[76,78] Deoxycorticosterone-induced sodium retention results in suppression of PRA and reduced secretion of aldosterone and 18-hydroxycorticosterone from the zona glomerulosa.[79,80] Glucocorticoid administration standardly results in reduction of DOC secretion and normalization of plasma volume; renin suppression ceases and PRA increases angiotensin II production, establishing glomerulosa function, with aldosterone levels eventually rising to normal. Suppression of DOC may not lower blood pressure in hypertensive 11β-hydroxylase deficiency patients, although this lack of response is a feature of long-standing hypertension of many causes.

Hypokalemia is also variable, and the degree of hypokalemia does not necessarily correlate with the severity of hypertension.[77] Low renin is a hallmark of this and other forms of mineralcocorticoid hypertension, but normal PRA has even been noted in two atypical 11β-hydroxylase deficiency cases.[81]

As in 21-hydroxylase deficiency, excess fetal androgen production causes prenatal virilization of females, resulting in ambiguous external genitalia with normal female internal reproductive organs. In newborn males with 11β-hydroxylase deficiency the external genitalia may be normal, but in either sex virilization ensues postnatally if the disorder is untreated. There is no direct correlation between the degree of virilization and hypertension.[77]

Hypertension Mechanisms. Deoxycorticosterone was recognized early in clinical studies to have significant mineralocorticoid potency, causing sodium retention, plasma volume expansion, and suppression of PRA,[82–84] yet intravenous DOC infusion does not uniformly induce hypertension in control subjects. In 11β-hydroxylase deficiency, patients may have elevated DOC and be normotensive,[85,86] and DOC may be normal or only mildly elevated in patients with hypertension.[87,88]

While studies with DOC have not consistently confirmed a central place for it alone in the development and maintenance of hypertension,[77,85–88] abnormal serum elevation of DOC is clearly an important factor in the clinical picture in 11β-hydroxylase deficiency.[76,78] New and Seaman[80] documented DOC secretion rates in two congenital 11β-hydroxylase patients that were 30 to 70 times those found in normal children; aldosterone secretion and excretion rates that prior to initiation of glucocorticoids were only $\frac{1}{10}$th those of normal controls were observed to rise even above normal range with the increase of PRA during dexamethasone suppression. Presenting clinically at a younger age, these patients presumably represented virtually complete blocks of the 11β-hydroxylase enzyme. Deoxycorticosteroid elevation alone has been shown in other studies not to be sufficient cause for suppression of PRA. Other determinants of hypertension in 11β-hydroxylase deficiency remain to be identified.

Adrenal 18-hydroxylation is deficient in 11β-hydroxylase deficiency[89]; parallel activity of these two enzyme functions has been shown also in normal subjects in adrenal inhibition studies using metyrapone.[90] Kater and Biglieri[91] reported low plasma 18-OH-DOC, 18-OH-B, and aldosterone in two adult patients with 11β-hydroxylase deficiency with concomitant marked elevation of DOC. In a clinical study by Levine et al.[79] examining excretion rates of these same steroids in four 11β-hydroxylase deficiency patients with suppression/stimulation tests controlling zonal activity, 11β-/18-hydroxylating activity was found to be intact in the zona glomerulosa, suggesting that the defect was specific to the zona fasciculata.

17α-Hydroxylase Deficiency. A defect in 17α-hydroxylase results in diminished production of cortisol and also of sex steroids, whose production requires the 17,20-lyase function of the same 17-α-hydroxylase enzyme. The enzyme defect is shared by adrenals and gonads and reduces production of all androgens and estrogens. Genitalia appear female in both genetic males and females.[92] Puberty fails to occur.

The diagnosis is confirmed by marked elevations of the serum steroids DOC and compound B. The exception is aldosterone, whose production, while not enzymatically blocked, is very low secondary to the suppressed renin resulting from the excess DOC.

Since the first description of a female patient with 17α-hydroxylase deficiency by Biglieri et al.,[93] and in a male by New,[94] reported cases in females and males now number about 50. Most males have been phenotypically female. Males have no evidence of internal genital formation: embryologically, blocked androgen production precludes any wolffian duct development, while intact testicular Sertoli cell production of AMH inhibits formation of female structures. Gynecomastia is a feature in males as a result of nonsuppression of the breast anlage.

Diagnosis is often made with the young female or apparent female presenting at pubertal age with primary amenorrhea or lack of development of secondary sex characteristics. The disorder may be revealed earlier in 46,XY karyotype cases presenting in infancy or childhood with inguinal hernia or mass. These patients are hypokalemic and hypertensive at the time of diagnosis. Alternately, hypokalemia and hypertension may be the first manifestations of the disorder. In long-standing cases that are un-

treated or undertreated, hypertension of considerable severity may develop.

Massive overproduction of compound B with serum concentrations 30 times normal and higher appears to provide for adequate physiologic response to infection or other stress. Plasma ACTH levels are less elevated than in other conditions of impaired cortisol production, perhaps as a result of limited feedback response to presence of this marginal glucocorticoid activity. Gonadotropin production is extremely high in both sexes because of absence of any sex steroid feedback.

Treatment consists of glucocorticoid replacement in prepuberty, and sex steroid replacement as appropriate for the phenotypic sex starting at pubertal age. In 46,XY patients the testes may be abdominal, inguinal, or labial; if therapy is directed toward phenotypic development as a male, the gonads may be preserved by orchiopexy. Estrogen replacement induces the breasts to develop satisfactorily and menstrual cycles may be established in genetic females.

A recent study has suggested an ACTH test in family studies of 17α-hydroxylase deficiency patients to detect heterozygotes.[95]

Lipoid Adrenal Hyperplasia (Cholesterol Desmolase Deficiency)

Limited conversion of cholesterol to pregnenolone at the initial step in steroid synthesis (involving the enzyme cytochrome P450scc, or cholesterol desmolase) leads to negligible production of all steroids. Massive accumulations of cholesterol in the adrenocortical tissue leads to the characteristic fatty appearance of the glands to which the name of this condition refers. First described by Prader[96,97] and also known as Prader syndrome, it is extremely rare. Affected individuals exhibit gonadal hypogenesis or agenesis, severe fluid and electrolyte disturbances, susceptibility to infection, and addisonian pigmentation, and they often do not survive beyond infancy.

Following early histologic examinations[98–100] and clinical descriptions,[101,102] including the first report of a less severe form of deficiency,[103] one study seeking to clarify the biochemistry of the defect (using the action of adrenal enzyme preparations on reaction intermediates in vitro) was able to identify a specific block at the step of cholesterol 20-hydroxylation in adrenal tissue from one patient.[104] Further biochemical examinations established that the component steps were reactive complexes and not free hydroxylated intermediates[17] and that the cholesterol-to-pregnenolone net conversion is catalyzed by a single mitochondrial cytochrome P450.[105,106]

A recent clinical case report described a patient diagnosed in the newborn period and successfully treated for 18 years, and also reviewed 32 cases from the literature[107]; cholesterol desmolase deficiency seems to occur with less severity and somewhat more frequently among Japanese.

Nonclassical (Late-Onset) Enzyme Defects

Classical and Nonclassical Forms

Total or near-total blocks in the activity of the steroidogenic enzymes result in genital ambiguity and abnormalities of salt retention in three fourths of cases.[35] These comprise the classical forms of CAH. Improved biochemical assessment of adrenal function allows the identification now of lesser enzyme defects that cause milder endocrine disturbance and absence of genital ambiguity. Called nonclassical forms, such partial defects have been confirmed for steroid 21-hydroxylase,[108,109] steroid 11β-hydroxylase,[110] and 3β-hydroxysteroid dehydrogenase,[111,112] and are presumed to exist for the other enzymes. As might be expected, nonclassical defects are much more common than occurrences of the corresponding classic defects. Epidemiologic studies have shown that nonclassical 21-hydroxylase deficiency is in fact the most common autosomal-recessive disorder in man.[62]

Nonclassical 21-Hydroxylase Deficiency

An attenuated, late-onset form of adrenal hyperplasia was first suspected in the early 1950s by gynecologists in clinical practice who used glucocorticoids for the treatment of women with physical signs of hyperandrogenism, including infertility.[113,114] The first documentation of suppression of 21-hydroxylase precursors in the urine of such individuals after glucocorticoid therapy was by Baulieu and coworkers in 1957.[115] During the next two decades, the empirical use of glucocorticoids for the treatment of virilized women became commonplace, because it was assumed that adrenal androgens were often elevated in those patients. Diagnosis of a 21-hydroxylase defect by serum measurement became possible in the early 1970s with the development of a radioimmunoassay specific for 17-hydroxyprogesterone (17-OHP).[116] Based on this radioimmunoassay, findings of family members with increases in serum concentrations of 17-OHP, the enzyme substrate in the 17-hydroxy pathway, led to speculation that these individuals were "expressing heterozygotes" of a severe 21-hydroxylase deficiency gene.[117,118] Many family studies of classic 21-hydroxylase deficiency followed the initial report by Dupont et al.[53] of genetic linkage of CAH (21-hydroxylase deficiency) with HLA. Through such studies it became apparent that the nonclassical 21-hydroxylase deficiency was also genetically transmitted as an autosomal recessive.[108,119,120] Linkage of nonclassical 21-hydroxylase deficiency to HLA was established,[121,122] confirming that this disorder was allelic with the classical defect.[120,123] The HLA associations for the nonclassical defect[122,124,125] are distinct from those found in the classical forms (see "HLA Linkage" earlier in this chapter) and differ by ethnicity.[62,121]

Clinical symptomatology of nonclassical 21-hydroxylase deficiency is variable, and may present at any age (Fig. 6–9). Certain individuals—males and females—affected with nonclassical 21-hydroxylase deficiency have no overt symptoms of disease while demonstrating biochemical abnormalities comparable with those with symptoms. Longitudinal follow-up of these cases (usually detected as part of a family study) often shows signs of hyperandrogenism to wax and wane with time.

Nonclassical 21-hydroxylase deficiency can result in premature development of pubic hair in children; to our knowledge, the youngest such patient noted had developed pubic hair at 6 months of age (see Table 6-2).[108] In a review of 23 cases presenting to The New York Hospital–Cornell Medical Center (NYH-CMC) for evaluation of premature pubarche, 7 children demonstrated a 17-OHP response to ACTH stimulation consistent with the diagnosis of nonclassical 21-hydroxylase deficiency, a prevalence of 30 per cent in this preselected group of pediatric patients at high risk.[126] Other investigators found only 1 of 15 children with premature adrenarche demonstrating an ACTH-stimulated 17-OHP re-

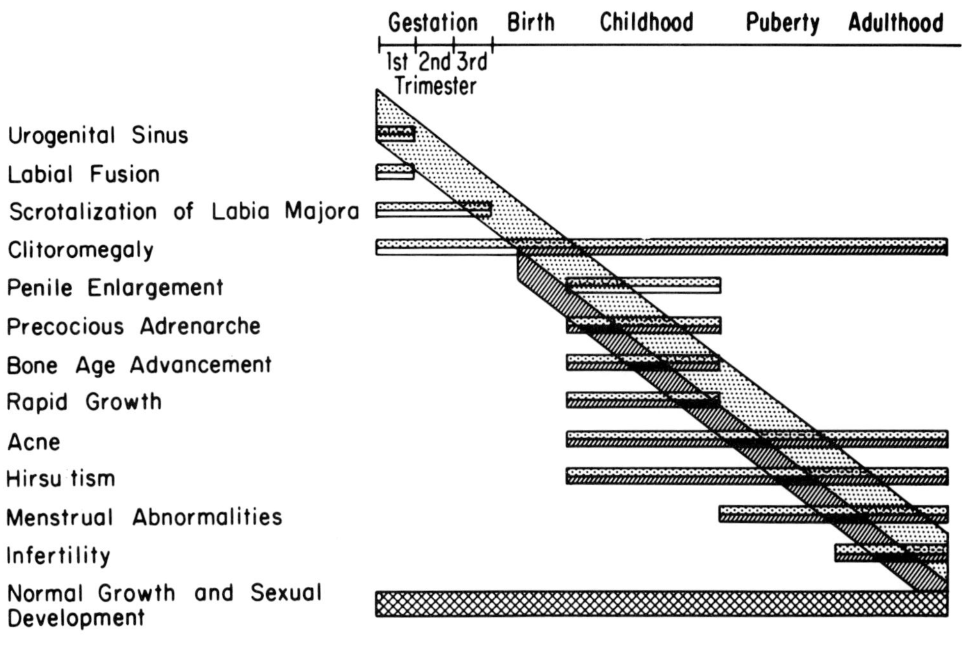

FIGURE 6–9. Clinical spectrum of HLA-linked steroid 21-hydroxylase deficiency. (From New MI, Dupont B, Grumbach K, Levine LS: Congenital adrenal hyperplasia and related conditions. *In* Stanbury JB, et al. (eds): The Metabolic Basis of Inherited Disease. 5th ed. New York, McGraw-Hill, 1983.)

TABLE 6–2. GENOTYPIC CHARACTERIZATION OF THE FORMS OF 21-HYDROXYLASE DEFICIENCY

Form of 21-Hydroxylase Deficiency	Clinical Phenotype	Hormonal Phenotype (in Response to ACTH)	Genotype
Classic	Prenatal virilization; fully symptomatic	Marked elevation of precursors (serum 17-OHP and Δ^4-A)*	$21\mathrm{OHdef}^{\mathrm{SEVERE}}$ / $21\mathrm{OHdef}^{\mathrm{SEVERE}}$
Nonclassic	Symptomatic: later development of virilization; milder symptoms	Moderate elevation of precursors	$21\mathrm{OHdef}^{\mathrm{SEVERE}}$ / $21\mathrm{OHdef}^{\mathrm{mild}}$
	Asymptomatic: no virilization other symptoms		$21\mathrm{OHdef}^{\mathrm{mild}}$ / $21\mathrm{OHdef}^{\mathrm{mild}}$
Carrier	Asymptomatic	Precursor level greater than normal	$21\mathrm{OHdef}^{\mathrm{SEVERE}}$ / $21\mathrm{OHase}$ (normal)
			$21\mathrm{OHdef}^{\mathrm{mild}}$ / $21\mathrm{OHase}$ (normal)
Normal	(Asymptomatic)	Lowest levels—some overlap seen with carriers	$21\mathrm{OHase}$ (normal) / $21\mathrm{OHase}$ (normal)

* 17-OHP, 17α-hydroxyprogesterone; Δ^4-A, Δ^4-androstenedione.

sponse greater than that of obligate heterozygote carriers of the 21-hydroxylase deficiency gene.[127] High serum concentrations of adrenal androgens promote the early fusion of epiphyseal growth plates, and children with this disorder commonly have advanced bone age and accelerated linear growth velocity, and ultimately are shorter than the final height prediction based on midparental height and on linear growth percentiles before the apparent onset of excess androgen secretion.

Severe cystic acne refractory to oral antibiotics and retinoic acid has been attributed to nonclassical 21-hydroxylase deficiency. In one study comparing the responses of 11 female patients with acne and 8 (female) control subjects to a 24-hour infusion of ACTH, elevated urinary excretion of pregnanetriol suggestive of a partial 21-hydroxylase deficiency was found in 6 patients.[128] In another study of 31 young female patients with acne and/or hirsutism tested with low-dose ACTH stimulation after overnight dexamethasone suppression, no cases of 21-hydroxylase deficiency were found.[129] Male-pattern baldness has been noted in other cases as the sole presenting symptom in young women with nonclassical 21-hydroxylase deficiency.

Menarche in females may be normal or delayed, and secondary amenorrhea is a frequent occurrence. Women with polycystic ovarian disease may in fact be patients with nonclassical 21-hydroxylase deficiency. An initial-phase adrenal sex steroid excess, disrupting the usual cyclicity of gonadotropin release and/or with direct effects on the ovary, is probable in the pathophysiology of this syndrome, leading ultimately to the formation of ovarian cysts, which then may continue to produce androgens autonomously.

In retrospective analysis it was revealed that 16 of 108 (14 per cent) women presenting to this institution (NYH-CMC) for evaluation of hirsutism and oligomenorrhea demonstrated a partial 21-hydroxylase defect.[112] The prevalence of nonclassical 21-hydroxylase deficiency as an etiology of these endocrine complaints in women in other published series ranges from 1.2 to 30 per cent.[130–135] The wide range of frequencies in these reports may relate to differences in ethnic makeup of the groups studied since the disease frequency varies in different ethnic groups.

Although the androgen profiles in serum and urine in either the basal or ACTH-stimulated state may not be markedly different overall from those demonstrated by women with the syndrome of polycystic ovaries from other causes, the serum 17-OHP response on ACTH stimulation clearly differentiates the patients with an adrenal 21-hydroxylase defect.[112,136] In six women with nonclassical 21-hydroxylase deficiency who underwent sonography or laparoscopic visualization of the ovaries, four had polycystic ovaries.[112] Thus even sonograms of the ovary do not distinguish women with excess androgens due to polycystic ovarian disease from those with nonclassic 21-hydroxylase deficiency. Adrenocorticotropin tests are required for the differential diagnosis. The response of the hypothalamic-pituitary-gonadal axis to luteinizing hormone–releasing hormone (LHRH) has been observed to be variably abnormal in virilized women with nonclassical 21-hydroxylase deficiency.[137,138] Similarly, ACTH tests are necessary to differentiate polycystic ovarian disease from nonclassical 21-hydroxylase deficiency after LHRH testing of pituitary gonadotropin secretion.

In boys, early beard growth, acne, and growth spurt may be detected. In cases of pubic hair growth and enlarged phallus from an androgen excess condition in boys, a reliable indication of an adrenal (as opposed to testicular) source of androgens is the proportionately small size of the testes that results from suppression of the hypothalamic-pituitary-gonadal axis. In men signs of androgen excess are difficult to appreciate, and the manifestations of this excess may be limited to short stature or oligozoospermia and diminished fertility from this same adrenal sex steroid–induced gonadal suppression.

Treatment with glucocorticoids is effective in suppressing adrenal androgen production, and, with time, clinical signs of androgen excess show improvement. With a 9-month life expectancy of established hair follicles, remission of hirsutism generally takes at least 1 to 2 years. An exact timetable for regression of each clinical sign has yet to be established.

Fertility in Nonclassical 21-Hydroxylase Deficiency. Since the presumptive identification of the first nonclassical patients some 30 years ago, it has been recognized that infertility in women may be reversed during glucocorticoid therapy.[113–115,139] Riddick and Hammond[140] reported that five patients with postmenarchal onset of 21-hydroxylase deficiency resumed regular menses and demonstrated adequate suppression of 17-ketosteroids and pregnanetriol within 2 months after beginning therapy with glucocorticoids alone. Birnbaum and Rose[139] found that of 18 infertile women with acne and/or facial hirsutism and hormonal criteria consistent with 21-hydroxylase deficiency, 5 conceived after 2 months and one after 7 months of prednisone treatment alone; 4 more women conceived within 2 months of the addition of clomiphene to the therapeutic regimen. Hormonal profiles after initiation of therapy were not reported in this study. Oligospermia and subfertility have been reported in men with nonclassical 21-hydroxylase deficiency[141,142] and reversal of infertility with glucocorticoid treatment in two men.[143,144] In the only published study of response to ACTH stimulation in a population of men with infertility and idiopathic oligospermia, none of the 50 subjects tested by Ojeifo and colleagues demonstrated a 17-OHP response consistent with the diagnosis of nonclassical 21-hydroxylase deficiency.[143] As stated previously, it is conceivable that reported variations in disease frequency when small populations are studied are attributable to sampling error in a disorder that has varying prevalence in different ethnic groups (see "Population Genetics of Nonclassical 21-Hydroxylase Deficiency" later in this chapter).

Nonclassical 3β-Hydroxysteroid Dehydrogenase Deficiency

As with 21-hydroxylase, nonclassical 3β-ol dehydrogenase is an attenuated enzyme defect with no major development abnormalities.[112] With postadrenarchal or peripubertal onset,[145] it appears to affect the fasciculata-reticularis zones, the spared functioning of the glomerulosa ensuring adequate salt retention.[66] Signs of virilization in females appearing postnatally are similar to those in patients with a 21-hydroxylase defect. Sixty-minute ACTH testing (serum sampling at before and 60 min after administration of Cortrosyn (synthetic $ACTH_{1-24}$) 0.25 mg I.V.) that shows serum Δ^5-17-hydroxypregnenolone (Δ^5-17P) and DHEA levels and serum ratios Δ^5-17P:17-OHP and Δ^5-17P:cortisol more than 2 SD above the normal mean values confirms the existence of a 3β-HSD defect.[66]

Nonclassical 11β-Hydroxylase Deficiency

Mild, late-onset, and even cryptic forms of 11β-hydroxylase deficiency have been reported.[110,146–150] As in 21-hydroxylase deficiency, this clinical variability may be due to allelic variation at the 11β-hydroxylase structural gene locus.

Heterozygote Detection

Adrenocorticotropin stimulation reliably evokes hormonal responses indicating heterozygous or affected status in tests subjects in nonclassical 21-hydroxylase deficiency; although the test is simple as an endocrine diagnostic procedure, it is too expensive for prospective screening. Alternatively, baseline 17-OHP concentrations, while these may not differ from normal values in heterozygotes or patients when measured randomly, are significantly higher at the time of the diurnal peak of concentration in the serum. Early morning serum values, therefore, may be informative. A screening protocol has recently been established that measures early morning (by 8 AM) 17-OHP in saliva by radioimmunoassay.[151] Adrenocorticotropin stimulation tests are necessary to confirm the diagnosis of heterozygosity for 21-hydroxylase deficiency, however.

In nonclassical 3β-ol dehydrogenase and 11β-hydroxylase deficiencies, investigations so far have not demonstrated a consistent measurable biochemical defect in obligate heterozygote parents either in the baseline state or with ACTH stimulation.

Population Genetics of Nonclassical 21-Hydroxylase Deficiency. A high prevalence of nonclassical 21-hydroxylase deficiency has been determined in a number of ethnic groups.[62] (See also section on "HLA Linkage" earlier in this chapter.) In this analysis, heterozygote (carrier) and (homozygous) affected status were established in family members by HLA typing, correlating HLA-B types with known HLA-B associations, in conjunction with ACTH testing using criteria provided by reference hormone data.[136] By counting the incidence of nonclassical deficiency genes relative to the presumed normal genes among allowed parental haplotypes, the frequency of nonclassical 21-hydroxylase deficiency was calculated. This was carried out for each ethnic group. The gene frequency for nonclassical 21-hydroxylase deficiency was highest in

Ashkenazic Jews and was also high in Hispanics, Yugoslavs, and Italians. Disease frequencies were .037 (1:27) for Ashkenazic Jews, 0.019 (1:53) for Hispanics, .016 (1:63) for Yugoslavs, .003 (1:333) for Italians, and .001 (1:1000) for other caucasoids (40 per cent of whom had an Anglo-Saxon background).[62]

Analysis by counting is validated by the affected sibling pair method of Thomson and Bodmer.[152] More recently, independent confirmation of the results has been provided by a computer-aided analysis of an expanded data base including the same families.[153] Employing the statistical method of commingling distributions in order to avoid certain assumptions in the counting method, this study arrived at the same ethnic-specific and overall gene and disease frequencies. Nonclassical 21-hydroxylase deficiency is thus the most frequent autosomal-recessive disorder in man.

Related Syndromes

Aldosterone Defects

Specific salt-losing syndromes may result from defects in well-defined steps in aldosterone synthesis. Ulick has resolved these into two types termed *corticosterone methyloxidase types I and II*.[154,155] Type I is the result of deficient 18-hydroxylation wherein the urinary levels of corticosterone metabolites are elevated. In type II the subsequent dehydrogenation is defective and 18-hydroxycorticosterone and its urinary metabolites are elevated, which is best perceived by increased ratios of 18-hydroxytetrahydro-11-dehydrocorticosterone (18-OH-THA; 11-dehydrocorticosterone = compound A) to tetrahydroaldosterone in the urine. Sexual ambiguity is not a feature of 18-hydroxylase (CMO I) or 18-dehydrogenase (CMO II) deficiency, since these distal blocks have quantitatively small effects on the steroid economy and adrenal sex steroid secretion is thus unaffected.

Corticosterone Methyloxidase Type I. The first patients identified with selective aldosterone deficiency (by Visser and Cost[156]) were determined on biochemical reexamination to exhibit a specific defect at the 18-hydroxylase (CMO I) step. This defect appears to occur even more rarely than the CMO II defect. Ulick pointed out that identification of a glomerulosa CMO II defect is made difficult by the fact that normal concentrations of compound B and suppressed concentrations of 18-OH-B and aldosterone are the expected pattern of selective, depressed glomerulosa function, the majority of substance B representing the contribution of the zona fasciculata rather than increased accumulation of precursor proximal to a block in the zona glomerulosa enzyme.

Corticosterone Methyloxidase Type II. The Type II deficiency presents at birth with hyponatremic hyperkalemia and dehydration. The disorder was first described by Royer (1961) and Russell (1963) (reviewed by Ulick[154]). Diagnosis is established by increased precursor-product ratios of 18-hydroxycorticosterone (18-hydroxycompound B; 18-OH-B) to aldosterone in serum, or of the metabolites 18-OH-THA to tetrahydroaldosterone (THaldo) measured in urine. A cluster of cases among Jews of Iranian origin was described by Rosler et al.,[157] but American pedigrees have been described as well.[158,159]

Biochemical studies[160] continue to support the proposal of Hall[22] that steroid 11β-hydroxylase, CMO I (18-hydroxylase), and CMO II (18-oxidase or aldosterone synthetase) are all enzyme activities of the same protein (cytochrome P450c11). Clinical studies have shown parallel 11β- and 18-hydroxylation defects in 11β-hydroxylase deficiency.[79,110] Corticosterone methyloxidase type II deficiency may represent an allelic variant of the 11β-hydroxylase deficiency. A recent molecular genetic study of affected and unaffected members of six families concluded that the CMO II defect is caused by a mutation at or very near the structural gene for cytochrome P450c11.[161]

17,20-Lyase Deficiency

17,20-Lyase activity resides in the same protein as 17α-hydroxylase.[18] Deficiency of 17,20-lyase causes an isolated defect in the synthesis of C_{19} sex steroids.[162–164] Urinary pregnanetriolone, a metabolite of 17-hydroxyprogesterone, is increased and increases further after ACTH and human chorionic gonadotropin (hCG) stimulation, the latter observation indicating concordance for the gene defect in both adrenal gland and testes.[165] Testosterone or DHEA excretion does not rise appreciably. Seven patients in a total of three different kindreds with this disorder have been reported[162–167]; all seven were genetic males.

Therapy, Prenatal Diagnosis, and Molecular Genetics

Therapy in CAH

Therapy in Classical CAH. The fundamental aim of endocrine therapy in CAH is to provide replacement of the deficient hormones. Since 1949, when Wilkins et al.[168] and Bartter et al.[169] discovered the efficacy of cortisone therapy for CAH due to 21-hydroxylase deficiency, glucocorticoid therapy has been the keystone of treatment for this disorder. Glucocorticoid administration both replaces the deficient cortisol and reduces ACTH release and overstimulation of the adrenal cortex, suppressing excessive adrenal androgen production. Proper glucocorticoid replacement therapy in 21- and 11β-hydroxylase deficiency ameliorates the noxious effects of oversecreted adrenal androgens, averting further virilization, slowing accelerated growth and bone age advancement to a more normal rate, and allowing a normal onset of puberty. Glucocorticoid treatment also leads to remission of hypertension in 11β- and 17α-hydroxylase deficiency, by diminishing oversecretion of hormonal precursors with mineralocorticoid activity. Excessive glucocorticoid administration should be avoided since this produces cushingoid facies, growth retardation, and inhibition of epiphyseal maturation. In the enzyme deficiencies impairing mineralocorticoid synthesis, the inclusion of a salt-retaining steroid in the replacement therapy is required to maintain adequate sodium balance.

Hydrocortisone (cortisol) is most often used, it is the physiologic hormone and does not introduce the complication of adjustment for potency, biologic half-life, or altered profile of steroid action. Oral administration is the preferred and usual mode of treatment; it has conventionally been believed that better suppression of adrenal androgen production is achieved with divided doses, although this has been questioned[170]; 10 to 20 mg/m^2 hydrocortisone divided equally in two daily doses by tablet is adequate for the otherwise healthy child. In non-life-threatening illness or stress, increased dosage of two to three times the maintenance regimen is indicated for a few days. Each family must be given injection kits of hydrocortisone (50 mg for young children; 100 mg for older patients) for emergency use. In the event of a surgical procedure, a total of five to 10 times the daily maintenance dose (depending on the nature of the operative procedure) may be required over the first 24 hours, and can then be rapidly tapered.

If there is poor response to hydrocortisone at the standard dose, dosage may be increased to 20 to 30 mg/m^2/day, or the regimen may be changed to either one of the hormone analogs, prednisone (17α,21-dihydroxypregna-1,4-diene-3,11,20-trione) or dexamethasone (9α-fluoro-16α-methylprednisolone). These agents are more potent and are longer acting, although their relative glucocorticoid and mineralocorticoid effects differ and the smaller amounts used make dosage adjustment more critical. Classical 21-hydroxylase patients with salt losing additionally require mineralocorticoid replacement. The cortisol analog (21-acetyloxy)-9α-fluorohydrocortisone (Florinef; 9α-FF) is used for its potent mineralocorticoid activity. In an adrenal crisis a patient unable to ingest medication or take fluids is administered parenteral DOC along with liberal infusions of isotonic saline.

Normalization of PRA. In 21-hydroxylase deficiency, although aldosterone levels may not be deficient in simple virilizing cases, PRA is often elevated, as in salt-wasting 21-hydroxylase deficiency.[171,172] Rosler et al.[171] showed that the PRA in 21-hydroxylase deficiency patients was closely correlated to the ACTH level and that when PRA was normalized by the administration of 9α-FF, the ACTH level fell and excessive adrenal androgen secretion diminished. Thus, inclusion of a salt-retaining steroid in the therapeutic management of non-salt-wasting 21-hydroxylase deficiency patients with elevated PRA does in fact improve hormonal control. The glucocorticoid dose in these patients could often be decreased, and normalization of PRA also often resulted in improved statural growth.[171,172]

Specific radioimmunoassays for steroids in serum, useful for the initial diagnosis of CAH, have also improved monitoring of hormonal control once therapy has been instituted. Serum 17-OHP and Δ^4-androstenedione levels provide a sensitive index of biochemical control in 21-hydroxylase deficiency.[173–175] In females and prepubertal males the serum testosterone level is also a useful index—but not in newborn and pubertal males.[173] The combined determinations of PRA, 17-OHP, and serum androgens together, as well as the clinical assessment of growth and pubertal status, must all be considered in adjusting the dose of glucocorticoid and salt-retaining steroids for optimal therapeutic control. Hydrocortisone and 9α-FF combinations have proved to be highly effective both in our clinic and in others.[174]

Plasma renin activity is useful as a therapeutic index not only in 21-hydroxylase deficiency but in the other salt-losing forms of CAH (cholesterol desmolase and 3β-ol dehydrogenase deficiencies) as well as in those forms of CAH with mineralocorticoid excess and suppressed PRA (11β-hydroxylase and 17α-hydroxylase deficiencies). When control is poor, PRA is elevated in the salt-losing forms and suppressed in the mineralocorticoid excess forms.

Sex Assignment.   Sexual ambiguity at birth characteristic of male or female pseudohermaphroiditism is a common presenting sign of CAH (Table 6–1). In such cases, a rational and judicious choice of sex assignment is a critical aspect of treatment, since the decision of sex assignment has obvious lifelong implications. Determination of genetic sex by karyotype or buccal smear and the accurate diagnosis of the specific underlying enzymatic defect are essential in assessing a patient's potential for future sexual activity and fertility.

In cases of female pseudohermaphroditism due to 21- or 11β-hydroxylase deficiency, female sex assignment is appropriate. When medical treatment is begun early in life, the initially large and prominent clitoris shrinks slightly and, as the surrounding structures grow normally, it becomes much less prominent so that surgery may not be required. When the clitoris is conspicuously enlarged or when the abnormal genitalia interfere with parent-child bonding, surgical revision to correct the appearance of the clitoris should be carried out. Definitive vaginoplasty should be performed by an experienced gynecologic surgeon.[176] Because of the normal internal genitalia, gonadal structure, and karyotype in these patients, normal puberty, fertility, and child-bearing are possible when there is early therapeutic intervention. In view of this potential for normal female sexual development, it is unfortunate when, as a result of a hasty delivery room examination of the virilized external genitalia, affected females are improperly assigned and reared as males.

In cases of male pseudohermaphroditism due to enzyme deficiencies impairing androgen synthesis, sex assignment consistent with the genetic sex (i.e., male sex assignment) is not always advisable. Virilization of the genitalia in these children is frequently so extremely and irrevocably incomplete as to make it impossible for the individual to function as a normal male. There are certain physiologic capabilities that are considered intrinsic to "normal" male sexual development: a capacity for urinating in a standing position in prepuberty, and a capacity for relatively normal, albeit infertile sexual activity and sexual development. In cases of impaired androgen synthesis, administration of sex steroids is usually required to induce development of appropriate sex characteristics at puberty—either estrogens if the patient is to be reared as a female or androgens if reared as a male.

Society sees phenotype, not genotype. Accordingly, the genetic sex is of less importance in the assigning of a sex of rearing for a male or female pseudohermaphrodite infant than the physiologic and anatomic character of the genitalia and their potential for development and function. Because of the wide individual variability in the presentation of ambiguous genitalia, there are no all-inclusive rules for sex assignment of these patients solely on the basis of genetic sex or type of enzyme deficiency.

Psychoendocrine Treatment.   Psychologists and psychiatrists well acquainted with these endocrine disorders provide a vital component of the treatment regimen, and one of the major goals of therapy is to ensure that gender role, gender behavior, and gender identity are isosexual with the sex of assignment.[177,178]

Prenatal Diagnosis

Amniocentesis.   Since the report by Jeffcoate et al.[179] of the successful identification of an affected fetus by elevated concentrations of 17-ketosteroids and pregnanetriol in the amniotic fluid, several investigators have undertaken prenatal diagnosis for congenital adrenal hyperplasia by similar measurements of hormone levels in pregnancy.[180] The most specific hormonal diagnostic test for 21-hydroxylase deficiency is amniotic fluid 17-OHP[181–185]; Δ4-androstenedione may be employed as an adjunctive diagnostic assay.[184] It has been suggested that elevated amniotic fluid 21-deoxycortisol may also be a marker for 21-

hydroxylase deficiency.[186] Amniotic fluid testosterone levels may not be outside the normal range in the case of an affected male.[184,187]

Human leukocyte antigen genotyping of a fetus in a family with an affected sibling provides an additional method for prenatal diagnosis of 21-hydroxylase deficiency.[188,189] Fetal HLA typing is done by standard serologic testing of cells cultured from the amniotic fluid. Whether or not the fetus is affected is determined by comparison with the HLA genotypes of the parents and affected sibling(s) as in family studies. Exceptions are found in cases of intra-HLA recombination. Because class II (HLA-DR) antigens are not expressed in these cell cultures, recombination on either fetal haplotype occurring in the B to DR segment and possibly including the 21-hydroxylase locus will not be detected. Possible homozygosity at the HLA-B locus in either parent and antigen sharing between parents are factors limiting categorization of the fetal 21-hydroxylase genotype by this method.

Amniotic fluid assay for 17-OHP should thus still be performed, since anomalous hormone levels may in some cases call into question the HLA result. Forest et al.,[190] in evaluating 17 pregnancies at risk for CAH, found in 2 cases in which HLA-A and -B typing of amniotic cell cultures predicted an affected fetus that amniotic fluid hormone levels were normal. These pregnancies were terminated, and while the inconsistency of test results could have been due to recombination between HLA-B and -DR, the authors postulated also that there may have been an enzyme defect not expressed in midgestation. Pang et al.[191] have reported normal amniotic fluid 17-OHP and Δ^4-androstenedione levels in simple virilizing fetuses. If the diagnosis of the index case is erroneous and the index case is really a normal child (Fig. 6–10), then the HLA typing is irrelevant and only hormonal analysis for 17-OHP in the amniotic fluid will indicate the normalcy of the fetus. In the case where the fetus has nonclassical CAH, the 17-OHP concentration in amniotic fluid will be normal and the diagnosis of nonclassical 21-hydroxylase deficiency must rest on HLA identity with the index patient with nonclassical 21-hydroxylase deficiency (Fig. 6–11).

Chorionic Villus Biopsy. With the advent of chorionic villus biopsy (CVB), evaluation of the fetus at risk is now possible in the first trimester at 8 to 11 weeks' gestation. Because normative standards for hormonal levels measurable at this early stage remain to be established, CVB diagnosis at present depends on HLA typing of the chorionic tissue. A new option is HLA typing by molecular genetic techniques, which identifies HLA polymorphisms in the genes for antigens of both class I (HLA-A, -B, -C) and class II (HLA-DR) with the aid of specific probes.[192] This technique is more exact (it has already begun to resolve subgroups of

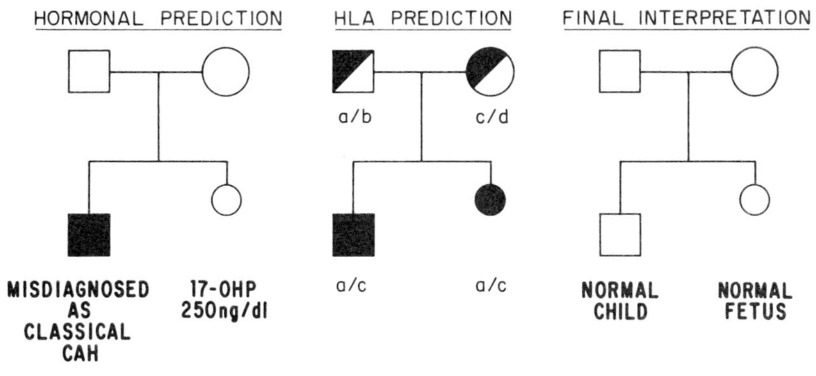

FIGURE 6–10. Misdiagnosis of CAH in the index case led to an erroneous prenatal diagnosis of CAH. Hormonal data indicated that the index case did not have CAH. Amniotic fluid hormone levels accurately predicted a nonaffected fetus, while HLA typing of amniotic cells was irrelevant since the index case did not have CAH. (From Pang S, Pollack MS, Loo M, et al: Pitfalls of prenatal diagnosis of 21-hydroxylase deficiency congenital adrenal hyperplasia. J Clin Endocrinol Metab 61:89, 1984.)

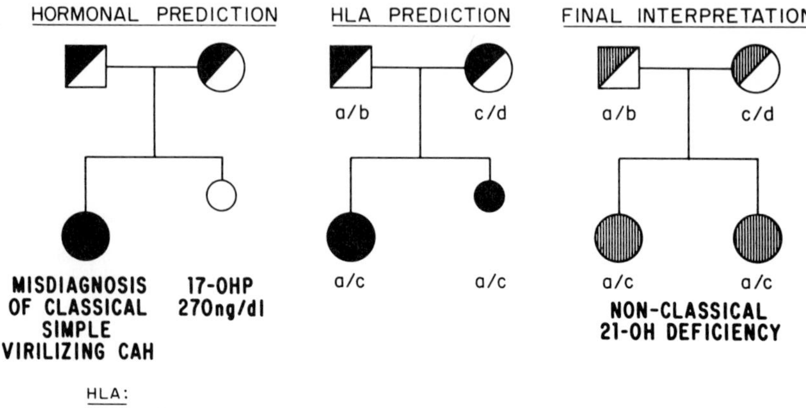

FIGURE 6–11. Pitfalls of prenatal diagnosis of nonclassical 21-hydroxylase deficiency. The fetus was prenatally predicted to be affected with 21-hydroxylase deficiency based on HLA typing and to be unaffected based on normal amniotic fluid 17-OHP concentration. Postnatally, the fetus presented with nonclassic 21-hydroxylase deficiency. The pitfalls in this case are: (1) index case was misdiagnosied as having classical simple virilizing CAH; and (2) amniotic fluid 17-OHP concentration was normal in a fetus affected with nonclassic, late-onset 21-hydroxylase deficiency. Human leukocyte antigen typing of amniotic cells is useful in prediction of fetuses affected with nonclassical CAH, whereas hormonal measurement in amniotic fluid is not useful in prenatal diagnosis of nonclassical, late-onset 21-hydroxylase deficiency. (From Pang S, Pollack MS, Loo M, et al: Pitfalls of prenatal diagnosis of 21-hydroxylase deficiency congenital adrenal hyperplasia. J Clin Endocrinol Metab 61:89, 1984.)

the standard serologic specificities), and the availability of class II probes makes possible the identification of B/DR recombinations. It is interesting to note that in the report from France amniotic fluid 17-OHP was clearly elevated even at 10 to 13 weeks gestation in three affected pregnancies and there was no discordance between hormonal results and restriction fragment length polymorphism-based diagnostic prediction in seven families studied.[192]

It is currently estimated that 25 per cent of classical 21-hydroxylase deficiency alleles carry a deletion of the active 21-hydroxylase B gene.[193] Identification of the presumed sequence aberrations occurring in the remaining 80 per cent of cases will depend on the appearance of characteristic restriction fragment length polymorphisms (RFLPs) in digests of genomic DNA samples. It is hoped with the characterization of specific nondeletional mutations that a growing panel of oligonucleotide probes informative in the resolution of 221-OHD genotypes may be used in prenatal diagnosis.

Prenatal Treatment. Treatment with dexamethasone has recently been employed in pregnancies at risk for 21-hydroxylase deficiency.[194–196] In pregnancies at risk for 21-hydroxylase deficiency where treatment was begun at 3 to 10 weeks' gestation (dexamethasone 0.5 mg orally twice daily) complete suppression of adrenocortical hormones was found in fluid obtained at amniocentesis. Only when dexamethasone therapy was discontinued before amniotic fluid sampling were the amniotic fluid hormone levels abnormally high. Masculinization of genitalia was completely prevented in one of three affected female fetuses and partially prevented in another female. In the third case, where treatment failed, the mother had begun dexamethasone at 10 weeks and terminated therapy at 28 weeks. No congenital malformations were found in any of the 21 treated fetuses.[196] Other successfully treated cases have been observed since publication of the 1987 report. The failure of one group of investigators to find evidence of suppression of the fetal pituitary-adrenal axis after short-term administration of dexamethasone at midterm[197] has little bearing on the likelihood of success when long-term therapy is begun in the first trimester. German investigators[195] also found high amniotic fluid 17-OHP levels in two pregnancies at risk for CAH treated with dexamethasone from the 10th to the 17th week, although therapy was stopped 5 days before the amniocentesis. The latter group postulated that there was increased metabolic clearance of dexamethasone, or that the dosage was inadequate.

Theoretically, institution of such therapy at 6 to 7 weeks of gestation—before onset of adrenal androgen secretion—should effectively suppress adrenal androgen production, and allow normal separation of the vaginal and urethral orifices in addition to preventing clitoromegaly. Obviously, if dexamethasone is to be administered at such an early date, it must be without knowledge of whether the fetus is affected. Following HLA and/or hormonal testing by either chorionic villus biopsy or amniocentesis, prenatal therapy may be discontinued if the fetus is male, or if it is an unaffected female (Fig. 6–12).

To date, no fetus of a mother treated with dexamethasone in low doses has been found to have any congenital malformation. Specifically, no cases have been reported of cleft palate, placental degeneration, intrauterine growth retardation, or fetal death, which have been observed in a rodent model of in utero exposure to high-dose glucocorticoids.[198]

FIGURE 6–12. Example of methods for prenatal diagnosis and treatment of congenital adrenal hyperplasia due to 21-hydroxylase deficiency. (From Speiser PW, New MI: An update of congenital adrenal hyperplasia. *In* Lifshitz F (ed): Pediatric Endocrinology. 2nd ed. New York, Marcel Dekker (in press 1989).)

1. **Pre-pregnancy:**

   Blood samples from <u>mother,</u> <u>father</u> and <u>affected sib</u> for:

   a) SEROLOGIC TESTING for HLA antigens.

   b) HYBRIDIZATION ANALYSIS using
      1. HLA Class I and II cDNA probes. Characteristic RFLPs (restriction fragment length polymorphisms) detected by molecular probes identify HLA antigens with greater specificity.
      2. Oligonucleotide probes synthesized to correspond to and directly identify the occurrence of known mutations in the active 21-hydroxylase gene sequence.

      Molecular analysis is becoming increasingly available but is not yet a part of standard laboratory evaluation. Oligonucleotide probes are still highly experimental.

   c) ACTH STIMULATION TESTING measuring 17α-hydroxyprogesterone in serum (or saliva) at 0 min (baseline) and 60 min after administration of Cortrosyn (0.25 mg i.v.) will reveal distinct hormonal responses according to 21-hydroxylase genotype.

      Once the 21-hydroxylase deficiency-linked HLA types for the pedigree have been determined, the detection of both marker haplotypes together in a genotype is presumptive diagnosis of affected status.

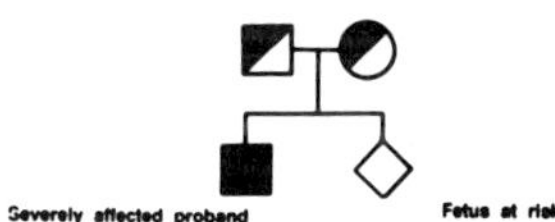

2. **In pregnancy:**

	FETAL AGE	DIAGNOSTIC TEST	THERAPY
a)	8 to 10 days	Pregnancy test (β-hCG assay)	start: dexamethasone 20 μg/(kg·d)
b)	9 or 10 weeks	CHORIONIC VILLUS BIOPSY	
		i) HLA serotypes (Class I) of cultured villus cells	If affected: continue
		ii) Hybridization analysis	
		iii) Metabolic assay (hormonal testing)	
		iv) Cell culture karyotype to ascertain fetal sex	If M: stop
c)	15 to 18 weeks	AMNIOCENTESIS (if CVB risk is unacceptable; also if genotyping by CVB has been equivocal)	
		i) HLA serotyping of cultured amniotic fluid (fetal) cells	(as above)
		ii) sex determination	(as above)
		iii) hormonal testing (17-hydroxyprogesterone RIA) if not under treatment	

Molecular Genetics in CAH

Steroid 21-Hydroxylase

Molecular Genetics of HLA (Human MHC). A 1000-kb segment contains the loci for HLA antigens A, B, and C (the main components of class I), expressed on most somatic cell types, whereas HLA-D (class II) antigens, expressed by activated lymphocytes, are coded for in a more proximally situated 800- to 1000-kb segment.[199] From a recently prepared restriction map of the MHC, a length of about 3500 kb has been established and the entire region is presumed to contain at least 50 genes.[200]

Approximately 20 genes have been identified occupying the class I regions in addition to the well-characterized HLA-A, -B and -C genes; some are pseudogenes and some appear to be expressed. The class II region in man has been subdivided into three major subregions, DP, DQ, and DR, each encoding both α and β chains.[201] Genetic studies have clarified the original D/DR serologic distinctions and have led to the further identification of expressed and unexpressed HLA class II genes. Cloning from DNA libraries has identified seven expressed genes per haplotype: one DR-α and two DR-β genes, one DQ-α and one DQ-β gene, and one DP-α and one DP-β gene. In addition, RNA has been found in some cell lines for genes termed DO-β and DZ-α.

In the HLA class III region, situated between classes I and II, are found the gene loci for properdin factor B (Bf) and the second and fourth components of serum complement (C2, and C4A and C4B); for tumor necrosis factors TNF-α (cachectin) and TNF-β (lymphotoxin); and the two genes for adrenal steroid 21-hydroxylase.[201]

Deleted Steroid 21-Hydroxylase and C4 in HLA. Initial molecular studies of steroid 21-hydroxylase deficiency made use of occurrences of the 21-hydroxylase deficiency disorder in association with known specific HLA antigens and HLA-linked complement loci. In particular, patients with severe salt-wasting 21-hydroxylase deficiency are often found to carry an extended HLA haplotype, A3,Bw47,DR7, and to express only one of the C4 proteins of serum complement.[59–61] Classic linkage studies had placed the 21-hydroxylase deficiency gene between HLA-B and -D/DR, and because one of the closely neighboring C4 genes was also affected, it was thought that a single major DNA deletion or rearrangement involving both loci could be borne on the Bw47,DR7 haplotype.

In order to establish that the HLA-linked defect in 21-hydroxylase deficiency involved the structural gene for the enzyme protein (cytochrome P450c21), bovine adrenal complementary DNA (cDNA) representing part of the (bovine) P450c21 coding sequence was used to probe DNA samples both from salt-wasting 21-hydroxylase deficiency patients carrying the Bw47,DR7 haplotype and normal individuals. Digests with restriction endonuclease enzymes Eco RI or Taq I produced two hybridizing fragments from normal DNA (Eco RI, 12 and 14 kb; Taq I, 3.2 and 3.7 kb). In both cases, one band (12 kb and 3.7 kb) was diminished or absent in DNA from all HLA-Bw47,DR7 21-hydroxylase deficiency patients. This was consistent with a deletion of one of two P450c21 (i.e., steroid 21-hydroxylase) genes.[202]

Restriction Mapping of Steroid 21-Hydroxylase and C4. Restriction analysis of overlapping long (40-kb) cosmid clones carrying C4A and C4B allowed precise determination of the steroid 21-hydroxylase/C4 gene arrangement.[203,204] The restriction map revealed that there are two 21-hydroxylase genes, tandemly 3′ and adjacent to the two C4 genes, C4A and C4B, and correspondingly termed 21-hydroxylase A and B genes. Current nomenclature names these genes CYP21A and CYP21B.

The 3.2-kb Taq I fragment is from the A gene and the 3.7-kb fragment from the B gene. The severe salt-wasting phenotype that occurs in Bw47,DR7 individuals, who are lacking one or both 3.7-kb fragments, suggested that expression of the B gene product is necessary for steroid 21-hydroxylation. By contrast, hormonally normal individuals homozygous for the extended haplotype HLA-A1,B8,DR3 (also with one null C4—now confirmed to be C4A) show no Taq I 3.2-kb band on hybridization analysis, and the A gene thus does not encode active P450c21. From the absence of any other clinical effect, the A gene was considered possibly to be a pseudogene[203,205] (see Fig. 6–13).

The boundaries of these deletions were determined by detailed mapping of restriction sites and by hybridization analysis using cloned cDNA encoding C4. The HLA-A1,B8,DR3 haplotype carries a deletion of both C4A and CYP21A, consistent with the null allele for C4A that is known to occur on

Chromosome 6p :

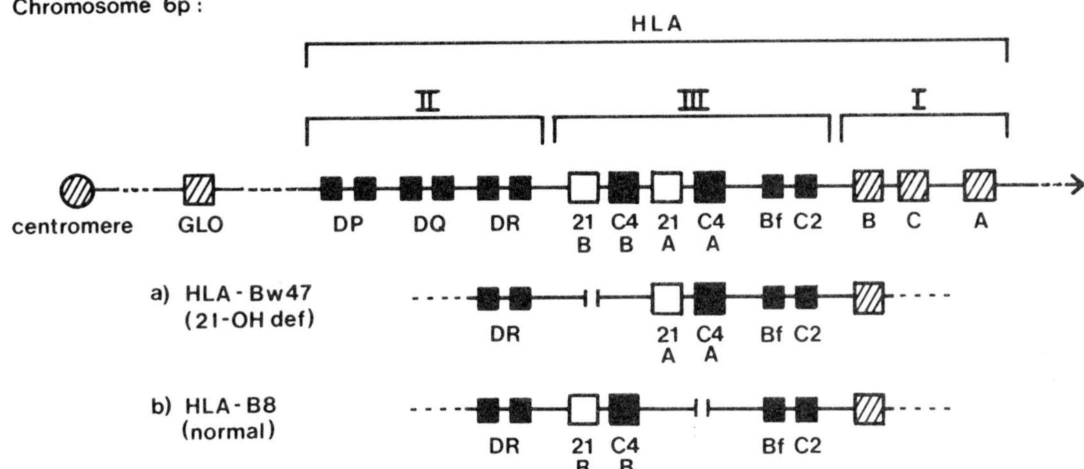

FIGURE 6–13. Arrangement of 21-hydroxylase and C4 genes within HLA. In association with HLA-Bw47 the active gene is deleted, whereas in association with B8 the pseudogene is deleted. Each of these haplotypes also has a null allele of one C4. (a) Deletion encompassing C4B and 21B (active gene, CYP21B); (b) deletion encompassing C4A and 21A (pseudogene, CYP21A). (From Speiser PW, Amor M, New MI, White PC: Molecular genetic basis for nonclassical 21-hydroxylase deficiency. N Engl J Med 319:19, 1988.)

this haplotype.[205–207] This haplotype occurs in about 5 per cent of all normal chromosomes.[55] In contrast, the A3,Bw47,DR7 haplotype has deleted C4B as well as CYP21B, explaining the null C4B allele on this haplotype.[56] This latter deletion splices the chromosomal region 3′ of the CYP21B gene onto the CYP21A gene, causing the A gene to migrate like a B gene on electrophoresis after DNA is digested with certain restriction endonucleases. Accurate identification of deletions is difficult in such cases[192] and may lead to errors of interpretation of Southern blots.

Nucleotide Sequence Analysis. The apparent lack of function of the A gene has been explained by nucleotide sequence analysis.[208,209] The A and B genes are about 98 per cent homologous in their coding regions. A nearly full-length cDNA clone derived from human fetal adrenal glands is identical with the reading sequence of B, whereas the exonic sequence of the A gene shows significant small differences, some of which (frame-shift and nonsense mutations) would alone be sufficient to prevent an active protein from being synthesized. It is concluded that CYP21A is a pseudogene.

Reciprocal Deletion/Duplication. The tandem duplication of C4 and 21-hydroxylase creates the possibility of misalignment and unequal crossing-over between chromatids during meiosis, resulting in comple-

mentary chromosomes with single or triple arrangements of C4/21-hydroxylase gene sets. The rearrangements observed in the HLA-A1,B8,DR3 and A3,Bw47,DR7 haplotypes, resulting in deletion of the C4A-CYP21A and C4B-CYP21B gene pairs may have come about by this type of mechanism.[204]

In the haplotype HLA-B14,DR1, associated with nonclassical 21-hydroxylase deficiency, a third C4 protein is expressed in serum[61] and analysis of DNA has indeed identified a third set of genes, consisting of an extra C4B gene[210] and an extra CYP21A or A-like gene.[193,205] If the extra A gene is a pseudogene like the normally present A gene, it should not contribute to the development of the nonclassical 21-hydroxylase deficiency phenotype, but instead merely travel with the presumed causative lesion in the CYP21B gene sequence.

While the HLA-B14,DR1 haplotype and nonclassical 21-hydroxylase deficiency are very common, the HLA-A3,Bw47,DR7 haplotype is extremely rare in the normal population and only comprises perhaps 20 per cent of classical 21-hydroxylase deficiency alleles. Additional patients with classical 21-hydroxylase deficiency who do not carry the HLA-Bw47 haplotype have been examined by hybridization analysis using 21-hydroxylase and/or C4 probes.[193,211] Approximately one fourth of the alleles in these patients have deletions of the CYP21B gene; the majority of such alleles also have a deletion of C4B. In one family, on one chromosome a second A gene has been substituted for CYP21B.[212] All patients with homozygous deletions of the B gene have salt-wasting 21-hydroxylase deficiency.

Gene Conversions between the CYP21 A and B Genes.   The remaining three fourths of classical alleles do not have associated restriction fragment polymorphisms and cannot be detected by Southern blot hybridization. Small exchanges of sequences between homologous genes, termed *gene conversions*, could cause many of these alleles by transferring one of the deleterious mutations from the CYP21A pseudogene to the B gene. Gene conversion has been previously documented in other cytochrome P450 genes.[213] Thus far, a number of gene conversions have been documented in mutant CYP21B genes.[214–217] One of these transfers the point mutation producing a stop codon (nonsense mutation) at position 318 from the CYP21A gene into CYP21B,[215] and another causes a radical AA change at a conserved position (isoleucine-172 to asparagine),[214] possibly affecting interactions between the P450 protein and the membrane of the endoplasmic reticulum (see Fig. 6–14). In contrast, a conservative change be-

tween nonpolar amino acids, substituting leucine for valine at position 281 in the P450c21 peptide sequence, appears to produce a milder alteration in enzyme function, and is observed in cases of nonclassical 21-hydroxylase deficiency.[217]

Both the stop condon[215] and the nonconservative AA substitution[217] point mutations were noted in 3 of 20 patients with classical 21-hydroxylase deficiency. All patients with the nonsense mutation have salt-wasting disease, whereas the patients with the asparagine-172 mutation have retained the ability to synthesize aldosterone (two have simple virilizing disease and one has an elevated plasma renin-aldosterone ratio without clinical salt wasting). One patient with salt-wasting disease carries a larger rearrangement involving exons 3 through 6 that transfers an 8-kb deletion from CYP21A to CYP21B, shifting the reading frame of translation and preventing synthesis of a functional protein.[216]

These data suggest that gene conversions are about as common as deletions as causes of 21-hydroxylase deficiency alleles.

Other alleles may carry point mutations affecting transcription of the gene or processing of RNA, or resulting in amino acid substitutions altering enzymatic function. One mutant gene from an individual with

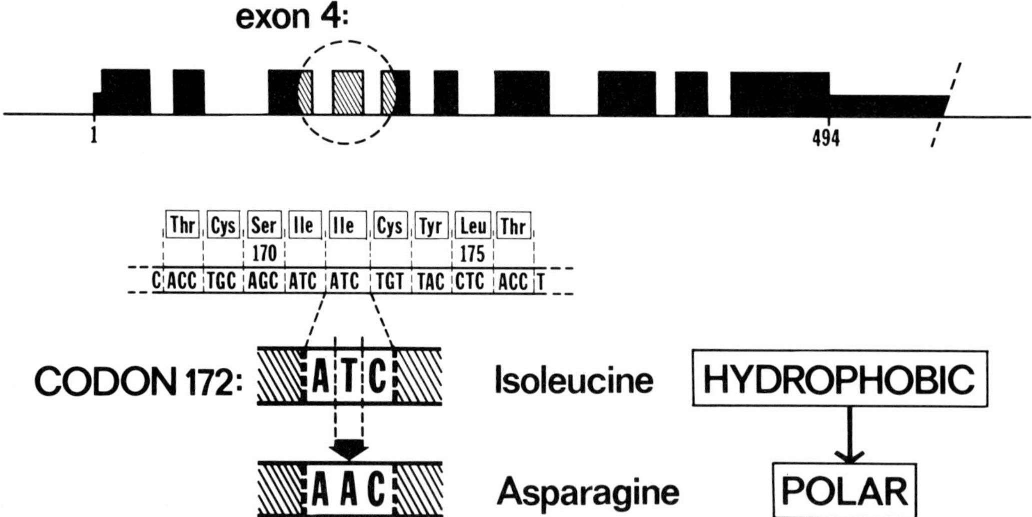

FIGURE 6–14.   Example of point mutation resulting in classical 21-hydroxylase deficiency (simple virilizing type). Schematic (*top*) depicts exon/intron organization of the gene CYP21B (nucleotide sequence approximately 3.1 kb) coding for cytochrome P450c21 (494 amino acids). Isoleucine at this position is highly conserved, not only in 21-hydroxylase in other species but in diverse cytochromes P450 as well, and a radical AA substitution would be expected significantly to disrupt enzyme function.[214] In contrast, a point mutation at codon 281 in exon 7, resulting in a conservative change (substituting an AA of similar characteristics), causes nonclassical 21-hydroxylase deficiency.[217] (From New MI, White PC, Pang S, Dupont B, Speiser PW: The adrenal hyperplasias. *In* Scriver CR, et al. (eds): The Metabolic Basis of Inherited Disease. 6th ed. New York, McGraw-Hill, 1989.)

salt-wasting 21-hydroxylase deficiency has two mutations: serine-269 is changed to threonine, and asparagine-494 is changed to serine. However, neither of these residues is conserved in P450c21 from other species, and so the functional significance of these mutations is unclear.

Correlation of Mutation with Phenotype. In general, the molecular characterization of the underlying mutations in patients with different forms of 21-hydroxylase deficiency suggests that clinical severity is roughly correlated with the extent or severity of the DNA lesion. Thus, deletions, stop codon (nonsense) mutations, frameshifts, and presumably some amino acid substitutions result in salt-wasting classical alleles, one nonconservative substitution results in a simple virilizing classical allele,[214] and a conservative amino acid substitution results in a nonclassical allele.[217] It should be pointed out that the distinctions between these diagnostic categories are not absolute; some males diagnosed as having simple virilizing 21-hydroxylase deficiency by hormonal testing in fact carry the presumed nonclassic allele associated with HLA-B14,DR1.

Steroid 17α-Hydroxylase/17,20-Lyase. The P450c17 structural gene (CYP17) has now been located on chromosome 10,[218] but thus far has not been regionally localized. Apparently the same gene is expressed in both the adrenal and the testis.[219] Second and third copies have been reported but not mapped. Initial hybridization studies of DNA samples from patients with 17α-hydroxylase deficiency did not disclose the presence of any gross deletions or rearrangements of this gene.[220] Most recently, however, molecular characterization of specific mutations in the structural gene coding for the P450c17 enzyme has been reported in Amish[221] and Japanese[222] pedigrees.

Other Steroidogenic Enzymes

Steroid 11β-Hydroxylase. If this disorder follows the model of 21-hydroxylase deficiency and 17α-hydroxylase deficiency, then presumably mutations in the structural gene for the 11β-hydroxylase/CMO I/II enzyme complex can produce the spectrum of clinical symptoms from hypertension and virilism (11β-OHD) to salt wasting without virilism. Because no mutations causing any of the clinical syndromes of 11β-hydroxylase or CMO I or II deficiency have yet been

identified, future studies will be needed to elucidate whether the clinical polymorphism results from genetic allelism.

A cDNA clone encoding human P450c11 has been isolated and used to locate the corresponding structural gene, CYP11B, on the long arm of chromosome 8.[223] Other genes of interest in this chromosomal region include the MYC and MOS cellular oncogenes and the gene (TG) for thyroglobulin. Further studies will be required to establish a linkage map relating these genes. While it appears that CYP11B is present in the haploid genome in a single copy, the possibility of two closely linked homologs, as in the case of the 21-hydroxylase A and B genes, has not been ruled out.

Globerman et al.,[161] studying the CMO II variant defect of 11β-hydroxylase, have postulated that CMO II deficiency will be allelic with the gene for the known cytochrome P450c11. Using a partial P450c11 cDNA probe and testing six families carrying the disorder, they detected a unique RFLP that specifically and uniformly identified affected members.[161] This polymorphism mapped either on or very near to the locus for CYP11B, with a total lod score of 3.74 (at θ = 0.00) in the six families examined.

3β-ol Dehydrogenase. In contrast with the other adrenal steroidogenic enzymes, the 3β-ol dehydrogenase enzyme, a dehydrogenase typically requiring NAD^+ as a cofactor, is not a cytochrome P450. Closely associated with 3β-ol dehydrogenase is the enzyme activity 3-ketosteroid Δ^{5-4} isomerase, which requires NAD^+ or NADH.[224] In mammalian species these two functions appear to reside within the same protein, but the enzyme generally has not been well characterized.

The gene encoding 3β-ol dehydrogenase/Δ^{5-4} isomerase has not been cloned. Deficiency of 3β-ol dehydrogenase is not linked to the HLA complex.[66] A recent study showed in several strains of mouse that 3β-ol dehydrogenase is encoded by the same structural gene in the adrenals and gonads, and is under separate regulatory control genetically in these two tissues.[225]

Cholesterol Desmolase (P450scc). The gene (CYP11A) for this mitochondrial P450 enzyme (P450scc) has been isolated, cloned, and localized to chromosome 15.[226] Mutation of the structural gene has not yet been identified in lipoid adrenal hyperplasia[227]; remote lesions affecting other cellular com-

ponents fundamental to early steroidogenesis could have similar effects.

CUSHING SYNDROME

Cushing syndrome is the consequence of
excessive cortisol secretion. The course of
the disease is variable, with an abrupt or
gradual onset, and signs may be subtle or
obvious.[228–230]

In the cases first studied, adrenal hyperfunction and increased cortisol were secondary to ACTH secretion by a pituitary basophilic adenoma. The name Cushing
disease is properly reserved for this specific
form of the disorder. It was subsequently
found that hypercortisolism from cortisol-
producing adrenal tumors produced the
same clinical picture. In addition to originating from tumors, which could be adenomas or carcinomas, autonomous adrenal
overproduction of cortisol was shown also to
originate possibly from hyperplasia of one
or both adrenals. Apart from these causes,
there are rare instances of ectopic ACTH
production by other tumors in childhood.

Symptoms and Signs

Cushing syndrome is relatively rare in
childhood, but may occur at any age, even
in early infancy.[231] Obesity is the most common presenting sign in all age groups, the
metabolic derangements of glucocorticoid
excess distinguishing it from simple obesity.[232] Fat distribution is centripetal, with
most fat accumulation in the face and neck
and on the trunk and abdomen (Fig. 6–15)
and not on the extremities, which instead
develop a wasted appearance because of increased protein catabolism and loss of muscle mass.[233] The effect on muscle in the
limbs is less evident in childhood, however,
and children with Cushing syndrome are
more likely to show generalized obesity.[231]
Whether central or generalized, the obesity
of Cushing syndrome is most often recognized by a typical facial appearance
("moon" facies) with chubby cheeks and
double chin (Fig. 6–15), often accompanied
by facial plethora, and also by hypertrophy
of the supraclavicular and dorsocervical fat
pad (the so-called buffalo hump).

Retardation of growth and skeletal maturation is a constant feature of the disease in
children.[231] Growth may decrease long before the appearance of obesity or other

symptoms, so that sometimes, growth retardation can be the only presenting sign.[234,235]
There is controversy, however, about mech-
anism(s) of inhibition of growth from glucocorticoid excess. It has been reported that
glucocorticoid effect is exerted at the peripheral level,[236] and also that glucocorticoids inhibit pituitary secretion of growth
hormone.[237–239] Delay of pubertal development has also been observed. The association of obesity and slowed growth or development suggests Cushing syndrome,
since exogenous obesity is usually accompanied by accelerated advances in height
and pubertal development.[231]

Thinning of the skin with appearance of
the typical purple striae on the abdomen,
buttocks, thighs, and axillae, and easy bruis-
ability are frequent signs. Mucocutaneous
fungal infections can occur. Hyperpigmentation is a rare feature in pituitary Cushing
disease, but is more common in patients
with ectopic ACTH-producing lesions, re-
flective of the higher ACTH levels in the
latter cases.[240] Excessive hair growth is also
commonly present in children. The hairline
is often low over the front and temples, with
the appearance of fine downy hair over the
back and limbs. There also may be more obvious signs of androgen excess, such as premature pubarche and acne. However, signs
of true virilization, such as clitoromegaly or
penile enlargement, are usually associated
with an androgen-producing adrenal
tumor.[241]

Muscular weakness, due to proximal myopathy,[242] and osteoporosis, especially of
the spine, are commonly observed also in
the pediatric age group.[231,232] Children are
susceptible to steroid-induced osteopenia
because of their lower bone mass and higher
initial bone turnover.

Hypertension is a common finding in
Cushing syndrome in childhood as in adulthood; the incidence in children has been
reported to be as high as 80 per cent.[243] The
evolution of increased blood pressure in the
hypercortisolemic state appears to occur via
a number of mechanisms distinct from the
hypertensive effects induced by mineralocorticoids. Mineralocorticoid secretion[244]
and PRA[245] are normal in most patients with
Cushing syndrome. Cortisol has been postulated to influence angiotensin levels by
increasing renin substrate formation, and
also to enhance pressor responses to both
angiotensin and catecholamines. A role for
cortisol acting itself as a mineralocorticoid,

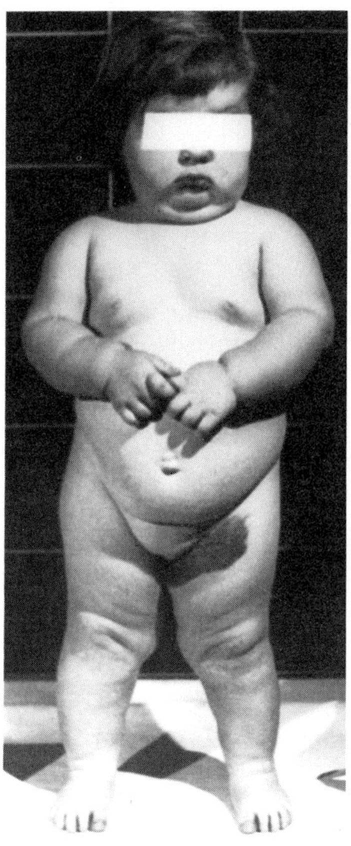 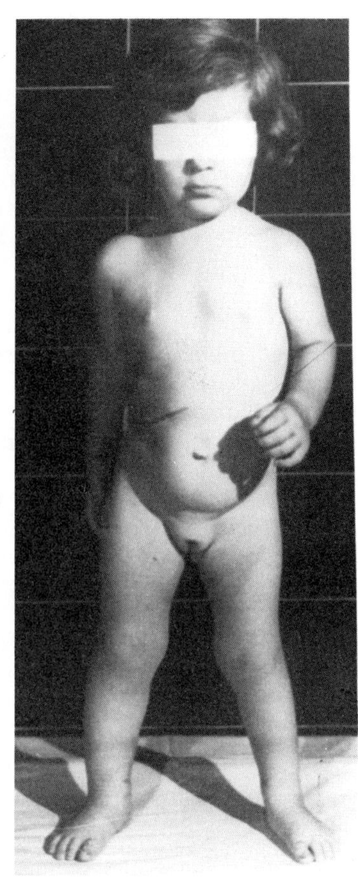

FIGURE 6–15. Cushing syndrome caused by adrenocortical carcinoma in a child. Patient is shown (*A*) prior to and (*B*) 3 months after surgery.

causing sodium retention and expansion of extracellular fluid volume, has been suggested,[246] although restriction of dietary sodium intake in Cushing syndrome does not affect blood pressure, in contrast to the effect observed in mineralocorticoid excess syndromes.

Frank diabetes mellitus is uncommon in children, but an impaired glucose tolerance is frequently observed. Psychological disturbances, from mild personality changes to severe psychosis, rarely occur in children.

Diagnosis

Several routine laboratory examinations, although not of major utility in the diagnosis of Cushing syndrome, may support the diagnosis. Of the blood constituents, hemoglobin, hematocrit, and red cell count are in the high-normal range; lymphopenia and eosinopenia are commonly present. Serum sodium level is usually normal; serum potassium level may occasionally be slightly reduced because of the mineralocorticoid

effect of the high cortisol levels. Severe hypokalemia is usually an indicator of an ACTH-producing tumor or adrenocortical carcinoma. Serum calcium and phosphorus levels also may be normal, although hypercalciuria occurs in 40 per cent of patients. The majority of patients are hyperinsulinemic and plasma lipoproteins [high, low, and very low density (HDL, LDL, and VLDL)] tend to be elevated.

Hormonal Tests

Of the many hormonal tests devised to identify abnormal production of cortisol and to distinguish the causes of Cushing syndrome, no test has 100 per cent sensitivity or specificity, and multiple testing is often necessary to confirm a specific diagnosis.

Plasma Cortisol. The normal plasma cortisol concentration is 5 to 25 µg/dl (140 to 690 nmol/l) in early morning, dropping to less than 50 per cent of that value in the late evening (11 PM to midnight). Loss of diurnal variation is typical of Cushing syndrome.

The false-negative rate of this test is only 3 per cent provided the evening sampling is performed late enough. This pattern of diurnal variation may not yet be established in children under 3 years of age, and the test in this young age group is not useful.

Urinary Free Cortisol. Measurement of urinary free cortisol reflects the integrated 24-hour plasma free cortisol concentrations.[247] In most cases, this is preferred to measuring urinary 17-hydroxycorticoids (cortisol metabolites) because it permits a better separation of normal from abnormal values. Normal values of urinary free cortisol in children are in the range of 25 to 75 $\mu g/m^2/24$ hour.[248] Three per cent of normal individuals have levels of urinary free cortisol exceeding the normal range on a single determination. Also, normal values have been reported in patients with confirmed Cushing syndrome.

Urinary 6β-Hydroxycortisol (6β-OHF). Measurement of 6β-hydroxycortisol, the major unconjugated urinary metabolite of cortisol, has been shown to be a reliable test in the evaluation of hypercortisolemic states. Levels of urinary 6β-OHF and the ratio of urinary 6β-OHF to free cortisol have been reported to be increased in patients with Cushing syndrome with urinary free cortisol and 17-hydroxycorticoid levels within the normal range.[249,250]

Stimulation and Suppression Tests

Once hypercortisolism is confirmed, further workup is required (see Fig. 6–16) to differentiate between a pituitary ACTH-secreting adenoma and an autonomous adrenal source of the abnormal cortisol production (ectopic ACTH-producing tumors are extremely rare in children). Basal plasma levels of ACTH (and of the related peptides β-lipotropin and β-endorphin) are elevated in cases of pituitary disturbance—but often only into the range of high normal, because negative feedback exercised by the increased cortisol levels is still capable of par-

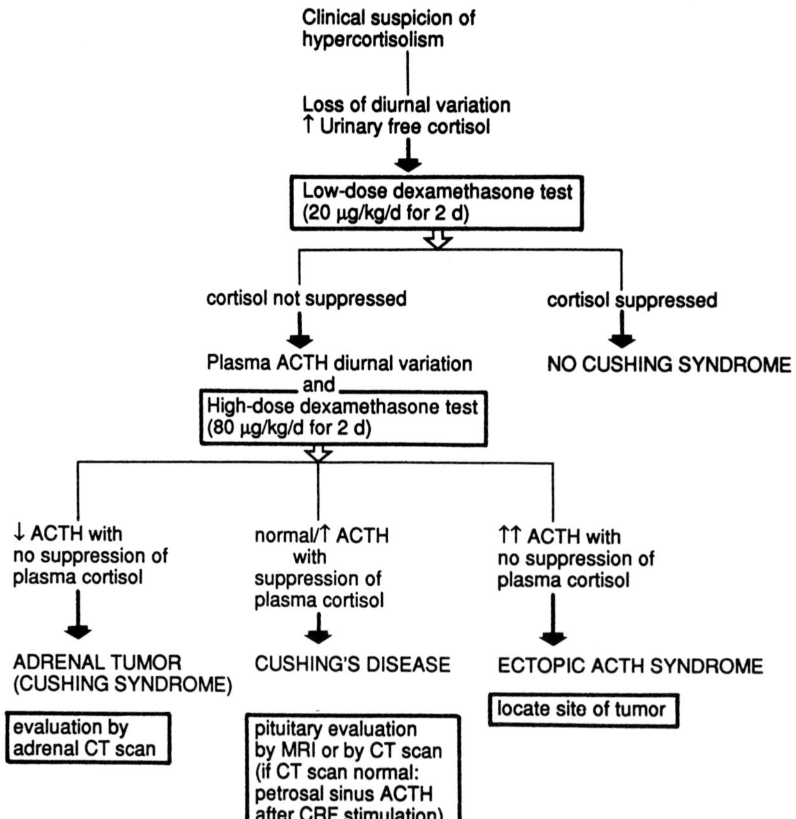

FIGURE 6–16. Flow chart indicating test procedures and results leading to specific diagnosis of the forms of suspected hypercortisolism. (From New MI, Del Balzo P: Disorders of the adrenal. *In* Eichenwald HF, Stroder J (eds): Current Pediatric Therapy. 2nd ed. Philadelphia, Brian C Decker, 1988.)

tially suppressing ACTH, establishing a new steady state.[251] The finding of a high-normal ACTH level in the face of hypercortisolemia is thus strongly suggestive of Cushing disease. In contrast, if the primary disturbance is in the adrenals, the pituitary is suppressed and ACTH levels are consistently low. Ectopic ACTH-producing tumors usually present with the highest levels of ACTH [greater than 200 pg/ml (44 pmol/L)].

Adrenal Suppression Tests. The overnight dexamethasone adrenal suppression test is used as an initial screening test in cases of suspected hypercortisolism. Dexamethasone 0.3 mg/m^2 orally is administered at 11 PM and an 8 AM plasma cortisol measurement is made the next morning[252]; suppression of adrenal cortisol output to a plasma value less than 5 µg/dl is considered normal. The presence of obesity, or of depression in depressive or bipolar affective disorders, may confuse the evaluation since cortisol levels are high and relatively nonsuppressible in these conditions also.

The low- and high-dose 48-hour dexamethasone tests (20 and 80 µg/kg/day, respectively, divided in four doses, administered for two consecutive days[253]) permit differentiation between a central and an adrenal cause of hypercortisolemia. In the case of corticotrophin-producing pituitary adenoma, but not of adrenal tumor, the higher dose of dexamethasone will cause a significant suppression of the urinary free cortisol or 17-hydroxycorticoids to less than 50 per cent of the baseline. Serum cortisol should decrease to less than 7 µg/dl.

The degree of suppression accepted as normal is not absolute, however; in addition to individual variations in metabolism of dexamethasone itself (i.e., slow metabolizers and fast metabolizers), other pharmacologic agents (e.g., anticonvulsants) can alter dexamethasone clearance. If there is any doubt concerning the results obtained, measurement both of serum dexamethasone and of cortisol concentrations during a repeat test will help in ascertaining the degree of suppression.

Cortrosyn and Metyrapone Tests. Testing with administered ACTH and with the steroidogenic inhibitor metyrapone may give results supporting a presumed diagnosis.

Cortrosyn testing (Cortrosyn [synthetic ACTH$_{1-24}$] 25 U/m^2 I.V.) will produce a further exaggerated cortisol response in pa-tients with pituitary Cushing disease, since the adrenals are not maximally stimulated. Patients with adrenal tumors generally show no change in plasma cortisol since the normal ACTH-responsive glandular tissue is suppressed and does not respond.

Metyrapone acts by blocking the 11β-hydroxylation of cortisol; the consequent fall in plasma cortisol levels results in increased ACTH secretion, which stimulates production of 11-deoxycortisol by the adrenals. In the standard metyrapone test, a dose of 450 mg/m^2 is given every 4 hours for 24 hours. A short metyrapone test has also been standardized, consisting of a single oral dose of 30 mg/kg at midnight; the latter may be associated with an impaired response secondary to poor absorption of the drug. In Cushing disease an exaggerated rise in 11-deoxycortisol is usually observed, whereas no response is expected if an adrenal or ectopic ACTH tumor are the cause of hypercortisolism.

Corticotropin-Releasing Factor (CRF) Test. The recently introduced CRF test has not proved to offer any particular advantage over the well-established procedures in diagnostic evaluation. Although the CRF response in patients with pituitary adenoma statistically produces an exaggerated increase in ACTH and cortisol levels compared with the response in patients with adrenal tumors or ectopic ACTH tumors, the variability in the individual responses remains quite high. Chrousos estimated that 20 per cent of patients with an ACTH-secreting pituitary adenoma do not respond to CRF stimulation, and that 8 per cent of patients with ectopic ACTH do respond.[254] A useful application of CRF testing is in special investigative procedures such as inferior petrosal sinus blood sampling, in which ACTH levels are measured simultaneously in the left and right inferior petrosal sinus. Corticotropin-releasing factor–stimulated ACTH values have been useful in lateralization, that is, in aiding in localizing pituitary microadenomas not demonstrable radiologically.[255]

Radiologic procedures for tumor localization should always be preceded by biochemical diagnosis. Standard skull x-rays rarely show an abnormality of the sella (only 10 to 15 per cent of patients with pituitary macroadenoma show evidence of sellar enlargement), and in patients with pituitary microadenoma high-resolution computed tomography (CT) scan of the sella is abnormal in only approximately 50 to 70 per cent of cases.[256,257] On the other hand, false-positive CT scans may be found in cases of interpituitary cyst, coincidental nonfunctioning adenoma, or empty sella syndrome. Magnetic resonance imaging (MRI) seems to offer better resolution and to have fewer false-negative results[258]; in a recent report the accuracy of diagnosis by MRI was greater than 80 per cent.[259] If an adrenal tumor is suspected, an abdominal CT scan is the most common procedure used. Ultrasonography and iodocholesterol scan of the adrenal are also used.[260,261]

Pituitary (Cushing Disease) and Ectopic ACTH

Excess ACTH of pituitary origin with bilateral adrenal hyperplasia is the usual cause of Cushing syndrome after 6 or 7 years of age. The inappropriate pituitary secretion of ACTH is most often from microadenomas (diameter less than 10 mm) located within the anterior pituitary. The adenomas in Cushing disease are characteristically basophilic; chromophobe adenomas may also occur. The presence of neuronal cells within the pituitary adenoma tissue has been reported, indicating an intermediate rather than anterior lobe origin in these cases of Cushing disease.[262]

In some instances of Cushing disease the basis of excess pituitary corticotropin (ACTH) secretion has been considered not to be a primary autonomous ACTH-secreting tumor, but rather the excessive stimulation of the corticotroph cell population by high levels of CRF from an underlying hypothalamic abnormality. Complicating the distinction, sustained CRF stimulation may lead to secondary pituitary adenoma formation.[263] However, some evidence supports the primary pituitary origin of the disease. The high remission rate obtained after surgical removal of the adenoma, the transient ACTH deficiency commonly observed postoperatively, and the restoration of diurnal cortisol variation all give evidence of intact hypothalamic function.[264-266]

The rare cases of ectopic ACTH production in childhood have been described in association with such tumors as thymoma, Wilm tumor, adrenal rest tumor, and pancreatic neoplasm.

Treatment

Bilateral adrenalectomy has been largely used in the past to resolve hypercortisolism in children, although Cushing disease is a disorder primarily of the pituitary and/or hypothalamus. This procedure was followed in up to 45 per cent of the patients by the appearance of Nelson syndrome, characterized by progressive hyperpigmentation and enlarged sella, presumably due to the progressive growth of a preexisting pituitary adenoma.[267] Currently, Cushing disease is treated either surgically or with pituitary irradiation, the latter being administered externally or by implanation of radioactive gold or yttrium in the pituitary.

Transsphenoidal microsurgery is the current procedure of choice; the remission rate following neurosurgery is approximately 85 to 95 per cent in children as well as in adults.[268,269] Glucocorticoid coverage is recommended during surgery; a residual transient hypoadrenalism is often observed postoperatively, lasting up to 30 months.

Conventional irradiation of the pituitary, in doses of 3500 to 5000 rad, has been widely used; the success rate in children has been reported to be higher than in adults, reaching 80 per cent of treated patients[270]; however the risk of hypopituitarism and consequent growth failure has to be considered.[271] Moreover, there is a lag period usually of 6 to 12 months before the effects of treatment become apparent. During this interval of time, hypercortisolism may have to be managed by medication such as metyrapone or cyproheptadine.[272]

Interstitial irradiation of the pituitary seems to be associated with a high remission rate in juveniles.[273] No recurrences were reported in a large group of patients followed for 3 to 26 years after receiving irradiation,[274] but hypopituitarism developed in 40 to 50 per cent of the cases. Although conventional irradiation has been until recently considered the treatment of choice in children with Cushing disease, the overall cure rate following pituitary microsurgery recently reported in a large series, and the safety of the procedure, argue for this therapeutic approach in children as well as in adults.[266]

Pharmacologic agents affecting neurotransmitter control of ACTH secretion represent a second choice of treatment in Cushing disease. Their use is associated with poor results and frequent side effects. Accordingly they are mostly used as supportive therapy in the interval before surgery or in conjunction with pituitary irradiation. Cyproheptadine,[275] a serotoninergic antagonist, causes increased appetite and worsening of obesity; bromocriptine, a dopamine agonist, is frequently associated with gastrointestinal disturbances.[276]

Adrenal

A tumor of the adrenal, either adenoma or carcinoma, is more likely to be the basic lesion in Cushing syndrome presenting in infancy or during the first few years of life. Females are more frequently affected, and age of appearance is mostly between 1 and 8 years. Pigmented adrenocortical micronodular dysplasia is a rare cause of Cushing syndrome. It occurs mostly in the first two decades of life, predominantly in girls. Familial cases have been reported.[277] Hormonal testing yields results compatible with an ACTH-independent adrenal source of abnormal cortisol production. Radiologic studies reveal normal-sized or slightly enlarged adrenals. Recently, a role for circulating immunoglobulins with stimulatory effects on adrenal steroidogenesis has been postulated to explain the pathogenesis of this syndrome.[278]

Treatment

Treatment of Cushing syndrome due to adrenal adenoma or carcinoma is by surgical removal of the affected gland followed by glucocorticoid replacement until normal function in the contralateral gland is restored. This usually takes 6 to 12 months, but suppression from the tumor can persist for up to 2 years. Malignant tumors of the adrenal gland often present with metastasis at diagnosis; prognosis in these cases is poor. Sometimes only partial surgical excision of the tumor is possible, but a reduction in the mass of the tumor is followed by decreased cortisol production and amelioration of symptoms. In case of metastasis or partial removal of the tumor, treatment with the adrenolytic agent mitotane (o,p'-DDD) is recommended.[279] Clinical remission is obtained in up to 80 per cent of cases, but the rate of relapse after discontinuation of treatment is high. Frequent side effects are skin rash, nausea, vomiting, somnolence, and adrenal atrophy. Metyrapone and aminoglutethimide,[280,281] which inhibit cortisol biosynthesis, can also be used. The major side effects of these agents are gastrointestinal disturbances and hirsutism (metyra-

pone) and somnolence, skin rash, and goiter (aminoglutethimide).

Recently, ketoconazole,[282] a steroidogenic enzyme inhibitor, and the glucocorticoid antagonist RU 486[283] have been employed in order to control the clinical symptoms secondary to hypercortisolism in patients with both pituitary Cushing disease and Cushing syndrome.

Exogenous Glucocorticoids (Iatrogenic)

Prolonged exposure to supraphysiologic concentrations of glucocorticoids results in suppression of the hypothalamus-pituitary-adrenal (HPA) axis. Individual susceptibility to development of suppression of the HPA axis is variable. If the patient has received such doses of glucocorticoids as can cause signs and symptoms of Cushing syndrome, adrenal suppression is always present. With glucocorticoid therapy lasting less than 2 weeks, regardless the dose administered, adrenal suppression is not expected. In circumstances between these extremes, the degree of adrenal suppression is variable. The preparation used, the dose and schedule of administration (e.g., daily or alternate-day regimen), and the duration of treatment are the major factors influencing the degree of HPA axis suppression and the time to recovery.

Symptoms of adrenal insufficiency, such as weakness, fatigue, hypotension, or even an acute adrenal crisis, can occur either after cessation of glucocorticoid therapy or, in case of major stress occurring during chronic glucocorticoid administration, without appropriate increase in the dosage.

To diagnose suppression of the HPA axis or to document recovery of the system following prolonged glucocorticoid administration, a standard ACTH stimulation test (Cortrosyn 25 U/m^2 I.V.) can be performed and the plasma cortisol response evaluated.[284] Plasma cortisol levels that fail to reach 20 μg/dl following maximal stimulation with ACTH strongly suggest adrenal insufficiency.

ADRENAL INSUFFICIENCY

Etiology

Inadequate secretion of the adrenal hormones can result from disease of the adrenal cortex (primary adrenal insufficiency or Addison disease), or from deficient secretion of ACTH from the pituitary (secondary adrenal insufficiency). The latter is usually associated with multiple anterior pituitary hormone deficiencies. Isolated pituitary ACTH deficiency is unusual. Prolonged administration of glucocorticoids causes suppression of the HPA axis and is a common cause of secondary adrenal insufficiency. In primary adrenal insufficiency all three classes of corticosteroids—glucocorticoids, mineralocorticoids, and adrenal androgens—are inadequately secreted, and the adrenal glands are atrophic. In adrenal insufficiency secondary to ACTH deficiency, mineralocorticoid secretion is not impaired, because of primary regulation of aldosterone synthesis by the renin-angiotensin system, among other stimuli.

Primary Adrenal Insufficiency (Addison Disease)

Primary adrenal insufficiency is a rare disease in children. Etiology varies with the age of presentation. Hypoadrenocorticism presenting during childhood or adolescence may be familial or sporadic. In the early part of the century tuberculosis was the most common cause, but in recent years this infection has accounted for less than 20 per cent of all cases.[285]

Rare conditions that have been associated with acquired adrenal insufficiency include fungal infections such as coccidioidomycosis, blastomycosis, histoplasmosis, and torulosis, as well as sarcoidosis, hemochromatosis, amyloidosis, metastatic malignancy, and hemorrhage (usually due to meningococcal or *Pseudomonas* septicemias), all of which may cause destruction of the adrenals. Adrenal failure has also been reported in the acquired immune deficiency syndrome (AIDS).[286]

Since the first description of circulating antibodies to adrenal and thyroid tissues was reported in a patient with Addison disease,[287] subsequent repeated observations of an increased prevalence of antibodies to different tissues have established disordered organ-specific immunity as a cause for this disorder. It now appears that most cases may represent the outcome of an autoimmune process,[288] and autoimmune adrenalitis or "idiopathic" Addison disease now accounts for approximately 80 per cent of all cases.

Polyglandular Autoimmune Syndromes. Adrenal insufficiency attributed to autoimmune phenomena is associated with disease of other endocrine glands as well. These polyendocrine syndromes may be divided into two types[289]: type I and type II polyglandular autoimmune syndrome (PGA). Type I PGA is usually seen in early life and is associated with mucocutaneous candidiasis and hypoparathyroidism with a low frequency of insulin-dependent diabetes mellitus or thyroid deficiency. Pernicious anemia, chronic active hepatitis, alopecia, malabsorption, and gonadal failure are occasionally seen in this form. Type II PGA occurs in middle life with a strong association with insulin-dependent diabetes mellitus and/or thyroid deficiency. Both types may occur in familial and sporadic forms. In type II PGA, there is an association with HLA-B8 within the major histocompatibility complex, which is not the case with type I.[290]

ACTH Unresponsiveness. A rare form of adrenal insufficiency occurring in childhood is the syndrome of familial unresponsiveness to ACTH.[291] Since the first description by Shepard et al.,[292] the ACTH insensitivity syndrome has been described in 30 families with 63 subjects affected. A defect of the ACTH receptor at the adrenal level was first demonstrated by Migeon et al.[293]; recently an associated defect in the lymphocyte ACTH receptor has been demonstrated in a patient with the syndrome.[294] Corticoid levels are very low in these patients, but aldosterone secretion is preserved. Clinically, the syndrome presents in early childhood with hypoglycemia and hyperpigmentation without salt loss. It may be associated with alacrima and achalasia. Lack of circulating antibodies and presence of normal mineralocorticoid activity exclude an adrenal autoimmune disease.

Adrenoleukodystrophy. Another rare cause of adrenal failure is an X-linked recessive familial disorder known as adrenoleukodystrophy (ALD).[295] This is a progressive disease of childhood that is manifest in the latter part of the first decade of life, and it is associated with progressive central demyelination resulting in blindness, deafness, dementia, quadriparesis, and death. Occasionally, Addison disease may be the only manifestation of the disease. Adrenal cortical cells and Schwann cells of patients with ALD contain characteristic lamellar cytoplasmic inclusions, consisting of cholesterol esterified with very long-chain saturated fatty acids (VLCFAs). All patients show increased plasma levels of saturated unbranched VLCFAs because of impaired capacity to degrade these lipids at the peroxisomal level. Apart from the childhood form of ALD, other forms of ALD have been described: the adult form, adrenomyeloneuropathy (AMN), is a variant of ALD usually presenting in young adulthood. Both phenotypes may occur in a kindred. The neurologic symptoms in AMN include progressive spastic paraparesis and polyneuropathy. The neonatal form of ALD is a distinct entity with autosomal-recessive inheritance, presenting during the first year of life with hypotonia, severe developmental delay, and seizure disorders. In contrast to X-linked ALD and AMN, absence of peroxisomes in body cells has been reported in neonatal ALD. Identification of female heterozygotes and prenatal diagnosis is possible by use of biochemical assays of VLCFAs in plasma, skin fibroblasts, and amniotic cells.[296]

Congenital Adrenal Hypoplasia. Congenital adrenal hypoplasia is a rare disease, causing a severe salt-wasting syndrome in the neonatal period without the clinical and hormonal findings characteristic of congenital adrenal hyperplasia.[297] Two different forms have been described: the miniature and the cytomegalic forms. In the miniature form, the adrenals have normal structure but are extremely small; this form is usually associated with cerebral malformations and can be sporadic or autosomal recessive. In the cytomegalic form, an X-linked disease, the normal adrenal architecture is replaced by large vacuolated cells resembling those of the provisional zone of the fetal adrenal cortex. This form is regularly associated with hypogonadotropic hypogonadism,[298,299] and rarely it may be associated with glycerol kinase deficiency and congenital dystrophic myopathy. In connection with the latter, a deletion of closely linked independent genetic loci on the X chromosome has recently been described.[300]

Acute adrenal insufficiency accompanying certain overwhelming infections in the neonatal period has been repeatedly described through the years. Fulminating meningococcemia, accompanied by adrenal hemorrhage (probably a generalized Schwartzman phenomenon), is known as the Waterhouse-Friderichsen syndrome. Rarely, cytomegalovirus or herpesvirus infections have been recognized as causes of adrenal failure.

Adrenal insufficiency seen in the early months of life is often the result of adrenal aplasia, hypoplasia, or hemorrhage.[228] Hemorrhage may be associated with a history of a traumatic or complicated delivery. Early adrenal insufficiency may also be observed in anencephaly and in congenital hypoplasia of the pituitary gland.

Symptoms and Signs

The manifestations of adrenal insufficiency may have gradual or sudden onset. Acute presentation with a classical addisonian crisis will result, for example, from hemorrhage into the adrenal gland, or from congenital aplasia (in which the crisis will be manifest in the early days of life). Apparent acute presentation may also be the result of a gradual deterioration of adrenocortical function whose earlier, subtle signs were not perceived. A characteristic early sign is a sense of weakness with undue fatigue, a matter that is not always easy to elicit in the young child. There is usually anorexia, loss of weight, pigmentation, (especially at pressure points and scarred areas of the skin), abdominal pain, vomiting, and sometimes diarrhea. Salt craving may be present despite anorexia; symptomatic hypoglycemia is a common finding in children. Vitiligo, due to immunologic destruction of melanocytes, is occasionally associated with idiopathic Addison disease.

On physical examination the most striking finding is the abnormal pigmentation of the skin (Fig. 6–17), which is most pronounced at the lip borders, on the buccal mucosa, nipples, scarred areas, and pressure points, and in the palmar (Fig. 6–18), axillary, and groin creases. Blood pressure may be low or normal, depending on the stage of the deficiency. Height has been reported to be below average at diagnosis, but normal growth and pubertal development are usually observed in well-treated children with Addison disease.[301]

Laboratory Tests

Laboratory tests may reveal diminished serum sodium, elevated serum potassium, and low fasting blood glucose levels. Neutropenia with relative lymphocytosis and eosinophilia are commonly observed. Elevation of blood urea nitrogen and serum cre-

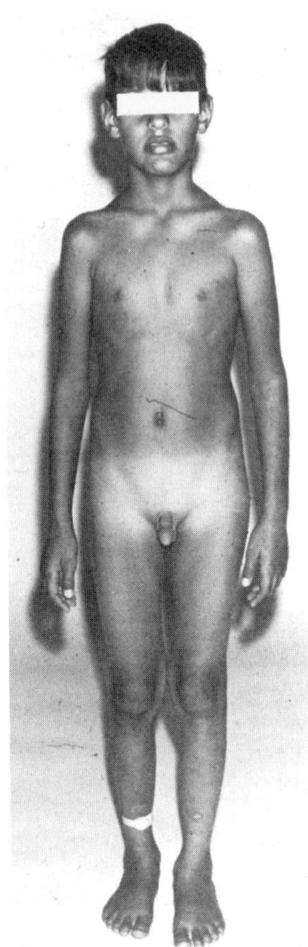

FIGURE 6–17. Twelve-year-old white male child with Addison disease. The chief complaint was limited to pigmentation and fatiguability.

atinine levels is secondary to dehydration and hemoconcentration.

Hormonal Tests

More useful is the assessment of pituitary and adrenal secretory functions. In adrenal insufficiency early morning serum cortisol concentration is low, usually less than 5 μg/dl, as is the urinary excretion of 17-hydroxycorticoids (generally less than 1.5 mg/m^2 in 24 hours). Serum or urinary C_{19} steroids (17-ketosteroids) are not of much value in making the diagnosis in children, because these are normally low. Primary and secondary forms can be differentiated by measurement of the plasma ACTH levels. In primary adrenal insufficiency, plasma ACTH levels are usually higher than 200 pg/ml, whereas in secondary adrenal insufficiency the ACTH level is inappropriately low when compared to circulating cortisol levels.

To further substantiate cortisol defi-ciency, the rapid ACTH stimulation test (Cortrosyn 25 U/m^2 I.V. bolus; serum sample obtained at 0 and 60 min) is a sensitive test of adrenal reserve. Response to ACTH depends upon the degree of adrenal destruction, but a serum cortisol value after ACTH stimulation of no greater than 15 μg/dl confirms insufficiency. However, a normal cortisol response to ACTH does not exclude a partial pituitary ACTH deficiency; for this reason, if secondary adrenal insufficiency is strongly suspected, pituitary responsiveness can be assessed by metyrapone testing (metyrapone 450 mg/m^2 P.O. every 4 hours for 24 hours) or insulin tolerance test (insulin 0.05 U/kg I.V.). On the other hand, cortisol response may be subnormal in long-standing secondary adrenal insufficiency. In this case, a prolonged ACTH simulation test (Synacthen depot 1 mg I.M. daily for 3 days) may be needed to determine if there is an abnormal increase in plasma cortisol levels.

Aldosterone secretion and excretion rates as well as serum levels are low and accompanied by elevated PRA in primary adrenal insufficiency. The renin-aldosterone axis remains normal in secondary adrenal insufficiency and in the ACTH insensitivity syndrome. Circulating adrenal antibodies can be detected in a high percentage of patients with idiopathic Addison disease.[285] Antibodies to other tissues (thyroid, parathyroid, gastric mucosa, islet cells) may occasionally be present.

Computed tomography scans may show enlargement of the adrenals, possibly with calcifications in the case of tuberculosis or hemorrhage; in the idiopathic form the adrenals are usually not enlarged.

Treatment

Treatment of the various forms of adrenal insufficiency entails replacement of deficient adrenal cortical hormones. A regimen for long-term management is oral hydrocortisone 15 to 20 mg/m^2/24 hour divided in three doses. The lowest dosage sufficient to control symptoms of hypoadrenocorticism should be administered, in order to permit normal growth. Mineralocorticoid treatment is recommended in all forms of primary adrenal failure to compensate for aldosterone deficiency. A synthetic mineralocorticoid, 9α-fluorocortisol (Florinef) is used at the dose of 0.05 to 0.1 mg/day orally.

The adequacy of treatment is monitored

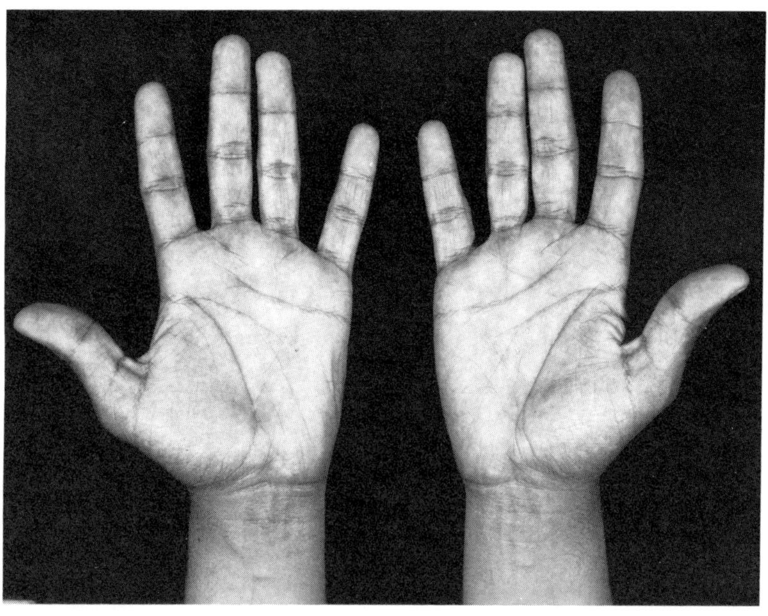

FIGURE 6–18. Hands of a boy with Addison disease. Note pigmented creases.

by observation of reduced hyperpigmentation, absence of hypotension and weakness, normalization of electrolytes (especially potassium), and reduction of plasma renin levels. Serum ACTH determinations are not helpful in evaluating the adequacy of therapy in primary adrenal insufficiency.

Intercurrent illness or stress requires an adjustment of glucocorticoid but generally not mineralocorticoid dosage because the high levels of glucocorticoid usually provide adequate mineralocorticoid activity. For minor stress such as fever or upper respiratory tract infections, the dosage of glucocorticoid should be doubled or tripled until the illness has resolved. If vomiting or diarrhea are present, hospitalization is required. In cases of major stress, such as surgical procedure or serious illness, the daily requirement of parenteral hydrocortisone is 40 to 100 mg/m^2 in three or four divided doses.

Adrenal Crisis

On occasion the child with adrenal insufficiency will suffer from acute crisis with prostration. This may be triggered by an intercurrent illness or injury but, at times, may have no discernible cause. Indeed, in some patients this may represent the first presentation of the disorder. The clinical signs include weakness, fever, abdominal pain, hypotension, dehydration, and shock. Hyponatremia, hyperkalemia, and hypoglycemia are commonly observed.

Treatment consists of fluid replacement and glucocorticoid administration to restore fluid volume and electrolyte balance. Mineralocorticoid replacement may not be necessary in the initial period of treatment because of the mineralocorticoid activity provided by the large amount of administered glucocorticoids and the saline infusion.

The associated or precipitating condition, usually infection, should be adequately treated. Fluids (0.15 M saline with 5 per cent dextrose) are infused at a rate of 1.5 to 2 times maintenance requirements (2250 to 3000 ml/m^2/day). If the patient is in shock, plasma (10 to 20 ml/kg) or normal saline (20 ml/kg) should be infused during the first hour of treatment. Cortisol as a soluble ester (either the 21-hemisuccinate or 21-phosphate) should be given as an I.V. bolus (50 mg for small children and 100 to 150 mg for larger children and adolescents), followed by 100 mg/m^2/24 hour added to the fluid infusion. Once the clinical condition begins to improve, this dose should be gradually tapered (decreased by one third every day to return to the maintenance dose within 5 days). When the daily hydrocortisone dose is below 100 mg, 9α-fluorocortisol should be added to the regimen.

It is of utmost importance to alert the patient and the parents to the risk of acute episodes and to issue the patient a Medic Alert tag. Moreover, all patients on replacement glucocorticoid treatment should be given an emergency kit of hydrocortisone injection (100-mg vial) to be used in case of accident or any severe stress.

TUMORS OF THE ADRENAL CORTEX

Symptoms and Signs

Tumors of the adrenal cortex have been described with onset from birth (Fig. 6–19) into adolescence.[302,303] They may be benign but are often malignant. They are of various types,[304] and the clinical manifestations will depend upon the nature of the hormones secreted. Most frequently in childhood they are virilizing. Cushingoid signs from glucocorticoid overproduction, less frequent in tumors, are usually part of a mixed picture that includes virilization (Fig. 6–20). On rare occasions tumors may be feminizing. A few instances of primary aldosteronoma have been reported in children as young as 3 years of age. A small percentage of tumors are nonfunctioning.

The virilizing tumors produce masculin-

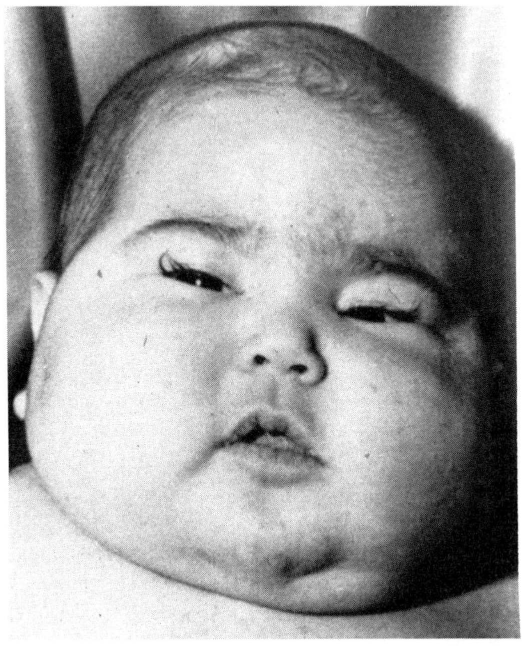

FIGURE 6–19. Face of infant suffering from Cushing syndrome arising from mixed congenital adrenocortical carcinoma. (From Giombetti R, et al: Cushing's syndrome in infancy: a case complicated by monilial endocarditis. Am J Dis Child 122:264, 1971.)

ization in girls and in a few instances, the tumor must be presumed to be congenital because of clitoral enlargement and labial fusion at birth. In boys they cause pseudoprecocious puberty. A large number of these tumors are associated with hypertension, and sometimes a mixed tumor will cause a picture of Cushing disease together with significant virilization. In both sexes, there will be an increase in the rate of linear growth and advancement of skeletal maturation. These tumors are more common in the first decade of life, and approximately 50 per cent are encapsulated adenomas. Others show invasion of the capsule and of blood vessels, with an increase of mitosis and extreme pleomorphism. They may metastasize to the lungs, kidneys, liver, or brain.

The virilizing tumors have been associated with hemihypertrophy, Beckwith syndrome, congenital malformations of the genitourinary tract, an array of hamartomatous disorders, and brain tumor (astrocytoma[305]).

Laboratory Tests

The occurrence of inappropriate virilization in a child merits investigation for the possibility of an adrenal tumor. The urinary 17-ketosteroids are distinctly elevated for age in most cases, and sometimes may exceed 100 mg/day. Often, DHEA will predominate among the 17-ketosteroids upon chromatographic separation, and this has proved to be a helpful tumor marker in these cases. The serum DHEA concentration may also be well elevated above the normal adult range. A rare adenoma has been reported to secrete only testosterone, under which circumstances there may not be an increased excretion of 17-ketosteroids or increased concentration of other steroids in the serum. It is therefore important to measure the serum level of testosterone if the other tests are not helpful. Some tumors are unusual in that they may respond to luteinizing hormone.

It is important to differentiate a virilizing tumor from congenital adrenal hyperplasia. Very high levels of 17-ketosteroid excretion are usually not seen in the latter, but, suppression tests are usually necessary to distinguish the two disorders. Administration of dexamethasone (0.5 mg four times daily) should reduce urinary 17-ketosteroid excretion to normal levels within 3 to 4 days in patients with adrenal hyperplasia but

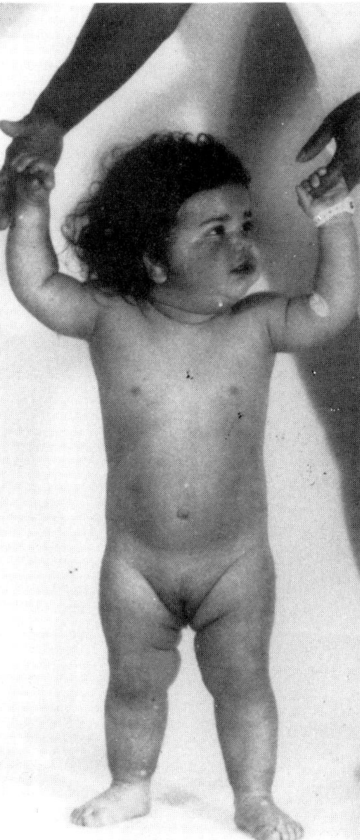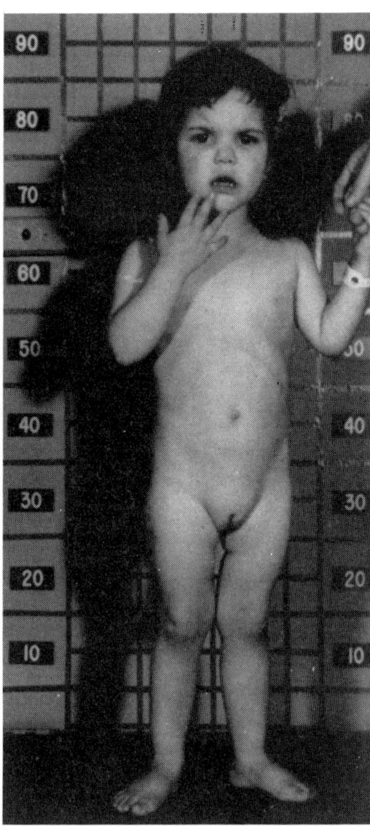

FIGURE 6–20. Infant with Cushing syndrome and masculinizing features resulting from the simultaneous occurrence of an adrenal cortical adenoma and a ganglioneuroblastoma. Child is shown prior to (*left*) and 10 months after (*right*) surgery. (From Dahms WT, Gray G, Vrana M, et al: Adrenocortical adenoma and ganglioneuroblastoma in a child. A case presenting as Cushing syndrome with virilization. Am J Dis Child 125:608, 1973.)

usually not in those with tumor. Failure of tumors to resond to ACTH with any further rise in 17-ketosteroid excretion is of limited value and reliability. It is important to locate the tumor, and the various methods have been discussed under Cushing disease. These tumors are usually unilateral.

Treatment

The treatment of choice is surgical extirpation. It is traditional to employ corticoid treatment during and for a few days after surgery until it can be determined that sufficient functioning adrenal tissue is present. There are few reports of absence of the contralateral gland. While the particular surgical approach will depend upon the circumstances, and the experience of the surgeon, we prefer a transabdominal approach in order that a thorough examination of both adrenals may be conducted in preparation for extensive extirpation when this is necessary.

For steroid coverage at the time of surgery the following is recommended, the dose varying with the size of the child. On the day before and on the day of surgery, 50 mg of hydrocortisone is given intramuscularly once daily. This has a long duration of action and is sufficient to make the intravenous administration of glucocorticoids unnecessary except in the face of unforeseen complications during surgery. The same dose is repeated on the first postoperative day and then reduced by 25 per cent on each subsequent day provided the patient's progress is satisfactory. Assessment of endogenous reserve may be made by measurement of serum cortisol in the early morning.

After surgical removal of the tumor, urinary 17-ketosteroids should be measured for a few days; they will fall to normal levels if the tumor has been entirely removed. Thereafter the test should be repeated every 6 months in order to detect recurrence. Somewhat more than 50 per cent of these tumors may recur. The drug o,p'-DDD has been employed for inoperable tumors or for recurrence but its use has not led to cures. It may induce regression of metastases and inhibit androgen production. Irradiation appears to be of no value. There is reason to believe that prognosis is better when the tumors are recognized and removed early in their course and when the urinary 17-ketosteroid excretion falls to within normal limits immediately after surgery.

Feminizing Tumors

Feminizing tumors of the adrenal cortex are rare in childhood.[306–308] They may, however, be responsible for a significant percentage of cases of prepubertal gynecomastia and need to be considered in the differential diagnosis whenever signs of feminization such as gynecomastia occur in boys before the onset of puberty. In girls they lead to signs of pseudoprecocious puberty, and ovarian tumors are often suspected before serious consideration is given to the possibility of an adrenal tumor. Ultrasonography has been refined to the point where adrenal masses can usually be detected, and if this imaging technique is inadequate CT scanning may be used. C_{21} steroids are produced in large quantities in this disorder and are converted to androstenedione, which serves as the precursor both for estrone and testosterone.[307] Estrone is converted to estradiol, but the concentrations of the former in the serum are frequently much higher than those of estradiol. Because testosterone is often produced in large quantities, enlargement of the penis and premature growth of sexual hair is often seen in addition to the feminizing signs. High serum concentrations of estrone and androstenedione are not typically present in patients with precocious feminization and when found are suggestive of the presence of an adrenal tumor. Excretion of 17-ketosteroids is considerably increased in cases of adrenal tumors and their measurement is often helpful in confirming the diagnosis.[307]

OTHER CAUSES OF ENDOCRINE HYPERTENSION

High-Renin Hypertension

Renovascular

Secondary hyperaldosteronism in children occurs secondary to an oversecretion of renin by the juxtaglomerular apparatus. This occurs in the presence of renovascular abnormalities, resulting in renal ischemia.[309,310] The renovascular abnormality may occur in the main renal artery, a segmental renal artery,[311] or as a result of coarctation of the aorta. Fibromuscular dysplasia is the most common renovascular ab-

normality in children.[312] Renal involvement in the extensive vascular changes characteristic of Takajasu arteritis may produce hypertension.[313] Secondary hyperaldosteronism associated with hypertension may also occur after renal transplantation,[314] with genitourinary tract obstruction,[315] or with fibrous encapsulation of the kidney.[316] The recently developed technique of percutaneous transluminal renal angioplasty (PTRA) has been a successful alternative to surgery in the correction of renal artery stenosis in children.[317]

Primary Reninism

Primary reninism or hyperreninemia is rare. It occurs in association with two types of kidney tumors, Wilms tumor (nephroblastoma) and tumors of the juxtaglomerular cell apparatus. Hyperreninemia and hypertension have been reported also in a case of congenital mesoblastic nephroma in an infant.[318]

Wilms Tumor. In patients with Wilms tumor or nephroblastoma, blood pressure is elevated in a significant percentage, but severe hypertension is unusual. The mechanism of excess renin production in this condition remains uncertain. Hyperreninemia may be secondary to renal artery occlusion by the tumor mass; progressive vascular involvement with hemorrhage into the tumor has also resulted in hypertension. In other cases there has been evidence of increased renin production by tumor cells.

Juxtaglomerular Cell Tumor. Juxtaglomerular cell tumors (renal hemangiopericytoma) have been reported rarely since the first case description (in 1967).[319] All tumors of this type have been single and benign; approximately one half have been in pediatric-age patients. The small size of these tumors (down to 8 mm) makes proper diagnosis difficult.

Bilateral Endocrine Dysfunction of the Kidney

In this syndrome, there is severe hypertension, marked hyperreninemia, and hyperaldosteronism.[320,321] Frequently there is associated hypertensive encephalopathy. The etiology of the disorder is unclear; however, hypersecretion of renin is contributed to equally by both kidneys. Absence of bilateral juxtaglomerular cell tumors may be determined by arteriographic studies and biopsy. Long-term follow-up has shown that there is complete spontaneous remission of the disorder. Treatment is symptomatic, directed at lowering the blood pressure until remission occurs.

Aldosteronism

Primary hyperaldosteronism (autonomous overproduction of aldosterone) results in high serum aldosterone levels producing hypertension with low PRA and hypokalemia. In children, primary hyperaldosteronism is very rare. To date, less than 25 cases have been reported.[322–329]

In the majority of cases of primary hyperaldosteronism bilateral adrenal hyperplasia is found, but adrenal adenoma or carcinoma can also be found. Complete and rapid suppression of aldosterone secretion by administration of dexamethasone characterizes the separate disorder called dexamethasone-suppressible hyperaldosteronism (DSH). The failure of administered dexamethasone to cause any reduction in serum aldosterone levels distinguishes primary hyperaldosteronism from DSH.

Magnetic resonance imaging, CT scan, radioiodocholesterol scans, and bilateral adrenal vein sampling are the diagnostic tools used in the identification and characterization of primary hyperaldosteronism.

In cases in which an adrenal adenoma is found, surgery is the treatment of choice. This mode of treatment is less satisfactory in cases of bilateral adrenal hyperplasia; in these cases, spironolactone at times achieves a better therapeutic result. Recently Armanini et al. reported that the concentration of mineralocorticoid binding sites on mononuclear leukocytes in patients with primary hyperaldosteronism was significantly lower than in normal subjects.[330] This suggests that the mineralocorticoid receptor is down-regulated in primary hyperaldosteronism. This has been described in other disorders of chronic hormone excess[331,332] but only recently in hyperaldosteronism. Mineralocorticoid receptor activity was normal in tested cases of DSH.

Dexamethasone-Suppressible Hyperaldosteronism

Dexamethasone-suppressible hyperaldosteronism is an autosomal dominant form of low-renin hypertension.[333] The adrenal and biochemical features are similar to those in primary hyperaldosteronism. However, the unique feature of this familial disorder is complete and rapid suppression of aldosterone secretion with dexamethasone administration. While remission of hypertension occurs readily in young patients, the blood pressure response is variable in adults. In addition, although cortisol dynamics are normal, there is a lack of aldosterone escape with continuous administration of ACTH.

The cause of the hyperaldosteronism remains obscure. However, extensive studies performed by New et al.[334] revealed that neither aldosterone nor any other known mineralocorticoid was responsible for the low-renin hypertension. Infusions of high doses of DOC, 18-hydroxydeoxycorticosterone (18-OH-DOC), dihydrocortisol, and aldosterone in the dexamethasone suppressed, normotensive state were ineffective in inducing hypertension in a patient with DSH.[335]

Further, ACTH infusion increased blood pressure and suppressed PRA to pretreatment ranges in dexamethasone-suppressed DSH patients, while chemical adrenalectomy lowered blood pressure and increased PRA values. These data suggest that the hypertension could be caused by an unidentified adrenal steroid (1) with mineralocorticoid properties that is (2) stimulated by ACTH and (3) suppressed by dexamethasone. In addition, mineralocorticoid receptor studies by Lan et al.[336] and Speiser et al.[337] using a rat renal slice receptor assay (RRA) demonstrated that mineralocorticoid activity was increased by ACTH administration and decreased by dexamethasone. The mineralocorticoid activity as measured by RRA in DSH patients was greater than radioimmunoassay-measurable DOC, compound, B, cortisol, and aldosterone, indicating the presence of an unidentified steroid that is dexamethasone-suppressible and stimulable by ACTH. The possibility that this steroid arises from a transitional region in the adrenal displaying biochemical features of both the zona glomerulosa and the zona fasciculata was put forth by Ulick et al.[338,339] Gomez-Sanchez,[340] and Connell et al.[341] Gomez-Sanchez et al. have reported that excretion of 18-hydroxycortisol and 18-oxocortisol is increased in the urine of patients with DSH.[342] Although these steroids have not been demonstrated to induce hypertension either in normotensive controls or in patients with DSH, they may nevertheless prove to serve reliably as markers for the disorder.

11β-Hydroxysteroid Dehydrogenase Deficiency (Apparent Mineralocorticoid Excess)

There are under two dozen cases of apparent mineralocorticoid excess (AME) known to date. This syndrome appears equally in males and females and in all racial groups. It is characterized by severe hypertension, hypokalemia, and hypoaldosteronism. Almost all patients present with accelerated end-organ damage, resulting in a morbidity of 19 per cent.[343] Presentation in almost all cases has been in childhood.

A genetic defect of the 11β-hydroxysteroid dehydrogenase enzyme system results in inadequate conversion of cortisol (substance F) to cortisone (substance E).[344] The 11β-HSD enzyme consists of two components, 11-oxidase (cortisol to cortisone) and 11-reductase (cortisone to cortisol)[345]; the 11-oxidase component is defective in AME. Because of the altered enzyme kinetics, the serum half-life of cortisol is prolonged. Normal free and bound cortisol levels are maintained by normal cortisol-binding globulin (CBG; transcortin) levels in conjunction with low cortisol secretion rates. Adrenocorticotropin is suppressed, possibly as a result of the abnormal cortisol-cortisone ratio at the level of the pituitary receptor.

Diagnosis of the disorder is made on the basis of an abnormally low serum E:F ratio, or low ratio of the tetrahydro metabolites THE and THF (THE:THF) in the urine. Monder et al.,[346] in a study comparing AME patients with normal controls, recently documented an associated defect in fibroblastic 5β-reductase activity in AME patients, causing an abnormally high ratio of allo-THF (5α-hydro) to the 5β metabolite, THF. It is not known what relation this may have to the primary 11β-HSD enzyme defect in this condition.

This condition of AME is difficult to treat and shows a high degree of morbidity/mortality. This may be due to a combination of two factors: (1) unusually malignant hypertension, and (2) severe potassium depletion. Renal damage is attested to by the occurrence of nephrocalcinosis in some cases; AME occurring with hypophosphatemic rickets, the first association with abnormal bone metabolism, was recently reported.[347] Changed accessibility of plasma steroids to

the mineralocorticoid receptor clearly is able to cause a fundamental disturbance of cellular action. Mineralocorticoid receptor blockade with spironolactone, usually in quite high doses, results in an initial lowering of blood pressure and increase in serum potassium. Addition of a diuretic may improve management, but patients may unfortunately become refractory to therapy.

The hypertension in this disorder is more severe than in other syndromes of mineralocorticoid excess, leading often to early end-organ damage. Neither the reason for the unusual malignancy nor the primary mechanism of the hypertension is clear. It has been proposed by New et al.[348] that the defect in the cortisol-cortisone shuttle is directly responsible for the hypertension seen in patients with AME. The proposed mechanism is that an abnormal cortisol-cortisone ratio increases availability and binding of cortisol at the mineralocorticoid receptor, allowing cortisol to act potently as a mineralocorticoid agonist. This theory is supported by the low levels observed of all circulating mineralocorticoids and by the absence of any increased mineralocorticoid activity as tested on several different bioassays. Clinical studies have also noted increased blood pressure and lowered serum potassium level in response to infusion of ACTH and/or hydrocortisone.[349] In our laboratories, mineralocorticoid receptor assays conducted on lymphocytes isolated from peripheral blood revealed levels 50 per cent of normal in a recently diagnosed AME patient. The suggested down-regulation of the mineralocorticoid receptor, pointing to a mineralocorticoid agonist effect, again implicates cortisol, which is the only corticosteroid present in the plasma in normal levels in these patients.

Recent examination of the mechanisms of action of the pharmacologic agent carbenoxolone (18β-glycyrrhetinic acid sodium hemisuccinate) has opened new avenues of speculation on aspects of mineralocorticoid action. It was initially supposed that this drug and other glycyrrhetinic acid congeners had an intrinsic aldosterone-like activity, and that this explained the hypertensinogenic effects of licorice ingestion, and proposed also that it might act by displacing aldosterone from nonspecific binding sites, thereby increasing effective aldosterone levels. In addition, carbenoxolone appeared to act by a separate nonmineralocorticoid receptor–dependent mechanism to enhance the electrolyte activity of aldosterone already present. Related modes of action have been noted also for the steroids 19-hydroxy-androstenedione (increasing subthreshold levels of aldosterone), 19-norandrostenedione (after Na[+] loading), 6β-hydroxyandrostenedione (kaliuresis only), and 5α-dihydrocortisol (intrinsically a weak mineralocorticoid agonist).[350] A very recent report by Stewart et al. on the observed effects of licorice ingestion[351] showed that altered cortisol metabolism indicating inhibition of the 11β-hydroxysteroid dehydrogenase enzyme results in sodium retention, further supporting the postulate that defective cortisol-cortisone interconversion, especially at the site of the distal collecting tubule of the kidney, is causative in the syndrome of AME. Just as identification of this rare hypertensive disorder (as indeed for the other adrenocortical low-renin disorders already discussed) has opened speculation on little-understood aspects of steroid hormonal functions, further characterization of the disorder will increase understanding of the physiologic processes.

Bartter Syndrome

Bartter syndrome is a rare disorder in which several of the features of hyperaldosteronism are present.[352] The nature of the primary defect is unknown but it appears to be a defect in reabsorption of chloride and sodium in the loop of Henle. The increased sodium load impairs potassium absorption distally and there is increased synthesis of prostaglandins in the kidney that impair the vascular responsiveness to the renin-angiotensin system. As a consequence, while many of the typical manifestations of hyperaldosteronism such as hypokalemic metabolic alkalosis are present, hypertension does not occur. The disorder may be inherited as an autosomal-recessive trait. The complaints include growth failure and dehydration because of impaired renal concentrating ability as well as muscular weakness and constipation. The diagnosis is confirmed by finding evidence of increased production of renin, angiotensin, aldosterone, and prostaglandin E_2 in the plasma; hypokalemia; hypochloremia; and metabolic alkalosis. Specific treatment is not available and the long-term outlook is uncertain. Therapeutic measures that are recommended include administration of potassium supplements, potassium-sparing diuretics, and inhibitors of prostaglandin synthesis. In the differential diagnosis of patients with renal wasting of potassium and metabolic alkalosis consideration should be given to the Liddle syndrome, a rare disorder that is distinguished by the underproduction of aldosterone, hypertension, and normal stature.[353]

ACKNOWLEDGMENTS: Supported by USPHS National Institutes of Health grants HD 00072, AM 07029, and by a grant (RR47) from the General Clinical Research Centers Program. Support is also acknowledged from the Horace Goldsmith Foundation and the Harold and Juliet Kalilow Foundation.

REFERENCES

1. Le Goascogne C, Robel P, Gouezou M, et al: Neurosteroids: Cytochrome P450scc in rat brain. Science 237:1212, 1988.
2. Ganong WF, Alpert LC, Lee TC: ACTH and the regulation of adrenocortical-secretion. N Engl J Med 290:1006, 1974.
3. Krieger DT, Liotta AS, Brownstein MJ, Zimmerman EA: ACTH, β-lipotropin and related peptides in brain, pituitary, and blood (review). Recent Prog Horm Res 36:277, 1980.
4. Al-Dujaili EAS, Hope J, Estivariz FE, Lowry PJ, Edwards CRW: Circulating human pituitary pro-γ-melanotrophin enhances the adrenal response to ACTH. Nature 291:156, 1981.
5. Vale W, Spiess J, Rivier C, Rivier J: Characterization of a 41-residue ovine hypothalamic peptide that stimulates secretion of corticotropin and β-endorphin. Science 213:1394, 1981.
6. Ganong WF: The central nervous system and the synthesis and release of adrenocorticotropic hormone. In Nalbandov AV (ed): Advances in Neuroendocrinology. Urbana, University of Illinois Press, 1963, p 92.
7. Guillemin R, Schally AV: Recent advances in the chemistry of neuroendocrine mediators originating in the central nervous system. In Nalbandov AV (ed): Advances in Neuroendocrinology. Urbana, University of Illinois Press, 1963, p 314.
8. Rivier CL, Plotsky PM: Mediation by corticotropin releasing factor (CRF) of adenohypophyseal hormone secretion. Annu Rev Physiol 48:475, 1986.
9. Ganong WF: Neurotransmitters and pituitary function: Regulation of ACTH secretion. Fed Proc 39:2923, 1980.
10. Gillies G, van Wiemersma TB, Lowry PJ: Characterization of rat stalk median eminence vasopressin and its involvement in adrenocorticotropin release. Endocrinology 103:528, 1978.
11. Jones MT, Gillham B: Factors involved in the regulation of adrenocorticotropic hormone/β-lipotropic hormone. Physiol Rev 68:743, 1988.
12. Davis JO: The renin-angiotensin system in the control of aldosterone secretion. In Page IH, Bumpus FM (eds): Handbook of Experimental

Pharmacology. New York, Springer-Verlag, 1974, vol 37, p 322.

13. Laragh JH: Aldosteronism in man: Factors controlling secretion of the hormone. *In* Christy NP (ed): The Human Adrenal Cortex. New York, Harper & Row, 1971, p 483.

14. Reid IA, Ganong WF: Control of aldosterone secretion. *In* Genest J, Koiw E, Kuchel O (eds): Hypertension: Physiopathology and Treatment. New York, McGraw-Hill, 1977, p 265.

15. Ganong WF: Control of aldosterone secretion. *In* Martini L, Gordan GS, Sciarra F (eds): Steroid Modulation of Neuroendocrine Function, Sterols, Steroids and Bone Metabolism. New York, Elsevier, 1984, p 111.

16. Koushanpour E, Kriz W: Tubular processing of glomerular ultrafiltrate: Mechanisms of electrolyte and water transport. *In* Renal Physiology: Principles, Structure, and Function. 2nd ed. New York, Springer-Verlag, 1986, p 196.

17. Hochberg RB, McDonald PD, Feldman M, Lieberman S: Studies on the biosynthetic conversion of cholesterol into pregnenolone. J Biol Chem 249:1277, 1974.

18. Kominami S, Shinzawa K, Takemori S: Purification and some properties of cytochrome P-450 specific for steroid 17α-hydroxylation and C17–C20 bond cleavage from guinea pig adrenal microsomes. Biochem Biophys Res Commun 109:916, 1982.

19. Nakajin S, Shinoda M, Haniu M, Shively JE, Hall PF: C21 steroid side-chain cleavage enzyme from porcine adrenal microsomes. J Biol Chem 259:3971, 1984.

20. Kominami S, Ochi H, Kobayashi Y, Takemori S: Studies on the steroid hydroxylation system in adrenal cortex microsomes. J Biol Chem 255:3386, 1980.

21. Suhara K, Gomi T, Sato H, et al: Purification and immunochemical characterization of the two adrenal mitochondrial cytochrome P-450 proteins. Arch Biochem Biophys 190:290, 1978.

22. Yanagibashi K, Haniu M, Shively JE, Shen WH, Hall P: The synthesis of aldosterone by the adrenal cortex: Two zones (fasciculata and glomerulosa) possess one enzyme for 11 beta-, 18-hydroxylation, and aldehyde synthesis. J Biol Chem 261:3556, 1986.

23. Wada A, Okamoto M, Nonaka Y, Yamano T: Aldosterone biosynthesis by a reconstituted cytochrome P-45011 beta system. Biochem Biophys Res Commun 119:365, 1984.

24. Jost A: Embryonic sexual differentiation. *In* Jones HW, Scott WW (eds): Hermaphroditism, Genital Anomalies and Related Endocrine Disorders. 2nd ed. Baltimore, Williams & Wilkins, 1971, p 16.

25. Jost A: Problems of fetal endocrinology: The gonadal and hypophyseal hormones. Recent Prog Horm Res 8:379, 1953.

26. Picard JY, Tran D, Josso N: Biosynthesis of labelled anti-Mullerian hormone by fetal testes: Evidence for the glycoprotein nature of the hormone and for its disulfide-bonded structure. Mol Cell Endocrinol 12:17, 1978.

27. Blanchard MG, Josso N: Source of the anti-Müllerian hormone synthesized by the fetal testis: Müllerian-inhibiting activity of fetal bovine Sertoli cells in tissue culture. Pediatr Res 8:968, 1974.

28. Page DC, Brown LG, de la Chappelle A: Exchange of terminal portions of X- and Y-chromosomal short arms in human XX males. Nature 328:437, 1987.

29. Simpson E, Chandler P, Goulamy E, et al: Separation of the genetic loci for the H-Y antigen and for testis, determination on the human Y chromosome. Nature 326:876, 1987.

30. Josso N: Anti-Müllerian hormone: New perspectives for a sexist molecule. Endocr Rev 7:421, 1978.

31. George FW, Catt KJ, Neaves WB, et al: Studies on the regulation of testosterone synthesis in the fetal rabbit testis. Endocrinology 102:665, 1978.

32. Siiteri PK, Wilson JD: Testosterone formation and metabolism during male sexual differentiation in the human embryo. J Clin Endocrinol Metab 38:113, 1974.

33. Peterson RE, Imperato-McGinley J, Gautier T, et al: Male pseudohermaphroditism due to steroid 5α-reductase deficiency. Am J Med 62:170, 1977.

34. Federman DD: Disorders of fetal endocrinology: Female pseudohermaphroditism. *In* Abnormal Sexual Development. Philadelphia, WB Saunders Company, 1979, p 121.

35. New MI, White PC, Pang S, Dupont B, Speiser PW: The adrenal hyperplasias. *In* Scriver CR, Beaudet AL, Sly WS, Valle D (eds): The Metabolic Basis of Inherited Disease. 6th ed. New York, McGraw-Hill, 1989.

36. White PC, New MI, Dupont B: Congenital adrenal hyperplasia. N Engl J Med 316:1519, 1580, 1987.

37. Wilkins L: The Diagnosis and Treatment of Endocrine Disorders in Childhood and Adolescence. 3rd ed. Springfield, IL, Charles C Thomas, 1962, p 410.

38. Prader A, Spahr A, Neher R: Erhöhte aldosteronausscheidung beim kongenitalien adrenogenitalen syndrom. Schweiz Med Wochenschr 85:45, 1955.

39. Klein R: Evidence for and against the existence of a salt-losing hormone. J Pediatr 57:452, 1960.

40. Kowarski AA, Finkelstein JW, Spaulding JS, et al: Aldosterone secretion rate in congenital adrenal hyperplasia. A discussion of the theories of the pathogenesis of the salt-losing form of the syndrome. J Clin Invest 44:1505, 1965.

41. Kuhnle U, Land M, Ulick S: Evidence for the secretion of an antimineralocorticoid in congenital adrenal hyperplasia. J Clin Endocrinol Metab 62:934, 1986.

42. Luetscher JA: Studies of aldosterone in relation to water and electrolyte balance in man. Recent Prog Horm Res 12:175, 1956.

43. Stoner E, DiMartino J, Kuhnle U, et al: Is salt wasting in congenital adrenal hyperplasia genetic? Clin Endocrinol 24:9, 1986.

44. Verkauf BS, Jones HW: Masculinization of the female genitalia in congenital adrenal hyperplasia: Relationship to the salt-losing variety of the disease. South Med J 63:634, 1970.

45. Prader A: Vollkommen männliche aussere Genitalentwicklung und Salzverlustsyndrom bei mädchen mit kongenitalem adrenogenitalem Syndrom. Helv Pediatr Acta 13:231, 1958.

46. Rosenbloom AL, Smith DW: Varying expression for salt losing in related patients with congenital adrenal hyperplasia. Pediatrics 38:215, 1966.

47. Kuhnle U, Chow D, Rapaport R, et al: The activity of the 21-hydroxylase (21-OH) enzyme in the glomerulosa and fasciculata of the adrenal cortex in congenital adrenal hyperplasia (CAH). J Clin Endocrinol Metab 52:534, 1981.
48. Baur MP, Sigmund S, Sigmund M, Rittner C: Analysis of MHC recombinant families. In Albert ED, Baur MP, Mayr WR (eds): Histocompatibility Testing 1984. Berlin, Springer-Verlag, 1984, p 324.
49. New MI: Congenital adrenal hyperplasia. In Farid N (ed): The Immunogenetics of Endocrine Disorders. 2nd ed. New York, Alan R. Liss, 1988, p 305.
50. Möller G (ed): Molecular genetics of class I and II MHC antigens. 1. Immunol Rev 84:1, 1985.
51. Möller G (ed): Molecular genetics of class I and II MHC antigens. 2. Immunol Rev 85:1, 1985.
52. Möller G (ed): Molecular genetics of class III MHC antigens. Immunol Rev 87:1, 1985.
53. Dupont B, Oberfield SE, Smithwick EM, et al: Close genetic linkage between HLA and congenital adrenal hyperplasia (21-hydroxylase deficiency). Lancet 2:1309, 1977.
54. Levine LS, Zachmann M, New MI, et al: Genetic mapping of the 21-hydroxylase deficiency gene within the HLA linkage group. N Engl J Med 299:911, 1978.
55. Dupont B, Pollack MS, Levine LS, et al: Congenital adrenal hyperplasia and HLA: Joint report from the Eighth International Histocompatibility Workshop. In Terasaki PI (ed): Histocompatibility Testing 1980. Los Angeles, HLA Tissue Typing Laboratory, 1981, p 693.
56. Awdeh ZL, Raum D, Yunis EJ, Alper CA: Extended HLA complement allele haplotypes: Evidence for T/t-like complex in man. Proc Natl Acad Sci (USA) 80:259, 1983.
57. Klouda PT, Harris R, Price DA: Linkage and association between HLA and 21-hydroxylase deficiency. J Med Genet 17:337, 1980
58. Dupont B, Virdis R, Lerner AJ, et al: Distinct HLA-B antigen associations for the salt-wasting and simple virilizing forms of congenital adrenal hyperplasia due to 21-hydroxylase deficiency. In Albert ED, Baur MP, Mayr WR (eds): Histocompatibility Testing 1984. Berlin, Springer-Verlag, 1984, p 660.
59. O'Neill GJ, Dupont B, Pollack MS, et al: Complement C4 allotypes in congenital adrenal hyperplasia due to 21-hydroxylase deficiency: Further evidence for different allele variants at the 21-hydroxylase locus. Clin Immunol Immunopathol 23:312, 1982.
60. Fleischnick E, Raum D, Alosco SM, et al: Extended MHC haplotypes in 21-hydroxylase deficiency congenital adrenal hyperplasia. Lancet 1:152, 1983.
61. Raum DL, Awdeh ZL, Anderson J, et al: Human C4 haplotypes with duplicated C4A or C4B. Am J Hum Genet 36:72, 1984.
62. Speiser PW, Dupont B, Rubinstein P, et al: High frequency of nonclassical steroid 21-hydroxylase deficiency. Am J Hum Genet 37:650, 1985.
63. Kaštelan A, Brkljacic-Surkalovič Lj, Dumič M: The HLA associations in congenital adrenal hyperplasia due to 21-hydroxylase deficiency in a Yugoslav population. Ann NY Acad Sci 458:36, 1985.
64. Bongiovanni AM: The adrenogenital syndrome with deficiency of 3β-hydroxysteroid dehydrogenase. J Clin Invest 41:2086, 1962.
65. Kenny FM, Reynolds JW, Green OC: Partial 3β-hydroxysteroid dehydrogenase (3β-HSD) deficiency in a family with congenital adrenal hyperplasia: Evidence for increasing 3β-HSD activity with age. Pediatrics 48:756, 1971.
66. Pang S, Levine LS, Stoner E, et al: Nonsalt-losing congenital adrenal hyperplasia due to 3β-hydroxysteroid dehydrogenase activity with normal glomerulosa function. J Clin Endocrinol Metab 56:808, 1983.
67. Hamilton W, Brush MG: Four clinical variants of congenital adrenal hyperplasia. Arch Dis Child 39:66, 1964.
68. Jänne O, Perheentupa J, Vihko R: Plasma and urinary steroids in an eight year old boy with 3β-hydroxysteroid dehydrogenase deficiency. J Clin Endocrinol Metab 31:162, 1970.
69. Parks GA, Bermudez JA, Anast CS, et al: Pubertal boy with ther 3β-hydroxysteroid dehydrogenase defect. J Clin Endocrinol Metab 33:269, 1971.
70. Schneider G, Genel M, Bongiovanni AM, et al: Persistent testicular Δ^5-isomerase-3β-hydroxysteroid dehydrogenase (Δ^5-3β-HSD) deficiency in the Δ^5-3β-HSD form of congenital adrenal hyperplasia. J Clin Invest 55:681, 1975.
71. de Peretti E, Forest MG, Feit JP, David M: Endocrine studies in two children with male pseudohermaphroditism due to 3β-hydroxysteroid dehydrogenase defect. In Genazzani AR, Thijssen JHH, Siiteri PK (eds): Adrenal Androgens. New York, Raven Press, 1980, p 141.
72. Zachmann M, Völlmin JA, Mürset G, et al: Unusual type of congenital adrenal hyperplasia probably due to deficiency of 3β-hydroxysteroid dehydrogenase. Case report of a surviving girl and steroid studies. J Clin Endocrinol Metab 30:719, 1970.
73. Cathro DM, Birchall K, Mitchell FL, Forsyth CC: 3β:21-Dihydroxypregn-5-ene-20-one in urine of normal human infants and in third day urine of child with deficiency of 3β-hydroxysteroid dehydrogenase. Arch Dis Child 40:251, 1965.
74. Kogut MD: Adrenogenital syndrome. Am J Dis Child 110:562, 1965.
75. Eberlein WR, Bongiovanni AM: Congenital adrenal hyperplasia with hypertension: Unusual steroid pattern in blood and urine (letter). J Clin Endocrinol 15:1531, 1955.
76. Eberlein WR, Bongiovanni AM: Plasma and urinary corticosteroids in the hypertensive form of congenital adrenal hyperplasia. J Biol Chem 223:85, 1956.
77. Rosler A, Leiberman E, Sack J, et al: Clinical variability of congenital adrenal hyperplasia due to 11β-hydroxylase deficiency. Horm Res 16:133, 1982.
78. New MI, Levine LS: Congenital adrenal hyperplasia. In Harris H, Hirschhorn K (eds): Advances in Human Genetics, Vol. 4. New York, Plenum Press, 1973, pp 251–376.
79. Levine LS, Rauh W, Gottesdiener K, et al: New studies of the 11β-hydroxylase and 18-hydroxylase enzymes in the hypertensive form of congenital adrenal hyperplasia. J Clin Endocrinol Metab 51:223, 1980.
80. New MI, Seaman MP: Secretion rates of cortisol and aldosterone precursors in various forms of

congenital adrenal hyperplasia. J Clin Endocrinol Metab 30:361, 1970.

81. New MI, Nemery RL, Chow DM, et al: Low-renin hypertension of childhood. *In* Biglieri EG, et al (eds): The Adrenal and Hypertension: From Cloning to Clinic (Ares Serono Symposia). New York, Raven Press, (in press 1989).

82. Ferrebee JW, Ragan C, Atchley, Loeb RF: Deoxycorticosterone esters. Certain effects in the treatment of Addison's disease. JAMA 113:1725, 1939.

83. Soffer RJ, Engle FL, Oppenheimer BS: Treatment of Addison's disease with desoxycorticosterone acetate by intramuscular injection and subcutaneous implantation of pellets. JAMA 115:1860, 1940.

84. Perera GA, Knowlton AI. Lowell A, Loeb RF: Effect of deoxycorticosterone acetate on the blood pressure of man. JAMA 125:1030, 1944.

85. Gandy HLM, Keutmann EH, Isso AJ: Characterization of urinary steroids in adrenal hyperplasia: Isolation of metabolites of cortisol, compound S, and deoxycorticosterone from a normotensive patient with adrenogenital syndrome. J Clin Invest 39:364, 1960.

86. Blunck W: Die α-ketolischen Cortisol und Corticosteronmetaboliten sowie die 11-Oxy- und 11-Desoxy-17-ketosteroide im Urin von Kindern. Acta Endocrinol 59(Suppl 134):9, 1968.

87. Green OC, Migeon CJ, Wilkins L: Urinary steroids in the hypertensive form of congenital adrenal hyperplasia. J Clin Endocrinol Metab 30:929, 1960.

88. Glenthøj A, Nielsen MD, Starup J: Congenital adrenal hyperplasia due to 11β-hydroxylase deficiency: Final diagnosis in adult age in three patients. Acta Endocrinol 93:94, 1980.

89. Ulick S: Adrenocortical factors in hypertension. 1. Significance of 18-hydroxy-11-deoxycorticosterone. Am J Cardiol 38:814, 1976.

90. Sonino N, Levine LS, Vecsei P, New MI: Parallelism of 11β- and 18-hydroxylation demonstrated by urinary free hormones in man. J Clin Endocrinol Metab 51:557–560, 1980.

91. Kater CE, Biglieri EG: Distinctive plasma aldosterone, 18-hydroxycorticosterone and 18-hydroxydeoxycorticosterone production in the 21-, 17α-, and 11β-hydroxylase deficiency types of congenital adrenal hyperplasia. Am J Med 75:43–48, 1983.

92. Mantero F, Scaroni C: Enzymatic defects of steroidogenesis: 17α-Hydroxylase deficiency. *In* New MI, Levine LS (eds): Adrenal Diseases in Childhood (Pediatric and Adolescent Endocrinology, vol 13). Basel, S. Karger, 1984, p 83.

93. Biglieri EG, Herron MA, Brust N: 17-Hydroxylation deficiency in man. J Clin Invest 45:1946, 1966.

94. New MI: Male pseudohermaphroditism due to 17α-hydroxylase deficiency. J Clin Invest 49:1930, 1970.

95. Wit JM, van Roermund HPC, Oostdik W, Baenraad ThJ, Thijssen JHH, Boer P, Janssen M, Spit M, van dem Brande JL: Heterozygotes for 17α-hydroxylase deficiency can be detected with a short ACTH test. Clin Endocrinol 28:657, 1988.

96. Prader A, Gurtner HP: Das syndrom des Pseudohermaphroditismus masculinus bei kongenitaler Nebennierenrinden-Hyperplasia ohne Androgenüberproduktion (adrenaler pseudoherm. masc.). Helv Paediatr Acta 10:397, 1955.

97. Prader A, Siebenmann RE: Nebenniereninsuffizienz bei kongenitaler Lipoid-hyperplasie der Nebennieren. Helv Paediatr Acta 12:569, 1957.

98. Dhom G: Zur Morphologie und Genese der Kongenitalen Nebennierenrindenhyperplasie beim männlichen Scheinzwitter. Z Allgem Pathol Anat 97:346, 1958.

99. Sasano N, Furuyama M, Yamazaki M: Congenital adrenal hyperplasia associated with gonadal agenesis. Endocrinol Jpn 10:215, 1963.

100. Roidot M, Menuel M-C, Coiffard N, et al: Hyperplasie lipoidique cerebriforme congenitale des surrenales. Etude anatomo-clinique de la premiere observation francaise du syndrome de Prader. Ann Anat Path 9:363, 1963.

101. O'Doherty NJ: Lipoid adrenal hyperplasia. Guy Hosp Rep 113:364, 1964.

102. Camacho AM, Kowarski A, Migeon CJ, Brough AJ: Congenital adrenal hyperplasia due to a deficiency of one of the enzymes involved in the biosynthesis of pregnenolone. J Clin Endocrinol Metab 28:153, 1968.

103. Kirkland RT, Kirkland JL, Johnson C, Horning MH, Librick L, Clayton GW: Congenital lipoid adrenal hyperplasia in an eight-year-old phenotypic female. J Clin Endocrinol Metab 36:488, 1973.

104. Degenhart HJ, Visser HKA, Boon H: A study of the cholesterol splitting enzyme system in normal adrenals and in adrenal lipoid hyperplasia. Acta Paediatr Scand 60:611, 1971.

105. Shikita M, Hall PF: Cytochrome P-450 from bovine adrenocortical mitochondria: An enzyme for the side chain cleavage of cholesterol. I. Purification and properties. II. Subunit structure. J Biol Chem 248:5598, 5605, 1973.

106. Takikawa O, Gomi T, Suhara K, et al: Properties of an adrenal cytochrome P450 (P450scc) for the side chain cleavage of cholesterol. Arch Biochem Biophys 190:300, 1978.

107. Hauffa BP, Miller WL, Grumbach MM, Conte FA, Kaplan SL: Congenital adrenal hyperplasia due to deficient cholesterol side-chain cleavage activity (20,22 desmolase) in a patient treated for 18 years. Clin Endocrinol 23:481, 1985.

108. Kohn B, Levine LS, Pollack MS, Pang S, Lorenzen F, Levy D, Lerner A, Rondanini GF, Dupont B, New MI: Late-onset steroid 21-hydroxylase deficiency: A variant of classical congenital adrenal hyperplasia. J Clin Endocrinol Metab 55:817, 1982.

109. New MI, Levine LS: Steroid 21-hydroxylase deficiency. *In* New MI, Levine LS (eds): Adrenal Diseases in Childhood (Pediatric and Adolescent Endocrinology, vol 13). Basel, S Karger, 1984, p 9.

110. Rosler A, Leiberman E: Enzymatic defects of steroidogenesis: 11β-Hydroxylase deficiency congenital adrenal hyperplasia. *In* New MI, Levine LS (eds): Adrenal Diseases in Childhood (Pediatric and Adolescent Endocrinology, vol 13). Basel, S. Karger, 1984, p 47.

111. Bongiovanni AM: Congenital adrenal hyperplasia due to 3β-hydroxylase deficiency. *In* New MI, Levine LS (eds): Adrenal Diseases in Childhood (Pediatric and Adolescent Endocrinology, vol 13). Basel, S Karger, 1984, p 72.

112. Pang S, Lerner AJ, Stoner E, Levine LS, Ober-

field SE, Engel I, New MI: Late-onset adrenal steroid 3β-hydroxysteroid dehydrogenase deficiency. A cause of hirsutism in pubertal and postpubertal women. J Clin Endocrinol Metab 60:428, 1985.

113. Jones HW, Jones GES: The gynecological aspects of adrenal hyperplasia and allied disorders. Am J Obstet Gynecol 68:1330, 1954.

114. Jefferies WM, Weir WC, Weir DR, Prouty RL: The use of cortisone and related steroids in infertility. Fertil Steril 9:145, 1958.

115. Decourt MJ, Jayle MF, Baulieu E: Virilisme cliniquement tardif avec excretion de pregnanetriol et insuffisance de la production du cortisol. Ann Endocrinol (Paris) 18:416, 1957.

116. Abraham GE, Swerdloff RS, Tulchinsky D, Hopper K, Odell WD: Radioimmunoassay of plasma 17-hydroxyprogesterone. J Clin Endocrinol Metab 33:42, 1971.

117. Zachman M, Prader A: Unusual heterozygotes of congenital adrenal hyperplasia due to 21-hydroxylase deficiency. Acta Endocrinol (Copenh) 87:55, 1978.

118. Zachman M, Prader A: Unusual heterozygotes of congenital adrenal hyperplasia due to 21-hydroxylase deficiency confirmed by HLA tissue typing. Acta Endocrinol (Copenh) 92:542, 1979.

119. Rosenwaks Z, Lee PA, Jones GS, Migeon CJ, Wentz AC: An attenuated form of congenital virilizing adrenal hyperplasia. J Clin Endocrinol Metab 49:335, 1979.

120. Levine LS, Dupont B, Lorenzen F, et al: Cryptic 21-hydroxylase deficiency in families of patients with classical congenital adrenal hyperplasia. J Clin Endocrinol Metab 51:1316, 1980.

121. Laron Z, Pollack MS, Zamir R, et al: Late onset 21-hydroxylase deficiency and HLA in the Ashkenazi population; a new allele at the 21-hydroxylase locus. Hum Immunol 1:55, 1980.

122. Pollack MS, Levine LS, O'Neill GJ, Pang S, Lorenzen F, Kohn B, Rondanini GF, Chiumello G, New MI, Dupont B: HLA linkage and B14,DR1,BfS haplotype association with the genes for late onset and cryptic 21-hydroxylase deficiency. Am J Hum Genet 33:540, 1981.

123. Levine LS, Dupont B, Lorenzen F, et al: Genetic and hormonal characterization of cryptic 21-hydroxylase deficiency, J Clin Endocrinol Metab 53:1193, 1981.

124. Blankstein J, Faiman C, Reyes FI, Schroeder ML, Winter JSD: Adult-onset familial adrenal 21-hydroxylase deficiency. Am J Med 68:441, 1980.

125. Migeon CJ, Rosenwaks Z, Lee PA, Urban MD, Bias WB: The attenuated form of congenital adrenal hyperplasia as an allelic form of 21-hydroxylase deficiency. J Clin Endocrinol Metab 51:647, 1980.

126. Temeck JW, Pang S, Nelson C, New MI: Genetic defects of steroidogenesis in premature pubarche. J Clin Endocrinol Metab 64:609, 1987.

127. Granoff AB, Chasalow FI, Blethen SL: 17-Hydroxyprogesterone responses to adrenocorticotropin in children with premature adrenarche. J Clin Endocrinol Metab 60:409, 1985.

128. Rose LI, Newmark SR, Strauss JS, Pochi PE: Adrenocortical hydroxylase deficiencies in acne vulgaris. J Invest Dermatol 66:324, 1976.

129. Lucky AW, Rosenfield RL, McGuire J, Rudy S, Helke J: Adrenal androgen hyperresponsiveness to adrenocorticotropin in women with acne and/or hirsutism: Adrenal enzyme defects and exaggerated adrenarche. J Clin Endocrinol Metab 62:840, 1986.

130. Child DF, Bu'lock DE, Anderson DC: Adrenal steroidogenesis in hirsute women. Clin Endocrinol 12:595, 1980.

131. Gibson M, Lackritz R, Schiff I, Tulchinsky D: Abnormal adrenal responses to adrenocorticotropic hormone in hyperandrogenic women. Fertil Steril 33:43, 1980.

132. Lobo RA, Goebelsmann U: Adult manifestation of congenital adrenal hyperplasia due to incomplete 21-hydroxylase deficiency mimicking polycystic ovarian disease. Am J Obstet Gynecol 138:720, 1980.

133. Chrousos GP, Loriaux DL, Mann DL, Cutler GB: Late-onset 21 hydroxylase deficiency mimicking idiopathic hirsutism or polycystic ovarian disease. An allelic variant of congenital virilizing adrenal hyperplasia with a milder enzymatic defect. Ann Intern Med 96:143, 1982.

134. Chetkowski R, DeFazio J, Shamonki I, Judd HL, Chang RJ: The incidence of late-onset congenital adrenal hyperplasia due to 21-hydroxylase deficiency among hirsute women. J Clin Endocrinol Metab 58:595, 1984.

135. Kuttenn F, Couillin P, Girard F, et al: Late-onset adrenal hyperplasia in hirsutism. N Engl J Med 313:224, 1986.

136. New MI, Lorenzen F, Lerner AJ, Kohn B, Oberfield SE, Pollack MS, Dupont B, Stoner E, Levy DJ, Pang S, Levine LS: Genotyping steroid 21-hydroxylase deficiency: Hormonal reference data. J Clin Endocrinol Metab 57:320, 1983.

137. Gangemi M, Benato M, Guacci AM, Menghetti G: Stimulation tests in adrenogenital syndrome induced by 21-hydroxylase deficit. Clin Exp Obstet Gynecol 10:127, 1983.

138. Speiser PW, Drucker S, New MI: Hypothalamic-pituitary-gonadal axis in nonclassical 21-hydroxylase deficiency. In: Program and Abstracts, 69th Annual Meeting of the Endocrine Society, Indianapolis, Indiana, June, 1987.

139. Birnbaum MD, Rose LI: The partial adrenocortical hydroxylase deficiency syndrome in infertile women. Fertil Steril 32:536, 1979.

140. Riddick DH, Hammond CB: Adrenal virilism due to 21-hydroxylase deficiency in the postmenarchial female. Obstet Gynecol 45:21, 1975.

141. Chrousos GP, Loriaux DL, Sherins RJ, Cutler GH Jr: Bilateral testicular enlargement resulting from inapparent 21-hydroxylase deficiency. J Urol 126:127, 1981.

142. Wischusen J, Baker HWG, Hudson B: Reversible male infertility due to congenital adrenal hyperplasia. Clin Endocrinol 14:571, 1981.

143. Ojeifo JO, Winters SJ, Troen P: Basal and ACTH-stimulated serum 17α-hydroxyprogesterone in men with idiopathic infertility. Fertil Steril 42:97, 1984.

144. Bonaccorsi AC, Adler I, Figueiredo JG: Male infertility due to congenital adrenal hyperplasia: Testicular biopsy findings, hormonal evaluation, and therapeutic results in three patients. Fertil Steril 47:664, 1987.

145. Rosenfield RL, Rich BH, Wolfsdorf JI, Cassorla F, Parks JS, Bongiovanni AM, Wu CH, Shackleton CHL: Pubertal presentation of congenital

Δ^5-3β-hydroxysteroid dehydrogenase deficiency. J Clin Endocrinol Metab 51:345, 1980.

146. Gabrilove JL, Sharma DC, Dorfman R: Adrenocortical 11β-hydroxylase deficiency and virilism first manifest in the adult woman. N Engl J Med 272:1189, 1965.

147. Newmark S, Dluhy RG, Williams GH, Pochi P, Rose L: Partial 11- and 21-hydroxylase deficiencies in hirsute women. Am J Obstet Gynecol 127:594, 1977.

148. Cathelineau G, Brerault JL, Fiet J, Julien R, Dreux C, Canivet J: Adrenocortical 11β-hydroxylation defect in adult women with postmenarchial onset of symptoms. J Clin Endocrinol Metab 51:287, 1980.

149. Birnbaum MD, Rose LI: Late onset adrenocortical hydroxylase deficiencies associated with menstrual dysfunction. Obstet Gynecol 63:445, 1984.

150. Hurwitz A, Brautbar C, Milwidsky A, Vecsei P, Milewicz A, Navot D, Rosler A: Combined 21- and 11β-hydroxylase deficiency in familial congenital adrenal hyperplasia. J Clin Endocrinol Metab 60:631, 1985.

151. Zerah M, Pang S, New MI: Morning salivary 17-hydroxyprogesterone is a useful screening test for nonclassical 21-hydroxylase deficiency. J Clin Endocrinol Metab 65:277, 1987.

152. Thomson G, Bodmer W: The genetic analysis of HLA and disease associations. In Dausset J, Svejgaard A (eds): HLA and Disease. Baltimore, Williams & Wilkins, 1977, p 84.

153. Sherman SL, Aston CE, Morton NE, Speiser PW, New MI: A segregation and linkage study of classical and nonclassical 21-hydroxylase deficiency. Am J Hum Genet 42:830, 1988.

154. Ulick S: Diagnosis and nomenclature of the disorders of the terminal portion of the aldosterone pathway. J Clin Endocrinol Metab 43:92, 1976.

155. Ulick S: Selective defects in the biosynthesis of aldosterone. In New MI, Levine LS (eds): Adrenal Diseases in Childhood (Pediatric and Adolescent Endocrinology, vol 13). Basel, S Karger, 1984, p 145.

156. Visser HKA, Cost WS: Corticosteroid excretion pattern in a familial salt-losing syndrome (abstract). Endocrinology 89[suppl]:81, 1964.

157. Rosler A, Rabinowitz D, Theodor R, et al: The nature of the defect in a salt-wasting disorder in Jews of Iran. J Clin Endocrinol Metab 44:279, 1977.

158. Veldhuis JD, Kulin HK, Santen RJ, Wilson TE, Melby JC: Inborn error in the terminal step of aldosterone biosynthesis. Corticosterone methyl oxidase type II deficiency in a North American pedigree. N Engl J Med 303:117, 1980.

159. Lee PDK, Patterson BD, Hintz RL, Rosenfeld RG: Biochemical diagnosis and management of corticosterone methyl oxidase type II deficiency. J Clin Endocrinol Metab 62:225, 1986.

160. Blanchouin-Emeric N, Defaye G, Toury R, Vonarx V, Aupetit B: The reoxidation of cytochrome P-450 by paraquat inhibits aldosterone biosynthesis from 18-hydroxycorticosterone. J Steroid Biochem 31:331, 1988.

161. Globerman H, Rösler A, Theodor R, New MI, White PC: An inherited defect in aldosterone biosynthesis caused by a mutation in or near the gene for steroid 11-hydroxylase. N Engl J Med 319:1193, 1988.

162. Zachmann M, Vollmin JA, Hamilton W, Prader A: Steroid 17,20-desmolase deficiency: A new cause of male pseudohermaphroditism. Clin Endocrinol 1:369, 1972.

163. Zachmann M, Werder EA, Prader A: Two types of male pseudohermaphroditism due to 17,20-desmolase deficiency. J Clin Endocrinol Metab 55:487, 1982.

164. Zachmann M, Prader A: 17,20-Desmolase deficiency. In New MI, Levine LS (eds): Adrenal Diseases in Childhood (Pediatric and Adolescent Endocrinology, vol 13). Basel, S Karger, 1984, p 95.

165. Forest MG, Lecornu M, De Peretti E: Familial male pseudohermaphroditism due to 17,20-desmolase deficiency I. In vivo endocrine studies. J Clin Endocrinol Metab 50:826, 1980.

166. Goebelsmann U, Zachmann M, Davajan V, Israel R, Mestman JH, Mishell DR: Male pseudohermaphroditism consistent with 17–20 desmolase deficiency. Gynecol Invest 7:138, 1976.

167. David M, Forest MG, Zachmann M, DePeretti E: 17,20-Desmolase deficiency in two unrelated prepubertal and adolescent boys previously diagnosed as simple hypospadias (abstract). Pediatr Res 15:83, 1981.

168. Wilkins L, Lewis RA, Klein R, Rosemberg E: The suppression of androgen secretion by cortisone in a case of congenital adrenal hyperplasia. Bull Johns Hopkins Hosp 86:249, 1950.

169. Bartter FC, Albright F, Forbes AP, Leaf A, Dempsey E, Carroll E: The effects of adrenocorticotropic hormone and cortisone in the adrenogenital syndrome associated with congenital adrenal hyperplasia: An attempt to explain and correct its disordered hormone pattern. J Clin Invest 30:237, 1951.

170. Winterer J, Chrousos GP, Loriaux DL, Cutler GB: Effect of hydrocortisone dose schedule on adrenal steroid secretion in congenital adrenal hyperplasia. J Pediatr 106:137, 1985.

171. Rosler A, Levine LS, Schneider B, Novogroder M, New MI: The interrelationship of sodium balance, plasma renin activity and ACTH in congenital adrenal hyperplasia. J Clin Endocrinol Metab 45:500, 1977.

172. Kuhnle U, Rosler A, Pareira JA, Gunczler P, Levine LS, New MI: The effects of long term normalization of sodium balance on linear growth in disorders with aldosterone deficiency. Acta Endocrinol 102:577, 1983.

173. Golden MP, Lippe BM, Kaplan SA, Lavin N, Slavin J: Management of congenital adrenal hyperplasia using serum dehydroepiandrosterone sulfate and 17-hydroxyprogesterone concentrations. Pediatrics 61:867, 1978.

174. Winter JSD: Maximal comment: Current approaches to the treatment of congenital adrenal hyperplasia. J Pediatr 97:81, 1980.

175. Korth-Schutz S, Virdis R, Saenger P, Chow DM, Levine LS, New MI: Serum androgens as a continuing index of adequacy of treatment of congenital adrenal hyperplasia. J Clin Endocrinol Metab 46:452, 1978.

176. Nihoul-Fekete C: Feminizing genitoplasty in the intersex child. In N Josso (ed): The Intersex Child (Pediatric and Adolescent Endocrinology, vol 8). Basel, S Karger, 1981, p 247.

177. Money J, Ehrhardt AA: Man and Woman, Boy and Girl. Differentiation and Dimorphism of

Gender Identity. Baltimore, Johns Hopkins University Press, 1972, p 89.

178. Baker SW: Psychological management of intersex children. *In* Josso N (ed): The Intersex Child (Pediatric and Adolescent Endocrinology, vol 8). Basel, S Karger, 1981, p 261.

179. Jeffcoate TNA, Fleigner JRH, Russell SH, Davis JC, Wade A: Diagnosis of the adrenogenital syndrome before birth. Lancet 2:553, 1965.

180. Levine LS: Prenatal detection of congenital adrenal hyperplasia. *In* Milunsky A (ed): Genetic Disorders and the Fetus. 2nd ed. New York, Plenum Press, 1986, p 369.

181. Frasier SD, Thorneycroft IH, Weill BA, Horton R: Elevated amniotic fluid concentration of 17-hydroxyprogesterone in congenital adrenal hyperplasia. J Pediatr 86:310, 1975.

182. Nagamani M, McDonough PG, Ellegood JO, Mahesh VB: Maternal and amniotic fluid 17-hydroxyprogesterone levels during pregnancy: Diagnosis of congenital adrenal hyperplasia *in utero*. Am J Obstet Gynecol 130:791, 1978.

183. Hughes IA, Laurence KM: Antenatal diagnosis of congenital adrenal hyperplasia. Lancet 2:7, 1979.

184. Pang S, Levine LS, Cederqvist LL, Fuentes M, Riccardi VM, Holcombe JH, Nitowsky HM, Sachs G, Anderson CE, Duchon MA, Owens R, Merkatz IR, New MI: Amniotic fluid concentration of Δ^5 and Δ^4 steroids in fetuses with congenital adrenal hyperplasia due to 21-hydroxylase deficiency and in anencephalic fetuses. J Clin Endocrinol Metab 51:223, 1980.

185. Hughes IA, Laurence KM: Prenatal diagnosis of congenital adrenal hyperplasia due to 21-hydroxylase deficiency: Amniotic fluid steroid analysis. Prenat Diagn 2:97, 1982.

186. Blankstein J, Fujieda K, Reyes FI, Faiman C, Winter JSD: Cortisol, 11-deoxycortisol and 21-desoxycortisol concentrations in amniotic fluid during normal pregnancy. Am J Obstet Gynecol 137:781, 1980.

187. Frasier SD, Weiss BA, Horton R: Amniotic fluid testosterone: Implications for the prenatal diagnosis of congenital adrenal hyperplasia. J Pediatr 84:738, 1974.

188. Couillin P, Nicolas H, Boue J, Boue A: HLA typing of amniotic-fluid cells applied to prenatal diagnosis of congenital adrenal hyperplasia. Lancet 1:1076, 1979.

189. Pollack MS, Levine LS, Pang S, et al: Prenatal diagnosis of congenital adrenal hyperplasia (21-hydroxylase deficiency) by HLA typing. Lancet 1:1107, 1979.

190. Forrest MG, Betuel H, Couillin P, Boue A, David M, Floret D, Francois R, Guibaud P, Plauchu H, Rappaport R: Prenatal diagnosis of congenital adrenal hyperplasia (CAH) due to 21-hydroxylase deficiency by steroid analysis in the amniotic fluid of mid-pregnancy: Comparison with HLA typing in 17 pregnancies at risk for CAH. Prenat Diagn 1:197, 1981.

191. Pang S, Pollack MS, Loo M, Green O, Nussbaum R, Clayton G, Dupont B, New MI: Pitfalls of prenatal diagnosis of 21-hydroxylase deficiency congenital adrenal hyperplasia. Ann NY Acad Sci 458:111, 1985.

192. Mornet E, Boue J, Raux-Demay M, Couillin P, Oury JF, Dumez Y, Dausset J, Cohen D, Boue A: First trimester prenatal diagnosis of 21-hydroxylase deficiency by linkage analysis of HLA-DNA probes and by 17-hydroxyprogesterone determination. Hum Genet 73:358, 1986.

193. Werkmeister JW, New MI, Dupont B, White PC: Frequent deletion and duplication of the steroid 21-hydroxylase genes. Am J Hum Genet 39:461, 1985.

194. Evans MI, Chrousos GP, Mann DW, Larsen JW, Green I, McCluskey J, Loriaux DL, Fletcher JC, Koons G, Overpeck J, Schulman JD: Pharmacologic suppression of the fetal adrenal gland in utero. JAMA 253:1015, 1985.

195. Dörr HG, Sippell WG, Haack D, Bidlingmaier F, Knorr D: Pitfalls of prenatal treatment of congenital adrenal hyperplasia (CAH) due to 21-hydroxylase deficiency (abstract no. 26). *In*: Program and Abstracts of the 25th Annual Meeting of the European Society for Paediatric Endocrinology, Zurich, August 31–September 3, 1986, p 55.

196. Forest MG, Betuel H, David M: Traitement antenatal de l'hyperplasie congenitale des surrenales pare deficit en 21-hydroxylase: Etude multicentrique. Ann Endocrinol (Paris) 48:31, 1987.

197. Charnvises S, Fencl MdeM, Osathanondh R, Zhu M-G, Underwood R, Tulchinsky D: Adrenal steroids in maternal and cord blood after dexamethasone administration at midterm. J Clin Endocrinol Metab 61:1220, 1985.

198. Goldman AS, Shapior BH, Katsumata M: Human foetal palatal corticoid receptors and teratogens for cleft palate. Nature 272:464, 1978.

199. Hardy DA, Bell JI, Long EO, et al: Genomic organization of the HLA class II region genes. Nature 323:453, 1986.

200. Carroll MC, Katzman P, Alicot EM, et al: Linkage map of the human major histocompatibility complex including the tumor necrosis factor genes. Proc Natl Acad Sci (USA) 84:8535, 1987.

201. Bell JI, Denney DW, McDevitt HO: Structure and polymorphism of murine and human class II major histocompatibility antigens. Immunol Rev 84:51, 1985.

202. White PC, New MI, Dupont B: Cloning and expression of cDNA encoding a bovine adrenal cytochrome P-450 specific for steroid 21-hydroxylation. Proc Natl Acad Sci (USA) 81:1986, 1984.

203. White PC, Grossberger D, Onufer BJ, Chaplin D, New MI, Dupont B, Strominger JL: Two genes encoding steroid 21-hydroxylase are located near the genes encoding the fourth component of complement in man. Proc Natl Acad Sci (USA) 82:1089, 1985.

204. Carroll MC, Campbell RD, Porter RR: Mapping of steroid 21-hydroxylase genes adjacent to complement component C4 genes in HLA, the major histocompatibility complex in man. Proc Natl Acad Sci (USA) 82:521, 1985.

205. Garlepp MJ, Wilton AN, Dawkins RL, White PC: Rearrangement of 21-hydroxylase genes in disease-associated MHC supratypes. Immunogenetics 23:100, 1986.

206. Carroll MC, Palsdottir A, Belt KT, Porter RR: Deletion of complement C4 and steroid 21-hydroxylase genes in the HLA class III region. EMBO J 4:2547, 1985.

207. Donohoue PA, Jospe N, Migeon CJ, McLean RH, Bias WB, White PC, Van Dop C: Restriction maps and restriction fragment length polymor-

phisms of the human 21-hydroxylase genes. Biochem Biophys Res Commun 136:722, 1986.

208. White PC, New MI, Dupont B: Structure of the human steroid 21-hydroxylase genes. Proc Natl Acad Sci (USA) 83:5111, 1986.

209. Higashi Y, Yoshioka H, Yamane M, Gotoh O, Fujii-Kuriyama Y: Complete nucleotide sequence of two steroid 21-hydroxylase genes tandemly arranged in human chromosome: A pseudogene and a genuine gene. Proc Natl Acad Sci (USA) 83:2841, 1986.

210. Carroll MC, Campbell RD, Bentley DR, Porter RR: A molecular map of the major histocompatibility complex class III region linking the complement genes C4, C2 and factor B. Nature 307:237, 1984.

211. Rumsby G, Carroll MC, Porter RR, Grant DB, Hjelm M: Deletion of the steroid 21-hydroxylase and complement C4 genes in congenital adrenal hyperplasia. J Med Genet 23:204, 1986.

212. Donohoue PA, Van Dop C, McLean RH, White PC, Jospe N, Migeon CJ: Gene conversion in salt-losing congenital adrenal hyperplasia with absent complement C4 protein. J Clin Endocrinol Metab 62:995, 1986.

213. Atchison M, Adesnik M: Gene conversion in a cytochrome P-450 gene family. Proc Natl Acad Sci (USA) 83:2300, 1986.

214. Amor M, Parker KL, Globerman H, New MI, White PC: Amino acid substitution in the CYP21B gene causing steroid 21-hydroxylase deficiency. Proc Natl Acad Sci (USA) 85:1600, 1988.

215. Globerman H, Amor M, New MI, White PC: Nonsense mutation causing steroid 21-hydroxylase deficiency. J Clin Invest 82:139, 1988.

216. Rodrigues NR, Dunham I, Yu C-Y, Carroll MC, Porter RR, Campbell R: Molecular characterization of the HLA-linked steroid 21-hydroxylase B gene from an individual with congenital adrenal hyperplasia. EMBO J 6:1653, 1987.

217. Speiser PW, Amor M, New MI, White PC: Molecular genetic basis for nonclassical 21-hydroxylase deficiency. N Engl J Med 319:19, 1988.

218. Matteson KJ, Picado-Leonard J, Chung B-C, Mohandas TK, Miller WL: Assignment of the gene for adrenal P450c17 (steroid 17α-hydroxylase/17,20-lyase) to human chromosome 10. J Clin Endocrinol Metab 63:789, 1986.

219. Chung B-C, Picado-Leonard J, Haniu M, Bienkowski M, Hall PF, Shively JE, Miller WM: Cytochrome P450c17 (steroid 17α-hydroxylase/17,20-lyase): Cloning of human adrenal and testis cDNAs indicates the same gene is expressed in both tissues. Proc Natl Acad Sci (USA) 84:407, 1987.

220. Bradshaw KD, Waterman MR, Couch RT, Simpson ER, Zuber MX: Characterization of complementary deoxyribonucleic acid for human adrenocortical 17α-hydroxylase: A probe for analysis of 17-hydroxylase deficiency. Mol Endocrinol 1:348, 1987.

221. Winter JSD, Couch RM, Muller J, Perry YS, Ferreira P, Baydala L, Shackleton CHL: Combined 17-hydroxylase and 17,20-desmolase deficiencies: Evidence for synthesis of a defective cytochrome P450c17. J Clin Endocrinol Metab 68:308, 1989.

222. Kagimoto M, Winter JSD, Kagimoto K, Simpson ER, Waterman MR: Structural characterization of normal and mutant human steroid 17α-hydroxylase genes: Molecular basis of one example of combined 17α-hydroxylase/17,20-lyase deficiency. Molec Endocrinol 2:564, 1988.

223. Chua SC, Szabo P, Vitek A, Grzeschik K-H, John M, White PC: Cloning of cDNA encoding steroid 11β-hydroxylase (P450c11). Proc Natl Acad Sci (USA) 84:7193, 1987.

224. Ishii-Ohba H, Inano H, Tamaoki B-I: Testicular and adrenal 3β-hydroxy-5-ene-steroid dehydrogenase and 5-ene-4-ene isomerase. J Steroid Biochem 27:775, 1987.

225. Stalvey JRD, Meisler MH, Payne AH: Evidence that the same structural gene encodes testicular and adrenal 3β-hydroxysteroid dehydrogenase-isomerase. Biochem Genet 25:181, 1987.

226. Chung BC, Matteson KJ, Voutilainen R, Mohandas TK, Miller WM: Human cholesterol side-chain cleavage enzyme, P450scc: cDNA cloning, assignment of the gene to chromosome 15, and expression in the placenta. Proc Natl Acad Sci (USA) 83:8962, 1986.

227. Matteson KJ, Chung B-C, Urdea MS, Miller WL: Study of cholesterol side-chain cleavage (20,22 desmolase) deficiency causing congenital lipoid adrenal hyperplasia using bovine-sequence P450scc oligodeoxyribonucleotide probes. Endocrinology 118:1296, 1986.

228. Kaplan SA: Disorders of the adrenal cortex. Pediatr Clin North Am 26:65, 1979.

229. McArthur RG, Hayles AB, Salassa RM: Childhood Cushing's disease. Results of bilateral adrenalectomy. J Pediatr 99:214, 1979.

230. Tyrrell JB, Brooks RM: Cushing's disease. N Engl J Med 298:753, 1978.

231. McArthur RG, Cloutier MD, Hayles AB, Sprague RE: Cushing's disease in children. Findings in 13 cases. Mayo Clin Proc 47:318, 1972.

232. Ross EJ, Marshall-Jones P, Friedman M: Cushing's syndrome. Diagnostic criteria. Q J Med 35:149, 1966.

233. Plotz CM, Knowlton AI, Kagan C: The natural history of Cushing's syndrome. Am J Med 13:597, 1952.

234. Lee PA, Weldon VV, Migeon CJ: Short stature as the only clinical sign of Cushing's syndrome. J Pediatr 86:89, 1975.

235. Streeten DHP, Faas FH, Elders MJ, et al: Hypercortisolism in childhood: Shortcomings of conventional diagnostic criteria. Pediatrics 56:797, 1975.

236. Unterman TG, Phillips LS: Glucocorticoid effects on somatomedin and somatomedin inhibitors. J Clin Endocrinol Metab 61:618, 1985.

237. Morris HG, Jorgensen JR, Jenkins SA: Plasma growth hormone concentration in corticosteroid-treated children. J Clin Invest 47:427, 1968.

238. Krieger DT, Glick SM: Growth hormone and cortisol responsiveness in Cushing's syndrome. Am J Med 52:25, 1972.

239. Strickland AL, Underwood LE, Joina SJ, et al: Growth retardation in Cushing's syndrome. Am J Dis Child 123:207, 1972.

240. Friedman M, Marshall-Jones P, Ross EJ: Cushing's syndrome: Adrenocortical hyperactivity secondary to neoplasma arising outside the pituitary-adrenal system. Q J Med 35:193, 1966.

241. Hutter AM, Kayhoe DE: Adrenal cortical carcinoma. Clinical features in 138 patients. Am J Med 41:572, 1966.

242. Khaleeli AA, Edwards HT, Gohil K, et al: Corticosteroid myopathy: A clinical and pathological study. Clin Endocrinol 18:155, 1983.
243. Loridan L, Senior F: Cushing's syndrome in infancy. J Pediatr 75:349, 1969.
244. Biglieri EG, Howe S, Slaton PE, Forsham PH: In vivo and in vitro studies of adrenal secretions in Cushing's syndrome and primary aldosteronism. J Clin Invest 42:516, 1963.
245. Krakoff L, Nicolis G, Acusel B: Pathogenesis of hypertension in Cushing's syndrome. Am J Med 58:216, 1975.
246. New MI, Oberfield SE, Carey R, et al: A genetic defect in cortisol metabolism as the basis for the syndrome of apparent mineralocorticoid excess. *In* Mantero F, Biglieri EG, Edwards CRW (eds): Endocrinology of Hypertension. New York, Academic Press, 1982, p 85.
247. Burke CW, Beardwell CG: Cushing's syndrome. An evaluation of the clinical usefulness of urinary free cortisol and other urinary steroid measurements in diagnosis. Br J Med 42:175, 1973.
248. Migeon C: Physiology and pathology of adrenocortical function in infancy and childhood. *In* Collu R, Ducharme JR, Guyda H (eds): Pediatric Endocrinology. New York, Raven Press, 1981, p 475.
249. Voccia E, Saenger P, Peterson RE, Rauh W, et al: 6β-Hydroxycortisol excretion in hypercortisolemic states. J Clin Endocrinol Metab 48:67, 1979.
250. Nakahura J, Yakata M: Determination of urinary cortisol and 6β-hydroxycortisol by high-performance liquid chromatography. Clin Chim Acta 149:215, 1985.
251. Reader SCJ, Daly JR, Alaghband-Zadeh J, Robertson WR: Negative feedback effects on ACTH secretion by cortisol in Cushing's disease. Clin Endocrinol 18:43, 1983.
252. Hindmarsh PC, Brook CGD: Single dose dexamethasone suppression test in children: Dose relationship to body size. Clin Endocrinol 23:67, 1985.
253. Liddle GW: Tests of pituitary adrenal suppressibility in the diagnosis of Cushing's syndrome. J Clin Endocrinol Metab 12:1539, 1960.
254. Chrousos G: Clinical applications of corticotropic-releasing factor. Ann Intern Med 102:344, 1985.
255. Landolt AM, Valavanis A, Girard J, Eberle AN: Corticotrophin-releasing factor-test used with bilateral, simultaneous inferior petrosal sinus blood-sampling for the diagnosis of pituitary-dependent Cushing's disease. Clin Endocrinol 25:687, 1986.
256. Turski PA, Damm M: Role of computed tomography in the evaluation of pituitary disease. Semin Ultrasound CT MR 6:276, 1985.
257. Saris JC, Patronas NJ, Doppman JL, et al: Cushing syndrome: Pituitary CT scanning. Radiology 162:775, 1987.
258. Dwyer AJ, Frank JA, Doppman JC, et al: Pituitary adenomas in patients with Cushing disease: Initial experience with Gd-DTPA-enhanced MR imaging. Radiology 163:421, 1987.
259. Mampalam TJ, Tyrrel B, Wilson CB: Transsphenoidal microsurgery for Cushing disease. A report of 216 cases. Ann Intern Med 109:487, 1988.
260. Sample WF, Sarti DA: Computed tomography and gray scale ultrasonography of the adrenal gland. A comparative study. Radiology 128:327, 1978.
261. Thrall JH, Freitas JE, Beirwaltes WH: Adrenal scintigraphy. Semin Nucl Med 8:23, 1978.
262. Lamberts SWJ, de Lange SA, Stefanko SZ: Adrenocorticotropin-secreting pituitary adenomas originate from the anterior or the intermediate lobe in Cushing's disease: Differences in the regulation of hormone secretion. J Clin Endocrinol Metab 54:286, 1982.
263. Krieger DT: Physiopathology of Cushing's disease. Endocrinol Rev 4:22, 1983.
264. Boyar RM, Witkin M, Carruth A, et al: Circadian cortisol secretory rhythms in Cushing's disease. J Clin Endocrinol Metab 48:760, 1979.
265. Fitzgerald PA, Aron DC, Findling JW, et al: Cushing's disease: Transient secondary adrenal insufficiency after selective removal of pituitary tumors. Evidence for a pituitary origin. J Clin Endocrinol Metab 54:413, 1982.
266. Melby JC Therapy of Cushing disease: A consensus for pituitary microsurgery. Ann Intern Med 109:445, 1988.
267. Hopwood NJ, Kenny FM: Incidence of Nelson's syndrome after adrenalectomy for Cushing's disease in children. Am J Dis Child 131:1353, 1977.
268. Styne DM, Grumbach MM, Kaplan SL, et al: Treatment of Cushing's disease in childhood and adolescence by transsphenoidal microadrenalectomy. N Engl J Med 310:889, 1984.
269. Guilhaume B, Bertagna X, Thomsen M, et al: Transsphenoidal pituitary surgery for the treatment of Cushing's disease: Results in 64 patients and long term follow-up studies. J Clin Endocrinol Metab 66:1056, 1988.
270. Jennings AS, Liddle GW, Orth DN: Results of treating childhood Cushing's disease with pituitary irradiation. N Engl J Med 297:957, 1977.
271. Schecine GE: Role of conventional radiation therapy in the treatment of functional pituitary tumors. *In* Linfoot JA (ed): Recent Advances in Diagnosis and Treatment of Pituitary Tumors. New York, Raven Press, 1979, p 289.
272. Couch RM, Winter JSD: Cushing's disease in childhood. J Pediatr Endocrinol 1:191, 1985.
273. Cassar J, Doyle FH, Mashiter K, Joplin GF: Treatment of Cushing's disease in juveniles with interstitial pituitary irradiation. Clin Endocrinol 11:313, 1979.
274. Sandler LM, Richards NT, Carr DH, Mashiter S, Joplin GF: Long term follow-up of patients with Cushing's disease treated by interstitial irradiation. J Clin Endocrinol Metab 65:441, 1987.
275. Krieger DT, Amorosa L, Linick F: Cyproheptadine-induced remission of Cushing's disease. N Engl J Med 293:893, 1975.
276. Lamberts SWJ, Klijn JGM, deQuijada M, et al: The mechanism of the suppressive action of bromocriptine on adrenocorticotropin secretion in patients with Cushing's disease and Nelson's syndrome. J Clin Endocrinol Metab 51:307, 1980.
277. Larsen JL, Cathey WJ, Odell WD: Primary adrenocortical nodular dysplasia, a distinct subtype of Cushing' syndrome. Case report and review of the literature. Am J Med 80:976, 1986.
278. Wulffraat NM, Drexhage HA, Wiersinga RD, et al: Immunoglobulins of patients with Cushing's syndrome due to pigmented adrenocortical mi-

cronodular dysplasia stimulate in vitro steroidogenesis. J Clin Endocrinol Metab 66:301, 1988.

279. Luton JP, Mahoudeau JA, Bouchard PH, et al: Treatment of Cushing's disease by o,p'-DDD. Survey of 62 cases. N Engl J Med 300:459, 1979.

280. Orth DN: Metyrapone is useful only as adjunctive therapy in Cushing's disease. Ann Intern Med 89:129, 1978.

281. Zachmann M, Gitzelmann RP, Zagalak M, Prader A: Effect of aminoglutethimide on urinary cortisol and cortisol metabolite in adolescents with Cushing's syndrome. Clin Endocrinol 7:63, 1977.

282. McLance DR, Hadden DR, Sheridan B, Atkinson AB: Clinical experience with ketoconazole as a therapy for patients with Cushing's syndrome. Clin Endocrinol 27:893, 1987.

283. Nieman LK, Chrousos GP, Kellner C, et al: Successful treatment of Cushing's syndrome with the glucocorticoid antagonist RU 486. J Clin Endocrinol Metab 61:536, 1985.

284. Kehlet H, Lindholm J, Bjerre P: Value of the 30 min ACTH test in assessing hypothalamic-pituitary-adrenocortical function after pituitary surgery in Cushing's disease. Clin Endocrinol 20:349, 1984.

285. Irvine WJ, Toft AD, Feek CM: Addison's disease. In James VHT (ed): The Adrenal Gland. New York, Raven Press, 1979, p 131.

286. Guenthmer EE, Rabinowe SL, Van Niel A, et al: Primary Addison's disease in a patient with the acquired immunodeficiency syndrome. Ann Intern Med 100:847, 1984.

287. Anderson JR, Goudie RB, Gray KG, Timbury GC: Autoantibodies in Addison's disease. Lancet 1:1123, 1957.

288. Neufeld M, MacLaren N, Blizzard RM: Autoimmune polyglandular syndromes. Pediatr Ann 9:154, 1980.

289. Neufeld M, MacLaren NK, Blizzard RM: Two types of autoimmune Addison's disease associated with different polyglandular autoimmune (PGA) syndromes. Medicine 60:355, 1981.

290. Eisenbarth G, Wilson P, Ward F, Lebovitz HE: HLA type and occurrence of disease in familial polyglandular failure. N Engl J Med 298:92, 1978.

291. Geffner ME, Lippe BM, Kaplan SA, et al: Selective ACTH insensitivity, achalasia, and alacrima: A multisystem system disorder presenting in childhood. J Pediatr Res 17:532, 1983.

292. Shepard TH, Landing BH, Mason DC: Familial Addison's disease: Case report of two sisters with corticoid deficiency unassociated with hypoaldosteronism. J Dis Child 97:154, 1959.

293. Migeon CJ, Kenny FM, Kowarski A, et al: The syndrome of congenital adrenocortical unresponsiveness to ACTH: Report of six cases. Pediatr Res 2:501, 1968.

294. Smith EM, Brosnan P, Meyer WJ, Blalock JE: An ACTH receptor on human mononuclear leukocytes. N Engl J Med 317:1266, 1987.

295. Davis LE, Synder RD, Orth DN, et al: Adrenoleukodystrophy and adrenomyeloneuropathy associated with adrenal insufficiency in three generations of a kindred. Am J Med 66:342, 1979.

296. Moser HW, Moser AE, Singh I, O'Neill BP: Adrenoleukodystrophy: Survey of 303 cases: Biochemistry, diagnosis and therapy. Ann Neurol 16:628, 1984.

297. Sperling MA, Wolfsen AR, Fisher DA: Congenital adrenal hypoplasia. J Pediatr 82:444, 1973.

298. Prader A, Zachmann M, Illig R: Luteinizing hormone deficiency in hereditary congenital adrenal hypoplasia. J Pediatr 86:421, 1975.

299. Kruse K, Sippell WG, Schnakenburg KV: Hypogonadism in congenital adrenal hypoplasia: Evidence for a hypothalamic origin. J Clin Endocrinol Metab 58:12, 1984.

300. Francke U, Harper JF, Darras BT, et al: Congenital adrenal hypoplasia, myopathy and glycerol kinase deficiency: Molecular genetic evidence for deletions. Am J Hum Genet 40:212, 1987.

301. Grant DB, Barres ND, Moncrieff MW, Savage MO: Clinical presentation, growth and pubertal development in Addison's disease. Arch Dis Child 60:925, 1985.

302. Kenny FM, Hashida Y, Ascari A, et al: Virilizing tumors of the adrenal cortex. Arch Dis Child 115:445, 1968.

303. Zaitoon MM, Mackie G: Adrenal cortical tumors in children. Neurology 12:645, 1978.

304. Symington T: The adrenal cortex. In Bloodworth JMB Jr (ed): Endocrine Pathology: General and Surgical. 2nd ed. Baltimore, Williams & Wilkins, 1982, p 419.

305. Fraumeni JF, Miller RW: Adrenocortical neoplasms with hemihypertrophy, brain tumors and other disorders. J Pediatr 70:129, 1967.

306. Bhettay E, Bonnier F: Pure oestrogen-secreting feminizing adrenocortical adenoma. Arch Dis Child 52:241, 1977.

307. Itami RM, Amundson GM, Kaplan SA, Lippe BM: Prepubertal gynecomastia caused by an adrenal tumor. Am J Dis Child 136:584, 1982.

308. Howard CP, Takahashi H, Hayles AB: Feminizing adrenal adenoma in a boy. Mayo Clin Proc 52:354, 1977.

309. Fry WJ, Ernst CB, Stanley JC, et al: Renovascular hypertension in the pediatric patient. Arch Surg 107:692, 1973.

310. Stockigt JR, Collins RD, Noakes CA, et al: Renal vein renin in various forms of renal hypertension. Lancet 1:1194, 1972.

311. Bennett SP, Levine LS, Siegal EJ, et al: Juvenile hypertension caused by overproduction of renin within a renal segment. J Pediatr 84:689, 1974.

312. Reintgen D, Wolfe WG, Osofsky S, Seigler HF: Renal artery stenosis in children. J Pediatr Surg 16:26, 1981.

313. Wiggenlinkhuizen J, Cremin BJ: Takajasu arteritis and renovascular hypertension in childhood. Pediatrics 62:209, 1978.

314. Potter DE, Schambelan M, Salvatierra O, et al: Treatment of high-renin hypertension with propanolol in children after renal transplantation. J Pediatr 90:307, 1977.

315. Carella JA, Silber I: Hyperreninemic hypertension in an infant secondary to pelviureteric obstruction treated successfully by surgery. J Pediatr 88:987, 1976.

316. Weinberger MH, Grim CE, Hollifield JW, et al: Primary aldosteronism. Ann Intern Med 90:386, 1979.

317. Fallo F, Oberfield SE, Levine LS, Stoner E, Greig F, New MI, Sniderman K, Saddekni S, Sos T: Evaluation of percutaneous transluminal

renal angioplasty in childhood hypertension. Int J Pediatr Nephrol 6:261, 1985.

318. Miles JH, Groshong T, Hakami N, Bauer J, Hensel J, Weinberger M: Congenital mesoblastic nephroma with hypertension, hypokalemia and hyperreninemia (abstract). J Pediatr 91:837, 1977.

319. Robertson PW, Klidjian A, Harding LK, Walters G, Lee MR, Robb-Smith AHT: Hypertension due to a renin-secreting renal tumor. Am J Med 43:963, 1967.

320. New MI, Laragh J: Hypertension with hyperaldosteronism and hyperreninemia in children: A clinical entity associated with subtle glomerulonephritis (abstract). Program and Abstract, Society for Pediatric Research 38th Annual Meeting, Atlantic City, NJ, 1968.

321. New MI, Laragh J: Childhood hypertension associated with bilateral endocrine dysfunction of the kidney. Acta Paediatr Scand 58:205, 1969.

322. Baer L, Sommers SC, Krakoff LR, Newton MA, Laragh JH: Pseudo-primary aldosteronism. An entity distinct from true primary aldosteronism. Circ Res 26,27(Suppl 1):203, 1970.

323. George JM, Wright L, Bell NH, Bartter FC: The syndrome of primary hyperaldosteronism. Am J Med 48:343, 1970.

324. Grim CE, McBryde AC, Glenn JF, Gunnells JC Jr: Childhood primary aldosteronism with bilateral adrenocortical hyperplasia: Plasma renin activity as an aid to diagnosis. Pediatrics 71:377, 1967.

325. Kelch RP, Connors MH, Kaplan SL, Biglieri EG, Grumbach MM: A calcified aldosterone-producing tumor in a hypertensive, normokalemic, prepubertal girl. J Pediatr 73:432, 1973.

326. New MI, Peterson RE: Aldosterone in childhood. In Levine SZ (ed): Advances in Pediatrics. Chicago, Year Book Medical Publishers, 1068, p 111.

327. Bryer-Ash M, Wilson D, Tune BM, Rosenfeld RG, Shochat SJ, Luetscher JA: Hypertension caused by an aldosterone-secreting adenoma. Am J Dis Child 128:673, 1986.

328. Oberfield SE, Levine LS, Firpo A, Lawrence D Sr, Stoner E, Levy DJ, Sen S, New MI: Primary hyperaldosteronism in childhood due to unilateral macronodular hyperplasia. Hypertension 6:75, 1984.

329. Decsi J, Soltesz G, Harangi F, Nemes J, Szabo M, Pinter A: Severe hypertension in a 10-year-old boy secondary to an aldosterone-producing tumor identified by adrenal sonography. Acta Pediatr Hung 27:233, 1986.

330. Armanini D, Witzgall H, Wehling M, Kuhnle U, Weber PC: Aldosterone receptors in different types of primary hyperaldosteronism. J Clin Endocrinol Metab 65:101, 1987.

331. Clayton RN: Hypothalamic releasing-hormone receptors. Clin Endocrinol Metab 12:175, 1983.

332. Schlechte JA, Ginsberg BH, Sherman BM: Regulation of the glucocorticoid receptor in human lymphocytes. J Steroid Biochem 16:69, 1982.

333. New MI, Siegal EJ, Peterson RE: Dexamethasone-suppressible hyperaldosteronism. J Clin Endocrinol Metab 37:93, 1973.

334. New MI, Peterson RE, Saenger P, Levine LS: Evidence for an unidentified ACTH induced hormone causing hypertension. J Clin Endocrinol Metab 43:1283, 1976.

335. New, MI, Levine LS: An unidentified ACTH-stimulable adrenal steroid in childhood hypertension. In New MI, Levine LS (eds): Juvenile Hypertension. New York, Raven Press, 1977, p 143.

336. Lan NC, Matulich DT, Stockigt JR, Biglieri EG, New MI, Baxter JD: Role of steroids in various states in mineralocorticoid-excess hypertension. In Giovannelli G, New MI, Gorini S (eds): Hypertension in Children and Adolescents. New York, Raven Press, 1981, p 165.

337. Speiser PW, Martin KO, Kao-Lo G, New MI: Excess serum mineralocorticoid binding activity in patients with dexamethasone-suppressible hyperaldosteronism (DSH) estimated by the rat renal receptor technique. J Clin Endocrinol 61:297, 1985.

338. Ulick S, Land M, Chu M: 18-Oxocortisol, a naturally occurring mineralocorticoid agonist. Endocrinology 113:2320, 1983.

339. Ulick S, Chu M, Land M: Biosynthesis of 18-oxocortisol by aldosterone-producing adrenal tissue. J Biol Chem 258:5498, 1983.

340. Gomez-Sanchez CE: 18-Hydroxycortisol and 18-oxocortisol, steroids from the transitional zone. Endocrine Res 10:609, 1985.

341. Connell J, Kenyon C, Corrie JET, Froser R, Watt R, Lever AF: Dexamethasone-suppressible hyperaldosteronism, adrenal cell hyperplasia? Hypertension 8:669, 1986.

342. Gomez-Sanchez CE, Montgomery M, Ganguly A, Holland OB, Gomez-Sanchez EP, Grim CE: Elevated urinary excretion of 18-oxocortisol in glucocorticoid-suppressible aldosteronism. J Clin Endocrinol Metab 59:1022, 1984.

343. Downey MK, Riddick L, New MI: Apparent mineralocorticoid excess; a genetic form of low-renin hypertension (abstract). Program and Abstract, American Society for Hypertension 2nd World Congress on Biologically Active Atrial Peptides, New York, May 1987.

344. Ulick S, Levine LS, Gunczler P, Zanconato G, Ramirez LC, Rauh W, Rosler A, Bradlow HL, New MI: A new syndrome of apparent mineralocorticoid excess associated with defects in the peripheral metabolism of cortisol. J Clin Endocrinol Metab 44:757, 1979.

345. Lakshmi V, Monder C: Evidence for independent 11-oxidase and 11-reductase activity of 11β-hydroxysteroid dehydrogenase: Enzyme latency, phase transitions, and lipid requirements. Endocrinology 116:552, 1985.

346. Monder C, Shackleton CHL, Bradlow HL, New MI, Stoner E, Iohan F, Lakshmi V: The syndrome of apparent mineralocorticoid excess; its association with 11β-dehydrogenase and 5β-reductase deficiency and some consequences for corticosterone metabolism. J Clin Endocrinol Metab 63:550, 1987.

347. Batista MC, Mendonca MD, Kater CE, Arnhold JP, Rocha A, Nicolau W, Bloise W: Spironolactone-reversible rickets associated with 11β-hydroxysteroid dehydrogenase deficiency syndrome. J Pediatr 87:989, 1986.

348. New MI, Oberfield SE, Carey RM, Greig F, Ulick S, Levine LS: A genetic defect in cortisol metabolism as the basis for the syndrome of apparent mineralocorticoid excess. In Mantero F, Biglieri EG, Edwards CRW (eds): Endocrinology of Hypertension (Serono Symposia No 50). New York, Academic Press, 1982, p 85.

349. Oberfield SE, Levine LS, Carey RM, Greig F, Ulick S, New MI: Metabolic and blood pressure responses to hydrocortisone in the syndrome of apparent mineralocorticoid excess. J Clin Endocrinol Metab 56:332, 1983.
350. Armanini D, Karbowiak I, Krozowski Z, Funder JW, Adam WR: The mechanism of mineralocorticoid action of carbenoxolone. Endocrinology 111:1683, 1982.
351. Stewart PM, Wallace AM, Valentino R, Burt D, Shackleton CHL, Edwards CRW: Mineralocorticoid activity of liquorice: 11β-Hydroxysteroid dehydrogenase deficiency comes of age. Lancet 2:821, 1987.
352. Gill JR: Bartter's syndrome. Annu Rev Med 31:405, 1980.
353. Aarskog D, Stea KF, Thorsen T, Wefring KW: Hypertension and hypokalemic alkalosis associated with underproduction of aldosterone. Pediatrics 39:884, 1966.

7

DISORDERS OF THE ADRENAL MEDULLA AND MULTIPLE ENDOCRINE ADENOMATOSIS SYNDROMES

Mary L. Voorhess

The Adrenal Medulla and the Sympathoadrenal System

At 6 to 7 weeks of embryonic life, neural crest cells that have been transformed into chromaffin cells migrate into the substance of the developing adrenal cortex and become the adrenal medulla. Other chromaffin cells remain close to the neural tube and give rise to extra-adrenal chromaffin masses such as the organ of Zuckerkandl. The extra-adrenal chromaffin tissue dominates during fetal life and for the first 1 to 2 years after birth, when it involutes. The adrenal medulla enlarges until about the age of 3 years, when it reaches maximum size and accounts for 10 per cent of the weight of each adrenal gland. The chromaffin cells of the adrenal medulla are innervated by preganglionic sympathetic fibers from the splanchnic nerves and are bathed by high concentrations of glucocorticoids contained in the venous drainage from surrounding adrenal cortical cells. They synthesize, store, and secrete catecholamines.

The sympathetic nervous system also is derived from cells of neural crest origin, and sympathetic nerve endings also have the ability to synthesize, store, and secrete catecholamines. The sympathetic nervous system and the adrenal medulla, together, compose the sympathoadrenal system, wherein neurochemical transducers (the catecholamines) convert neuronal activity into physiologic responses. The sympathoadrenal system is under direct control of the central nervous system.

The primary disorders of the adrenal medulla and the sympathetic nervous system in children are neoplasms. The highly undifferentiated neuroblastoma develops from intra- or extra-adrenal sympathetic nervous tissue; the pheochromocytoma, rarely malignant in young people, arises from chromaffin cells anywhere in the body. Abnormally high levels of catecholamines are found in the plasma and urine of affected individuals and serve as tumor markers.

Adrenal medullary insufficiency is not associated with any specific clinical disorder. Epinephrine deficiency has been described in some patients with hypo-glycemia, but it is likely that other factors were responsible since the adrenal medulla is not necessary for euglycemia.

The Catecholamines

The important catecholamines in man are dopamine, norepinephrine, and epinephrine (Fig. 7–1). *Dopamine* is a transmitter in the central nervous system and is the precursor for norepinephrine and epinephrine in the sympathetic nerves and the adrenal medulla. The quantity of dopamine in sympathoadrenal tissue is small, however. Homovanillic acid (HVA) is the principal metabolite of dopamine in the urine. *Norepinephrine* is a chemical neurotransmitter in brain and in sympathetic nerves, where

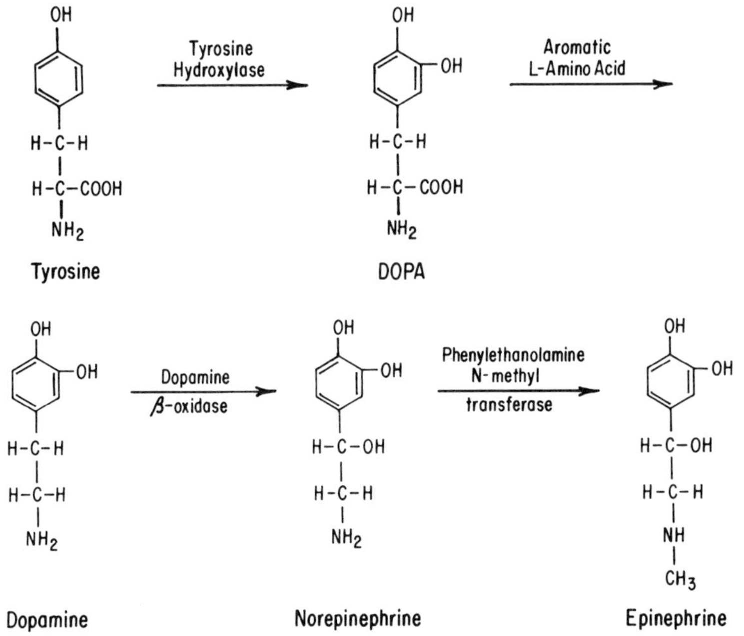

Tyrosine — Tyrosine Hydroxylase → DOPA — Aromatic L-Amino Acid →

Dopamine — Dopamine β-oxidase → Norepinephrine — Phenylethanolamine N-methyl transferase → Epinephrine

FIGURE 7–1. The principal pathway for the biosynthesis of catecholamines.

it is synthesized and stored in peripheral nerve endings and released in response to sympathetic nerve impulses in innervated tissues throughout the body. Some norepinephrine also is found in the adrenal medulla, but the primary medullary catecholamine is *epinephrine.* In fact, synthesis of epinephrine is essentially limited to the adrenal medulla (small amounts have been found in brain and sympathetic neurons), where activity of the epinephrine-forming enzyme phenylethanolamine-N-methyltransferase (PNMT) depends on glucocorticoids. Epinephrine is stored in chromaffin cells and in response to splanchnic nerve impulses is released into the circulation, where its effect is exerted in tissues far removed from the site of release.

The physiologic effects of the catecholamines are mediated by receptors on the surface of the target cell plasma membrane. The hormone-receptor interaction triggers the events that lead to the specific biologic action of each amine. There are two classes of adrenergic receptors, α and β, which have been subdivided into α_1 and α_2 and β_1 and β_2 subtypes. Activation of β_1 and β_2 stimulates the adenylate cyclase system while α_2 receptors inhibit it. α_1 Receptors are involved with increases in intracellular calcium ion and phosphoinositol hydrolysis. In general, activation of α receptors is excitatory and activation of β receptors is inhibitory except that stimulation of α receptors

relaxes gut muscle and stimulation of β receptors is excitatory in the myocardium. β_1 Receptor activity enhances myocardial contractility, heart rate, and atrioventricular conduction. β_2 Receptors are concerned with bronchodilation and vasodilation. Dopaminergic (DA) receptors in blood vessels also are divided into two classes; DA-1 receptors induce vasodilation primarily in renal, mesenteric, coronary, and cerebral arterial beds while DA-2 receptor activity causes inhibition of norepinephrine release from sympathetic nerve endings.

Norepinephrine is primarily an α receptor stimulator, whereas epinephrine induces both α and β receptor activity. Thus, norepinephrine causes constriction of blood vessels and rise in systolic and diastolic blood pressure. In addition to its cardiovascular effects, adrenergic receptor activity mediates many other responses that regulate basic metabolic processes, including glycogenolysis, lipolysis, inhibition of insulin release, and electrolyte transport.[1] A review is beyond the scope of this chapter. The α receptor is blocked selectively by phentolamine or phenoxybenzamine, and propranolol blocks the β receptor.

The activity of the sympathoadrenal system continuously changes to regulate metabolic function in many tissues and to maintain constancy of the internal environment. The physiologic effects of the catecholamines are rapidly dissipated, however. Circulating norepinephrine and epinephrine have a half-life in plasma of less than 1 min. Norepinephrine released from sympathetic nerve endings is inactivated primarily by reuptake into the sympathetic nerves. The remainder enters the general circulation where, with epinephrine, it is cleared principally by metabolism in the liver, gut, and kidney, with formation of metanephrines and 3-methoxy-4-hydroxymandelic acid (vanillylmandelic acid, or VMA), which are excreted in the urine (Fig. 7–2). Free norepinephrine and epinephrine also are actively secreted by the renal tubules and appear in the urine.

Assay of Sympathoadrenal Function

It is difficult to accurately assess physiologic and pathophysiologic function of the sympathetic nervous system in man. As noted, the greater part of norepinephrine released from sympathetic nerve endings is inactivated by reuptake into sympathetic nerve granules, and a portion of the remainder is metabolized to metanephrines and VMA. The rate of these changes can be variable, as is renal excretion of amines and metabolites. Thus, measurement of plasma and/or urinary norepinephrine does not necessarily reflect sympathetic activity. Adrenal medullary function can be estimated by determining plasma or urinary epinephrine levels, however. Despite the episodic nature of epinephrine release from chromaffin granules and the small amounts of this cate-cholamine that appear in plasma and urine, current analytical techniques permit epinephrine determination with reasonable accuracy.[2]

Regardless of these limitations, measurements of urinary catecholamines and metabolites can be used in the diagnosis and follow-up care of patients with neuroblastoma, ganglioneuroblastoma, and pheochromocytoma. The quantity of these compounds excreted in association with tumors of neural crest origin generally is abnormally high, and experience over the past three decades has demonstrated the validity of the analyses.

It is critically important that each clinical laboratory establish the normal range for excretion of urinary catecholamines and metabolites by healthy children of various ages for its particular assay procedure and publish a list of interfering compounds. Drugs and diet often hamper the analyses when nonspecific methods are used. Methyldopa (Aldomet), quinine, tetracyclines, intravenous vitamin preparations, medications containing catecholamine derivatives (nose drops and bronchodilators), and iodinated dyes are among the offending substances. Determination of free norepinephrine and epinephrine and use of chromatographic techniques for analysis of the metabolites are best. Collection of 24-hour urine specimens is most desirable, but this may be difficult in infants and young children. Standards have been developed, and values are expressed as micrograms of metabolite per

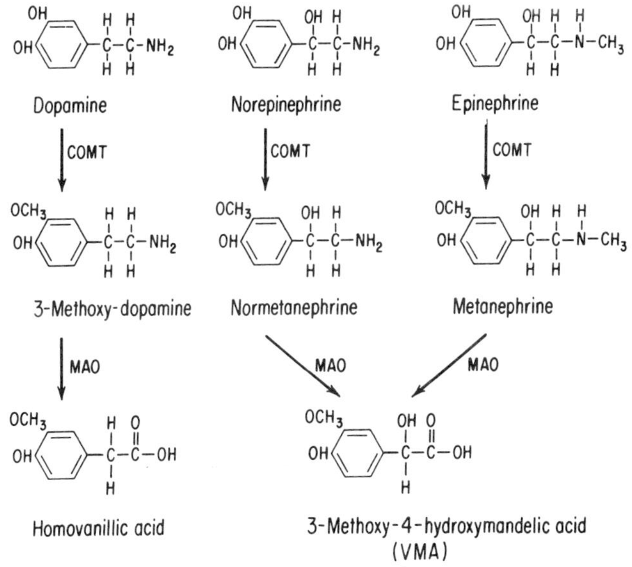

FIGURE 7–2. Schematic diagram illustrating formation of homovanillic acid, the metanephrines, and VMA from the catecholamines. COMT, catechol-*o*-methyl transferase; MAO, monoamine oxidase.

TABLE 7–1. URINARY EXCRETION OF CATECHOLAMINES AND VMA BY HEALTHY CHILDREN*·†

| | μg per 24 hours | | | | | | μg per sq M per 24 hours | | | | | |
| | NE | | E | | VMA | | NE | | E | | VMA | |
Age	Mean	SD	Mean	SD	Mean	SD	Mean	SD	Mean	SD	Mean	SD
birth to 1 year	10.6	3.4	1.3	1.2	569	309	41.1	15.3	4.7	3.3	2021	1121
1 through 5 years	18.8	7.0	3.2	2.7	1348	443	27.9	8.9	4.9	4.4	2001	571
6 through 15 years	37.4	16.6	4.8	2.4	2373	698	31.2	15.7	4.3	1.9	2133	378
over 15 years	50.7	15.7	7.1	3.3	3192	669	30.5	8.1	4.3	1.9	1931	389

* From Voorhess ML: Urinary catecholamine excretion by healthy children: Daily excretion of dopamine, norepinephrine, epinephrine, and 3-methoxy-4-hydroxymandelic acid. Pediatrics 39:252, 1967.

† NE, norepinephrine; E, epinephrine; VMA, vanillylmandelic acid (3-methoxy-4-hydroxymandelic acid).

milligram of creatinine excreted. Although creatinine excretion is not always constant during a 24-hour period, expression of the data in this manner is helpful,[3–5] (see Tables 7–1 and 7–2).

Measurements of plasma dopamine, norepinephrine, and epinephrine concentrations using a single isotope radioenzymatic assay or high-performance liquid chromatography are available in some laboratories. Collection of blood samples and preparation for analysis requires meticulous attention to detail. Interpretation of results may be difficult because stress, acute illness, drugs, and a host of other factors influence plasma catecholamine concentrations. After 12 hours of age, supine, resting concentrations of plasma catecholamines are similar among children and adults.[6]

NEUROBLASTOMA

General Characteristics

Neuroblastoma is a common malignant neoplasm of early life that arises from primitive neuroblasts derived from the neural crest. It may be found wherever sympathetic nervous tissue is located, but it most often arises in the adrenal medulla or from the autonomic ganglia in the chest or abdomen. Olfactory neuroblastomas (esthesioneuroblastomas),[7] primary cerebral neuroblastomas,[8] and peripheral nerve neuroblastomas,[9] although rare, do occur. Neuroblastoma of the newborn is a well-recognized entity.[10] Placental metastases have been identified in cases of congenital neuroblastoma, indicating intrauterine dissemination of malignant cells,[11] and the tumor can cause antenatal death.[12] Furthermore, mothers in late pregnancy whose fetuses had neuroblastoma have described signs and symptoms of catecholamine excess, suggesting that the amines entered the maternal circulation.[13] Peak incidence occurs before the age of 3 years, and the tumor is uncommon after childhood. Scattered cases have been recorded in adolescents and adults, however.[14–16]

Neuroblastoma occurs in both sexes, with a slight preponderance in males. A variety

TABLE 7–2. URINARY EXCRETION OF CATECHOLAMINE METABOLITES BY NORMAL CHILDREN*·†

| | μg per mg Creatinine | | | | | |
| | VMA | | HVA | | M + NM | |
Age	Mean	SD	Mean	SD	Mean	SD
1–12 months	6.9	3.2	12.9	9.58	1.64	1.32
1–2 years	4.7	2.22	12.6	6.26	1.68	1.13
2–5 years	3.95	1.72	7.58	3.56	1.25	0.77
5–10 years	3.3	1.40	4.7	2.66	1.13	0.78
10–15 years	1.91	0.77	2.5	2.42	0.60	0.48
15–18 years	1.4	0.61	1.0	0.65	0.24	0.23

* From Weetman RM, Rider PS, Oei TO, et al: Effect of diet on urinary excretion of VMA, HVA, metanephrine and total free catecholamine in normal preschool children. J Pediatr 88:46, 1976.

† VMA, vanillylmandelic acid (3-methoxy-4-hydroxymandelic acid); HVA, homovanillic acid; M, metanephrine; NM, normetanephrine.

of congenital malformations, such as heart disease, skeletal abnormalities, agangliosis, and pyloric stenosis, have been described in association with the tumor, but conclusive evidence of an association with specific defects has not been found.[17–19] Neuroblastoma usually is a sporadic disorder, but it may be familial.[20–23] The pattern of inheritance is not clear. Chromosome abnormalities, including double minute and abnormal banding patterns, have been described.[24] Triploid tumors and near-or pseudodiploid or hypotetraploid tumors have been reported, the former pattern almost always associated with stage I or II infant tumors and the latter with stage III or IV or relapsed tumors of children 1 year old or older.[25] Knudson and Meadows have suggested the formation of a neuroblastoma is a genetic disorder of normal development because of the relationships of neuroblastoma to neuroblastoma in situ and to ganglioneuroma.[26]

Beckwith and Perrin found microscopic, incidentally encountered, neuroblastomas in situ in the adrenal glands of infants less than 3 months of age at necropsy and estimated the incidence to be 40 times greater than the number of clinically diagnosed cases of neuroblastoma.[27] This suggests that for every 100 cases of overt neuroblastoma, 4000 "tumors" in newborn infants disappear without becoming clinically apparent. Spontaneous regression of the tumor has been noted many times in young infants with neuroblastoma in liver and bone marrow. Host defenses and cellular immunity appear to be important in this reaction.[28,29] Furthermore, neuroblastomas in vivo and in vitro are able to mature into ganglioneuroblastomas and into ganglioneuromas.[30,31] Neurofibromas and neurofibrosarcomas have been described with neuroblastoma.[32,33] The biologic bases for these phenomena are not completely understood. The hypothesis that mutant genes may be involved in these transformations is intriguing.[26,34]

The tumor metastasizes early to lymph nodes, liver, bone marrow, and skeleton, and widespread disease is present at the time of diagnosis in two thirds of cases.[35] Sometimes, retro-orbital, skin, or skeletal metastases suggest neuroblastoma before a primary site is evident. Subcutaneous metastatic nodules, which blanch on palpation, are common in neonates with neuroblastoma.[36] Rarely, the original tumor never is identified. There is an age-dependent cure

rate: most infants less than 1 year of age at the time of diagnosis of neuroblastoma survive, whereas children over 2 years of age at diagnosis almost always succumb to disseminated disease.

Symptoms and Signs

Neuroblastoma originating in the adrenal gland or in the spinal ganglia can reach a large size and metastasize before it encroaches on vital structures or otherwise causes clinical evidence of disease. Therefore, the first suspicion of the tumor frequently occurs when an abdominal mass is felt on routine physical examination or when a metastatic lesion heralds the presence of disease (Fig. 7–3). The clinical picture varies tremendously, and the presenting symptoms and signs may be unusual. Unilateral or bilateral periorbital swelling with ecchymosis and proptosis occur with orbital metastases. Acute cerebellar encephalopathy characterized by severe ataxia and opsoclonus has been reported several times. Although extremely rare, blindness can be the presenting symptom. Paresis of the extremities develops when neuroblastoma arises from dorsal root ganglia or when it extends intraspinally to compress the

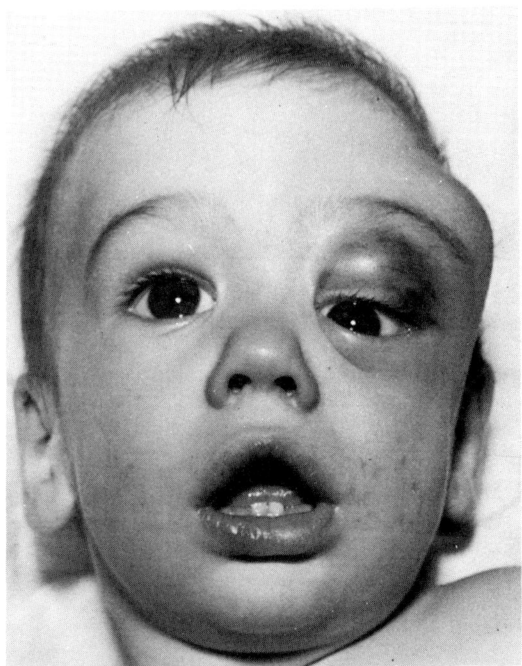

FIGURE 7–3. Five-month-old infant with unilateral proptosis, ecchymosis, and periorbital swelling due to metastases from a neuroblastoma of the right adrenal.

cord. Bone pain and a limp from osseous involvement may mimic arthritis. Hypertension, polydipsia, polyuria, flushing, and excessive perspiration occasionally are present when catecholamine production is abnormally high, although the incidence is remarkably low compared to that of children with pheochromocytoma. Interestingly, however, in one study of 59 children with neurogenic tumors (no pheochromocytoma), 19 per cent had hypertension and there was no correlation of hypertension with urinary catecholamine levels.[37] Chronic watery diarrhea and the hypokalemia syndrome can develop if the tumor cells secrete vasoactive intestinal peptide (see page 244). In advanced disease, irritability, anorexia, weight loss, fever, anemia, and other general symptoms and signs of extensive malignant disease are seen. Such diverse disorders as intravascular coagulation, Cushing syndrome, hypercalcemia, hypoglycemia, and fetal hydantoin-alcohol syndromes have been reported in association with neuroblastoma.[38–46]

Diagnosis

Imaging Studies

Most neuroblastomas arise from the adrenal gland or from the paravertebral sympathetic ganglia, so imaging studies of the abdomen generally will delineate the tumor (Fig. 7–4). Combined computed tomography (CT) and ultrasound provide better anatomic evaluation of the mass than plain films and intravenous urograms, and obviate the need for angiography in most cases.[47]

Recent experiences with magnetic resonance imaging (MRI) indicate it usually gives more information than CT. The selection of procedures should be individualized for each patient. Chest examination always should be done in a search for posterior mediastinal disease.

Bone marrow examination, including aspiration and biopsy, should always be done as part of the staging workup. Routine radiographs and radionuclide skeletal survey will help identify the extent of metastases. Liver and brain scans are additional adjuncts in defining dissemination of neuroblastoma. Angiography of the inferior vena cava and aorta as well as pedal lymphangiography may be required in selected cases. Since the extent of disease is important in staging the tumor, in selecting the treatment protocol, and in prognosis, detailed roentgenographic and isotopic studies are necessary in each case.

Whenever there is paresis of the extremities, loss of bladder control, or other neurologic symptoms of spinal cord compression imaging of the spine should be performed promptly. Magnetic resonance imaging is particularly useful in evaluating intervertebral extension. Emergency decompression may be required.

Biochemical Studies

A useful aid to preoperative diagnosis of neuroblastoma is measurement of catecholamines, their metabolites, or both. Numerous articles have been written in the past 25 years about this subject, and a variety of compounds have been found to be ab-

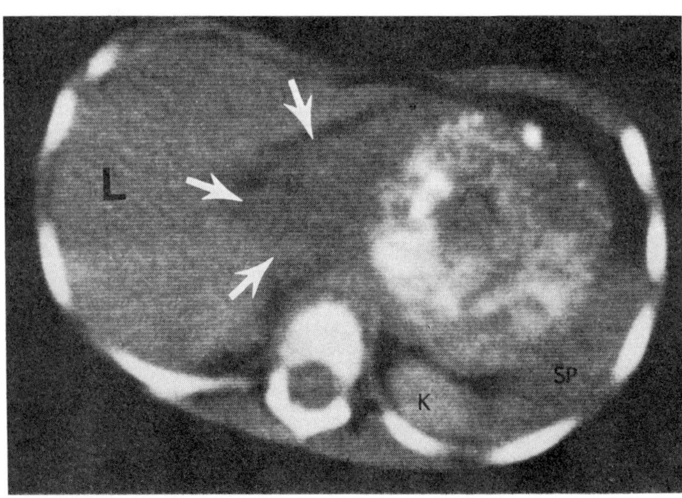

FIGURE 7–4. An abdominal CT scan delineating a calcified neuroblastoma as well as a noncalcified portion of tumor crossing the mdilein (arrows). Its relationship to the kidney (K), spleen (SP), and liver (L) is clearly visible. (From Berger PE, Kuhn G, Munschauer R: Computed tomography and ultrasound in the diagnosis and management of neuroblastoma. Radiology 128:663, 1978.)

normally high in the plasma or urine of patients with neuroblastoma. Discussion here will be limited to those substances that can be measured readily in general clinical chemistry laboratories or in reference laboratories.[48–51]

It has been well established that approximately 95 per cent of children with neuroblastomas excrete abnormally large amounts of dopamine, norepinephrine, and/or amine metabolites in their urine. After excision of tumor, the levels return to normal within a few days. Epinephrine output usually is not high because the tumor is unable to synthesize this amine. In patients treated by radiation therapy or chemotherapy, there is gradual reduction in catecholamine output over several weeks. If catecholamine or metabolite levels remain abnormally high or return from normal to abnormal levels, residual or recurrent tumor is present.[52] Both primary tumors and metastases are capable of producing catecholamines.

There is a spectrum of urinary excretion of catecholamines and metabolites by patients with neuroblastomas despite a similar histologic appearance among the tumors. Most children (75 to 80 per cent) excrete abnormally large amounts of dopamine, HVA, norepinephrine, and VMA. About 15 per cent have high dopamine, HVA, and norepinephrine output but *normal* VMA excretion. Thus, measurement of only VMA is not an appropriate diagnostic test for neuroblastoma because a value within the normal range does not rule out the presence of tumor. In rare cases, no abnormality in the urinary output of catecholamines or metabolites is detected, particularly when neuroblastoma arises from dorsal root or dorsal root ganglia.[53]

The highest probability of biochemically identifying a neuroblastoma occurs when both HVA and VMA levels are measured in the urine.[54] An abnormally large amount of either or both compound(s) is found in about 95 per cent of patients. Urinary metanephrine excretion is elevated in approximately 75 per cent of individuals. Dopamine and norepinephrine excretion levels are high in the urine of nearly all patients with neuroblastoma, but most routine clinical laboratories are not equipped technically to measure these compounds. When clinical suspicion of neuroblastoma is high but measurement of HVA and VMA is not diagnostic, determination of dopamine, norepinephrine, and other metabolites is indicated. When "free" urinary HVA is borderline, the measurement of total content of urinary HVA may be helpful.[55]

Caution is urged in the use of screening tests for neuroblastoma because a high number of false-positive and false-negative results have been reported.[56,57] Regardless, Japanese workers have been performing mass screening at age 6 months by measuring VMA on a spot urine; HVA was recently added to the test.[58,59] It is too early to determine the affect of this screening on overall survival.

In addition to the catecholamines, serum ferritin,[60] nervous system–specific enolase,[61,62] and a tumor-associated ganglioside appear to be useful tumor markers and beneficial in evaluating the success of therapy.[63] Metaiodobenzylguanidine (MIBG) scintigraphy and ^{31}P MRI spectroscopy also have potential in following growth of neuroblastoma.[64–66]

Histologic Studies

Definitive diagnosis depends on histologic identification of neuroblasts in primary tumor or metastases. In light microscopic sections, the cells resemble lymphocytes and may be confused with other neoplasms composed of small round cells, whereas the ultrastructure of neuroblastoma cells viewed by electron microscopy is distinctive and may complement routine cytologic studies.[67]

Differential Diagnosis

Intra-abdominal neoplasms, such as Wilms tumor, lymphomas, and sarcomas, as well as Ewing sarcoma, acute leukemia, and other disorders that involve bone, may mimic neuroblastoma. With rare exceptions, these disorders are not associated with abnormalities of the catecholamines, however. Pheochromocytomas synthesize catecholamines, but the plasma and urine levels of norepinephrine and epinephrine generally are much greater in patients with pheochromocytoma than those recorded in association with neuroblastoma. In addition, the clinical picture of the two disorders is quite different. (Table 7–3). Increased HVA and VMA have been reported in infants with failure to thrive, with neurodegenerative disorders and hypertension, and with severe heart failure,[65–70] but these conditions are

TABLE 7–3. A COMPARISION OF CLINICAL AND BIOCHEMICAL FINDINGS IN MOST PATIENTS WITH NEUROBLASTOMA OR PHEOCHROMOCYTOMA

Characteristic	Neuroblastoma	Pheochromocytoma
Age	Infancy and childhood	Any age
Hypertension	Uncommon	Nearly 100 per cent
Metastases	Common	Uncommon
Dopamine and HVA*	+ + + +	N to + +
Norepinephrine*	+ to + +	+ + + to + + + +
Epinephrine*	N	N to + + +
Metanephrine*	N to + + + +	+ + + +
VMA*	N to + + + +	+ + + +

* N = normal; + + + + = markedly elevated.

not likely to be confused with neuroblastoma.

Staging and Treatment

Surgery, radiation therapy, and chemotherapy are used in various combinations to treat patients with neuroblastoma. Accurate staging of the disease is important in planning the approach to therapy and in estimating the prognosis. Staging generally is based on the extent of disease, pattern of metastases, and surgical resectability. The system of Evans et al.[71] probably the most widely used, is as follows:

Stage I: tumor confined to the organ or structure of origin.
Stage II: regional spread that does not cross the midline.
Stage III: tumors extending in continuity beyond the midline.
Stage IV: remote disease involving the skeleton, brain, lung, distant lymph nodes, and so on.
Stage IVS: patients who would otherwise be stage I or II but who have remote disease confined to liver, spleen, or bone marrow without radiologic evidence of bone metastases.

Other staging systems have been recommended by Hayes, et al.[72] and other oncologists.[73]

Generally patients with localized disease should have the primary tumor removed as completely as possible, but radical extirpation, which places the patient at high risk, usually is not appropriate. Irradiation and chemotherapy can be used subsequently to shrink tumor size, perhaps permitting com-

plete excision at a later time.[74] When the patient has obvious distant metastases at diagnosis, it is unlikely that removal of the primary tumor will improve the course of disease. Chemotherapy is the primary treatment in this case. Multidrug therapy generally is of considerable symptomatic benefit to children with neuroblastoma and is more effective than single-agent treatment. Vincristine, cyclophosphamide, cisplatinum, doxorubicin (Adriamycin), and their analogs are being used in various combinations for their antitumor effect. Bone marrow transplantation currently is being evaluated for patients with poor prognosis and advanced disease if they can be placed into remission.[75] Metaiodobenzylguanidine also is being used therapeutically.

Infants at stage IVS of neuroblastoma who have small primary tumors and metastases only to liver or skin generally do well and have a good chance of experiencing regression of the tumor, either spontaneously or with minimal therapy. Treatment should be individualized, depending on the extent of disease. The primary tumor probably should be excised to avoid the rare complication of late recurrence at the site of the primary even when the remainder of disease has regressed. Massive hepatomegaly can be treated with small doses of irradiation or chemotherapy. Aggressive treatment should be avoided.[16]

Appropriate and timely treatment of neuroblastoma requires a team approach among the surgeon, radiation therapist, hematologist-oncologist, pathologist, and nursing care specialists at an oncology center. Detailed review of therapeutic measures is beyond the scope of this chapter. The reader is referred to the pediatric oncology literature for the latest advances in neuroblastoma treatment.

Prognosis and Follow-Up

Survival of neuroblastoma is age related. Generally the younger the patient at the time of diagnosis the better the prognosis, except patients less than 4 weeks of age with stage IVS disease do less well than older infants with comparable disease. Children with metastases to bone cortex usually have a dismal prognosis at any age. Despite vigorous attempts, the various therapeutic modalities that have been employed during the past 25 years have not changed the cure rate for neuroblastoma. Recent studies indicate that biologic characteristics may be as important as age and pattern of disease in predicting prognosis. Patients with actively growing neuroblastoma have increased levels of ferritin, a major iron-storage tissue protein, that return to normal when clinical remission is achieved.[60] Most children with stage IV neuroblastoma have elevated levels of ferritin, whereas those with stage IVS disease do not. E-rosette inhibitory factor (a substance that inhibits autologous lymphocyte formation of rosettes with sheep erythrocytes) has been detected in the serum of stage IV neuroblastoma patients but is absent in serum of stage IVS patients. Thus, stages IV and IVS neuroblastoma can be differentiated by serum ferritin determinations and lymphocyte E-rosette inhibition.[77] Serum levels of neuron-specific enolase above 100 ng/ml have been found more often in association with extensive metastases than in patients with stages I and II neuroblastoma.[62] There is a positive correlation between amplification of the N-myc oncogene and early tumor progression of neuroblastoma subsequent to diagnosis and absence of amplication in stage IVS tumors.[78]

Patients with stage IV disease may have a better prognosis when their VMA:HVA ratio is high, suggesting that tumors that are unable to make large amounts of norepinephrine are more malignant.[79] Additionally, a relatively lower HVA excretion has been reported in association with a more benign course in children less than 2 years of age.[80] These biologic observations together with the histopathologic prognostic factors in neuroblastic tumors described by Shimada et al.,[81] provide much-needed new information about the perplexing behavior of neuroblastomas. Indeed, Evans and colleagues have used these factors to predict outcome among a group of 124 children with disease.[82] Their analysis suggests that combinations of age, tumor stage, serum ferritin level, and histologic type may be able to define a favorable and an unfavorable group. Using serum ferritin level, age, and tumor stage, they found a 93 per cent 2-year survival in patients younger than 2 years of age with normal ferritin level; a 58 per cent 2-year survival in patients 2 years or older with normal ferritin level; and a 19 per cent 2-year survival in patients with an abnormal ferritin level. Survival was 100 per cent among 30 patients less than 2 years of age with normal ferritin level and stages I, II,

and IVS disease and 79 per cent among 18 children less than 2 years of age with normal ferritin level and stages III and IV disease. Obviously, this information will be very important in making decisions about the most beneficial treatment modalities for long-term survival.

Long-term, follow-up of the patients is required. Some will have a recurrence after 8 to 10 disease-free years. Late complications following radiation therapy, such as nephritis, abnormalities of bone growth, and bone tumor, may occur.[83] I have seen two patients with a thyroid adenoma, presumably caused by scatter from irradiation of a cervicothoracic neuroblastoma many years previous to the adenoma. Disturbances in gonadal function may result from radiation, chemotherapy, or both.[84]

Serial measurements of catecholamines and metabolites are very helpful in following the response to therapy. The values are normal following successful removal or destruction of all functioning tumor tissue, whereas the presence of residual or recurrent disease is indicated by abnormally high levels of the various compounds.

High levels of serum lactic dehydrogenase (LDH) have been found in most patients with neuroblastoma, and serial measurements are useful in following disease activity. Reduction of levels to normal is associated with survival, whereas an increase in values indicates recurrence of the tumor.[85] It appears that regular monitoring of the levels of serum ferritin, neuron-specific enolase, and LDH as well as urinary catecholamines and metabolites should provide useful markers of neuroblastoma activity.

GANGLIONEUROBLASTOMA

Neuroblastomas are able to mature and differentiate into ganglioneuroblastomas, which are tumors composed of clusters or sheets of neuroblasts together with mature neurons or ganglion cells. The number of each cell type varies considerably. The critical factors that promote this phenomenon are not well understood. Sometimes it happens spontaneously, and other times the process follows intensive chemotherapy. It occurs predominantly in extra-adrenal sites and in a higher proportion of girls than boys. Generally, the ganglioneuroblastoma is a much less aggressive neoplasm than the neuroblastoma and is associated with higher survival and cure rates.[81] Ganglioneuro-blastoma cannot be distinguished from neuroblastoma by biochemical analyses; patients with both tumors have abnormally high levels of catecholamines and/or their metabolites. The principles of treatment and follow-up care are similar to those for neuroblastoma.

GANGLIONEUROMA

The ganglioneuroma is a benign tumor composed of adult ganglion cells. Most originate in the chain of sympathetic ganglia, which extends from the base of the skull to the pelvis, including the adrenal medulla. Some have been reported in the gastrointestinal tract, peripheral joints, central nervous system, and other locations.[86] The ganglioneuroma most likely represents a neuroblastoma that has progressed through the ganglioneuroblastoma stage and become a fully mature and differentiated tumor. Serial section of the tissue is required to be certain nests of neuroblasts are not present.

Generally, the tumor grows slowly and causes few symptoms until it is large and encroaches on vital structures. (A tumor of any size may be associated with chronic diarrhea, however; see next section.) Ganglioneuromas frequently are found in the posterior mediastinum, or they may be located in the paravertebral gutters. I have not found abnormally high catecholamine levels associated with a pure ganglioneuroma except when it has been accompanied by the syndrome of chronic diarrhea.

Treatment consists of surgical excision. Irradiation and chemotherapy are not used.

Neural Tumors and Chronic Diarrhea

A small number of patients with ganglioneuroblastoma or ganglioneuroma have a syndrome of failure to thrive, intractable watery diarrhea, and hypokalemia. Flushing, abdominal distention, and metabolic acidosis also may be present. The diarrhea persists despite all types of dietary manipulation, including elimination of oral feedings. Water and electrolyte losses through the intestinal tract are excessive, and large amounts of parenteral fluids with potassium are required to correct dehydration and hypokalemia. When the tumor is excised, the diarrhea ceases abruptly and the patient dramatically improves.

The secretory diarrhea in these cases is due to production of vasoactive intestinal peptide (VIP) by the tumor and is similar to the water diarrhea syndrome associated with pancreatic tumors and other neoplasms in the adult. Most of the ganglioneuroblastomas and ganglioneuromas also secrete large amounts of catecholamines. Since VIP is a potent vasodilator and norepinephrine causes vasoconstriction, it is possible for the child to be normotensive or have hypertension, depending on the relative amounts of hormone production and release.[87,88]

Measurements of plasma VIP and catecholamine levels should be performed in children with severe, intractable watery diarrhea. If abnormally high levels of either or both hormones are found, a search should be made for a tumor of neural crest origin. Prostaglandins also can be abnormally high in some patients.[89]

Treatment consists of surgical excision of the tumor. Sometimes, even partial removal of the neoplasm will result in reduction of VIP levels and termination of diarrhea. When a nonresectable ganglioneuroblastoma is encountered, treatment with α-methyltyrosine might be helpful in controlling the diarrhea by causing a decrease in VIP.[87] The drug also is effective in reducing hypertension from catecholamine excess.

PHEOCHROMOCYTOMAS

General Characteristics

The pheochromocytoma is a rare tumor of childhood and can arise from chromaffin tissue anywhere in the body. Most commonly it is located in the adrenal medulla, especially on the right side. The majority of the rest occur along the abdominal sympathetic chain, particularly in the organ of Zuckerkandl and the renal hilus. However, cervical tumors, intrathoracic pheochromocytomas, and lesions of the bladder wall can be found. Bilateral adrenal and multiple neoplasms are frequent in children. Malignant tumors are rare. Boys are affected more often than girls, whereas in adults there usually is a female predominance. Symptoms of a pheochromocytoma have been described as early as 1 month of age, but the incidence in pediatric patients generally peaks at 9 to 12 years. Familial pheochromocytomas have been reported many times either as a single disorder or as part of the multiple endocrine adenomatosis syndromes[90–96] (see later in this chapter).

Symptoms and Signs

Most clinical manifestations are caused by the physiologic and pharmacologic effects of norepinephrine and epinephrine, which are synthesized and released by the pheochromocytoma into the circulation. The production and turnover of catecholamines vary from patient to patient, but sustained rather than paroxysmal hypertension is present in most children. The systolic blood pressure may reach levels of 250 mm Hg, with corresponding increases in diastolic pressure. Orthostatic hypotension is found in some older children and adolescents and is probably related to an inability to activate sympathetic reflexes.[97] Headache, sweating, nausea and vomiting, visual disturbances, and weight loss are the most common symptoms. The child often has an anxious expression, appears pale and weak, and is emotionally labile. Tremor and tachycardia can be present. Intermittent episodes of abdominal pain and distention occur, and chronic constipation is sometimes troublesome. Polydipsia, polyuria, and enuresis may simulate diabetes insipidus.[98] Rarely, an extra-adrenal pheochromocytoma causes ureteric obstruction. A peculiar reddish-blue discoloration, with edema of the tip of the nose and the fingers (acrocyanosis), and cool extremities develop when there is pronounced peripheral constriction of blood vessels.

Encephalopathy, with convulsions and retinopathy as well as cardiomegaly and cardiac failure, may be associated with severe, long-standing hypertension. In addition, cardiomyopathy and active myocarditis can be produced by catecholamine excess.[99–101] Abnormalities of glucose metabolism, with hyperglycemia and glucosuria as well as elevations of free fatty acids, often accompany catecholamine overproduction.[102]

Numerous other clinical findings have been observed in children with the tumor. Pheochromocytomas may masquerade as essential hypertension, renal disease, thyrotoxicosis, an emotional disorder, a gastrointestinal malady, and so on. Definitive diagnosis may be delayed for long periods, particularly in children and adolescents, in whom the index of suspicion is low. When-

ever recurrent or chronic hypertension is documented, pheochromocytoma should be considered in the diagnosis. Physicians caring for pregnant teenagers should be mindful that pheochromocytoma is a rare complication of pregnancy and associated with high maternal and fetal mortality.[103,104] It also may occur in association with neurofibromatosis, cerebellar hemangioblastoma, Cushing syndrome, multiple endocrine adenomatosis, intracerebral aneurysms, polycythemia, astrocytoma, sarcoidosis, and other disorders arising from cells of the diffuse endocrine system. Rarely the pheochromocytoma is an incidental finding at postmortem examination.[105–116]

Diagnosis

The most specific aid to diagnosis is finding abnormally high levels of catecholamines and normetanephrine-metanephrine or VMA in the urine. Generally the diagnosis can be confirmed or excluded by analysis of a 24-hour urine sample, for it is rare, indeed, to find normal levels of both norepinephrine, epinephrine, and metabolites in the presence of a hormone-producing pheochromocytoma.[117] The predominant catecholamine excreted by children is often norepinephrine, in contrast to adults in whom both norepinephrine and epinephrine output may be high. Urinary excretion of dopamine and HVA has been reported to be helpful in discriminating benign from malignant pheochromocytomas, but both compounds may be abnormally elevated with either lesion.[50,118]

In the rare circumstance in which the child has paroxysmal episodes suggesting intermittent release of catecholamines, carefully timed urine collections during and after an attack will identify whether the episode is associated with excess catecholamine production and release. Norepinephrine and epinephrine should be measured in these situations because they more accurately reflect dynamic changes in urinary catecholamine output than does determination of metanephrine or VMA excretion.

Measurement of urinary VMA or normetanephrine-metanephrine is a satisfactory screening test for the presence of a pheochromocytoma. Nearly all patients with the tumor will have an abnormally high urinary output of these metabolites.[119] It is recommended, however, that norepinephrine and epinephrine levels also be determined when metabolites are abnormally high, to confirm the presumptive diagnosis of a pheochromocytoma and to provide precise information about norepinephrine and epinephrine production. High epinephrine levels suggest that the tumor is intra-adrenal or in the organ of Zuckerkandl rather than elsewhere, although exceptions have been reported.[120] Furthermore, epinephrine has potent β-adrenergic effects, which may lead to tachyarrhythmias and hypermetabolic syndromes, so it is helpful to know if excessive amounts of this hormone are being released. When the index of suspicion for a pheochromocytoma is high and the levels of VMA or metanephrine are normal, catecholamine output always should be checked. Rarely, metabolite excretion will be normal when the parent amines are abnormally elevated.

The daily urinary excretion of catecholamines and metabolites is much less for healthy infants and children than for adults, so it is important to check all results against appropriate control data (Tables 7–1 and 7–2). In addition, the analytic methodology influences the "normal values." The physician must be certain that the clinical laboratory is using specific analytical techniques to avoid falsely elevated values.

Most patients with pheochromocytoma also have markedly elevated plasma norepinephrine and epinephrine levels. Although there is not an extensive literature about plasma catecholamine concentrations in children with pheochromocytoma, it is probable that they are similar to adults. It is important to emphasize the following points[121–124]:

1. Patients with pheochromocytomas may have normal plasma concentrations during asymptomatic, normotensive intervals.

2. There may be overlap of catecholamine levels between patients with pheochromocytoma and those without a tumor (i.e., essential hypertension).

3. Many medications interfere with plasma norepinephrine and epinephrine analysis measured by techniques used in most laboratories.

4. There is considerable variation in "normal" plasma catecholamine concentrations depending on blood glucose and serum sodium levels, emotional stress, position (supine or upright) and so forth.

Physicians who order plasma studies should be thoroughly familiar with the assay to avoid misinterpretation of test results. Measurement of catecholamines and metabolites in a 24-hour urine sample reflects output over a prolonged period of time, whereas plasma catecholamine concentrations can change from minute to minute because of the short half-life of the amines. There is general agreement that a single plasma catecholamine value should not be used as the sole diagnostic test. Confirmation of the plasma finding by repeat analysis and/or measurement of urinary catecholamines should be carried out. Duncan and colleagues[125] compared the value of plasma samples with 24-hour urine samples in identifying patients with pheochromocytoma and found that measurement of free norepinephrine in 24-hour urine samples provided the best index of pheochromocytoma.

Use of pharmacologic tests (histamine, phentolamine, tyrosine, or glucagon) to diagnose pheochromocytoma is primarily of historic interest. The tests lack a high degree of specificity and may provoke both false-positive and false-negative responses. More recently, the central-acting α_2-adrenergic agonist clonidine has been tried as a diagnostic aid because the drug suppresses the neurologically mediated plasma catecholamines released into the circulation whereas catecholamines from a pheochromocytoma are not suppressed. The clonidine test also is problematic. Hypotension is a potential risk in both types of patients, and false-negative and false-positive results have been reported.[121,126]

Hyperreninemia and secondary hyperaldosteronism, hypercalcemia and hypercalcuria, ectopic ACTH syndrome, polycythemia, and abnormalities in carbohydrate and fat metabolism may be found in association with pheochromocytomas. The tumor also can produce VIP, adrenorphin, serotonin, enolase enzymes, and growth hormone–releasing factor. Lactic acidosis has been described in patients with pheochromocytoma probably secondary to the effect of catecholamines on intermediary metabolism and the peripheral circulation.[127–144]

Localization of Tumors

Investigations should be directed toward localization of tumor(s) after documentation of abnormally high levels of catecholamines and metabolites in body fluids of patients with the clinical picture of pheochromocytoma has confirmed the diagnosis.

Computed tomography is the primary aid in localization of primary or recurrent pheochromocytomas. It will detect tumors larger than 1.0 cm with remarkable accuracy.[145] Metaiodobenzylguanidine scintigraphy also is helpful in imaging the adrenal medulla and pheochromocytomas since the uptake and storage of the compound simulates norepinephrine. It is the examination of choice for recurrent or metastatic disease because it permits whole-body imaging. Metaiodobenzyylguanidine may be labeled either with iodine-123 or iodine-131. Percentage uptake of M[^{123}-I]GB has been shown to correlate better with the catecholamine storage granules in pheochromocytoma than measurement of urine or plasma catecholamine levels. There is a false-negative rate of about 13 per cent with MIBG scintigraphy, primarily due to limited tracer uptake by tumor cells. False-positive scans may occur, especially when normal adrenal medullary uptake is misinterpreted as tumor.[64,146,147] Magnetic resonance imaging also is being used in localization of pheochromocytoma. A report by Quint et al. indicated that MRI and scintigraphy are probably superior to CT in demonstration of primary extra-adrenal tumors and MRI, CT, and M[^{131}I]BG scintigraphy are nearly equal in identifying primary adrenal pheochromocytomas.[148]

Use of the three techniques described above has largely eliminated the need for invasive procedures such as arteriography and venous sampling. Determination of plasma catecholamine concentrations at different levels of the inferior or superior vena cava or other veins may be helpful when the tumor cannot be located by other means or when multiple lesions are suspected. Venography usually is a safe procedure. The laboratory data must be interpreted with great care, since blood flow patterns and intermittent secretion of hormones by the tumor(s) or by the normal adrenal medullae influence plasma levels of norepinephrine and epinephrine and may lead to falsely high or normal values.[149,150] The contrast material that is used in arteriography can stimulate the release of catecholamines from a pheochromocytoma, so it is essential that this procedure only be performed by experienced physicians.[151,152] As mentioned previously, it is an excellent general

rule to achieve α blockade of the patient before angiography is carried out.

Treatment

The treatment of choice is surgical excision of the tumor(s). This should be done as soon as the patient has been adequately prepared for surgery, using α blockade alone or in combination with β blockade. Adequate preoperative treatment makes resection as safe a procedure as removal of other tumors in the abdomen or chest. When excision is not possible, pharmacologic agents can be used to inhibit catecholamine synthesis and to establish adrenergic blockade.

Preoperative Treatment

Generally, 2 weeks of preoperative therapy is required, depending on the general well-being of the patient as well as on the severity of the hypertension and the other effects of high levels of circulating catecholamines. The objective of therapy is to prevent the physiologic and metabolic consequences of the excess norepinephrine and/or epinephrine released by the tumor and to minimize the potentially serious intraoperative complications that can occur in the absence of adrenergic blockade.

α-Adrenergic blocking agents should be administered to control hypertension. The amount of drug required to achieved adequate blockade varies from patient to patient and is determined by progressively increasing the daily dose until the desired response is obtained. Titration is best performed in the hospital. Phenoxybenzamine hydrochloride (Dibenzyline) is a long-acting oral preparation that usually is well tolerated and provides a satisfactory control of the pressor effects of the catecholamines. Phenoxybenzamine, 5 mg every 12 hours orally, is an adequate starting dose for a young child; an older child may require 10 mg every 12 hours. The dose of phenoxybenzamine also may be calculated by weight (i.e., 0.25 to 1.0 mg/kg/day divided every 12 hours). The daily dose can be increased every 3 to 4 days, if necessary, but not to a level so high that significant side effects of blockade develop. These include nasal congestion, gastrointestinal irritation, and hypotension.

Phentolamine (Regitine) is also an α-adrenergic blocking agent. It is a short-acting drug and is particularly effective for intravenous use when acute control of blood pressure is necessary during hypertensive crises, diagnostic radiologic evaluations, or surgery. Phentolamine, 1 mg/dose intravenously or intramuscularly, is appropriate acute therapy for a child. The drug also can be titrated intravenously to provide short-term control of hypertension. Phentolamine also is effective orally, but its duration of action is short, compared to phenoxybenzamine, so it must be given every 4 to 6 hours. A therapeutic effect usually is obtained with phentolamine 5 mg/kg/day orally, in divided doses, every 4 to 6 hours. This preparation often causes nasal stuffiness, gastrointestinal disturbances, and weakness in children. Phenoxybenzamine is superior for long-term oral therapy. Prazosin (Minipress) has been used in the preoperative preparation of adults with pheochromocytoma, but information about its safety in children is lacking.

Patients whose tumors produce large amounts of epinephrine and/or who have serious tachyarrhythmias often require treatment with β-adrenergic blocking drugs. Generally, β blocking drugs should not be administered until adequate α blockade has been achieved, to protect the heart from unopposed α stimulation. Extreme care must be exercised in the use of β blocking drugs when myocardiopathy is present, because the negative inotropic effects of the drug may result in congestive heart failure. Propranolol is an effective drug for treatment of children with pheochromocytomas. It can be administered intravenously for acute control of a serious arrhythmia or can be given orally for chronic control. Propranolol, 1 mg given intravenously over 1 min, with electrocardiographic monitoring, may be used in an emergency. Propranolol, 5 to 10 mg given every 6 to 8 hours orally, generally results in a good response. The dose may be carefully titrated upward as necessary to achieve the desired effect.[153,154]

When adrenergic blockade does not control the effects of the excessive circulating norepinephrine and epinephrine, treatment with α-methyltyrosine (Demser, Merck) may be tried. This compound blocks the conversion of tyrosine to dopa in the biosynthesis of catecholamines by inhibiting tyrosine hydroxylase activity and thus reduces the production of dopamine, norepinephrine, and epinephrine. An initial starting dose of α-methyltyrosine, 5 to 10 mg/kg/day orally, in divided doses, every 6 hours, is appropriate for a child. The daily dose can be titrated upward as necessary to control the symptoms. Sedation usually is the only side effect of therapy unless high doses are prescribed.[155,156]

Some patients with pheochromocytoma have a reduced blood volume, apparently related to chronic constriction of the vascular bed and to a decreased red cell mass.[157] Phenoxybenzamine therapy preoperatively helps to correct this problem by reducing adrenergic activity and permitting expansion of the intravascular space. Failure to recognize the potential for hypovolemic shock following excision of a pheochromocytoma can create an emergency in the operating room. Volume-expanding fluids should be administered rapidly during surgery when postresection hypotension occurs.

Intraoperative Treatment

Opinions vary as to whether therapy with short-acting α-adrenergic blockers, such as phentolamine, should be substituted for long-acting phenoxybenzamine for 1 to 2 days prior to surgery. Regardless, it is imperative that the anesthesiologist and the surgeon understand the pathophysiology of the catecholamines and that there be careful monitoring of blood pressure and cardiac function from the beginning of induction of anesthesia to the end of the surgical procedure. Intravenous phentolamine can be titrated as necessary and is an effective drug for maintaining a stable and normal blood pressure. Sodium nitroprusside, a peripherally acting hypotensive agent with a short duration of action, has been found to be effective for intraoperative management of hypertensive episodes in patients with pheochromocytomas and may be used safely with adrenoreceptor blocking agents.[158] Intravenous propranolol in doses up to 1 mg generally is effective in controlling tachydysrhythmias. As noted above, if preoperative care has corrected blood volume depletion and if fluid therapy is adequate during surgery, hypotension should not occur after excision of the tumor. Intravenous infusion of norepinephrine seldom is required. Hydrocortisone for parenteral use should be available so that it can be administered if bilateral adrenalectomy is required for removal of bilateral adrenomedullary tumors. Bilateral tumors and concurrent intra- and extra-adrenal tumors are features of pheochromocytomas in childhood.

Postoperative Care

Hypertension may be present for 24 to 36 hours after excision of a pheochromocytoma because of transient hypervolemia associated with parenteral fluid therapy or because the sympathetic nerve endings contain abundant stored catecholamines. Continuing elevation suggests residual tumor or renovascular disease. If the hypertension is corrected by an intravenous infusion of phentolamine, it is likely another tumor is present. All patients, regardless of their blood pressure, should have plasma and/or urinary catecholamine levels checked prior to discharge to be certain the values are normal.

Hypoglycemia has been reported after excision of pheochromocytoma; it is probably due to hyperresponsive β cells and increased insulin production.[159] This transient finding is corrected by intravenous dextrose therapy.

Continued follow-up medical care is important because the tumor may recur years later. Likewise, the patient and family members should be observed for multiple endocrine adenomatosis.[160]

Malignant Pheochromocytoma

Malignant pheochromocytoma is very rare in childhood. Generally the diagnosis is difficult because benign tumors can be extra-adrenal and multicentric in origin and because histologic criteria alone are inadequate to establish malignancy. Pleomorphic cells, blood vessel involvement, and capsular invasion occur in benign tumors. There are no biochemical features that distinguish malignant from benign pheochromocytomas. A malignant tumor may be found many years after removal of a benign lesion.

Conclusive diagnosis of malignancy or metastases depends on the demonstration of functional pheochromocytomas in areas where chromaffin tissue is not normally found. Iodine-131–MIBG scintigraphy is useful in localization of metastatic disease.[64] These metastatic sites include bone, lymph nodes, liver, and lung. The tumor also may be found in brain, spinal cord, and pleura.

Malignant pheochromocytomas generally are resistant to radiation therapy and chemotherapy although combined therapy may be palliative. Recent reports indicate that M[^{131}I]BG may be useful as a radiotherapeutic agent. Chronic therapy with α and β blockers or with α-methyltyrosine can be used to control the clinical manifestations of catecholamine excess. Survival may last a few months to many years.[161,162]

MULTIPLE ENDOCRINE ADENOMATOSIS SYNDROMES

The multiple endocrine adenomatosis (MEA) syndromes are familial disorders characterized by hyperplasia or tumor involving more than one endocrine gland (Table 7–4). The clinical manifestations are variable and reflect the functional status of the involved hormone-producing tissue(s). Sometimes the clinical picture suggests a single-gland endocrinopathy for years and pluriglandular involvement is masked, while at other times the signs and symptoms of multiple organ involvement develop simultaneously. The disorders are inherited in a mendelian autosomal-dominant pattern with variable expressivity and high penetrance, but the pathogenesis of the syndromes is unknown.

Pearse noted that many endocrine cells in different tissues have similar histochemical properties (i.e., Amine content, amine Precursor Uptake and amino acid Decarboxylase activity).[163] The mnemonic APUD has been applied to these cells. The stored amine is usually dopamine or serotonin; the amine precursor is the amino acid L-dopa or 5-hydroxytryptophan; the decarboxylase activity is due to the enzyme aromatic-L-amino acid decarboxylase. The APUD cells produce more than 35 physiologically active peptides and a small number of active amines. Many of these peptides have been

TABLE 7–4. COMMON ABNORMALITIES FOUND IN THE MULTIPLE ENDOCRINE ADENOMATOSIS SYNDROMES

Abnormality	MEA I	MEA II	MEA III
Anterior pituitary tumors	+		
Pancreatic islet cell tumors	+		
Parathyroid hyperplasia or tumors	+	+	
Pheochromocytoma		+	+
Medullary thyroid carcinoma		+	+
Multiple neural tumors			+

identified jointly in endocrine cells and in neuron cell bodies or processes. Some of the cells are derived from the neural crest while the origin of others is not definite, but most are deemed to be "neuroendocrine programmed."[164] The diffuse neuroendocrine system is constituted by the cells of the central and peripheral divisions of the APUD series. The central division contains the neuroendocrine and endocrine cells of the hypothalamus-pituitary axis and the pineal gland, while the peripheral division contains all the cells outside these regions. Peptide and amine products from cells of the pancreas, stomach, intestine, lung, parathyroid, adrenal medulla, sympathetic nervous system, carotid body, and thyroid are included in the peripheral division. Most tumors of the MEA syndromes are derived from cells of the APUD series, so there appears to be a relationship between cell type and tumor, but the specific defect is not clear. The process of dedifferentiation may explain ectopic peptide hormone production in some neoplasms.[165] The observation that many tumors of APUD cells of both central and peripheral divisions contain neuron-specific enolase supports the unifying concept of the APUD system.[166]

Multiple Endocrine Adenomatosis I (Wermer's Syndrome or Multiple Endocrine Neoplasia Type I)

This disorder is characterized by simultaneous or successive tumors of the anterior pituitary gland, the islet cells of the pancreas, and the parathyroid glands, as well as adenomas or carcinomas of the thyroid and the adrenal cortex. Lipomas, bronchial and intestinal carcinoid tumors, schwannomas, and thymomas also have been reported, albeit infrequently.[167] Both sexes are affected with approximately equal frequency, and the disease has been described in all ages from late childhood on. Multiple endocrine adenomatosis I is rare before age 10 and typically begins between ages 20 and 40 years.

The pituitary tumors may be nonfunctional and lead to pituitary insufficiency; may produce growth hormone and cause acromegaly; or may produce ACTH and result in Cushing disease or cause hyperprolactinemia.[168] Surgical resection or radiation therapy is used for treatment.

The pancreatic tumors can be benign or malignant and secrete insulin, glucagon, or gastrin. Sequential production of all three different hormones from a single tumor has been demonstrated.[169] Pancreatic tumors that produce gastrin and are associated with intractable peptic ulceration constitute the Zollinger-Ellison syndrome. It is estimated that about one half of the patients with Zollinger-Ellison syndrome have or will develop other endocrine tumors. Total gastrectomy is required for treatment of the peptic ulceration, and total pancreatectomy often is necessary for the pancreatic lesions, since many are multiple rather than single.

Hypercalcemia due to parathyroid adenoma or hyperplasia is the most common abnormality in MEA I, especially in patients older than 18 years.[170,171] A circulating mitogenic factor may stimulate the rate of parathyroid cell division and lead to parathyroid dysfunction in affected individuals.[172,173] The hyperparathyroidism often is insidious, and many affected family members have been found by routine screening of serum calcium levels. Treatment is surgical. Since there is a high incidence of multiple parathyroid gland involvement and a high rate of recurrence, total or near-total parathyroidectomy is recommended during the initial exploration of the neck of patients from families with MEA.

Families of all patients with pituitary, pancreatic, and parathyroid tumors should be screened, especially if there is a history of other members with tumors. Every patient with a tumor of one of these glands should be screened for involvement of other endocrine glands, and follow-up studies should be done yearly.

Multiple Endocrine Adenomatosis II (Sipple Syndrome or Multiple Endocrine Neoplasia Type 2a)

Multiple endocrine adenomatosis II is composed of medullary carcinoma of the thyroid, pheochromocytoma, and parathyroid hyperplasia or tumor. The frequency with which the syndrome occurs is difficult to estimate, since medullary thyroid carcinoma or pheochromocytoma may appear as a sporadic case (? new mutation), as a familial disorder, or as part of a MEA syndrome. In their review of 85 cases of familial pheochromocytoma, Steiner and coworkers found that 77 per cent had pheochromocytoma alone, 16 per cent had pheochromocytoma and medullary thyroid carcinoma, and 6 per cent had pheochromocytoma, medullary thyroid carcinoma, and parathyroid disease.[174] Linkage studies using DNA probes have mapped the gene for MEA II to chromosome 10.[175,176]

Medullary thyroid carcinoma arises from the C cells of the thyroid gland and is inherited as an autosomal-dominant trait that is transmitted from generation to generation by parents of either sex to children of either sex. The other parts of the syndrome—parathyroid disease and pheochromocytoma—seem to show a lower degree of penetrance than medullary thyroid carcinoma (MTC).[177] Screening of relatives of patients with familial MTC has resulted in diagnosis at increasingly younger ages.[178] There is a recent report of an 18-month-old infant born to a mother with MTC and neuromata who was found to have both MTC and multiple neuromas of the lips.[179] The carcinoma usually is bilateral or multifocal when discovered.

A palpable thyroid nodule may be present, but most often the patient is asymptomatic, and there is no evidence of thyroid disease on physical examination. The tumor does not take up radioiodine, and it is not thyroid-stimulating hormone (TSH) dependent. Some patients will have dense, irregular calcifications visible radiographically in the thyroid carcinoma as well as in tumor metastases to cervical lymph nodes and liver. The C cells of the thyroid and MTC produce the hormone calcitonin. The occurrence of high basal plasma levels of calcitonin or abnormal calcitonin secretion in response to provocative testing seems to identify patients with medullary thyroid carcinoma. The calcium gluconate infusion test consists of the administration of 15 mg of elemental calcium per kilogram intravenously over a 4-hour period, with measurements of serum calcitonin at 0, 3, and 4 hours. The pentagastrin stimulation test consists of the administration of pentagastrin (Peptavlon, Ayerst), 0.5 μg/kg, as an intravenous bolus injected within 5 sec. Serum calcitonin is measured at 0 time and at 1, 2, 5, 10, and 15 min after pentagastrin injection. A basal calcitonin concentration in excess of 0.40 ng/ml or a stimulated value greater than 0.58 ng/ml is considered abnormal.[178]

Serum histaminase activity is elevated in many patients with MTC, and is useful in detecting residual carcinoma after surgery.[177] Some patients with MTC will have watery diarrhea and flushing episodes similar to those of the carcinoid syndrome. The tumor has been implicated in the ectopic secretion of ACTH, prostaglandins, and VIP.

Pheochromocytomas usually are bilateral or multifocal within the adrenal glands in MEA II. Diffuse hyperplasia of the adrenal medulla, which may be the precursor of pheochromocytoma, also has been described.[180] Because the clinical presentation and the biochemical detection of pheochromocytoma depend on the amount of catecholamine released by the tumor into the circulation, patients with MTC may harbor a pheochromocytoma long before it is detected. This can present a worrisome problem when an "undiagnosed" tumor releases excessive amounts of catecholamine during a surgical procedure (i.e., neck exploration for thyroid carcinoma and hyperparathyroidism). A careful search for a catecholamine-secreting tumor always should be made preoperatively in patients who have other components of the MEA syndrome so the pheochromocytoma can be excised first.

The incidence and the etiology of the hyperparathyroidism in MEA II is not clear. Parathyroid hyperplasia, rather than adenoma, seems to be more common, and it may be secondary to excess calcitonin secretion by MTC or to catecholamine-stimulated parathyroid hormone production. In their review of 45 patients, Keiser et al. found elevated serum Ca^{2+} in 19, hypercellularity of the parathyroid in 4, hyperplasia in 47, and adneomas in 4.[177]

Total thyroidectomy is the treatment for MTC. Even in a patient whose tumor is confined to the thyroid, immunoreactive calcitonin gradually falls into the undetectable range after surgery. The reason for the slow decline is not clear.[178] The parathyroid glands should be examined at the time of neck exploration. It is recommended that grossly abnormal tissue be biopsied and excised. Unless the patient is hypercalcemic, normal parathyroid tissue is best left in place.[181]

All family members should be screened for the presence of medullary thyroid carcinoma when one affected individual is identified. The pentogastrin and the calcium infusion tests are effective for detection of the tumor, and one of them should be performed yearly. Aggressive screening leads to early diagnosis and reduction in the occurrence of metastatic disease. Initial screening has been recommended as early as 1 year of age.[182,183] Likewise, all members of families with familial pheochromocytoma should be screened for MTC.

Patients with MTC and family members also should be screened for adrenal medullary hyperplasia and pheochromocytoma. A careful history looking for symptoms of catecholamine excess, a physical examination, and determination of urinary free norepinephrine and epinephrine are recommended yearly.

Multiple Endocrine Adenomatosis III (Multiple Endocrine Neoplasia Type 2b or 3)

The major components of this syndrome are multiple neuromas, medullary thyroid carcinoma, and pheochromocytoma. In addition, affected individuals generally have skeletal abnormalities, including dorsal kyphosis, pectus excavatum, pes cavus, and high-arched palate. Less commonly, scoliosis, lordosis, and valgus deformities of the knees and toes are present. They often have a marfanoid habitus but, in contrast to patients with Marfan syndrome, ectopia lentis and aortic abnormalities have not been described. The majority have characteristic facies because both lips are diffusely enlarged and may be "bumpy," probably as a result of neuromas (Fig. 7–5). The tumors also may be found in the tongue (Fig. 7–6) and buccal mucosa as well as the eyelids, conjunctiva, and cornea. Slit-lamp examination of the cornea often shows hypertrophied corneal nerves. Prognathism occasionally has been noted, and some patients have an acromegalic appearance. These features of the syndrome usually are present early in life but often escape notice until MTC or pheochromocytoma is diagnosed.[184]

Most patients have chronic, serious, and diverse gastrointestinal complaints, including feeding difficulty, projectile vomiting, crampy abdominal pain, constipation, and diarrhea. There may be abdominal distention, visible peristalsis, and x-ray evidence of megacolon or diverticulosis of the colon. These findings probably are related to alimentary tract ganglioneuromatosis, which may extend from the lips to the rectum, combined with hormones produced by MTC and/or pheochromocytoma.[185,186]

Most patients with MEA III have been reported as single cases. It is likely that some represent new gene mutations, but others

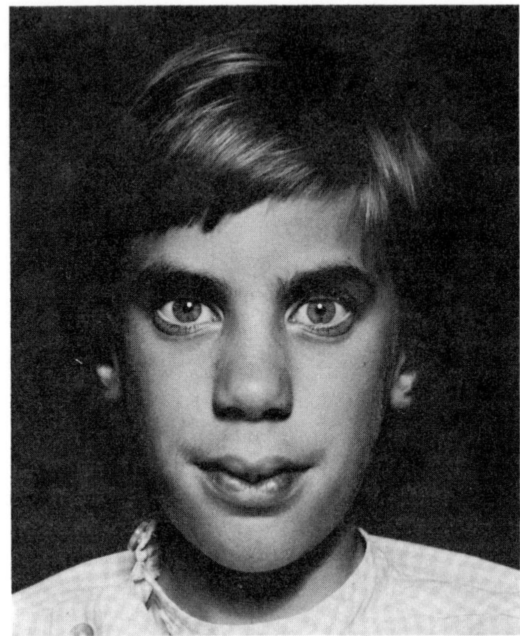

FIGURE 7–5. Typical facies of multiple endocrine enoplasia, type 2b, in an 11-year-old patient. The upper and lower lips are thickened. The broad base of the nose and the staring expression due to thickening of upper and lower tarsal plates are typical of the syndrome. (From Carney JA, Hayles AB: Alimentary tract manifestations of multiple endocrine neoplasia, Type 2b. Mayo Clin Proc 52:543, 1977.)

may have affected family members who have not yet been identified. In familial cases, the pattern of transmission has been consistent with an autosomal-dominant mode of inheritance. There is some overlap with the phakomatoses because neurofibromas and café-au-lait spots have been noted in patients with MEA III. In a review of 41 cases, Khairi et al. found neuromas, medullary thyroid carcinoma, and pheochro-

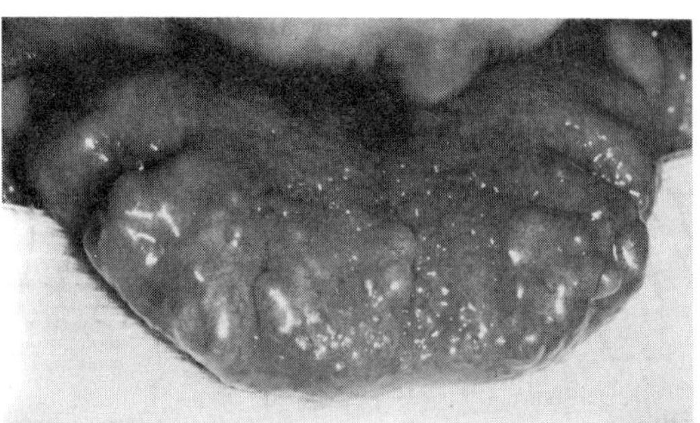

FIGURE 7–6. Large confluent nodules on the anterior portion of the tongue of the patient shown in Figure 7–5. (From Carney JA, Hayles AB: Alimentary tract manifestations of multiple endocrine neoplasia, Type 2b. Mayo Clin Proc 52:543, 1977.)

mocytoma in 48.7 per cent, neuroma and MTC in 43.9 per cent, and neuroma and pheochromocytoma in 7.3 per cent.[184] The diagnosis of multiple neuromas is suggested by the clinical findings and confirmed by biopsy and histologic examination. There is no specific treatment for the disorder. Mucosal neuromas are not subject to carcinomatous change and primarily are a cosmetic problem that may require plastic surgery. Descriptions of MTC and pheochromocytoma have been reviewed earlier in this chapter. Medullary thyroid carcinoma usually is diagnosed at a younger age than is pheochromocytoma in patients with MEA III. Once one component of the syndrome is identified, a search for others should be made. Screening for abnormal calcitonin levels is particularly important—as previously described—so that MTC can be diagnosed and total thyroidectomy can be performed before metastases have occurred. An absent flare response to intradermal histamine has been described in patients with MEA III, but the specificity of the test for diagnosis is not certain.[188]

Multiple Endocrine Adenomatosis of Mixed Type

Even though multiple endocrine adenomatosis syndromes I, II, and III are distinct disorders in most cases, it is clear that there is overlap. Hansen and colleagues have reviewed eight patients who had features of both MEA I and II.[189] The Zollinger-Ellison syndrome has been reported in a young adult with MEA II[190] and in a 13-year-old boy with neurofibromatosis.[191] These findings support the concept that the MEA syndromes may represent a spectrum of endocrine disorders arising from an abnormality of "neuroendocrine-programmed" cells.

REFERENCES

1. Landsberg L, Young JB: Catecholamines and the adrenal medulla. *In* Wilson JD, Foster DW (eds): Williams Textbook of Endocrinology. 7th ed. Philadelphia, WB Saunders Company, 1985, p 908.
2. Landsberg L: Catecholamines and the sympathoadrenal system. *In* Ingbar SH (ed): The Year in Endocrinology. New York, Plenum Medical Book Co, 1976, p 177.
3. Weetman RM, Rider PS, Oei TO, et al: Effect of diet on urinary excretion of VMA, HVA, metanephrine and total free catecholamine in normal preschool children. J Pediatr 88:46, 1976.
4. Gitlow SE, Mendlowitz M, Wilk EK, et al: Excretion of catecholamine catabolites by normal children. J Lab Clin Med 72:612, 1968.
5. Voorhess ML: Urinary catecholamine excretion by healthy children: Daily excretion of dopamine, norepinephrine, epinephrine and 3-methoxy-4-hydroxymandelic acid. Pediatrics 39:252, 1967.
6. Eliot RJ, Law R, Leake RD, et al: Plasma catecholamine concentrations in infants at birth and during the first 48 hours of life. J Pediatr 96:311, 1980.
7. Castro L, de la Pava S, Webster JH: Esthesioneuroblastomas. Am J Roentgenol Rad Therapy Nuc Med 105:7, 1969.
8. Horten BC, Rubinstein LJ: Primary cerebral neuroblastoma. A clinocopathological study of 35 cases. Brain 99:735, 1976.
9. Nesbitt KA, Vidone RA: Primitive neuroectodermal tumor (neuroblastoma) arising in sciatic nerve of a child. Cancer 37:1562, 1976.
10. Schneider KM, Becker JM, Krasna IH: Neonatal neuroblastoma. Pediatrics 36:359, 1965.
11. Anders D, Kindermann G, Pfeifer U: Metastasizing fetal neuroblastoma with involvement of the placenta simulating fetal erythroblastosis. J Pediatr 82:50, 1973.
12. Birner WF: Neuroblastoma as a cause of antenatal death. Am J Obstet Gynecol 82:1388, 1961.
13. Voûte PA Jr, Wadman SK, Van Putten WJ: Congenital neuroblastoma symptoms in the mother during pregnancy. Clin Pediatr 9:206, 1970.
14. Voorhess ML, Watkins ES: Intracranial neuroblastoma and abnormal catecholamine excretion in a 42 year old woman. Case report. J Neurosurg 31:358, 1969.
15. Tang C-K, Hajdu SI: Neuroblastoma in adolescence and adulthood. NY State J Med 75:1434, 1975.
16. Mackay B, Luna MA, Butlet JJ: Adult neuroblastoma. Electron microscopic observations in nine cases. Cancer 37:1334, 1976.
17. Reisman M, Goldenberg ED, Gordon J: Congenital heart disease and neuroblastoma. Am J Dis Child 111:308, 1966.
18. Sy WM, Edmonson JH: The developmental defects associated with neuroblastoma—etiologic implications. Cancer 22:234, 1968.
19. Miller RW, Fraumeni JF Jr, Hill JA: Neuroblastoma: Epidemiologic approach to its origin. Am J Dis Child 115:253, 1968.
20. Chatten J, Voorhess ML: Familial neuroblastoma. N Engl J Med 277:1230, 1967.
21. Griffin ME, Bolande RP: Familial neuroblastoma with regression and maturation to ganglioneurofibroma. Pediatrics 43:377, 1969.
22. Wagget J, Aherne G, Aherne W: Familial neuroblastoma: Report of two sib pairs. Arch Dis Child 48:63, 1973.
23. Pegelow CH, Ebbin AJ, Powars D, et al: Familial neuroblastoma. J Pediatr 87:763, 1975.
24. Malenbaum GB, Gilbert F: Double minute chromosomes and the homogeneously staining regions in chromosomes of a human neuroblastoma cell line. Science 198:739, 1977.
25. Kaneko Y, Kanda N, Maseki N, et al: Different karyotypic patterns in early and advanced stage neuroblastomas. Cancer Res 47:311, 1987.
26. Knudson AG Jr, Meadows AT: Development genetics of neuroblastoma. JNCI 57:675, 1976.

27. Beckwith JB, Perrin EV: In situ neuroblastomas: A contribution to the natural history of neural crest tumors. Am J Pathol 43:1089, 1963.

28. Bill AH: Studies of the mechanism of regression of human neuroblastoma. J Pediatr Surg 3:727, 1968.

29. Hellström KE, Hellström I: Immunity to neuroblastomas and melanomas. Annu Rev Med 23:19, 1972.

30. Greenfield LJ, Shelley WM: The spectrum of neurogenic tumors of the sympathetic nervous system: maturation and adrenergic function. JNCI 35:215, 1965.

31. Goldstein MN, Burdman JA, Journey LJ: Long-term tissue culture of neuroblastomas. II. Morphologic evidence of differentiation and maturation. JNCI 32:165, 1964.

32. Griffin ME, Bolande RP: Familial neuroblastoma with regression and maturation to ganglioneurofibroma. Pediatrics 43:377, 1969.

33. Bolande RP, Towler WF: A possible relationship of neuroblastoma to von Recklinghausen's disease. Cancer 26:162, 1970.

34. Knudson AG Jr, Meadows AT: Regression of neuroblastoma IV-S: A genetic hypothesis. N Engl J Med 302:1254, 1980.

35. Gross RE, Farber S, Martin LW: Neuroblastoma sympatheticum. A study and report of 217 cases. Pediatrics 23:1179, 1959.

36. Hawthorne HC Jr, Nelson JS, Witzleben CL, et al: Blanching subcutaneous nodules in neonatal neuroblastoma. J Pediatr 77:297, 1970.

37. Weinblatt ME, Heisel MA, Siegel SA: Hypertension in children with neurogenic tumors. Pediatrics 71:947, 1983.

38. Solomon GE, Chutorian AM: Opsoclonus and occult neuroblastoma. N Engl J Med 279:475, 1968.

39. Bray PF, Ziter FA, Lahey ME, et al: The coincidence of neuroblastoma and acute cerebellar encephalopathy. J Pediatr 75:983, 1969.

40. Bond JV: Unusual presenting symptoms in neuroblastoma. Br Med J 2:327, 1972.

41. Hrabovsky E, Jones B: Congenital intraspinal neuroblastoma. Am J Dis Child 133:73, 1979.

42. Thompson EN, Bosley A: Disseminated intravascular coagulation in association with congenital neuroblastoma. Postgrad Med J 55:814, 1979.

43. Dahms WT, Gray G, Vrana M, et al: Adrenocortical adenoma and ganglioneuroblastoma in a child. A case presenting as Cushing syndrome with virilization. Am J Dis Child 125:608, 1973.

44. Al-Rashid RA, Cress C: Hypercalcemia associated with neuroblastoma. Am J Dis Child 133:838, 1979.

45. Shapiro M, Simcha A, Rosenmann E, et al: Hypoglycemia associated with neonatal neuroblastoma and abnormal responses of serum glucose and free fatty acids to epinephrine injection. Isr J Med Sci 2:705, 1966.

46. Seeler RA, Israel JN, Royal JE, et al: Ganglioneuroblastoma and fetal hydantoin-alcohol syndromes. Pediatrics 63:524, 1979.

47. Berger PE, Kuhn G, Munschauer R: Computed tomography and ultrasound in the diagnosis and management of neuroblastoma. Radiology 128:663, 1978.

48. Von Studnitz W, Käser H, Sjoerdsma A: Spectrum of catecholamine biochemistry in patients with neuroblastoma. N Engl J Med 269:232, 1963.

49. Gitlow SE, Bertani LM, Ransen A, et al: Diagnosis of neuroblastoma by qualitative and quantitative determination of catecholamine metabolites in urine. Cancer 25:1377, 1970.

50. Voorhess ML: Neuroblastoma-pheochromocytoma: products and pathogenesis. Ann NY Acad Sci 230:187, 1974.

51. La Brosse EH, Comoy E, Bohuon C, et al: Catecholamine metabolism in neuroblastoma. JNCI 57:633, 1976.

52. Voorhess ML, Gardner LI: The value of serial catecholamine determinations in children with neuroblastoma. Report of a case. Pediatrics 30:241, 1962.

53. Voorhess ML: Neuroblastoma with normal urinary catecholamine excretion. J Pediatr 78:680, 1971.

54. Tuchman M, Morris CL, Ramnaraine ML, et al: Value of random urinary homovanillic acid and vanillylmandelic acid levels in the diagnosis and management of patients with neuroblastoma: Comparison with 24-hour urine collections. Pediatrics 75:324, 1985.

55. Tuchman M, Stoeckeler JS: Conjugated versus "free" acidic metabolites of catecholamines in random urine samples: Significance for the diagnosis of neuroblastoma. Pediatr Res 23:576, 1988.

56. Johnsonbaugh RE, Cahill R: Screening procedures for neuroblastoma: false negative results. Pediatrics 56:267, 1975.

57. Addanki S, Gombos RL, Hinnenkamp ER, et al: Screening tests for vanillylmandelic acid. J Pediatr 90:955, 1977.

58. Sawada T, Nakata T, Takasugi N, et al: Mass screening for neuroblastoma in infants in Japan. Lancet 2:271, 1984.

59. Sawada T, Kawakatu H, Sugimoto T: Screening for neuroblastoma. Lancet 2:1204, 1987.

60. Hann HL, Levy HM, Evans AE: Serum ferritin as a guide to therapy in neuroblastoma. Cancer Res 40:1411, 1980.

61. Ishiguro Y, Kato K, Ito T, et al: Nervous system-specific enolase in serum as a marker for neuroblastoma. Pediatrics 72:696, 1983.

62. Zeltzer PM, Parma AM, Dalton A, et al: Raised neuron-specific enolase in serum of children with metastatic neuroblastoma. Lancet 2:361, 1983.

63. Ladish S, Wu Z-L: Detection of a tumour-associated ganglioside in plasma of patients with neuroblastoma. Lancet 1:136, 1985.

64. Shulkin BL, Shen SW, Sisson JC, et al: Iodine-131 MIBG scintigraphy of the extremities in metastatic pheochromocytoma and neuroblastoma. J Nucl Med 28:315, 1987.

65. Bomanji J, Levison DA, Flatman WD, et al: Uptake of iodine-123 MIBG by pheochromocytomas, paragangliomas and neuroblastomas: A histopathological comparison. J Nucl Med 28:973, 1987.

66. Maris JM, Evans AE, McLaughlin AC, et al: 31-P nuclear magnetic resonance spectroscopic investigation of human neuroblastoma in situ. N Engl J Med 312:1500, 1985.

67. Mackay B, Masse SR, King OY, et al: Diagnosis of neuroblastoma by electron microscopy of bone marrow aspirates. Pediatrics 56:1045, 1975.

68. Hirschberger M, Kleinberg F: Failure to thrive and death in early infancy associated with raised

urinary homovanillic and vanillylmandelic acids. Arch Dis Child 51:977, 1976.

69. Young I, Hosking GP: Familial neurodegenerative disorders associated with raised urinary vanillylmandelic acid. Arch Dis Child 53:682, 1978.

70. Lees MH: Catecholamine metabolite excretion of infants with heart failure. J Pediatr 69:259, 1966.

71. Evans AE, D'Angio GJ, Randolph J: A proposed staging for children with neuroblastoma. Cancer 27:374, 1971.

72. Hayes FA, Green A, Hustu HO, et al: Surgicopathologic staging of neuroblastoma: Prognostic significance of regional lymph node metastases. J Pediatr 102:59, 1983.

73. Carlsen NLT, Christensen IJ, Schroeder H, et al: Prognostic value of different staging systems in neuroblastomas and completeness of tumour excision. Arch Dis Child 61:832, 1986.

74. Smith EI, Krous HF, Tunell WP, et al: The impact of chemotherapy and radiation therapy on secondary operations for neuroblastoma. Ann Surg 191:561, 1980.

75. Philip T, Bernard JL, Zucker JM, et al: High-dose chemoradiotherapy with bone marrow transplantation as consolidation treatment in neuroblastoma: An unselected group of stage IV patients over one year of age. J Clin Oncol 5:266, 1987.

76. Evans AE, Chatten J, D'Angio GJ, et al: A review of 17 IV-S neuroblastoma patients at the Children's Hospital of Philadelphia. Cancer 45:833, 1980.

77. Hann H-WL, Evans AE, Cohen IJ, et al: Biologic differences between neuroblastoma stages IV-S and IV. Measurement of serum ferritin and E-rosette inhibition in 30 children. N Engl J Med 305:425, 1981.

78. Seeger RC, Brodeur GM, Sather H, et al: Association of multiple copies of the N-myc oncogene with rapid progression of neuroblastomas. N Engl J Med 313:1111, 1985.

79. Laug WE, Siegel SE, Shaw KNF, et al: Initial urinary catecholamine metabolite concentrations and prognosis in neuroblastoma. Pediatrics 62:77, 1978.

80. Gitlow SE, Dziedzic LB, Strauss L, et al: Biochemical and histologic determinants in the prognosis of neuroblastoma. Cancer 32:898, 1973.

81. Shimada H, Chatten J, Newton WA Jr, et al: Histopathologic prognostic factors in neuroblastic tumors: Definition of subtypes of ganglioneuroblastoma and an age-linked classification of neuroblastoma. JNCI 73:405, 1984.

82. Evans A-E, D'Angio GJ, Propert K, et al: Prognostic factors in neuroblastoma. Cancer 59:1853, 1987.

83. O'Malley B, D'Angio GJ, Vawter GF: Late effects of roentgen therapy given in infancy. Am J Roentgenol Rad Ther 89:1067, 1963.

84. Parra A, Santos D, Cervantes C, et al: Plasma gonadotropins and gonadal steroids in children treated with cyclophosphamide. J Pediatr 92:117, 1978.

85. Quinn JJ, Altman AJ, Frantz CN: Serum lactic dehydrogenase, an indicator of tumor activity in neuroblastoma. J Pediatr 97:89, 1980.

86. Hamilton JP, Koop CE: Ganglioneuromas in children. Surgery Gynecol Obstet 121:803, 1965.

87. Kaplan SJ, Holbrook CT, McDaniel HG, et al: Vasoactive intestinal peptide secreting tumors of childhood. Am J Dis Child 134:21, 1980.

88. Voorhess ML: Functioning tumors. Am J Dis Child 134:14, 1980.

89. Sandler M, Karim SMM, Williams ED: Prostaglandins in amine-peptide-secreting tumors. Lancet 2:1053, 1968.

90. Hume DM: Pheochromocytoma in the adult and in the child. Am J Surg 99:458, 1960.

91. Stackpole RH, Melicow MM, Uson AC: Pheochromocytoma in children. J Pediatr 63:315, 1963.

92. Gifford RW Jr, Kvale WF, Maher FT, et al: Clinical features, diagnosis and treatment of pheochromocytoma. A review of 76 cases. Mayo Clin Proc 39:281, 1964.

93. Gibbs MK, Carney AJ, Hayles AB, et al: Simultaneous adrenal and cervical pheochromocytomas in childhood. Ann Surg 185:273, 1977.

94. Hodgkinson DJ, Telander RL, Sheps SG, et al: Extra-adrenal intrathoracic functioning paraganglioma (pheochromocytoma) in childhood. Mayo Clin Proc 55:271, 1980.

95. Albores-Saavedra J, Maldonado ME, Ibarra J, et al: Pheochromocytoma of the urinary bladder. Cancer 23:1110, 1969.

96. Melicow MM: One hundred cases of pheochromocytoma (107 tumors) at the Columbia-Presbyterian Medical Center, 1926–1976. A clinicopathological analysis. Cancer 40:1987, 1977.

97. Engelman K, Zelis R, Waldmann T, et al: Mechanism of orthostatic hypotension in pheochromocytoma. Circulation 38:(Suppl VI):VI-72, 1968.

98. Tevetoglu F, Lee C-H: Adrenal pheochromocytoma simulating diabetes insipidus. Am J Dis Child 91:365, 1956.

99. Van Vliet PD, Burchell HB, Titus JL: Focal myocarditis associated with pheochromocytoma. N Engl J Med 27:1102, 1966.

100. Schaffer MS, Zuberbuhler P, Wilson G, et al: Catecholamine cardiomyopathy: An unusual presentation of pheochromocytoma in children. J Pediatr 99:276, 1981.

101. Imperato-McGinley J, Gautier T, Ehlers K, et al: Reversibility of catecholamine-induced dilated cardiomyopathy in a child with pheochromocytoma. N Engl J Med 316:793, 1987.

102. Engelman K, Mueller PS, Sjoerdsma A: Elevated plasma free fatty acid concentrations in patients with pheochromocytoma. N Engl J Med 270:865, 1964.

103. Brenner WE, Yen SSC, Dingfelder JR, et al: Pheochromocytoma: Serial studies during pregnancy. Am J Obstet Gynecol 113:779, 1972.

104. Leak D, Carroll JJ, Robinson DC, et al: Management of pheochromocytoma during pregnancy. CMA J 116:371, 1977.

105. Bolande RP: The neurocristopathies. Hum Pathol 5:409, 1974.

106. Williams GA, Crockett CL, Butler WWS III, et al: The coexistence of pheochromocytoma and adrenocortical hyperplasia. J Clin Endocrinol Metab 20:622, 1960.

107. Spark RF, Connolly PB, Gluckin DS, et al: ACTH secretion from a functioning pheochromocytoma. N Engl J Med 301:416, 1979.

108. Beaser RS, Guay AT, Lee AK, et al: An adrenocorticotropic hormone-producing pheochromo-

cytoma: Diagnostic and immunohistochemical studies. J Urology 135:10, 1986.

109. Sakurai H, Yoshike Y, Isahaya S, et al: Case report: A case of ACTH-producing pheochromocytoma. Am J Med Sci 294:258, 1987.

110. Chapman RC, Diaz-Perez R: Pheochromocytoma associated with cerebellar hemangioblastoma. JAMA 182:1014, 1962.

111. DeSouza TG, Berlad L, Shapiro K, et al: Pheochromocytoma and multiple intracerebral aneurysms. J Pediatr 108:947, 1986.

112. Waldmann TA, Bradley JE: Polycythemia secondary to a pheochromocytoma with production of an erythropoiesis stimulating factor by the tumor. Proc Soc Exp Biol Med 108:425, 1961.

113. Nibbelink DW, Peters BH, McCormick WF: On the association of pheochromocytoma and cerebellar astrocytoma. Neurology 19:455, 1969.

114. Murray KM, Schillaci RF: Sarcoidosis and pheochromocytoma. West J Med 146:745, 1987.

115. Gaisie G, Oh KS, Young LW: Coexistent neuroblastoma and Hirschsprung's disease—another manifestation of the neurocristopathy? Pediatr Radiol 8:161, 1979.

116. St. John Sutton MG, Sheps SG, Lie JT: Prevalence of clinically unsuspected pheochromocytoma. Review of a 50-year autopsy series. Mayo Clin Proc 56:354, 1981.

117. Crout JR, Pisano JJ, Sjoerdsma A: Urinary excretion of catecholamines and metabolites in pheochromocytoma. Am Heart J 61:375, 1961.

118. Frier DT, Tank ES, Harrison TS: Pediatric and adult pheochromocytomas. Arch Surg 107:252, 1973.

119. Kaplan NM, Kramer NJ, Holland OB, et al: Single-voided urine metanephrine assays in screening for pheochromocytoma. Arch Intern Med 137:190, 1977.

120. Engelman K, Hammond WG: Adrenaline production by an intrathoracic pheochromocytoma. Lancet 1:609, 1968.

121. Bravo EL, Tarazi RC, Gifford RW, et al: Circulating and urinary catecholamines in pheochromocytoma. Diagnostic and pathophysiologic implications. N Engl J Med 301:682, 1979.

122. Ratge D, Baumgardt G, Knoll E, et al: Plasma free and conjugated catecholamines in diagnosis and localization of pheochromocytoma. Clin Chim Acta 132:229, 1983.

123. Bravo EL, Gifford RW Jr: Pheochromocytoma: Diagnosis, localization and management. N Engl J Med 311:1298, 1984.

124. Cryer PE: Phaeochromocytoma. Clin Endocrinol Metab 14:203, 1985.

125. Duncan MW, Compton P, Lazarus L, et al: Measurement of norepinephrine and 3,4-dihydroxyphenylglycol in urine and plasma for the diagnosis of pheochromocytoma. N Engl J Med 319:136, 1988.

126. Taylor HC, Mayes D, Anton AH: Clonidine suppression test for pheochromocytoma: Examples of misleading results. J Clin Endocrinol Metab 63:238, 1986.

127. Hung W, August G: Hyperreninemia and secondary hyperaldosteronism in pheochromocytomas. J Pediatr 94:215, 1979.

128. Miller SS, Sizemore GW, Sheps SG, et al: Parathyroid function in patients with pheochromocytoma. Ann Intern Med 82:312, 1975.

129. Passwell, J, Boichis H, Lotan D, et al: The metabolic effects of excess noradrenalin secretion from a pheochromocytoma. Am J Dis Child 131:1011, 1977.

130. Waldmann T, Bradley JE: Polycythemia secondary to a pheochromocytoma with production of an erythropoiesis stimulating factor by the tumor. Soc Exp Biol Med 108:425, 1961.

132. Brooks MH, Guha A, Danforth E Jr, et al: Pheochromocytoma: Observations on mechanism of carbohydrate intolerance and abnormalities associated with development of Goldblatt kidney following removal of tumor. Metabolism 18:445, 1969.

133. Vetter H, Vetter W, Warnholz C, et al: Renin and aldosterone secretion in pheochromocytoma. Effect of chronic alpha-adrenergic receptor blockade. Am J Med 60:866, 1976.

134. Sparagana M, Feldman JM, Molnar Z: An unusual pheochromocytoma associated with an androgen secreting adrenocortical adenoma. Evaluation of its polypeptide hormone, catecholamine and enzyme characteristics. Cancer 60:223, 1987.

135. Nigawara K, Suzuki T, Tazawa H, et al: A case of recurrent malignant pheochromocytoma complicated by watery diarrhea, hypokalemia, achlorhydria syndrome. J Clin Endocrinol Metab 65:1053, 1987.

136. Fisher BM, MacPhee GJA, Davies DL, et al: A case of watery diarrhoea syndrome due to an adrenal phaeochromocytoma secreting vasoactive intestinal peptide with coincidental autoimmune thyroid disease. Acta Endocrinol (Copenh) 114:340, 1987.

137. Yanase T, Nawata H, Kato K, et al: Studies on adrenorphin in pheochromocytoma. J Clin Endocrinol Metab 64:692, 1987.

138. O'Connor DT, Deftos LJ: Secretion of chromogranin A by peptide-producing endocrine neoplasms. N Engl J Med 314:1145, 1986.

139. Roth KA, Wilson DM, Eberwine J, et al: Acromegaly and pheochromocytoma: A multiple endocrine syndrome caused by a plurihormonal adrenal medullary tumor. J Clin Endocrinol Metab 63:1421, 1986.

140. Yoneda M, Takatsuki K, Yamanchi K, et al: Determination of enolase isozymes in various adrenal gland tumours. Clin Endocrinol 26:303, 1987.

141. Warner RRP, Blaustein AS: Coexistence of pheochromocytoma and carcinoid syndrome produced by metastatic carcinoid of the ileum. Mt Sinai J Med 36:536, 1970.

142. Osamura RY, Tsutsumi Y, Yanaihara N, et al: Immunohistochemical studies for multiple peptide-immunoreactivities and co-locatization of met-enkephalin-arg-gly-leu, neuropeptide Y and somatostatin in human adrenal medulla and pheochromocytomas. Peptides 8:77, 1987.

143. Yanase T, Nawata H, Kato K, et al: Catecholamines and opioid peptides in human phaeochromocytomas. Acta Endocrinol (Copenh) 113:378, 1986.

144. Bornemann M, Hill SC, Kidd GS II: Lactic acidosis in pheochromocytoma. Ann Intern Med 105:880, 1986.

145. Stewart BH, Bravo EL, Haaga J, et al: Localization of pheochromocytoma by computed tomography. N Engl J Med 299:460, 1978.

146. Sisson JC, Frager MS, Valk TW, et al: Scinti-

graphic localization of pheochromocytoma. N Engl J Med 305:12, 1981.

147. Swensen SJ, Brown ML, Sheps SC, et al: use of 131 I-MIBG scintigraphy in the evaluation of suspected pheochromocytoma. Mayo Clin Proc 60:299, 1985.

148. Quint LE, Glazer GM, Francis IR, et al: Pheochromocytoma and paraganglioma: Comparison of MR imaging with CT and I-131 MIBG scintigraphy. Radiology 165:89, 1987.

149. Davies RA, Pratt NL, Sole MJ: Localization of pheochromocytoma by selective venous catheterization and assay of plasma catecholamines. Can Med Assoc J 120:539, 1979.

150. Harrison TS, Freier DT: Pitfalls in the technique and interpretation of regional venous sampling for localizing pheochromocytoma. Surg Clin North Am 54:339, 1974.

151. Meaney TF, Buonocore E: Selective arteriography as a localizing and provocative test in the diagnosis of pheochromocytoma. Radiology 87:309, 1966.

152. Scott HW Jr, Oates JA, Nies AS, et al: Pheochromocytoma: Present diagnosis and management. Ann Surg 183:587, 1976.

153. Harrison TS, Dagher FJ, Beck L, et al: Rationale and indications for preoperative adrenergic receptor blockade in pheochromocytoma. Med Clin North Am 53:1349, 1969.

154. Gitlow SE, Pertsemlidis D, Bertani LM: Management of patients with pheochromocytoma. Am Heart J 82:557, 1971.

155. Jones NF, Walker G, Ruthven CRJ, et al: α-Methyl-p-tyrosine in the management of pheochromocytoma. Lancet 2:1105, 1968.

156. Robinson RG, De Quattro V, Grushkin CM, et al: Childhood pheochromocytoma. Treatment with alpha methyl tyrosine for resistant hypertension. J Pediatr 91:143, 1977.

157. Brunjes S, Johns VJ Jr, Crane MG: Pheochromocytoma. Postoperative shock and blood volume. N Engl J Med 262:393, 1960.

158. Daggett P, Verner I, Carruthers M: Intraoperative management of phaeochromocytoma with sodium nitroprusside. Br Med J 2:311, 1978.

159. Wilkins GE, Schmidt N, Doll WA: Hypoglycemia following excision of pheochromocytoma. Can Med Assoc J 116:367, 1977.

160. Freier DT, Tank ES, Harrison TS: Pediatric and adult pheochromocytomas. A biochemical and clinical comparison. Arch Surg 107:252, 1973.

161. James RE, Baker HL Jr, Scanlon PW: The roentgenologic aspects of metastatic pheochromocytoma. Am J Roentgenol Rad Ther Nuc Med 115:783, 1972.

162. Philipps AF, McMurtry RJ, Taubman J: Malignant pheochromocytoma in childhood. Am J Dis Child 130:1252, 1976.

163. Pearse AGE: The cytochemistry and ultrastructure of polypeptide hormone-producing cells of the APUD series and the embryologic, physiologic and pathologic implications of the concept. J Histochem Cytochem 17:303, 1969.

164. Pearse AGE, Takor TT: Embryology of the diffuse neuroendocrine system and its relationship to the common peptides. Fed Proc 38:2288, 1979.

165. Stevens RE, Moore GE: Inadequacy of APUD concept in explaining production of peptide hormones by tumours. Lancet 1:118, 1983.

166. Tapia FJ, Barbosa AJA, Marangos PJ, et al: Neuron-specific enolase is produced by neuroendocrine tumors. Lancet 1:808, 1981.

167. Schmike RN: Multiple endocrine adenomatosis syndromes. Adv Intern Med 21:249, 1976.

168. Prosser PR, Karam JH, Townsend JJ, et al: Prolactin secreting pituitary adenomas in multiple endocrine adenomatosis Type 1. Ann Intern Med 91:41, 1979.

169. Peurifoy JT, Gomez LG, Thompson JC: Separate pancreatic gastrin cell and beta-cell adenomas. Report of a patient with multiple endocrine adenomatosis Type 1. Arch Surg 114:956, 1979.

170. Benson L, Ljunghall S, Akerström G, et al: Hyperparathyroidism presenting as the first lesion in multiple endocrine neoplasia type 1. Am J Med 82:731, 1987.

171. Snyder G III, Scurry MT, Deiss WP Jr: Five families with multiple endocrine adenomatosis. Ann Intern Med 76:53, 1972.

172. Brandi ML, Aurbach GD, Fitzpatric LA, et al: Parathyroid mitogenic activity in plasma from patients with familial multiple endocrine neoplasia type 1. N Engl J Med 314:1287, 1986.

173. Brandi ML, Marx SJ, Aurbach GD, et al: Familial multiple endocrine neoplasia type 1: A new look at pathophysiology. Endocr Rev 8:391, 1987.

174. Steiner AL, Goodman AD, Powers SR: Study of a kindred with pheochromocytoma, medullary thyroid carcinoma, hyperparathyroidism and Cushings disease: Multiple endocrine neoplasia, Type 2. Medicine 47:371, 1968.

175. Mathew CGP, Chin KS, Easton DF, et al: A linked genetic marker for multiple endocrine neoplasia type 2A on chromosome 10. Nature 328:527, 1987.

176. Simpson NE, Kidd KK, Goodfellow PJ, et al: Assignment of multiple endocrine neoplasia type 2A to chromosome 10 by linkage. Nature 328:528, 1987.

177. Keiser HR, Beaven MA, Doppman J, et al: Sipple's syndrome: Medullary thyroid carcinoma, pheochromocytoma and parathyroid disease. Studies in a large family. Ann Intern Med 78:561, 1973.

178. Graze K, Spiler IJ, Tashjian AH Jr, et al: Natural history of familial medullary thyroid carcinoma. N Engl J Med 299:980, 1978.

179. Stjernholm MR, Freudenbourg JC, Mooney HS, et al: Medullary carcinoma of the thyroid before age 2 years. J Clin Endocrinol Metabol 51:252, 1980.

180. Carney JA, Sizemore GW, Tyce GM: Bilateral adrenal medullary hyperplasia in multiple endocrine neoplasia, Type 2. The precursor of bilateral pheochromocytoma. Mayo Clin Proc 50:3, 1975.

181. Brunt LM, Wells SA Jr: Advances in the diagnosis and treatment of medullary thyroid carcinoma. Surg Clin North Am 67:263, 1987.

182. Telander RL, Zimmerman D, van Heerden JA, et al: Results of early thyroidectomy for medullary thyroid carcinoma in children with multiple endocrine neoplasia type 2. J Pediatr Surg 12:1190, 1986.

183. Gagel RF, Tashjian AH Jr, Cummings T, et al: The clinical outcome of prospective screening for multiple endocrine neoplasia type 2a. An 18 year experience. N Engl J Med 318:478, 1988.

184. Khairi MRA, Dexter RN, Burzynski NJ, et al: Mu-

cosal neuroma, pheochromocytoma and medullary thyroid carcinoma: multiple endocrine neoplasia type 3. Medicine 54:89, 1975.

185. Carney JA, Go VLW, Sizemore GW, et al: Alimentary tract ganglioneuromatosis. N Engl J Med 295:1287, 1976.

186. Carney JA, Hayles AB: Alimentary tract manifestations of multiple endocrine neoplasia, Type 2b. Mayo Clin Proc 52:543, 1977.

187. Kukreja SC, Hargis GK, Rosenthal IM, et al: Pheochromocytoma causing excessive parathyroid hormone production and hypercalcemia. Ann Intern Med 79:838, 1973.

188. Baum JL: Abnormal intradermal histamine reaction in the syndrome of pheochromocytoma, medullary carcinoma of the thyroid gland and multiple mucosal neuromas. N Engl J Med 284:963, 1971.

189. Hansen OP, Hansen M, Hansen HH, et al: Multiple endocrine adenomatosis of mixed type. Acta Med Scand 200:327, 1976.

190. Cameron D, Spiro HM, Landsberg L: Zollinger-Ellison syndrome with multiple endocrine adenomatosis Type II. Letter to the editor. N Engl J Med 299:152, 1978.

191. Garcia JC, Carney JA, Stickler GB, et al: Zollinger-Ellison syndrome and neurofibromatosis in a 13 year old boy. J Pediatr 93:982, 1978.

8

THE OVARY AND FEMALE SEXUAL MATURATION

Robert L. Rosenfield

DEVELOPMENT OF THE FEMALE REPRODUCTIVE SYSTEM

Puberty (adolescence) is the stage of transition from the sexually immature to the potentially fertile stage during which secondary sexual characteristics appear.

By the mid-1960s a general concept of the major factors involved in the initiation of puberty was established (Fig. 8–1).[1,2] A decrease in sensitivity of the brain "gonadostat" to sex hormone negative feedback was thought to be the primary event. This signaled the hypothalamus to discharge neurohumors (then unidentified), which in turn stimulated the pituitary to release gonadotropins. The resultant rise in gonadotropin [luteinizing hormone (LH) and follicle-stimulating hormone (FSH)] secretion was thought to account straightforwardly for increased estrogen production by the ovary. A mature relationship was thought to develop in which the blood levels of estrogen and gonadotropins were regulated reciprocally via the gonadostat,[3] much as a furnace is regulated by a thermostat. The pineal had been identified as having gonadal suppressive properties. The increased adrenocortical secretion of 17-ketosteroids (17-KS), which begins at about the time of puberty ("adrenarche"), was thought to be due to a pituitary factor stimulating adrenal androgens in synergism with adrenocorticotropic hormone (ACTH).[4]

The rapid scientific advances since 1965 have permitted this concept to be tested in increasingly sophisticated ways. In the subsequent decade, radioimmunoassay, originally developed by Yalow and Berson, was applied to the measurement of gonadotropins and sex steroids; the gonadotropin-releasing hormone (GnRH) for both LH and FSH was isolated, identified, and synthesized by Guillemin's and Schally's groups. The adenylate cyclase system, postulated by Sutherland to mediate the action of peptide hormones, was found to mediate gonadotropin effects on the ovarian follicle. The initial steps in the mechanism of action of steroid hormones were defined by Jensen, Gorski, and their groups. The landmark nature of many of these discoveries has been recognized by the awarding of Nobel Prizes in Medicine to Sutherland in 1971 and to Yalow, Schally, and Guillemin in 1977.

Our present concept of the mechanisms controlling puberty is more refined and complex than it once was, although the above schema is correct in a general sense. The gonadostat is a patently oversimplistic concept for but one aspect of a complex system that regulates the hypothalamic pulse generator. The gonadostat setting seems to change throughout childhood in a biphasic manner. This model is illustrated in Figure 8–2.[5,6] During fetal life the gonadostat is insensitive to negative feedback by sex hormones; it matures during infancy, but does not become highly sensitive until mid childhood. During late prepuberty the gonadostat relinquishes its inhibition at first slowly, then with increasing rapidity. The changing set-point initially permits increasing, episodic secretion of GnRH. Increasing sensitivity of the pituitary gonadotropic cells to GnRH follows. The change in LH and FSH secretion is first detectable at night. Eventually the gonads become increasingly sensitized to gonadotropin stimulation, grow at an increased rate, and bring about sustained rises in plasma sex hormone levels. Some of these phenomena synergize with others, so that auto-amplification occurs and the pace of change accelerates. Eventually the set-

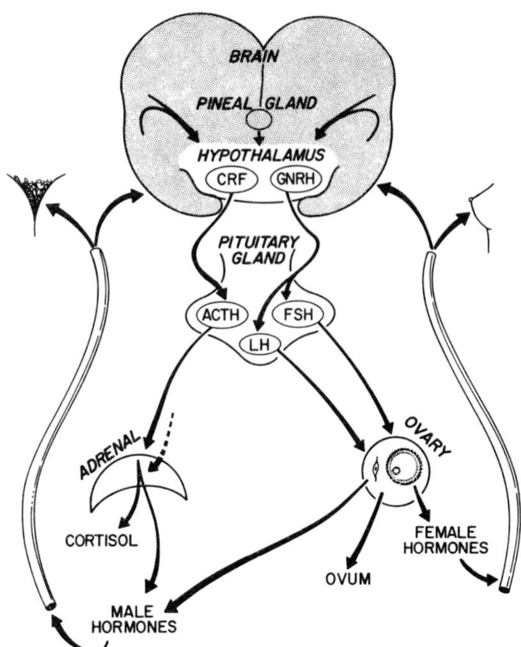

FIGURE 8–1. Diagrammatic representation or the neuroendocrine-ovarian axis involved in normal pubertal development.

point for gonadotropin release comes to vary sufficiently to encompass a positive feedback mechanism: that is, the pituitary acquires the ability to secrete a surge of LH when the ovary signals via increasing estrogen secretion that it is prepared for ovulation.

The data on which this model is based are presented below. The most recent data on the hormonal milieu and accompanying physical stages of normal puberty are then presented. Abnormal puberty is subsequently discussed: the causes, differential diagnosis, and management.

Maturation of the Neuroendocrine-Ovarian Axis

Fetus

Neuroendocrine Unit. The anterior lobe of the pituitary gland, of stomal ectodermal origin, and posterior lobe, of neural origin, differentiate by 11 weeks' gestational age.[7] Gonadotropin-releasing hormone is detectable in the hypothalamus, and LH and FSH are detectable in the pituitary gland by this time. Hypothalamic GnRH rises in parallel with fetal pituitary and serum LH and FSH.[8] All peak at about 20 to 24 weeks to levels not again seen until the mature midcycle surge.[9–12] The connections of the pituitary portal system reach completeness at about this time.[12]

Female fetuses have greater serum LH and FSH levels than males. It is disputed whether the hypothalamic GnRH of females is greater. Indirect evidence in favor of a possible difference between the sexes is the experimental evidence that GnRH-containing neurons develop earlier in female than in male rats[13] and that neonatal androgen exposure of the rat permanently diminishes the development of one of the major GnRH-

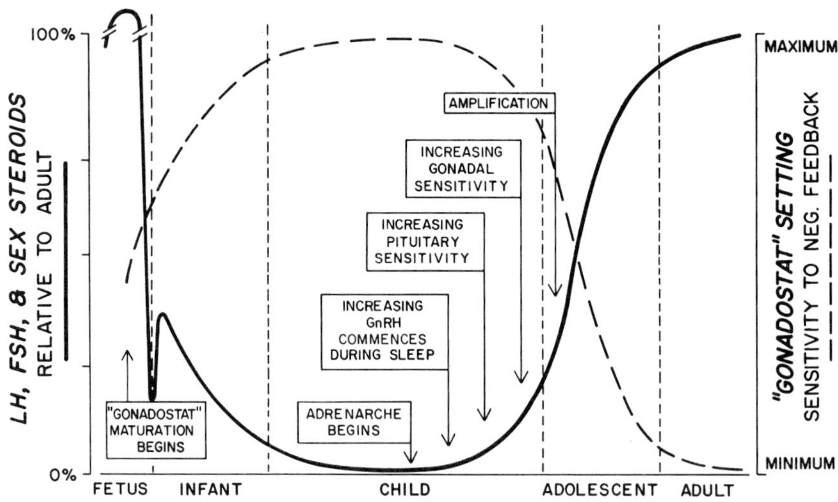

FIGURE 8–2. The changing pattern of serum gonadotropins and sex hormones from fetal life to maturity in relationship to the apparent sensitivity of the CNS "gonadostat" to the negative feedback effect of sex hormones and the underlying hormonal events. (Modified from Grumbach et al.[5] and Winter et al.[6])

containing areas (the preoptic-strial).[14,15] The androgen-mediated event may well occur in the human in early to midgestation, the stage at which the human fetal testes are actively secreting and completing phallic differentiation[16] and that corresponds to other maturational events in the neonatal rat.[11]

In late gestation hypothalamic GnRH and pituitary LH and FSH secretions begin to wane. These changes seem partly due to the hypothalamus coming under control of inhibitory central nervous system (CNS) influences and partly due to the increased sex steroids produced by the fetoplacental unit. If this maturation is not complete in utero, it goes to completion in postnatal life; prematurely born girls have higher serum LH and FSH levels than full-term ones.[12]

The production of gonadotropins by the fetal pituitary seems to be necessary for normal ovarian development. Hypophysectomy of rhesus fetuses has been reported to reduce the number of germ cells and oocytes as well as the integrity of the rete ovarii.[17] Therefore, it seems that survival of gametes depends upon the secretions of the fetal pituitary. The mechanism is unclear; this pituitary effect may be indirect, mediated through accelerated atresia, lack of support of the rete system, or lack of stimulation of the follicle.

Ovary. The ovaries differentiate in the urogenital ridge adjacent to the anlagen of adrenal cortex and the kidney. The granulosa cells are the homologues of the Sertoli cells. The theca, interstitial, and hilus cells are the homologs of the Leydig cells of the testes; hilus cells may even contain crystalloids like Leydig cells. Adrenocortical rests occasionally come to lie in the hilus of the ovary.[18] The ovaries are distinguishable from testes at about 40 days' gestation.[19]

The primitive germ cells migrate into the ovary from the yolk sac endoderm during the first month of gestation. The oogonia then go through mitotic division; this stage begins to wane at the third month, but continues up to the seventh month. They then undergo oogenesis, entering the prophase of meiosis to become oocytes,[20] during the final 5 to 6 months of gestation. The number of oocytes reaches a peak at the fifth month.[21] When oocytes enter the diplotene stage of meiotic prophase they must be furnished with granulosa cells to form a primordial follicle, or else they undergo atresia.[22] Primordial follicles appear in the fourth month—this is much later than the organization of the analogous structure in the testes, the tubules—and peak in number between the fifth and ninth months. Preantral follicles, with their increasing granulosa cell proliferation and organization of theca, appear in later gestation. The number of small preantral follicles is at its peak at term. After the seventh month, antral follicles appear.[23,24] Typically one or two antral follicles of 1 to 2 mm in diameter are present in the ovary by term. Thus, at birth ovarian follicle development is fully complete (Fig. 8–3),[25,26] and the complement of ova is greater than at any other time during postnatal life (Fig. 8–4).

This differentiation of the gonad along ovarian lines occurs in the absence of a testes-determining factor.[27]

The maintenance of the oocyte population is clearly dependent upon the presence of a normal X-chromosome complement within the germ cell. Studies of glucose-6-phosphate dehydrogenase (G6PD) electrophoretic patterns indicate that both X chromosomes of the oocyte are active, in contrast to the situation in somatic cells.[29] This interpretation is consistent with the finding that fetuses with a 45,XO karyotype have a normal number of early oocytes in the ovary, but a drastic reduction in the number of follicles.[30]

The initiation of meiosis and differentiation of the granulosa cell layer of the follicle have been postulated to be related to the interaction of the rete ovarii with the ovarian cortex.[31] The thymus may somehow be involved in follicular differentiation. Children with ataxia telangiectasia have decreased numbers of ovarian follicles.[22] Furthermore, thymectomy of the female mouse neonatally (equivalent to intrauterine thymectomy in man) interferes with subsequent sexual differentiation; there is evidence that this effect is independent of infection.[32]

The major source of sex hormones in the female fetus is the fetoplacental unit. The fetal ovary does not seem to contribute appreciably to the fetal hormonal milieu. Estradiol (E2) and testosterone have not been detected in fetal ovaries, although Goldman et al. and Winter et al. have shown that the capacity to synthesize some precursors exists.[22]

Infants and Children

Neuroendocrine Unit. The neonate undergoes a minipuberty. Serum FSH and

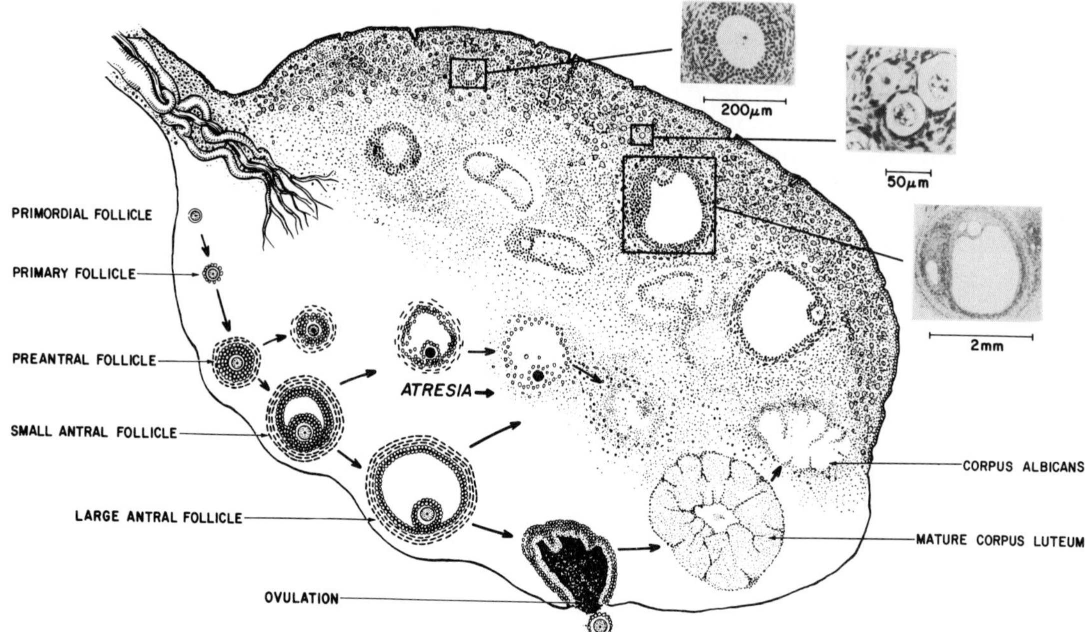

FIGURE 8–3. The human ovary. The lower portion of the figure shows the classification of follicles.[22] A primordial follicle consists of a "naked" germ cell. Primary follicles are enclosed by a ring of granulosa cells. Preantral (type 3–5, growing secondary, or medium) follicles are growing and have a thecal layer. They contain up to 300 granulosa cells. Their diameter ranges from 50 to 200 μm. The oocyte diameter increases from 25 or less to 80 microns. Antral (graffian, tertiary, or vesicular) follicles have a fluid-filled antrum and a full-grown oocyte, are lined by over 300 granulosa cells, and have a well-developed theca; they are over 200 μm in diameter. The dimensions of the mature ovary are about 1.25 × 2.75 × 4 cm. (Photomicrographs of ovarian details are reproduced from Peters H: The human ovary in childhood and early maturity. Eur J Obstet Gynecol Reprod Biol 9/3: 137, 1979.) The upper portion of the figure diagrammatically illustrates the histologic appearance of the perimenarchial ovary (modified from Ross and Schreiber[25]).

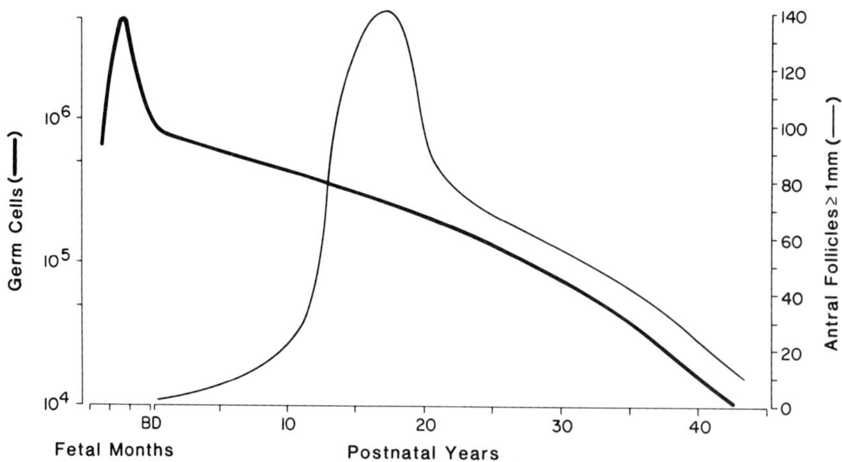

FIGURE 8–4. The development of ovarian follicles from fetal life to maturity. Curves for total number of germ cells (heavy line) and large antral follicles (thin line) smoothed from the data of Baker[21] and Block.[23] The loss of germ cells is exponential throughout postnatal life.[24] At puberty a marked shift occurs in the pattern of development of follicles: an increased fraction grows to large antral size.

LH are low in cord blood, then increase significantly (Fig. 8–5).[6,33,34] This neonatal rise in gonadotropins commences when the estrogen concentrations fall from inhibitory levels at birth because of disruption of the fetoplacental unit. Subsequently, serum LH rises for several months and serum FSH rises for much of infancy to levels greater than those of males. These phenomena seem to be related to a lack of maturation of CNS inhibitory tracts, as if the gonadostat were relatively insensitive to sex hormone levels. That the sensitivity of the gonadostat of young infants is akin to that of adults is indicated by the rise of serum gonadotropins to the postmenopasual range in congenital agonadism.[35]

In later infancy both FSH and LH begin to fall to low levels (Fig. 8–5). One cause of this fall may well be an increase in hypothalamic estrogen receptors. Hypothalamic E2 receptors increase in a pattern reciprocal to the fall in serum gonadotropins in the rat (Fig. 8–6).[36] A similar pattern has been reported for hypothalamic dihydrotestosterone (DHT) receptors.[37] These changes in the efficiency with which the hypothalamus can recognize sex hormones could account for its increasing sensitivity to the inhibitory effect of small amounts of circulating E2 and testosterone. However, it seems likely than an even more important mechanism for the fall in gonadotropins is the maturation of neural tracts that bring the hypothalamus under strong inhibitory influences from the CNS gonadostat.

The relatively high serum FSH levels of younger girls tend to persist into early childhood.[33,38] Immunoreactive GnRH excretion tends to be greater in girls than in boys at this time.[39]

A nadir in both serum gonadotropins occurs by about 6 years of age (Figs. 8–2 and

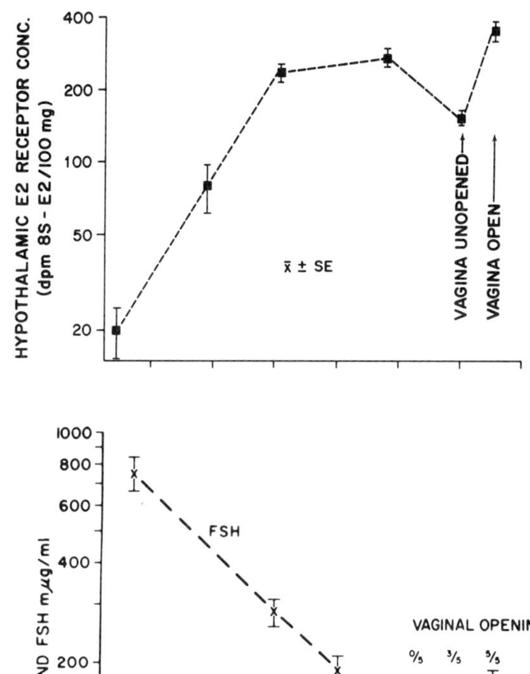

FIGURE 8–6. Relationship of maturation of hypothalamic estrogen receptors (*top*) to serum gonadotropin levels (*bottom*) in the developing female rat. (From data of Kato et al. and Odell et al.; reproduced with permission from Rosenfield RL: Hormonal events and disorders of puberty. *In* Gynecologic Endocrinology. Chicago, Year Book Medical Publishers, 1977.)

8–5). At this age the LH and FSH response to GnRH is also minimal and often undetectable. Furthermore, at this stage agonadism is seldom reflected in a rise in serum gonadotropins or gonadotropin reserve.[34,35] These data support the concept that the gonadostat sensitivity to negative feedback—by small amounts of gonadal and adrenal steroids—is at its maximum in midchildhood.

Although gonadotropin production is at its nadir in midchildhood, it is not completely suppressed.[40] Gonadotropin activity is detectable, at the limits of sensitivity of the mouse uterine weight assay, in 14 per cent of 24-hour urine specimens from young prepubertal children. Specific FSH and LH bioassays on concentrates of urine have revealed 2- to 6-year-old children to excrete

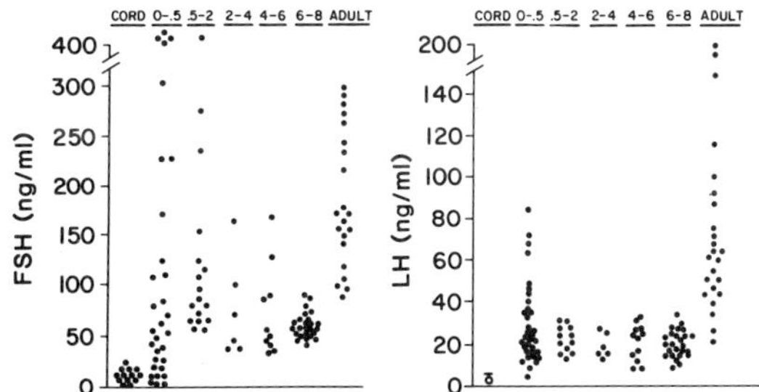

FIGURE 8–5. The distribution of serum FSH and LH levels from infancy through adulthood (data of Winter and Faiman[6,33,34]). Umbilical cord level of LH measured by β subunit–specific RIA from Kaplan et al.[9]

averages of 1.1 IU FSH/day and 0.22 IU LH/day. This amount of FSH is about 15 per cent of that excreted by the adult; this amount of LH is 3 per cent of that excreted by the adult. Immunoreactive LH and FSH have been detected by radioimmunoassay (RIA) in most 24-hour urine specimens from children, even those negative by bioassay. Rifkind et al. found the relatively tonic immunoreactive LH and FSH excretion to be punctuated by intermittent bursts of increased LH excretion.[41] Similarly, RIA detects FSH and LH in the serum of most prepubertal children.

Between 5 and 9 years of age, estimation of urinary FSH by radioimmunoassay indicates a doubling of production, with a less dramatic change in LH excretion. This change correlates with rising excretion of immunoreactive GnRH.[39] The findings indicate that hormonal changes signaling development of puberty are found late in the first decade of life. Close examination of the LH pattern in man suggests that GnRH is always secreted in an episodic fashion and that the increase in secretion commences at night in prepuberty. An episodic flux of LH serum levels at about 1- to 2-hour intervals[42] and a diurnal variation in LH excretion[43,44] have been discerned—albeit at low levels—in prepubertal children. Thus, the hormonal secretory pattern of the prepubertal 9-year-old child is different from that of the 6-year-old.

The gonadotropins detected by bioassay appear to be bioactive judging from the ovarian changes during childhood. Gonadotropins stimulate follicular growth in a dose-dependent way and are required for antrum formation,[45] which is observed in childhood.

Ovary. The ovary of the infant and child is not quiescent, contrary to earlier conceptions. The ovary develops responsiveness to gonadotropins very early.[46] Autopsy studies of older infants and children who have died suddenly and unexpectedly also indicate that the ovary is active at this time.[22]

Follicles start to grow and many reach the antral stage at all ages. The number of large antral follicles approximately doubles over that in infancy by 7 years, and quadruples by 9 years (Fig. 8–4). As many as six antral follicles normally occur in an ovary and reach a diameter as great as 7 mm.[22,47] However, all large antral follicles normally undergo atresia in childhood.[22] The ovary increases in size mainly because the stroma is augmented as atresia takes place in follicles that are continuously beginning to grow.

Plasma E2 levels parallel those of FSH, rising to early pubertal levels for the first several months of life and falling gradually thereafter (Fig. 8–7).[48]

Since FSH sometimes reaches the adult range in infant girls (Fig. 8–5), the reason why more ovaries do not go on to complete maturation is probably either because the FSH reaches adult height only episodically and/or because LH levels are not coincidentally high enough to stimulate sufficient synthesis of E2 precursors. However, on occasion there is detectable estrogen production.[33,48,49]

Puberty

The endocrinologic changes of puberty actually begin in late preadolescence before secondary sex characteristics appear. The underlying basic event is increasing secretion of hypothalamic GnRH.

Increased GnRH secretion in man was initially deduced when Kastin, Job, and Grumbach and their collaborators demonstrated that preadolescent children had GnRH-releasable pituitary stores of LH and FSH (Fig. 8–8).[50] Subsequently, it was reported that in man the excretion of an immunoreactive fragment of GnRH increases to adult levels during puberty.[39,51] Studies in the rat suggest that hypothalamic GnRH increases through puberty, with a greater fraction entering free granules from synaptosome stores with increasing age.[52]

Knobil subsequently showed that puberty can be induced in the immature female rhesus monkey by administering GnRH in hourly pulses that yield blood levels of about 2000 pg/ml.[53] Prolonged administration of GnRH according to this regimen first gradually brought about transient increases in LH and FSH. This then induced cyclic follicular development. The resultant moderate E2 surge was of such magnitude as to result in menarche due to withdrawal menstrual bleeding in an anovulatory cycle (Fig. 8–9). Continuation of the same GnRH regimen led to development of normal monthly ovulatory menstrual periods. Physiologic pulses of GnRH in man probably attain lower concentrations (200 pg/ml) and are less frequent (every 100 min) than in monkeys.[54]

The fact that the hormonal secretory pat-

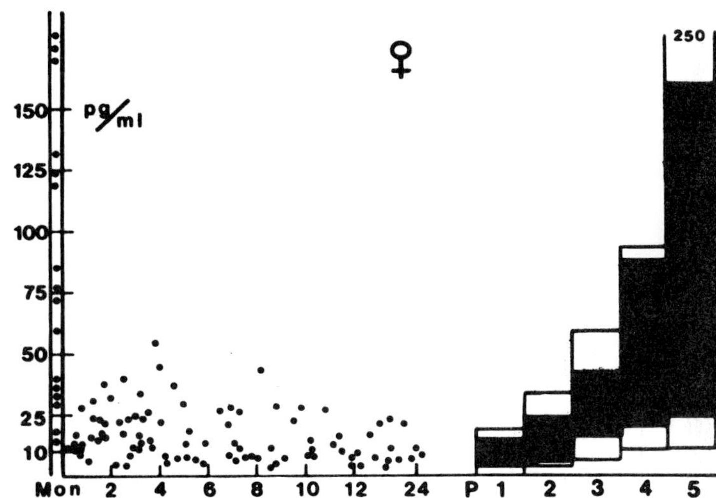

FIGURE 8–7. The distribution of plasma E2 levels in infant females, compared with pubertal and adult female levels. The columns represent the normal ranges for the various stages of puberty; the area between 10th and 90th percentiles is dark. Stage P1 includes all prepubertal girls older than 2 years. The values between the ordinates were found between 2 and 5 days of age. (from Bidlingmeier F, Knorr D: Oestrogens: Physiological and clinical aspects. Pediatr Adolesc Endocrinol 4:43, 1978.)

terns of puberty begin at night was first shown by Boyar et al. in 1972. They measured serum LH and FSH concentrations in blood drawn at 20-min intervals for 24 hours.[55] Prepubertal children have low LH levels around the clock. In early pubertal children, LH rises significantly with the onset of sleep and returns to prepubertal levels before awakening. With further maturation nocturnal LH rises further and

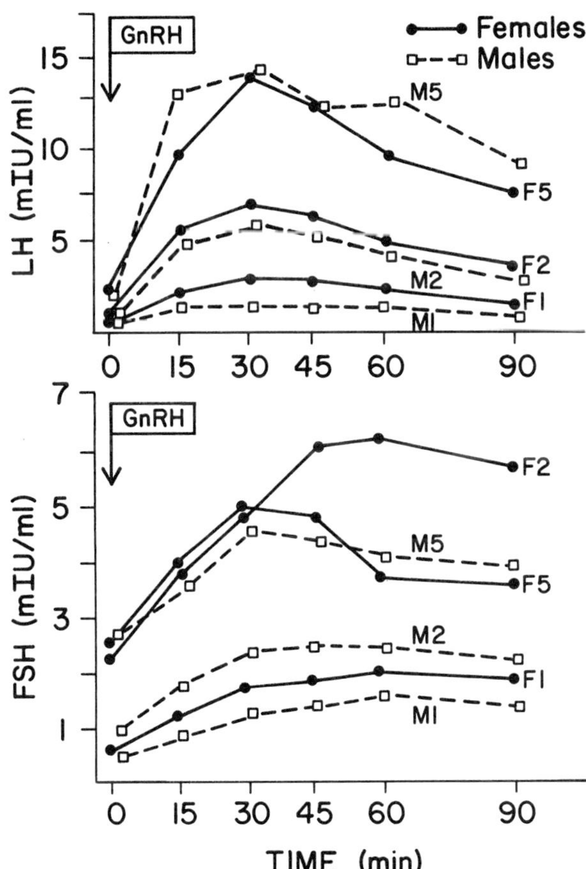

FIGURE 8–8. The LH and FSH responses to GnRH bolus (50 μg/m^2) in males (M) and females (F) in prepuberty (ages $\geq$ 5–6 yr; F1, M1), early puberty (F2, M2), and later puberty (F5, M5). The responses to GnRH tend to progress with advancing puberty; however, early pubertal girls have a readily releasable FSH pool that is greater than that of more advanced adolescents. The peak responses of girls tend to be somewhat greater than those of boys at comparable stages. (Redrawn from the data of Dickerman et al.[50])

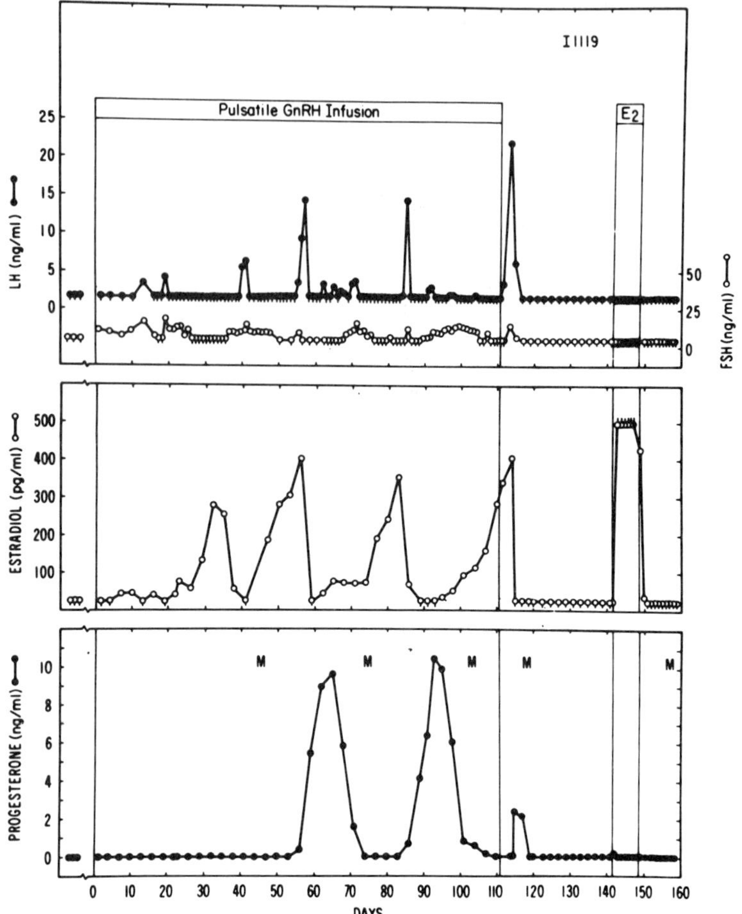

FIGURE 8–9. Induction of puberty in a 13-month-old prepubertal rhesus monkey by an unvarying, pulsatile GnRH regimen (1 μg/min × 6 min hourly). Luteinizing hormone, FSH, E2, and progesterone were undetectable prior to the GnRH infusion. Upon GnRH infusion, the duration of which is shown by the horizontal open bar, a rise in FSH was the first change detectable by midmorning sampling midway between GnRH pulses. A substantial E2 surge occurred about 1 month later. The subsequent LH surge was too modest to elicit ovulation, but menses (M) occurred a few days after subsidence of the week-long E2 surge—menarche resulting from an anovulatory cycle. Continuation of the GnRH led to the sustained occurrence of ovulatory menstrual cycles at 28-day intervals. An identical outcome results if an arcuate-lesioned adult animal undergoes this GnRH regimen. The third of the LH surges occurred 2 days after GnRH was discontinued. Progesterone secretion from the corpus luteum was blunted and transient in the absence of sustained LH secretion. A subsequent increase in plasma E2 produced by E2 implantation subcutaneously failed to elicit a gonadotropin surge, indicating that the animal had reverted to an immature state. Menarche eventually spontaneously recurred in such animals at the usual age (about 27 months). Small vertical lines beneath data points indicate values below the sensitivity of the assay. Note that gonadotropins and E2 were often undetectable ("prepubertal" range) during the induced puberty. (Reproduced from Knobil E: The neuroendocrine control of the menstrual cycle. Recent Prog Horm Res 36:53, 1980.)

longer; then the amplitude of daytime pulsations begins to increase. As the child approaches menarche, the daytime LH levels continue to increase until the mature adult pattern is achieved, in which this diurnal gonadotropin rhythm no longer persists. This pattern was subsequently shown to be true for FSH as well, although the FSH changes are less striking. The pubertal diurnal rhythm is more resistant to acute sleep reversal than is that of growth hormone.[56] These changes are shown together with the resultant E2 changes in a pubertal girl in Figure 8–10.[57]

These studies have led to the current concept that puberty results when the hypothalamus begins to release GnRH with increasing frequency and amplitude, first only at night, then around the clock. This concept also helps explain why FSH increases out

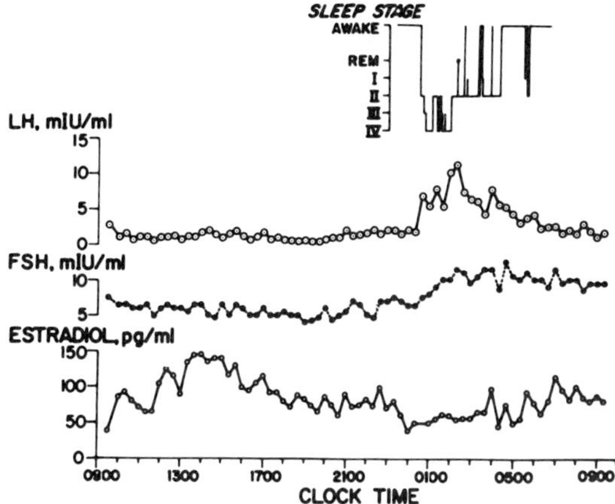

FIGURE 8–10. The patterns of serum LH, FSH and E2 typical of early female puberty. Note that daytime gonadotropin levels are in the "prepubertal" range. Note also the episodic nature of LH release at intervals of 1 to 3 hours. Estradiol levels are seen to fluctuate considerably in the course of the daytime, rising to peak levels about 12 hours after the maximum nocturnal gonadotropin surges. (Reproduced from Boyar RM, Wu RHK, Roffwarg H, et al: Human puberty: 24-hour estradiol patterns in pubertal girls. J Clin Endocrinol Metab 43:1418, 1976.)

of proportion to LH early in puberty.[33,40] When GnRH pulses are given infrequently, the FSH:LH ratio is high. This difference in FSH:LII ratios resulting from changing GnRH frequency is explicable at least in part by the differences in serum half-lives of LH and FSH. The latter is cleared much more slowly (see later in this chapter), and this leads to longer persistence of FSH in serum after its release.

This early predominance of FSH has important biologic consequences. It leads to relatively selective growth and development of the follicular compartment of the ovary. Furthermore, the gonadotropin changes seem to be cyclic from their very onset[34,58] and capable of inducing cyclic estrogen production.[33,49,53] Our working model of the nature of pituitary-ovarian dynamics in early puberty is illustrated in Figure 8–11.

Augmentation of the bioactivity of plasma gonadotropin(s) occurs during puberty. Plasma LH bioactivity rises nearly fivefold more during the course of puberty than does LH as measured by RIA (Fig. 8–12).[59] The reason for the disparity between bioactive LH (B-LH) and immunoreactive LH (I-LH) is unclear. Androgens increase[60] and estrogens decrease the LH biopotency by altering LH sialylation. In addition, during puberty there are changing proportions of

biologically inactive material within plasma radioimmunoassayable LH.[61] A change in the amount of substance(s) other than LH that affect LH bioactivity is unlikely. The heterogeneity of serum LH probably reflects altered production of intermediary LH metabolites.

A variety of auto-amplification phenomena occur that facilitate puberty, maturation of the dominant follicle, and ovulation. These are summarized in Table 8–1.[62-75] These phenomena occur at all levels of the axis. The CNS is stimulated by preovulatory levels of E2 to increase GnRH pulse size. At the pituitary level there is the self-priming effect of GnRH, whereby a pulse of GnRH sensitizes the pituitary to have a greater LH response to a subsequent identical GnRH pulse. Critical patterns of E2 and progesterone secretion enhance the pituitary LH and FSH responsiveness to GnRH. At the gonadal level, the cascade of events is augmented by the FSH induction of aromatase activity and progestin production in granulosa cells, phenomena in which androgens play a synergistic role. Furthermore, FSH stimulates granulosa cell meiosis and induces LH receptors, phenomena in which E2 plays a synergistic role. Subsequently, LH is able to further enhance the aromatase and progesterone effects. Progesterone itself plays a synergistic role in stimulating granulosa cell progesterone and prostaglandin synthesis in concert with both FSH and LH.

Just before ovulation in the rat, ovarian GnRH receptor sites diminish.[76] At about this time the ovary changes its pattern of metabolism so that the secretion of androstanediol-3β-monosulfate decreases to levels that are no longer inhibitory to LH secretion.[77] It is unknown whether such phenomena are important in other species.

The preovulatory gonadotropin surge occurs when all these interrelating, cascading processes culminate in activation of the positive feedback mechanism, the hallmark of sexual maturity. "Positive feedback" refers to the ability of female hormones to stimulate the mature midcycle surge of pituitary gonadotropins.

Menarche does not necessarily indicate full maturation of the neuroendocrine-ovarian axis. As the studies of Knobil illustrate (Fig. 8–9), the first menstruation can be due to estrogen-withdrawal bleeding—and usually is—but ovulatory cycles may follow in short order. General characteristics of the

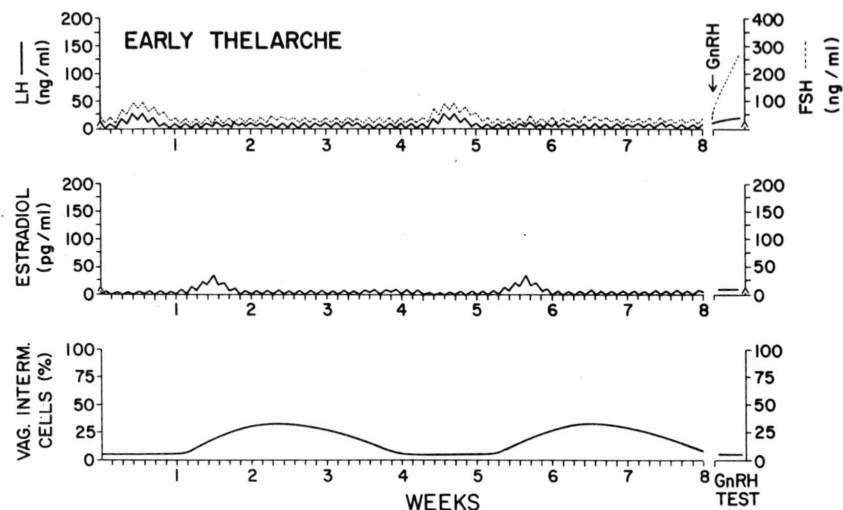

FIGURE 8–11. Diagram depicting our working hypothesis of the hormonal patterns in girls during very early puberty. We conceptualize this pattern as occurring both cyclically in the earliest stage of normal puberty and occasionally in unsustained sexual precocity (i.e., most U.S. cases of idiopathic premature thelarche). Day- and nighttime serum concentrations of hormones (gonadotropins relative to the LER-907 standard) and the percentage of intermediate cells on vaginal smear are shown. The typical response to a GnRH test is illustrated.

Subclinical hormonal cycles lasting about 1 month result from a few days of increased FSH and LH secretion. Because the drive to gonadotropin release is relatively weak, FSH and LH production are suppressed promptly and for long periods of time by the resultant modest amounts of E2 secretion. Estradiol is detectable in plasma for only a few days a month. Maturation of the vaginal mucosa, however, is detectable for about 2 weeks after E2 production has waned.

perimenarcheal ovary are shown in Figure 8–3.

Adult

Normal Menstrual Cycle: Hormone Patterns. In many respects, puberty is recapitulated during the follicular phase of each menstrual cycle. The pattern of gonadotropin and steroid hormone levels is shown in Fig. 8–13.[78,79] Gonadotropin and sex hormone levels are low during the premenstrual phase of the mature cycle (Fig. 8–13A). Gonadotropin concentrations then increase at the time of menstruation, FSH predominating while nocturnal LH pulsation is slow[80] (Fig. 8–13B). Luteinizing hormone pulsation increases to a stable circhoral pattern and E2 production slowly begins (Fig. 8–13C). Estradiol levels gradually increase and serum FSH levels fall reciprocally (Fig. 8–13D). The subsequent geometric increase in plasma E2 concentrations then selec-

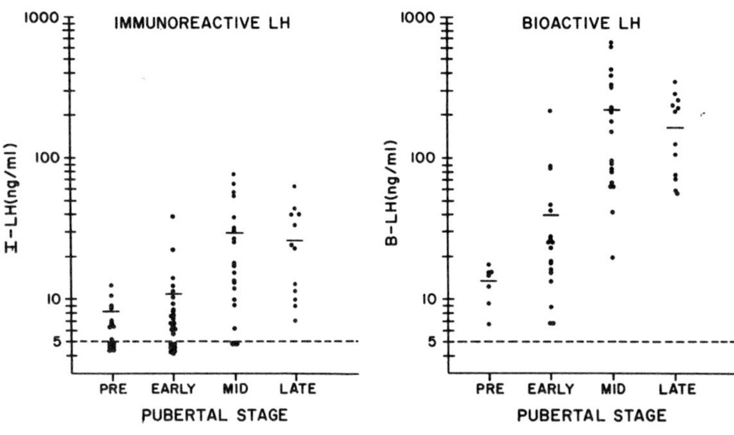

FIGURE 8–12. Bioactive LH (B-LH) (right panel) and immunoreactive LH (I-LH) (left panel) in the same daytime serum samples of girls 10 to 16 years of age at various pubertal stages. The dashed lines indicate the limit of sensitivity of the assays. Bioactive-LH rises relatively more than I-LH in the course of puberty. The peak in the apparent biopotency of LH, estimated from the ratio of B-LH to I-LH, occurs at about the time of menarche. Late = early follicular phase, normally menstruating, postmenarchial girls. (Data from Lucky et al.[59])

TABLE 8–1. AUTO-AMPLIFICATION PROCESSES INVOLVED IN PUBERTAL PROGRESSION, FOLLICLE MATURATION & OVULATION

1. Central nervous system GnRH secretion increases via:
   a. E2 inducing progesterone receptors[65]
   b. Progesterone synergizes with E2[64]
2. Pituitary LH and FSH responsiveness to GnRH increases via:
   a. GnRH self-priming[66]
   b. Critical patterns of E2 secretion stimulating LH/FSH responsiveness[67–69]; progesterone synergizes with E2[68–70]
   c. LH bioactivity increasing[59]
3. Gonadal responsiveness to FSH and LH increases via
   a. FSH-inducing aromatase and progesterone in granulosa cells; androgens and progesterone synergize with this effect[71–73]
   b. FSH-stimulated granulosa meiosis[74] and FSH-inducing granulosa LH receptors[75]; estrogens synergize with this effect[74]

tively amplifies the pituitary's LH response to GnRH as E2 reaches about 90 pg/ml for over 3 days[67–69] (Fig. 8–13E). When the plasma E2 rises to over 200 to 300 pg/ml, the positive feedback mechanism is activated and the midcycle gonadotropin surge commences (Fig. 8–13F). Estradiol then induces the progesterone receptor in the hypothalamus and pituitary.[65] Progesterone increasing to 100 ng/dl facilitates the LH surge, shortens the duration of time over which E2 is required for the surge from 36 to 24 hrs, and brings about an FSH surge. The mech-anism of progesterone action involves inhibition of GnRH cleavage.[70] Androgens may play a role in facilitating FSH[81] and GnRH[82] release. The LH surge is then primarily responsible for luteinizing the preovulatory ovarian follicle (Fig. 8–13F). At this time, LH pulses become larger and their apparent bioactivity increases. Then ovulation results.

Estrogen levels fall when the follicle is disrupted (Fig. 8–13G). As the corpus luteum begins to form, progesterone increases steadily, followed by increasing E2 and 17-hydroxyprogesterone levels (Fig. 8–13H). These steroids are all sustained at high levels for several days. In response to the high progesterone level, gonadotropin pulsation slows.[83] In the absence of increasing human chorionic gonadotropin (hCG) from a conceptus, the corpus luteum's life span is exhausted and its production of progesterone and E2 wanes. Subsequently, FSH begins to rise out of proportion to LH. Shortly after the sex steroids withdraw from the scene, the endometrium sloughs, giving rise to menstrual flow. Meanwhile, the FSH-induced follicular growth begins to gain momentum and the next cycle begins.

Follicular (Proliferative) Phase Ovary. The hormonal functions of the follicle have dual purposes that must be closely coordinated: to change the milieu of the ovum to prepare for ovulation and to signal the pituitary to send its ovulatory messenger (LH). Thus, the ovary is the *zeitgeber* for the cycle, the normal cyclic pattern of ovarian hormone secretion acting directly on pituitary gonadotrophs that are being stimulated by normal circhoral pulses of GnRH.[53] The processes that are triggered also auto-amplify the gonadotropin signal (Table 8–1). Ovarian hormones even play a facilitating role in this event by augmenting the amplitude of the GnRH response,[62–64] thereby "guaranteeing" a preovulatory gonadotropin surge.

Ovarian follicular steroid hormone biosynthesis seems best explained by a two-compartment model.[74,75,84] Figure 8–14 diagrammatically illustrates in detail our current concept of ovarian follicular development and sex steroid secretion in relationship to changing gonadotropin levels. Thecal-interstitial cells, which contain only LH receptors, secrete androgen and encircle granulosa cells. These contain only FSH receptors and aromatize androgen to estrogen (Fig. 8–14A).

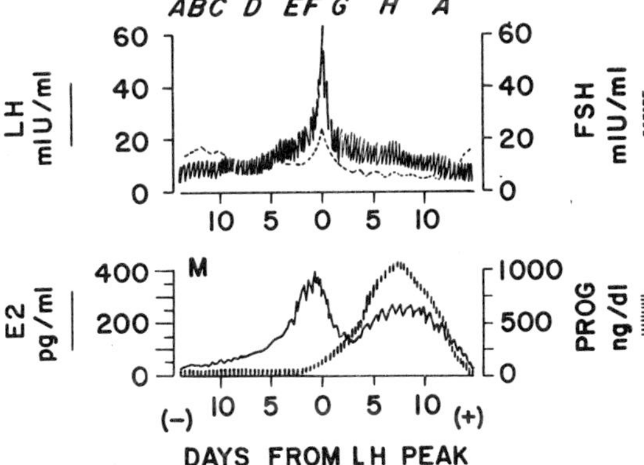

FIGURE 8–13. Mean gonadotropin and sex steroid levels during the normal menstrual cycle. The data are centered in reference to days before (−) or after (+) the day of the LH peak (day 0). Letters A through F above the top panel correspond to stages of follicular development in Figure 8–14. M (lower panel) shows time of menses. PROG, progesterone. (Drawn from the data of Abraham[78] and Ross et al.[79])

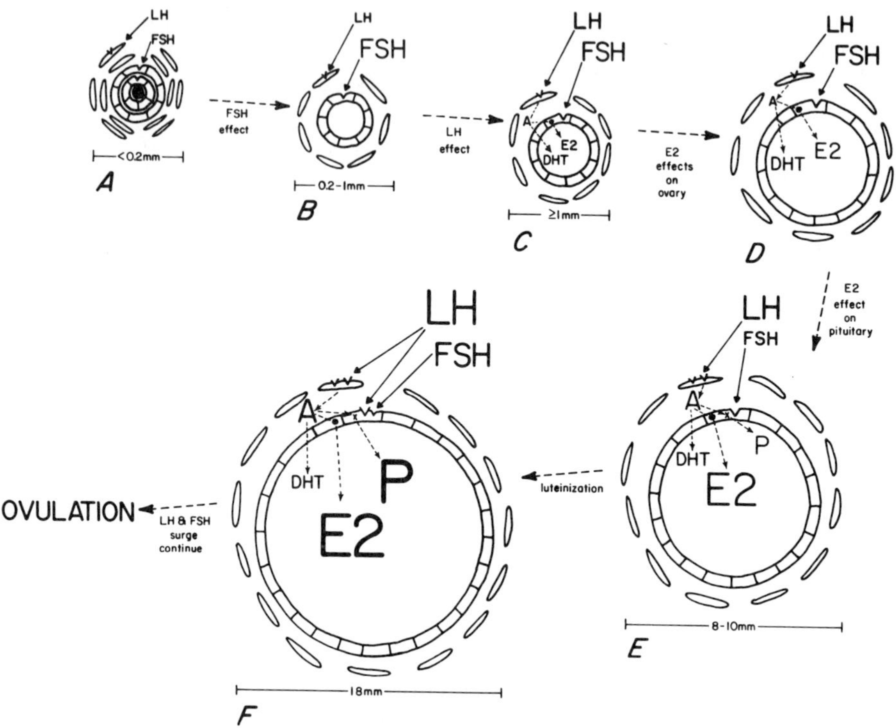

FIGURE 8–14. Relationships among gonadotropins, the ovarian follicle, and ovarian steroids. *A* through *F* depict stages of ovarian follicular development found during the times of the menstrual cycle designated by the corresponding letters on Figure 8–13. The size of the letters designating hormones relates to the magnitude of their serum and/or follicular concentrations. *A*, Preantral follicle with LH and FSH receptors in theca and granulosa cells, respectively; there is no antrum surrounding the ovum (stippled in center). *B*, Small antral follicle; this develops in response to an increase in FSH.[45] The ovum, which becomes eccentric, is not shown in any of the antral follicles. *C*, Large antral follicle (1 mm or larger). Aromatase activity (●) has been induced in granulosa cells. Interactions between theca and granulosa cells, the former producing androgens (androstenedione; A), result in estradiol (E2) and dihydrotestosterone (DHT) synthesis. *D*, Estradiol stimulates follicular growth, which in turn results in more E2 synthesis. *E*, Estradiol enhances pituitary LH secretion in response to GnRH, while at the same time inhibiting pituitary FSH secretion. The increased LH induces more theca LH receptors and stimulates androgen production. Androgens serve as substrate for E2 formation and synergize with FSH to stimulate progesterone (P) secretion. *F*, In the preovulatory follicle, FSH induces LH receptors on the granulosa cell, which completes luteinization. Steroid secretion is augmented further. Then increasing progesterone amplifies the positive feedback effect of E2 to initiate the preovulatory gonadotropin surge.

Follicle-stimulating hormone initiates granulosa cell proliferation and antrum formation,[45] which will eventually result in these cells developing the capacity to synthesize E2 (Fig. 8–14*B*). However, the small antral follicle does not produce substantial amounts of sex steroids. Luteinizing hormone stimulates the theca to develop and seems to enhance the activity of the thecal 17α-hydroxylase/lyase necessary for androgen biosynthesis.[72,85] Androgen production becomes great enough to synergize with FSH to stimulate aromatase activity within the granulosa cells[71] and to also serve as a substrate for E2 formation. As antral follicles grow to over 1 mm, their granulosa cells begin to produce E2 (Fig. 8–14*C*).[86–89]

By the midfollicular phase (Fig. 8–14*D*), the increasing local estrogenization stimulates proliferation of granulosa cells.[74] A recent study suggests that E2 may play a lesser role in primate follicular development than that deduced from studies in the rat.[90] This results in an accelerating rate of E2 production and preferential conversion of androstenedione to E2 rather than DHT by these cells.[86,87,90–93] At this time, the follicle irreversibly selected to become dominant to the exclusion of all others is the major source of E2.[94] Typically, there is only one such follicle. Only this follicle continues to grow so as to reach a diameter over 9 mm.

By the late follicular phase (Fig. 8–14*E*), pituitary LH responsiveness to GnRH is augmented by the rising E2 level. The increased LH causes further proliferation of thecal cells and an increase in their LH receptor content.[72] Androgen production is consequently increased. This synergizes with FSH—which is more effectively concentrated in the follicle in spite of its lower blood level[90]—to both augment aromatase activity and bring about increasing progesterone secretion by the well-estrogenized granulosa cells of these follicles. Progesterone then enhances the synthesis of both itself and E2.[72,73] The increased thecal androstenedione production is diverted much more to E2 than to dihydrotestosterone biosynthesis. Antral fluid steroid concentrations reflect these changes (Fig. 8–15).[86,87,90] As the gonadotropin surge commences, FSH induces LH receptors in the highly E2-primed granulosa cells.[75,84] The granulosa cells, now luteinized, augment E2 and progestin production in response to LH as well as FSH.

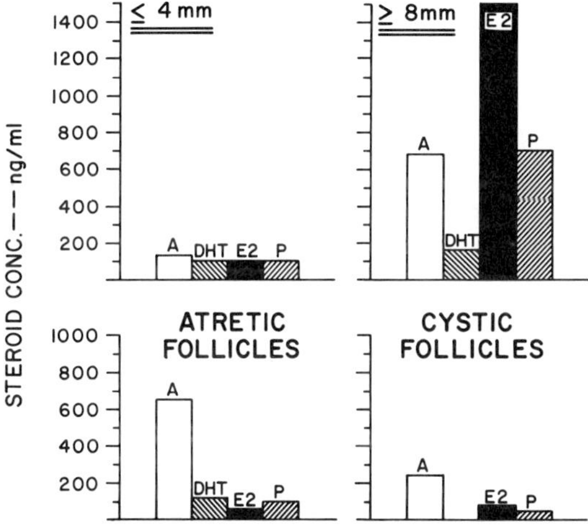

FIGURE 8–15. Normal human antral fluid steroid concentrations. Healthy follicles are well populated by granulosa cells (50 per cent or more of maximal complement). Healthy follicles seem capable of further development because many of them (75 per cent) contain healthy-appearing oocytes (histologically intact germinal vesicles), 96 per cent of which are viable in culture. Moderately large follicles (8 mm or larger diameter) only make their appearance in the midfollicular phase of the cycle and contain FSH. Data are shown only for those large follicles well populated by granulosa cells, only one of which usually arises in the follicular phase of each menstrual cycle. Atretic follicles are small follicles beginning to show degenerative changes in the number of granulosa cells and appearance of the oocyte. Cystic follicles tend to be larger follicles with only a sparse granulosa cell lining. The testosterone content of antral fluid is about one-third that of DHT, owing to the pattern of granulosa cell metabolism of androstenedione (A). P, progesterone. (Interpolated from data of McNatty et al.[86,87])

The final steps in follicle maturation happen rapidly: increasing progesterone production synergizes with increasing E2 production to stimulate a further surge of pituitary gonadotropins. Estradiol exerts this effect via positive feedback actions at both the CNS and pituitary levels. Thereafter, the follicle begins to prepare for ovulation by ceasing to grow—the mechanisms of growth arrest including desensitization of the response to LH and FSH,[95] inhibition of aromatase activity by androgen[71] and progesterone,[96,97] and production of increasing amounts of prostaglandin in response to the LH surge.[95]

Proteolytic activity then increases, the intercellular spaces fill with mucopolysaccharides, and cell junctions loosen.[74,98] Meiosis undergoes completion with the secondary oocyte being formed and the first polar body undergoing separation prior to ovulation.[99] (A premature LH surge in a subject with an unripe follicle will not result in ovulation.) Ovulation then occurs.

The processes stimulating follicular development are nicely balanced by those stimulating atresia. Androgens probably play a role in the normal process of atresia. It seems critical that the influence of androgens not become excessive or no viable follicle will develop beyond about the 6-mm stage.[89] Atretic follicles contain relatively high concentrations of androgens (Fig. 8–15). In vivo studies suggest that this is related to excessive quantities of ovarian androgens antagonizing the promotion of granulosa cell proliferation and development by E2.[100] Androgens, and progestins as well, also seem to have biphasic effects on aromatase activity such that, in contrast to the effect of low concentrations, large concentrations inhibit aromatase.[71] Furthermore, high androgen levels antagonize LH receptor formation and action.[73,101]

Inhibin is a nonsteroidal product of the granulosa cell that preferentially inhibits FSH secretion.[102] Its production is reciprocally stimulated by FSH.[103] Inhibin may not only inhibit FSH release at the pituitary level, but may act at a higher level as well.[104] Serum levels of inhibin parallel E2 levels and vary inversely with the plasma FSH.[105] Thus, suppression of FSH by inhibin acting in concert with E2 may be important in preventing more than one dominant follicle from emerging in each cycle.

Luteal (Secretory) Phase Ovary. Following ovulatory rupture of the graafian follicle, capillaries and fibroblasts from the theca proliferate and break down the separating basement membrane. The granulosa and theca cells then intermingle and complete the luteinization process; these cells together with their surrounding tissues comprise the corpus luteum.[25] Histologically, luteinization is a process of lipid accumulation. The biochemical hallmark of luteinization is the capacity for progesterone biosynthesis in response to LH; this is accompanied by increased estrogen secretion in man.[106,107]

During its functional life span the corpus luteum is normally the major source of the sex hormones secreted by the ovary. Corpus luteum function reaches its peak about 4 days after ovulation and begins to wane about 4 days before menstruation (Fig. 8–12H). Loss of sensitivity to LH and E2 herald luteal senescence. Regression of the corpus luteum—luteolysis—occurs if pregnancy does not provide chorionic gonadotropin. Luteolysis is probably mediated by prostaglandin. Transformation of the corpus luteum into an avascular scar, the corpus albicans, then occurs.

Early luteal increase in secretion of estrogens and progestins causes "secretory" transformation and hyperplasia of the endometrium. Later fall-off in secretion of female hormones to a level insufficient to maintain the endometrium results in menstruation. Withdrawal of progesterone is specifically responsible for constriction of spiral arteries, local prostaglandin accumulation, and subsequent ischemic necrosis of the endometrium. Normal menstrual flow then results from a complete slough of the vascular secretory endometrium.

A major determinant of normal corpus luteum formation and function is optimal development of the corpus luteum predecessor, the dominant follicle. Follicular phase FSH seems critically important for optimal development of this follicle. A wave of follicular growth is normally initiated in response to the midcycle FSH surge and regresses with increasing corpus luteum progesterone secretion. Another wave of growth commences in the late luteal phase, in response to the late luteal rise of FSH as luteal progesterone and E2 secretion wanes. Lowering of FSH levels in the early follicular phase, either spontaneously[63] or by inhibin administration,[102] impairs subsequent corpus luteum function.

Control of Puberty and the Reproductive Cycle

Factors Controlling the Onset of Puberty

Major factors involved in the initiation of puberty and the regulation of the reproductive cycle are shown at the top of Fig. 8–16. The essential element is maturation of the CNS centers that cause a reduction in the inhibition of hypothalamic GnRH secretion. The locale and nature of these center(s) are unclear. The major inhibitory influences are

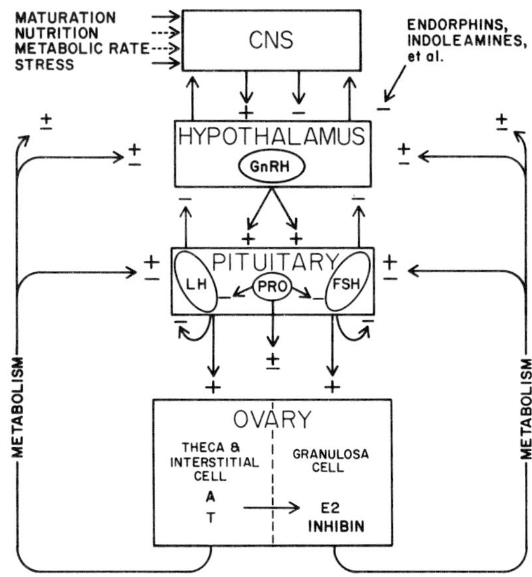

FIGURE 8–16. Diagram of the major mechanisms controlling the onset and maintenance of sex hormone secretion by the unripe antral follicle. The CNS influences GnRH secretion both negatively and positively. In order for the CNS to relinquish its inhibitory control over GnRH secretion, it must achieve a high level of maturity. Even after this is achieved, psychic influences may negatively influence the system. Nutrition and the basal metabolic rate must be optimal; their effects are reversible. The possibility cannot be excluded that these latter factors act directly at the hypothalamic level. Whether efferent tracts from the hypothalamus to the cerebrum play a role in reproductive function is unknown. Pineal secretion of melatonin and other substances is known to exert inhibitory influences on GnRH in lower animals. Gonadotropin-releasing hormone stimulates LH and FSH. Short-loop feedback and auto-feedback of the gonadotropins upon GnRH release and their own release, respectively, are shown. Prolactin (PRO) has multiple effects on gonadotropin synthesis. In unripe antral follicles LH acts on theca and interstitial cells, FSH on granulosa cells. Androstenedione (A) and testosterone (T) secreted by the theca are aromatized by the granulosa cell, under the influence of FSH, to E2. The granulosa cell is also the site of production of the FSH inhibitor, inhibin. Estradiol has a biphasic effect on the mature pituitary and on hypothalamic GnRH release as well. Testosterone itself seems normally to be of minor importance in regulating the female gonadotropin release.

thought to be routed through the posterior hypothalamus, and the stimulatory influences through the anterior hypothalamus.[1,109]

Pubertal maturation and skeletal maturation seem to have common determinants. Girls generally enter puberty when they achieve a pubertal bone age. The bone age correlates better than chronologic age with the various stages of puberty, particularly as menarche approaches.[110] Pubertal stage normally correlates better with the bone age ($r = .82$) than with the chronologic age ($r = .72$) (RL Rosenfield, unpublished data). Skeletal age correlates better with menarche than chronologic age, height, or weight, and its variance at menarche is half that of chronologic age.[111] The bone age at the onset of breast development averages about 10.75 years, and that at menarche averages about 13.0 years. Disorders that accelerate bone maturation, such as congenital adrenogenital syndrome or hyperthyroidism, tend to advance the age of onset of true puberty.[112] Disorders that retard skeletal maturation, such as growth hormone deficiency, hypothyroidism, or anemia, tend to delay the onset of puberty.[113]

Nutrition is obviously closely tied in with maturation and body mass. Weight was found to correlate significantly with initiation of the pubertal growth spurt, peak growth velocity, and menarche by Frisch and Revelle.[114] This was in contrast to chronologic age or height. Frisch hypothesized that some weight-related factor is a trigger for pubertal development. This hypothesis has been supported in many settings,[115] but it has been criticized on methodologic and statistical grounds.[116] Exceptions clearly exist, as in sexual precocity.

Nevertheless, optimal nutrition is clearly necessary for initiation and maintenance of normal menstrual cycles. The basis of the relationship is the subject of controversy. Increase in body fat and decrease in relative lean body weight and metabolic rate to critical levels have been postulated to be key events leading to puberty. Frisch et al. favor the theory that the amount of body fat is critical because in rats fed isocaloric high- and low-fat diets, the former group achieved estrus first.[117] Wilen and Naftolin could not confirm this relationship in food-restricted rats,[118] although the inclusion of gastrointestinal contents in their calculations of body composition could have affected their results. Energy expenditure seems to be an important factor, and may be independent of nutrition.[119] Candidate mediators include insulin[116] and aspartate, analogs of which stimulate sexual precocity.[120] At this time, the nature of the metabolic signal that initiates puberty is unknown.

The sensitivity of FSH and LH to negative feedback by E2 clearly diminishes during the teenage years.[121] Follicle-stimulating hormone suppressibility seems to wane independently of gonadal status, but the suppressive effect of E2 on LH production may fade partly as a consequence of E2 exposure. The failure of antiestrogens to stimulate gonadotropins in pre- or early puberty, as they do in the adult, has been attributed to the high sensitivity of the gonadostat to the weak estrogenic effect of such agents.[5,122] On the other hand, the apparent sensitivity of the "gonadostat" seems increasingly likely in most circumstances to simply be inversely proportional to the "drive" of the GnRH pulse generator.[120] In other words, when there is little stimulation of GnRH secretion the pulse generator is easily inhibited.

The pineal body exerts an inhibitory influence on GnRH, via its secretion of indoleamines, and perhaps peptides, in lower animals.[123] Serum melatonin levels fall with age,[124] but the pineal plays no obvious role in normal human reproduction.

Factors Controlling the Menstrual Cycle

A computer model describing the relationships among the major determinants of the menstrual cycle has been formulated.[125] However, this antedates current data on the dose- and time-related biphasic effects of female hormones and on the role of inhibin and similar factors. Endorphinergic, dopaminergic, noradrenergic, serotoninergic, and cholinergic tracts impinge upon GnRH neurons.[126] Opiates, dopamine, and norepinephrine have been reported to have inhibitory effects; norepinephrine, acetylcholine, and serotonin have stimulatory effects. However, the relation of the activity of these tracts to the status of hormonal cycles is only incompletely understood.

High CNS centers seem to be important to maintain tonic gonadotropin levels.[127] Some E2 effects seem mediated via CNS receptors. Luteal-phase progesterone levels seem to exert their inhibitory effect on the frequency of LH release here as well.[128]

Once the CNS has matured, nutrition and metabolic status, as discussed in the previous section, and stress state determine whether the GnRH is released from the hypothalamus in the normal, circhoral, pulsatile manner. The most important group of GnRH-containing neurons for maintenance of cyclic discharge are those of the arcuate (infundibular) nucleus (Fig. 8–17).[53] The secretion of GnRH neurons is inherently pulsatile.[129]

Pituitary gonadotrope GnRH receptors have been shown to be down-regulated by E2, as well as by high concentrations of progesterone and androgens.[130] Estrogen and progestin exert both their inhibitory and stimulating effects by modulating the relative and absolute amounts of LH and FSH released by the gonadotropic cell.[53,131,132] The inhibitory effect of modest levels of E2 is of rapid onset and sustained; the stimulatory effects of higher E2 levels are of later onset and short lived. Luteinizing hormone and FSH themselves inhibit GnRH release (short-loop feedback) and inhibit their own release (ultra-short-loop or auto-feedback).[133,134]

Prolactin has complex effects on gonadal function. Prolactin in low concentrations enhances E2 and progesterone secretion by increasing ovarian LH receptors.[135] High levels of prolactin are primarily inhibitory to ovarian function. Hyperprolactinemia inhibits gonadotropin release; at least in part this occurs by suppressing gonadotropin GnRH receptors.[136] High prolactin also inhibits ovarian E2 and progesterone biosynthesis,[137] while stimulating adrenal androgen production.[138]

A variety of other neural or hypophysial hormones have been reported to modulate gonadotropin secretion or action. Corticotropin-releasing hormone clearly inhibits gonadotropin release.[139] A LH release inhibiting factor has been reported.[140] α-Melanocyte-stimulating hormone[141] and neuropeptide Y[142] are stimulatory to LH release. Follicle-stimulating hormone metabolites antagonize FSH action.[143]

Likewise, it is becoming apparent that the ovaries produce numerous hormones that also modulate gonadotropin secretion and action. With the isolation of inhibin came the discovery that structurally related peptides had similar pituitary (e.g., follistatin) or ovarian (e.g., follistatin, transforming growth factor-β) effects—or opposing effects at the pituitary (e.g., activin) or ovarian (e.g., activin transforming growth factor-β) levels.[102] Transforming growth factor-β also stimulates meiotic maturation of the oocyte.[144] Many other growth factors or cytokines modulate ovarian cell growth or function.[145,146] Certain steroid metabolites (e.g., 3α-hydroxyprogesterone) have been claimed to selectively suppress FSH.[147] A GnRH-like protein has been described in the ovary[148] that may act through ovarian GnRH receptors to suppress steroidogenesis in the human ovary.[149,150] The impor-

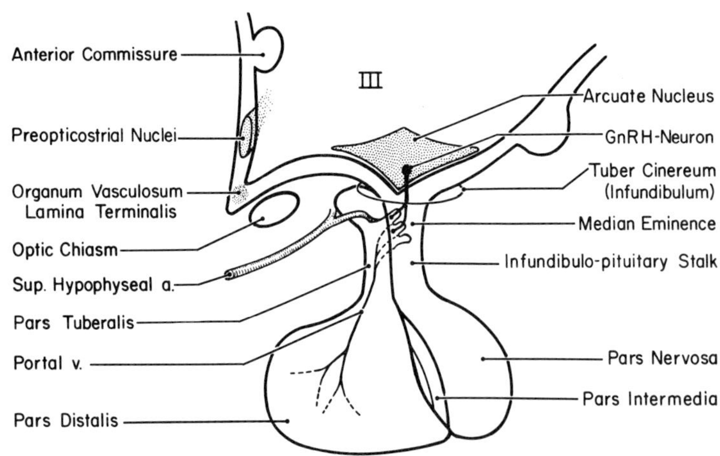

FIGURE 8–17. The location of major GnRH-containing neurons (shaded) in relation to the hypothalamus and pituitary gland. The neurons are of greatest density in the arcuate nuclei and in the periventricular wall of the medial basal hypothalamus; these neurons project to the adjacent median eminence. The second most dense population of GnRH neurons lies in the preoptico-strial area. The development of some is altered by early androgenization.[14] Some are connected by the stria terminalis to the amygdalae; other projections from this area appear to connect indirectly with the median eminence, perhaps via the organum vasculosum lamina terminalis, a midline structure that resembles the median eminence. The pituitary portal veins transport blood rich in releasing factors to sinusoids engulfing anterior pituitary cells.

tance of these factors in normal human reproductive physiology is unclear.

Maturation of Adrenal Androgen Secretion

Adrenarche is the maturational increase in adrenal 17-KS production and is related to the growth of sexual hair.[151,152] It is characterized by a disproportionate rise in Δ^5-3β-hydroxysteroids, particularly dehydroepiandrosterone sulfate (DHAS). Adrenarche represents a change in the pattern of adrenal secretory response to ACTH (Fig 8–18): the rise in DHAS production is accompanied by striking rises in 17-hydroxypregnenolone and dehydroepiandrosterone (DHEA) responsiveness to ACTH, whereas glucocorticoid production does not change.

The zona reticularis of the adrenal cortex is probably a major source of these adrenarchal changes.[153] This zone begins to form in the central adrenal cortex at 3 years of age. It has been postulated to originate from persistent cells of the fetal adrenocortical zone that have failed to undergo involution. The degree of its development as a continuous zone correlates with the increasing DHAS

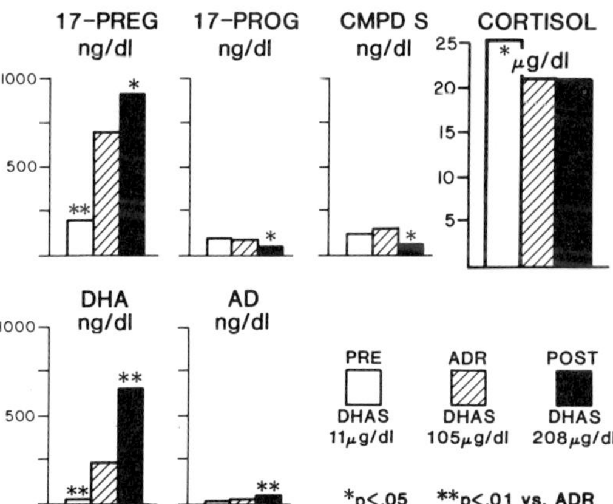

FIGURE 8–18. Changing pattern of adrenal steroidogenic response to ACTH with maturation. Shown are plasma steroid levels 30 min post-ACTH (10 µg/m²) in prepubertal children (PRE), children with premature adrenarche as an isolated phenomenon (ADR), and follicular-phase adult females (ADULT). The layout is organized according to the biosynthetic pathway (see Fig. 8–23). Note that 17-hydroxypregnenolone (17-PREG) and dehydroepiandrosterone (DHA) responses of children with premature adrenarche are intermediate between the prepubertal and adult responses. 17-PROG, 17-progesterone; CMPD S, compound S (11-deoxycortisol); AD, androstenedione. (Redrawn from the data of Rich BR, et al: Adrenarche: Changing adrenal response to ACTH. J Clin Endocrinol Metab 52:1129, 1981.)

production that commences at about 6 years of age. Cells of this zone possess sulfokinase activity[154] and have low Δ^5-3β-hydroxysteroid dehydrogenase (3β-HSD) activity judged from intra-adrenal steroid concentrations[155] and histochemistry. Thus, as ACTH is secreted in response to the body's demands for cortisol, the reticularis zone would seem to secrete DHEA and DHAS as by-products.

Both in vivo and in vitro data are consistent with maturational increases of C_{17-20} lyase and 17-hydroxylase activity.[151,155,156] Whether 3β-HSD is inhibited during adrenarche by substrate and products[157] or is instead low only in the zona reticularis cell population that contains the sulfokinase is unknown.

A pituitary hormone ("adrenarche factor") may well be required to bring about the adrenarchal change.[4] A distinct pituitary adrenal androgen-stimulating hormone has been postulated to exist by Grumbach et al. and Parker and Odell.[153] However, our data[151] and those of Winter et al.[155,157] suggest that an adrenarchal factor need only control the growth and differentation of a population of adrenocortical cells. Such a factor might alter the structure and function of a subgroup of preexisting steroid-secreting cells by altering the enzyme activity within. The latter is a particularly attractive hypothesis now that both C_{17-20} lyase and 17α-hydroxylase are known to be activities of a single cytochrome, P450.[158] This signifies that these two activities must be differentially regulated, otherwise cortisol secretion could not occur without 17-KS secretion in childhood. If this postulated trophic factor were suppressible by dexamethasone administration, the sluggish changes in DHAS concentration after dexamethasone administration[78] or withdrawal[159] would be explained. Candidates for a dexamethasone-suppressible adrenarchal factor include pro-ACTH related peptides. Adrenarche is not necessarily related to gonadarche[160] and, thus, seems independent of gonadotropin secretion. However, the ovary, independently of its estrogen output, seems to play a role in supporting DHAS production.[161]

Whether adrenarche plays a more fundamental role in puberty than contributing to the growth of sexual hair is unknown. It is conceivable that adrenal androgens normally play a role in maturing the neuroendocrine system,[111] increasing gonadotropin bioactivity,[60] or selectively promoting prepubertal or pubertal growth.[162]

Development of the Genital Tract and Secondary Sexual Organs

Uterus and Cervix

The müllerian system of the embryo gives rise to the uterus, cervix, upper vagina, and fallopian tubes in the absence of antimüllerian hormone secretion by fetal testes during the first trimester of gestation.[16] Diethylstilbestrol-induced dysplasia suggests that excessive estrogen in fetal life interferes with normal differentiation of these structures.[163]

The uterus and cervix are too small to be clearly palpable by bimanual examination per rectum prepubertally. They enlarge under the influence of estrogen during puberty. The endometrium and cervical glands then undergo cyclic changes in concert with cyclic ovarian function. In response to estrogen during the follicular phase of the cycle the endometrial epithelium and stroma proliferate. The uterine glands increase in number and lengthen. After ovulation, in response to progestins, the endometrium increases in thickness: stromal edema occurs, and the uterine glands enlarge, become sacculated, and secrete a glycogen-rich mucoid fluid. The coiled arteries lengthen further during this time and become increasingly spiral.

The major cyclic change in the cervix is in the secretion of the endocervical glands, which lubricate the vaginal vault. The mucus they secrete during the low-estrogen phase of the cycle is scanty and relatively thin. The mucus becomes more viscous and elastic as estrogens rise in the later follicular phase of the cycle—the extent to which it can be stretched into a long spindle, *spinnbarkeit*, is a function of the estrogen level.[164]

Vagina

The mucous membranes of the urogenital tract are comprised of hormone-responsive stratified squamous epithelium (Fig. 8–18).[2] The basal layer is the regenerative area. In the absence of estrogen there is only a parabasal layer of cells over this, and the vagina is thin, with a tendency to alkalinity, which predisposes it to local infection. In response to estrogen, epithelial proliferation occurs, with formation of successive intermediate and superficial layers. With this maturation the cytoplasm of each cell first expands, leading to formation of small intermediate cells. With further estrogenization, the nuclei become pyknotic and form large intermediate cells. Greater estrogenization brings about their transformation to superficial cells: the cytoplasm changes from basophilic to acidophilic with the accumulation of glycogen. Resistance to infection of the fully developed vaginal mucosa results from its thickness and from its acid pH, which occurs from the fermentation of the glycogen of the superficial cells. In response to progesterone, degenerative changes appear in vaginal mucosal cells: superficial cells decrease, the cytoplasm assumes a "crinkled" appearance, cells degenerate, and bacterial proliferation increases.

Vaginal smears show the characteristic cyclic changes in the cell types comprising the vaginal epithelium (Fig. 8–19).[165] In the prepubertal years parabasal cells predominate, and characteristically 10 per cent or less are small intermediate cells. A pattern

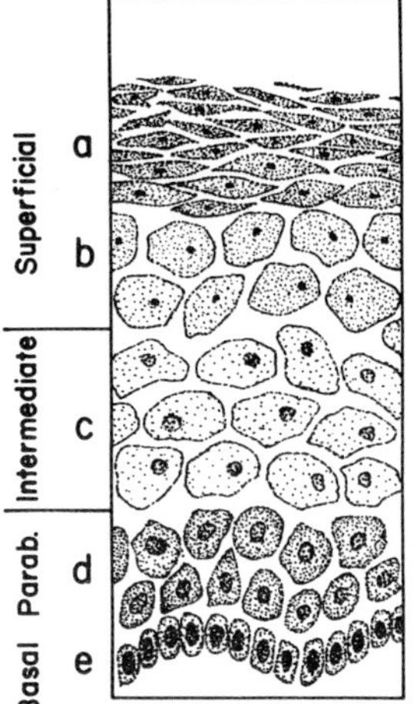
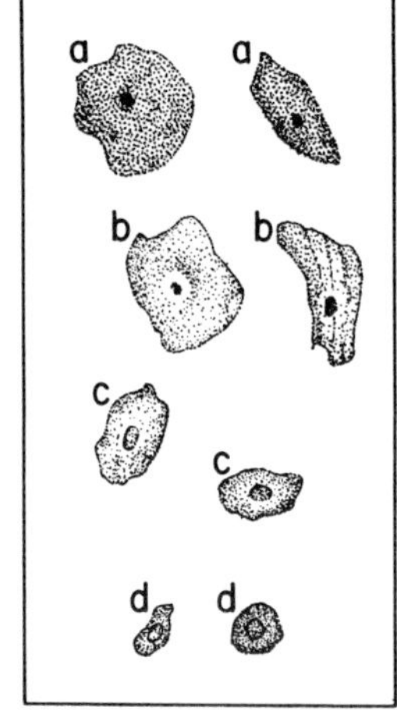

FIGURE 8–19. The layers of vaginal epithelium of the well-estrogenized adult. The superficial layer contains surface cells that are cornified (squamous) with eosinophilic cytoplasm and pyknotic nuclei (*a*) as well as large intraepithelial cells that are also karyopyknotic but basophilic (*b*). The intermediate zone contains basophilic cells that have less cytoplasm and intermediate-size nuclei (*c*). The basal and parabasal cells have a relatively small amount of basophilic cytoplasm and relatively vesicular nuclei (*d*). (Redrawn from Wilkins L: The Diagnosis and Treatment of Endocrine Disorders in Childhood and Adolescence. Springfield, ILL, CC Thomas, 1968.)

consisting entirely of intermediate cells is typical of early puberty. The early follicular phase of the menstrual cycle is characterized by the predominance of large intermediate cells with few, if any, superficial cells. Peak maturation is reached at midcycle, at which time 35 to 85 per cent of the cells seen on vaginal smear are superficial; the remainder are large intermediate cells. This peak develops over a 1-week period in response to E2 levels of about 70 pg/ml.[166]

Mammary Glands

Multiple rudimentary branching mammary ducts are found beneath the nipple in infancy; they grow and branch during the prepubertal years only slowly.[167] Under the influence of estrogen, the nipples grow, mammary terminal duct branching progresses to the stage at which ductules are formed, and fatty stromal growth increases until it constitutes about 85 per cent of the mass of the breast. Growth hormone (probably via insulin-like growth factors)[168] and glucocorticoids play a permissive role.[169] Lobulation appears around menarche, when multiple blind saccular buds form by branching of the terminal ducts. These effects are presumably due to the presence of progesterone. The breast stroma swells cyclically during each luteal phase. Full alveolar development normally only occurs during pregnancy under the influence of additional progesterone and prolactin. Prolactin is unlikely to play a role in breast growth without priming by female hormones.[169] Some increase in glandular parenchyma remains postpartum.

Pilosebaceous Apparatus

The pilosebaceous apparatus (PSA) with but few exceptions consists of both a piliary and a sebaceous component.[170] In androgen-dependent areas, the hair is fine and short (vellus) and the sebaceous gland poorly developed in the prepubertal child. Depending on the location, the PSA will develop into either a terminal hair follicle (in which a large medullated hair becomes the prominent structure) or a sebaceous follicle (in which the sebaceous gland becomes prominent and the hair remains vellus) as androgen levels rise (Fig. 8–20). Androgens seem to promote sexual hair growth by recruiting a population of PSAs with preset

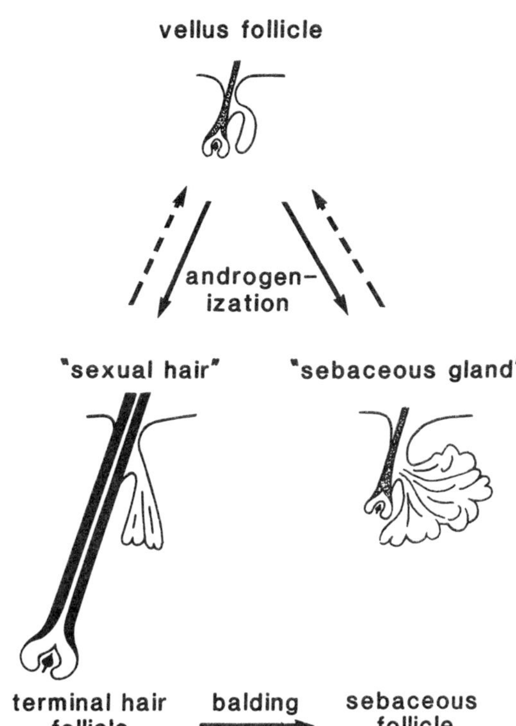

FIGURE 8–20. Role of androgen in the development of the pilosebaceous apparatus. Solid lines indicate effects of androgens. Dotted lines indicate the effects of antiandrogens.

genetic sensitivity to switch from producing vellus hairs to producing terminal hairs. Androgens promote sebaceous gland development by stimulating multiplication and differentiation of sebocytes. Sebaceous follicles are sensitive to relatively low levels of androgen and become relatively well developed at adult female levels of androgens. However, at these same androgen levels, terminal hairs develop in only the pubic and axillary areas. Greater amounts of androgen are required to successively recruit terminal hair development in less sensitive areas. All these processes are reversible by antiandrogens. Male-pattern alopecia occurs primarily because of the conversion of terminal hair to sebaceous follicles upon the exposure of genetically predisposed individuals to high androgen levels for a prolonged time. Growth hormone seems synergistic with androgen through the mediation of insulin-like growth factors. Estrogens have a modest stimulating effect on hair growth; this may well be due to induction of androgen receptors by estrogen. Estrogens are potent inhibitors of sebum secretion.

Hormonal Secretion, Transport, Metabolism, and Action

Peptide Hormones

Peptide hormones act by binding to specific receptors located in the plasma membranes of target cells (Fig. 8–21).[171] The receptor is coupled by the guanine nucleotide regulatory protein to adenylate cyclase. Cyclic adenosine-3′, 5′-monophosphate (cAMP) then activates protein kinase. Phosphorylation of various cytoplasmic and nuclear proteins is then thought to mediate the action of the peptide hormones. Calcium modifies the cAMP response.[172] The presumed diversity among target cells in their responses to protein kinase action may relate to diversity and type of kinase, intracellular compartmentalization, substrate availability, and other factors determined by the genome of the target cell.

Gonadotropin-releasing hormone is a decapeptide[173] — [pyro]Glu - His - Trp - Ser - Tyr-Gly-Leu-Arg-Pro-Gly-NH_2. One gene encodes the single precursor protein for both GnRH and prolactin release-inhibiting factor.[174] This provides a mechanism for coupled reciprocal regulation of gonadotropins and prolactin. Gonadotropin-releasing hormone not only effects prompt release of preformed gonadotropins (readily releasable pool), but also stimulates the synthesis of gonadotropins (reserve pool).[67,175] Al-

though GnRH stimulates the secretion of both LH and FSH, there is some evidence for possible GnRH-independent FSH secretion,[176] such as in response to the FSH-releasing protein activin.[102] Repeated administration of GnRH augments the pituitary responsiveness to subsequent GnRH pulses ("self-priming").[66] This has been ascribed partly to up-regulation of GnRH receptors[130] partly to postreceptor phenomena.[177] Steroid-induced changes in gonadotropin release may be mediated by modulation of pituitary receptors for GnRH. Gonadotropin-releasing hormone has recently been found to have some interesting paradoxical effects. First, upon protracted, continuous administration it down-regulates pituitary gonadotropin secretion.[53,173] Second, it has a variety of direct antigonadal properties.[75,84] It inhibits FSH induction of progesterone secretion, aromatase activity, and LH receptor in granulosa cells; down-regulates LH receptors and the induction of LH receptors by hCG; and inhibits the hCG stimulation of progesterone secretion by luteal cells. These effects are mediated by interaction with receptors perhaps "intended" for a local ovarian class of factors that have GnRH-like properties.[148–150]

Luteinizing hormone and FSH are glycoprotein hormones that consist of two chains.[171] The α chains of LH, FSH, hCG, and thyroid-stimulating hormone (TSH) are virtually identical, are functionally interchangeable, and have molecular weights of about 14,000.[178,179] The β chain of each hormone differs, particularly in configuration, with molecular weights of about 14,000 (LH) and 19,000 (FSH). Although β chains are inherently inactive, they confer biologic specificity when combined with an α chain. They are synthesized in a single type of cell, and both are sometimes identified within the same cell.[180] After synthesis of these hormones on the ribosomes, the carbohydrate moieties, constituting about 16 per cent of the weight, are successively added in the rough endoplasmic reticulum and Golgi apparatus. The oligosaccharides at the periphery of the molecules vary somewhat among the chains.

Gonadotropin standards are impure (Fig. 8–22). They contain not only LH and FSH, but varying amounts of free α or β subunits, which have no inherent bioactivity, molecules heterogeneous at least in part because of varying degrees of glycosylation, and other pituitary hormones.[181] Reported go-

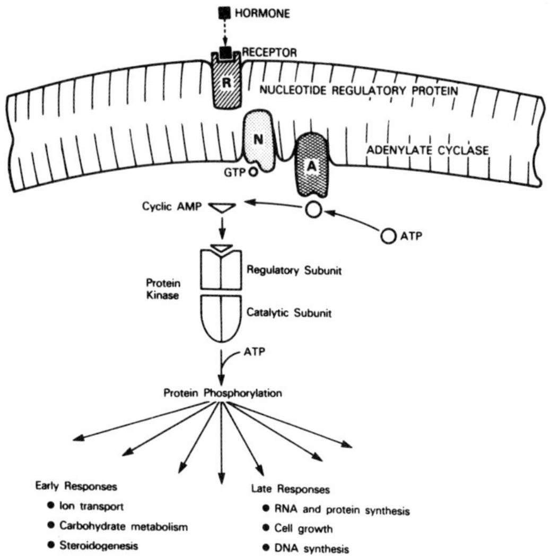

FIGURE 8–21. Role of cyclic AMP in peptide hormone mechanism of action. (From Catt KJ, Harwood JP, Clayton RN, et al: Regulation of peptide hormone receptors and gonadal steroidogenesis. Recent Prog Horm Res 36:557, 1980.)

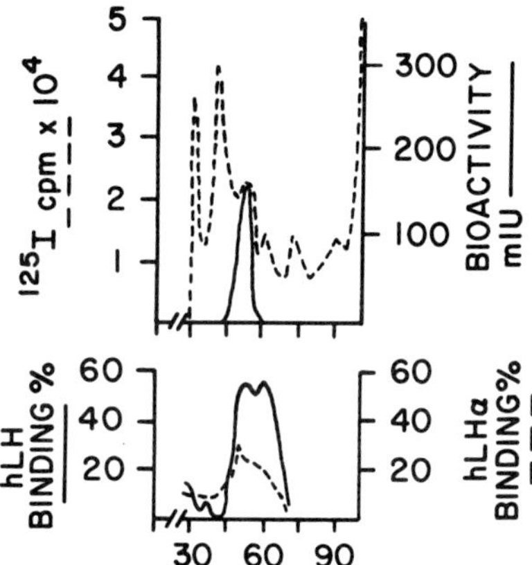

FIGURE 8–22. Gel filtration profile of a highly purified hLH standard (Kabi-1974). Only about 10 per cent of the protein in this preparation is bioactive (top panel). Radioimmunoassay for hLH (performed with National Pituitary Agency anti-hLH and ^{125}I-Kabi-1974 tracer) (bottom panel) detects immunoreactive material in nonbioactive areas. Much of this immunoreactive-nonbioactive materal has α-subunit immunoreactivity (bottom panel). Therefore, subunit-containing gonadotropin fragments probably constitute a significant portion of the immunoreactive LH. (Redrawn from data of Suginami et al.[181])

nadotropin levels vary from study to study because different antisera raised to these impure standards interact with various fractions of iodinated or plasma gonadotropin species to varying degrees, because of differing immunopotency of standards, and because of different bioassay procedures used for calibration. The most plentiful and widely used pituitary gonadotropin standard is LER-907. LER-907 is highly impure: it has only about 0.5 per cent the specific activity (IU/mg) of the current NIH standard I-2 or the purified LH standard shown in Figure 8–22. One hundred nanograms of LER-907 contains about 2.0 mIU of FSH according to in vivo bioassay and 4.8 mIU FSH according to RIA.[182] One hundred nanograms of LER-907 also contains 4.8 mIU of LH by in vivo bioassay and is equivalent in radioimmunoassay to an amount that contains 29 mIU of in vivo bioassayable LH (according to the 2nd IRP, Table 8-2).

The introduction of a sensitive in vitro bioassay has made it possible to extensively characterize the LH content of gonadotropin standards in terms of bioactivity and immunoreactivity. The biopotency of the immunoreactive LH is quite different in each available standard (Table 8–2). LER-907 and its repackaged form, WHO 69/104, are the least biopotent of the available LH standards. According to LH bioassay using in vitro interstitial cell testosterone production, 100 ng LER-907 is equivalent to 4.1 ng I-2 and 9.5 mIU of the 2nd IRP hMG. According to radioimmunoassay, 100 ng LER-907 is equivalent to 2.2 ng I-2 and an amount of the 2nd IRP hMG that has 22 mIU of LH activity in the in vitro bioassay. Consequently, the immunoreactive LH of I-2 is 5.2 times and that of the 2nd IRP hMG is 2.3 times more biopotent in the in vitro bioassay than is that of LER-907. Plasma immunoreactive LH has a biopotency similar to that of the relatively basic I-2, Kabi-1974, and LER-960 standards.[61] Therefore, the ratio of bioactivity to immunoreactivity (B:I) of plasma LH is about 1 in reference to these standards and about 5 in reference to LER-907.

FSH is similarly heterogeneous.[183] Sensitive in vitro bioassays for FSH based on stimulation of aromatase activity have recently been reported.[184] The B:I of serum FSH was recently reported to rise from 0.78 in puberty to 1.94 in the follicular phase to 6.2 in the ovulatory phase of the menstrual cycle[185] with respect to the NIH standard hFSH-3.

Hormonal production rates are given in Table 8–3.

Luteinizing hormone is cleared more rapidly from the blood than FSH or hCG.[194,195] Luteinizing hormone disappears from blood in an exponential pattern: RIA indicates that the half-life of the initial component is about 20 min and the half-life of the second component is about 4 hours (the bioactive LH

TABLE 8–2. BIOPOTENCY OF HUMAN LH STANDARDS RELATIVE TO hLH KABI-1974*

Standard	B-I†
Kabi-1974	1.00
LER-960	0.83
1st IRP 68/40‡	0.72
2nd IRP hMG§	0.45
LER-907**	0.20

* From Robertson and Diczfalusy, 1977 in Burstein S, et al.[61] Kabi-1974 has 7090 IU (relative to WHO 60/104)/mg by in vitro bioassay.

† B-I, ratio of bioassayable LH to immunoassayable LH. Bioassay: in vitro interstitial cell testosterone production. RIA: bioactive ^{125}I-Kabi-1974 tracer and WHO antiserum.

‡ 1st International Reference Preparation (IRP) of pituitary LH for RIA (Hartree).

§ 2nd IRP of human menopausal gonadotropins (hMG) for bioassay.

** LER-907 is 8 per cent more biopotent than its filtered and repackaged derivative, WHO 69/104, the 1st IRP of pituitary LH and FSH for bioassay.[182]

IRP, Internal Reference Preparation.

TABLE 8–3. AVERAGE HORMONE BLOOD PRODUCTION RATES IN MID-FOLLICULAR PHASE WOMEN*

Hormone	Production Rate	Pertinent References
LH	615 IU/day†	186
FSH	215 IU/day†	187
Androstenedione	3.4 mg/day	188
Dehydroepian-drosterone	7.0 mg/day	188
DHAS	7.0 mg/day‡	189, 190
Dihydrotes-tosterone	0.06 mg/day	188
Estradiol	0.1 mg/day	191
Estrone	0.1 mg/day	191
Progesterone	1.1 mg/day	192
17-OH-Proges-terone	1.2 mg/day	193
Testosterone	0.2 mg/day	188

* These production rates are roughly equivalent to those in midpuberty. The average daily production of those hormones that fluctuate cyclically is substantially greater. For example, E2 production transiently peaks to about 0.5 mg/day, so that the average production over the monthly cycle is about 0.2 mg/day or 6 mg/month.

† In terms of 2nd IRP hMG.

‡ Approximate urinary production rate, expressed as unconjugated DHEA.

half-life is about one-third faster[196]). These respective components for FSH are 4 and 70 hours; those for hCG are 11 and 23 hours. The metabolic clearance rate of LH is 35 and that of FSH is 20 L/day.[186,187] Gonadotropins are primarily metabolized by the liver after the removal of the terminal sialic acid residues, which retard clearance. About 10 to 15 per cent of gonadotropins are excreted in urine[197]; only about one third of this is in a biologically active form.[198]

The first step in gonadotropin action, binding to target cell receptor, is influenced by the carbohydrate portion of the hormone. Studies of Leydig cells indicate that only miniscule changes in the occupancy of gonadotropin receptors are required to elicit the steroidogenic effect of LH. The process seems to be mediated by adenylate cylase (although the LH effect is seen at doses too low to increase cell content of cAMP) because increased phosphorylation of cAMP-dependent protein kinases can be shown to be closely coupled to the LH effect.

Prolactin has structural and functional similarities to growth hormone and placental lactogen. Lactotroph growth and prolactin secretion are stimulated by estrogens. Prolactin release from the anterior pituitary is primarily under the control of hypothalamic inhibition: both dopamine[199] and pro-lactin release-inhibiting factor[174] are involved. The latter is contained within the same precursor protein as GnRH, thus providing a mechanism for their reciprocal control. Prolactin secretion also is inhibited by thyroxine and is responsive to thyrotropin-releasing hormone (TRH).

Inhibin is a glycoprotein hormone consisting of two disulfide-linked subunits that are highly homologous with transforming growth factor-β.[102] The α subunit is approximately 20 kilodaltons. The β subunit is 11 to 12 kilodaltons and occurs in two forms, β-A and β-B. These are homologous with the COOH-terminal portion of müllerian inhibiting substance. Dimers of the β subunit are termed activin. Activin-A is the homodimer of β-A; activin-B is the heterodimer consisting of β-A plus β-B. Whereas inhibin inhibits gonadotropin production, activin stimulates it. Follistatin has recently been identified as a protein made by the gonads that is about 50 per cent homologous with epidermal growth factor (EGF) and is also capable of inhibiting pituitary and gonadal function.

Steroid Hormones

The interrelationship of progestin, androgen, and estrogen biosynthesis is shown in Figure 8–23.[200] Low-density lipoprotein is a major source of steroidogenic substrate.[84] Steroid hormone biogenesis from cholesterol begins with 20α-hydroxylation and subsequent splitting off of the side chain between C_{20} and C_{22}, the "desmolase" step (A).[158] The Δ^5-isomerase-3β-hydroxysteroid dehydrogenase step (3β-ol) (B) may occur next and is obligatory for the synthesis of all potent steroid hormones. Progesterone, in the absence of 17α-hydroxylation, is the substrate for the synthesis of mineralocorticoids. 17α-Hydroxylation (B′) is required for biosynthesis of sex steroids as well as glucocorticoids. 17-Hydroxyprogesterone, via successive 21- and 11β-hydroxylations (C, D), is an obligatory intermediary in the biosynthesis of cortisol. 17-Hydroxyprogesterone is also an obligatory intermediate in the formation of androgens and estrogens, via enzymatic lysis of the side chain (G) to form 17-KS. Both 17α-hydroxylase and C_{17-20} lyase activity are now known to be mediated by a single cytochrome, P450c17. 17β-Reduction (H) of 17-KS must occur for the synthesis of testosterone and E2. Transformation of testosterone to other 17β-

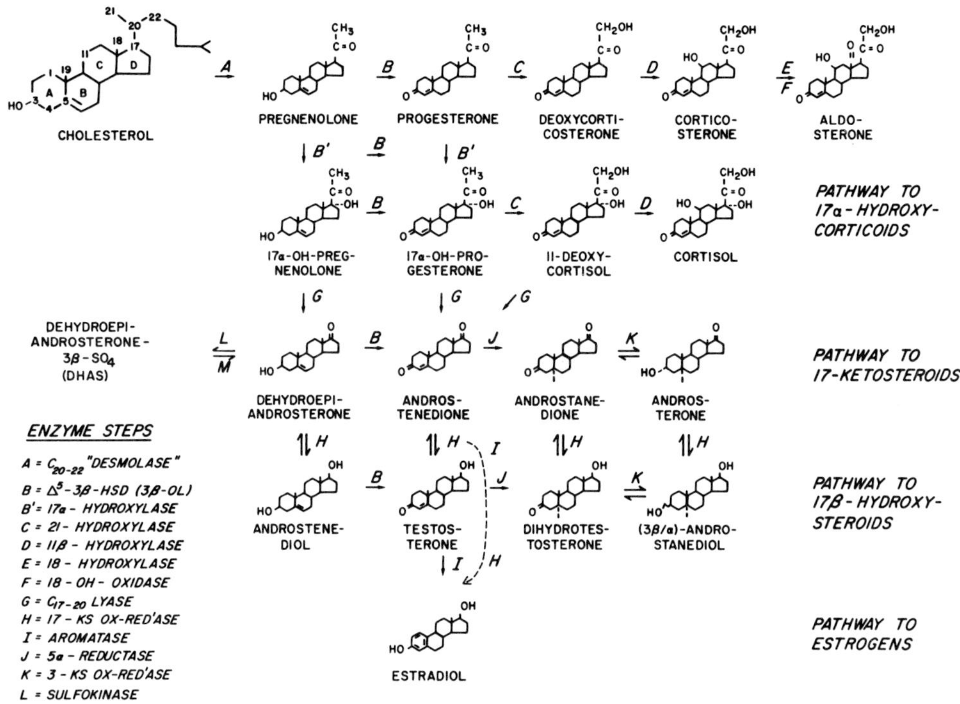

FIGURE 8–23. Major pathways of steroid hormone biosynthesis from cholesterol. Relevant carbon atoms of cholesterol are designated by conventional number, rings by letters. The flow of hormonogenesis is generally to the right and downward. The top line shows pathway from progesterone to mineralocorticoids; the second line, the pathway to glucocorticoids; the third line, that to 17-ketosteroids; the fourth line, that to potent androgens. The bottom and dotted lines indicate those pathways to estrogen (long dotted line involves the 17-keto estrogen estrone [not shown], as an intermediate). KS, ketosteroids; HSD, hydroxysteroid dehydrogenase; OH, hydroxy. The terms "desmolase" and "lyase" are often used interchangeably, as are the terms "hydroxysteroid dehydrogenase" and "ketosteroid (oxido) reductase." (Modified from Rosenfield et al.[16])

hydroxysteroid androgens, such as DHT, occurs via steps J and K. Estrogens are formed by aromatization of androstenedione and testosterone (I).

The ovary normally accounts for about 25 per cent of testosterone secretion in the mature female (0.06 mg daily), but it secretes about 30 times as much A (1.6 mg daily).[188] These amounts are similar to those secreted by the adrenal. However, the ovary secretes less than 10 per cent as much DHEA as the adrenal.

Potent sex hormones are produced not only by secretion, but by peripheral conversion of secreted prehormones by nonendocrine organs. The ovary and the adrenal cortex are the sources of prehormones as well as secreted hormones. About 50 per cent of plasma testosterone (0.1 mg daily) normally is formed indirectly by peripheral conversion. Although 85 per cent of normal estrogen production in the woman arises by secretion in midcycle, 50 per cent of estrogen production can arise from extraglandular sources during the low-estrogen phases of the menstrual cycle.[201] Peripheral formation of active steroids occurs in a wide number of sites, including liver, fat, and target organs.[202–204] For example, steps B, H, I, J, and K (Fig. 8–23) readily occur in the liver, and adipose tissue becomes a major site of aromatization in the obese individual.

The "production rate" of a hormone equals its secretion rate plus (in the case of hormones formed outside of endocrine glands) the rate of formation of the hormone by peripheral conversion of secreted precursors. The "blood production rate" is calculated as metabolic clearance rate (MCR) × plasma concentration; this is because in the steady state the amount of hormone irreversibly leaving the plasma compartment equals the amount entering it. The calculation of production rates from the urinary excretion of labeled metabolites is much more complex when a unique metabolite

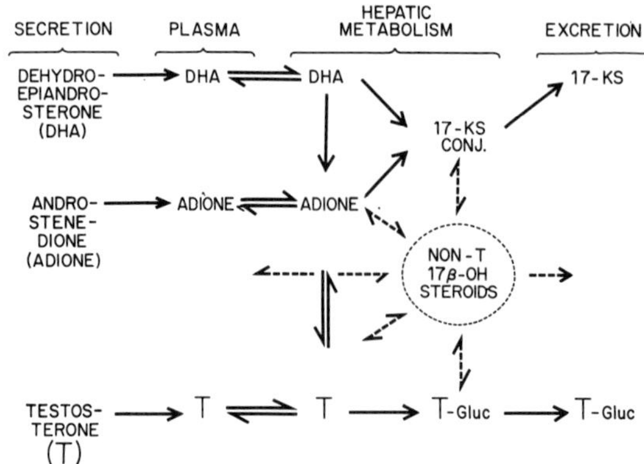

FIGURE 8–24. Diagram illustrating the relationship between secreted, plasma, and urinary steroids.[188] 17-Ketosteroid (17-KS) excretion does not reflect accurately the excretion of the most important plasma androgens. Only 25 per cent or less of testosterone is excreted as 17-KS metabolites; therefore, important changes in testosterone production may not appreciably affect urinary 17-KS excretion. Furthermore, even the major 17-KS, DHAS, is excreted poorly until its production rate becomes quite high. On the other hand, perhaps 50 per cent of the Zimmermann chromogens are not identifiable as 17-KS, and 2 mg daily results from hydrocortisone metabolism. In addition, 17-KS metabolism differs in the child and adult. Testosterone glucuronide excretion does not accurately reflect the plasma testosterone level. Less than 2 per cent of testosterone appears in the urine as such. In addition, plasma 17-KS, such as androstenedione, may be converted to testosterone glucuronide without ever circulating as unconjugated testosterone.

does not exist, as is usually the case.[205] Because of extensive steroid interconversions, the quantity of a hormone excreted in urine is not necessarily proportional to the amount reaching target tissues (Fig. 8–24). For example, so large a fraction of urinary testosterone glucuronide is formed directly from androstenedione by compartmentalized metabolism within the liver that the range of urinary excretion of testosterone in women overlaps the range in men to some degree. The blood production rates of steroid hormones are given in Table 8–3.

Plasma estrogens are regulated by LH and FSH in a log-dose, negative feedback relationship.[125] However, since inhibin seems to play a role in gonadotropin regulation, estrogen secretion may not be as finely tuned as widely regarded. Teleologically, it may be reasoned that this may be because estrogen secretion is in some respects a by-product of ovum maturation. Plasma androgen levels are certainly not finely regulated. This is because they are essentially by-products of adrenal cortisol and ovarian E2 secretion. Consequently, they play little role

in the regulation of the trophic hormones for these glands. In addition, peripheral steroid metabolism is not under negative feedback control; it seems determined to some extent both by the perinatal and by the adult androgenic milieu.[206]

Plasma steroids seem to reach their sites of action and metabolism by simple diffusion from the vascular compartment. About 98 per cent of plasma testosterone and E2 are bound to testosterone-estradiol binding globulin (TEBG) and albumin. TEBG is also called sex hormone binding globulin (SHBG). Differences between individuals in the plasma binding of testosterone and related 17β-hydroxysteroids are due to differences in their TEBG levels because albumin levels do not differ much among individuals and the albumin association constants for steroids are low.[207] TEBG is a major determinant of the egress of testosterone, E2, and other 17β-hydroxysteroids from plasma.[208] The relationship between TEBG binding and steroid ligand clearance is shown in Figure 8–25. However, it is controversial as to which fraction of the plasma E2 and testosterone is available to target organs; the biologically active portion of the plasma 17β-hydroxysteroids seems to be that which is free from TEBG and albumin[209] rather than that which is not

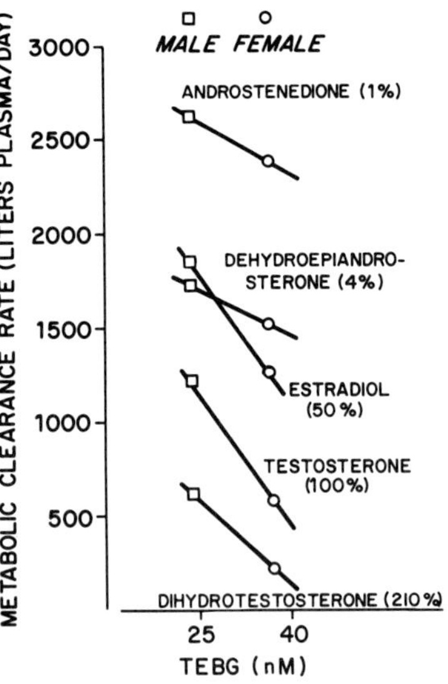

FIGURE 8–25. The relationship between the metabolic clearance rate (MCR) and binding of C_{19} steroids to testosterone estradiol binding globulin (TEBG). The MCR of each steroid has been related to the mean TEBG levels of men and women. The approximate affinity of each steroid for TEBG, relative to testosterone, is indicated in parenthesis. (Modified from Rosenfield.[208])

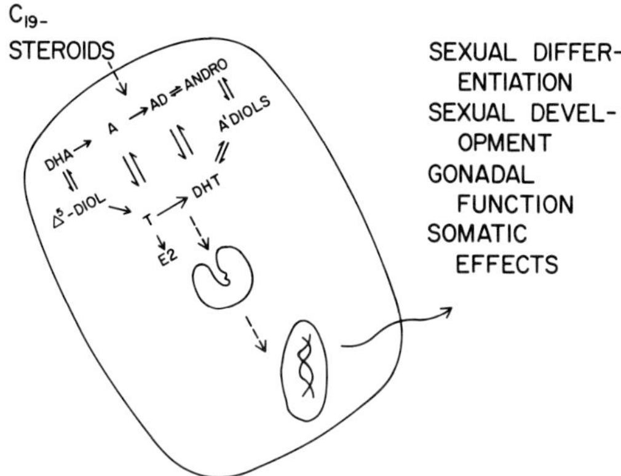

FIGURE 8–26. Model of the mechanism of androgen action, emphasizing the effect of steroid metabolism within a target cell on the mode of action. Solid arrows indicate pathways of steroid metabolism from 17-ketosteroid precursors as laid out in Figure 8–23. Broken arrow indicates transport. The cell-specific intracellular pattern of C_{19}-steroid metabolism determines the relative availability of testosterone or DHT to the cytosol receptor for translocation to the nucleus. In cells such as the rat granulosa cell in which Δ^5-3β-hydroxysteroid dehydrogenase activity is high, androstenediol (Δ^5-diol) is as potent as testosterone; the human sebaceous gland has a similar pattern of steroid metabolism. (Modified from Nimrod et al.[212])

bound to TEBG.[210] The velocity of passage of steroid hormones into cells is extremely rapid (about 10^{-4} cm/sec) and seems to parallel the solubility of the steroids in membrane lipids.[211]

Target cell metabolism influences the cell's response to the steroid hormones that reach it (Fig. 8–26).[212] Although transformation is not fundamental to the mode of action of E2, E2 effectiveness can be influenced by target cell metabolism. The induction of 17β-hydroxysteroid oxidation in target tissues by progesterone, resulting in conversion of E2 to the less potent estrogen estrone, serves to counterbalance estrogenization.[213] A recently postulated mode of estrogen action in the hypothalamus, pituitary, and CNS is through the formation of catechol estrogens.[213,214] For example, 2-hydroxylase and catechol-0-methyltransferase form 2-hydroxy- and 2-methoxy-E2 from E2. These compounds may act as unique neurotransmitters.

Whether testosterone or DHT is more active within a given type of target cell seems to be dependent upon the local pattern of steroid metabolism. For example, the granulosa cell of the rat is known to be more sensitive to testosterone than to DHT because of its pattern of metabolism: it is fairly low in 5α-reductase activity, which converts

testosterone to DHT, and exceedingly rapid in its catabolism of DHT[212]—therefore, the predominant nuclear form of androgen is testosterone. Conditions in the pituitary make it likely that testosterone and DHT are normally translocated to nuclear acceptor sites in about equal amounts and that E2 does not mediate testosterone action there.[215,216] A major mode of testosterone action within the hypothalamus is probably via E2 since the hypothalamus preferentially metabolizes testosterone to estrogen.[216,217] Although some testosterone effects on behavior in rats can be ascribed to aromatization by the CNS,[16] other effects are androgen specific[218] furthermore, aromatization by suprahypothalamic areas of the CNS has not been documented in primates.

Within target cells, the steroid hormones all have a similar basic mode of action (Fig. 8–27).[219,220] All undergo some degree of metabolism before binding to a specific cytosol receptor protein. This steroid-receptor complex is activated, and then translocated to nuclear DNA acceptor sites. Subsequently, DNA-dependent RNA polymerase activity increases, followed by enhanced production

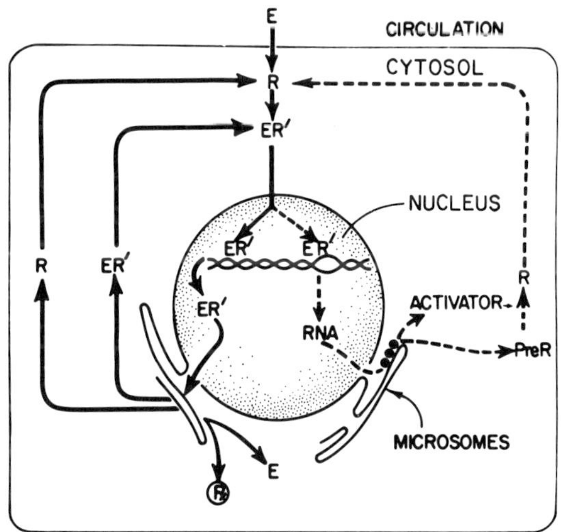

FIGURE 8–27. Estrogen mode of action, emphasizing receptor turnover. The dotted lines indicate the process of receptor synthesis or activator synthesis. Solid lines indicate the processes of reutilization of nuclear estradiol-receptor complexes and regeneration of free cytosolic receptor from the nucleus. E, estrogen; R, cytosolic receptor; ER', transformed estrogen-receptor complex; PreR, a postulated inactive receptor precursor existing in the cytosol; ®, receptor degradation, proposed as arising in the vicinity of the microsomes. (From Muldoon TG: Regulation of steroid hormone receptor activity. Endocr Rev 1:339, 1980.)

of protein. The gene structures of all steroid hormone receptors have been recently shown to be similar. The estrogen, progesterone, androgen, glucocorticoid, and thyroid receptors are highly homologous with one another and with the v-erbA oncogene product.[221,222] Progesterone and E2 modulate the actions of one another by effects on their specific receptors: increased estrogens in the preovulatory phase of the cycle induce target organ receptors for both E2 and progesterone; luteal phase levels of progesterone then suppress the production of both receptors.[220,223,224] Receptor replenishment is important for a sustained steroid effect (Fig. 8–27).

The properties of the cytosol receptor are determinants of steroid potency. Estradiol is a more potent estrogen than estrone and estriol because it binds to the steroid binding domain of the estrogen receptor best.[225] Dihydrotestosterone is an inherently more potent androgen than testosterone primarily because it does not dissociate from the androgen receptor as readily, although its association constant is only slightly greater.[221]

Antiestrogens (e.g., clomiphene) and antiandrogens (e.g., cyproterone acetate) act by blocking cytosol receptor sites. Since these block hormone action by weakly and transiently occupying receptor sites, they have weak agonistic effects, as well. For example, estriol, androgens, and clomiphene are short-acting estrogen agonists (they do not reside in the nucleus long enough to elicit the full array of responses mediated by the E2-receptor complex), yet they antagonize the action of E2 by preventing the association of the ligand—in this case, E2—most capable of complete interaction with the receptor and most capable of replenishing receptors. In a similar manner, progestins (e.g., medroxyprogesterone, cyproterone acetate) may act as weak androgen agonists and as antiandrogens.[226,227]

NORMAL SEXUAL MATURATION: HORMONAL AND PHYSICAL STAGES

The "Puberty" of the Fetus and Neonate

The fetus grows in a richer steroidal milieu than the pubertal female owing to the function of the fetoplacental unit. Concentrations of estrogens in fetal serum are extremely high (Table 8–4). The umbilical cord plasma free testosterone level is mod-

estly greater than that in normal adult females.[188] Dehydroepiandrosterone sulfate is at an adrenarchal-adult level. Daily 17-KS excretion may be as high as 2.5 mg at birth.

The newborn shows some signs of this hormonal stimulation. Hypertrophic labia minora and superficial cell transformation of the urogenital epithelium are consistently observed estrogen effects, and a palpable breast bud appears at term in 32 per cent of babies.[234] Menstrual bleeding and colostrum production sometimes occur in neonates as the baby is withdrawn from the estrogenic environment. Sebaceous gland hypertrophy results from the androgenic state,[235] and the clitoral shaft sometimes seems especially prominent.

The transient small neonatal surge in the function of the neuroendocrine-gonadal axis (Fig. 8–5) is associated with early pubertal hormone levels and responses to GnRH.[12,236] It may be sufficient to sustain breast development through early infancy. These phenomena then regress as the neuroendocrine-gonadal axis is maturing in the opposite direction to that of the pubertal child (Fig. 8–2).

Childhood

As the neuroendocrine-gonadal axis becomes quiescent and the fetal zone of the adrenal cortex regresses, steroid hormone levels fall through infancy to reach a nadir in midchildhood (Table 8–4). Although their levels fall, gonadotropins are usually detectable by RIA throughout childhood (Fig. 8–5). Gonadotropins are often detectable by biassay as well.[61] Although there is seldom obvious sexual development as a consequence of these changes, monitoring of vaginal smears has occasionally revealed evidence of transient estrogen secretion.[49] Thus, close monitoring of estrogen levels in normal prepubertal girls occasionally reveals them to be above typical prepubertal levels.[33,48]

Adolescence

Typical Developmental Pattern

The earliest hormonal changes of puberty occur in late preadolescence—clinically prepubertal 10-year-olds have greater average gonadotropin and sex hormone levels than do prepubertal 6-year-olds. The earliest change in the late preadolescent years is

TABLE 8–4. TYPICAL NORMAL RANGES FOR OVARIAN AND ADRENAL PLASMA STEROIDS*

	E2 (pg/ml)	Estrone (pg/ml)	17-OH-PROG (ng/dl)	A (ng/dl)	T (ng/dl)	DHAS (μg/dl)
Umbilical cord	5,000–15,000[a]	15,000–39,000[b]	1200–4200[a]	15–170[c]	5–50[a]	50–260[d]
0.1–1.0 yr	<75[a]	<20	<200[a]	<80[e]	<20[a]	<40[d]
1.0–4.0 yr	<10[a]	<40[a]	<60[e]	<70[e]	<15[a]	<40[d]
4.0–8.0 yr	<10[a]	<40[a]	<80[e]	<50[e]	<15[a]	<40[d]
Prepubertal >8 yr	<10[a]	<40[a]	<90[a]	<100[f]	<20[g]	10–95[d]
Pubertal	5–125[a]	10–95[b]	15–110[a]	15–150[a]	5–80[g]	40–400[d]
Postmenarchial†	25–250[g]	15–100[a]	25–120[g]	55–200[g]	15–80[g]	60–500[d]

* Actual values in any laboratory vary with assay method. 17-OH-PROG, 17-hydroxyprogesterone; A, androstenedione; T, testosterone.
† Follicular phase adult, exclusive of preovulatory period.
[a] References 6 and 228.
[b] Reference 229.
[c] Reference 230.
[d] Reference 152.
[e] Reference 231.
[f] Reference 232.
[g] References 151 and 233.

the adrenarchal rise in DHAS (see Table 8–4).

Serum gonadotropins begin to rise gradually after 8 years of age. The chronologic age at which this rise occurs varies considerably among children. Therefore, the pubertal rise in gonadotropins is best appreciated by relating gonadotropin levels to pubertal stage. Radioimmunoassay of daytime serum samples indicates that the serum FSH increases in girls about 2.5-fold in the course of puberty and LH about 4.5-fold, with levels among females at the various stages often overlapping (Fig. 8–5). To a great extent this overlap arises from the fact that the secretion of gonadotropins, particularly LH has episodic and diurnal rhythms: LH undergoes rapid excursions up to threefold about every 2 hours, and daytime sampling does not reflect overall gonadotropin production during early puberty (Fig. 8–10). Bioassay of urinary FSH indicates a fivefold rise at this time. In contrast, bioassay of serum LH shows a 23-fold rise from pre- to late puberty in daytime samples, with a clear, consistent distinction between prepubertal and postmenarchial females (Fig. 8–12).

The serum gonadotropin response to GnRH is characteristic of the pubertal status (Fig. 8–8). Gonadotropin excretion reflects the increasing gonadotropin production of puberty. Radioimmunoassay of urinary gonadotropins in timed (3- to 24-hr) urine collections before[237,238] and after[239,240] GnRH infusion has been reported to discriminate between prepubertal and sexually mature individuals. GnRH agonists add a dimension to GnRH testing: they are sufficiently potent stimuli to LH and FSH release to bring about an increase in ovarian secretion (Fig. 8–28).[241] These responses characteristically increase with sexual maturation.

Sex hormone levels rise further as the consequence of ovarian and adrenal maturation. Pubertal levels are intermediate between those of prepuberal and sexually mature individuals. Table 8–4 shows typical normal ranges for serum levels of most of the commonly measured steroid hormones. Progesterone levels are 30 ng/dl or less in childhood.[228] Once pubertal levels of estrogens or androgens are achieved, their effects become obvious within about 6 months.

Serum prolactin rises moderately in females at about 14 years of age.[242] This is presumably due to estrogen secretion, since it does not occur in boys.

The first physical sign of puberty may be either breast development (thelarche) or pubic hair development (pubarche). The stages of breast and pubic hair development are shown in Figure 8–29.[243,244] Tanner stage I is prepubertal. Breast development stage II (B II) is appreciated as a palpable subareolar bud before it can be seen as an elevation. Stage B III is obvious enlargement and elevation of the whole breast. Stage B IV, the phase of areolar mounding, is very transient and may not necessarily appear. Stage B V is the stage of attainment of mature breast contour. Presexual pubic hairs (PH II)—i.e., short, light, and straight—are often not obvious except upon close examination. Frank sexual pubic hair (PH III; long, dark, and curly hairs) subsequently appear, and actually usually commence on the labia majora before spreading to the pubis. Pubic hair then gradually progresses to maturity (stage V), the full female

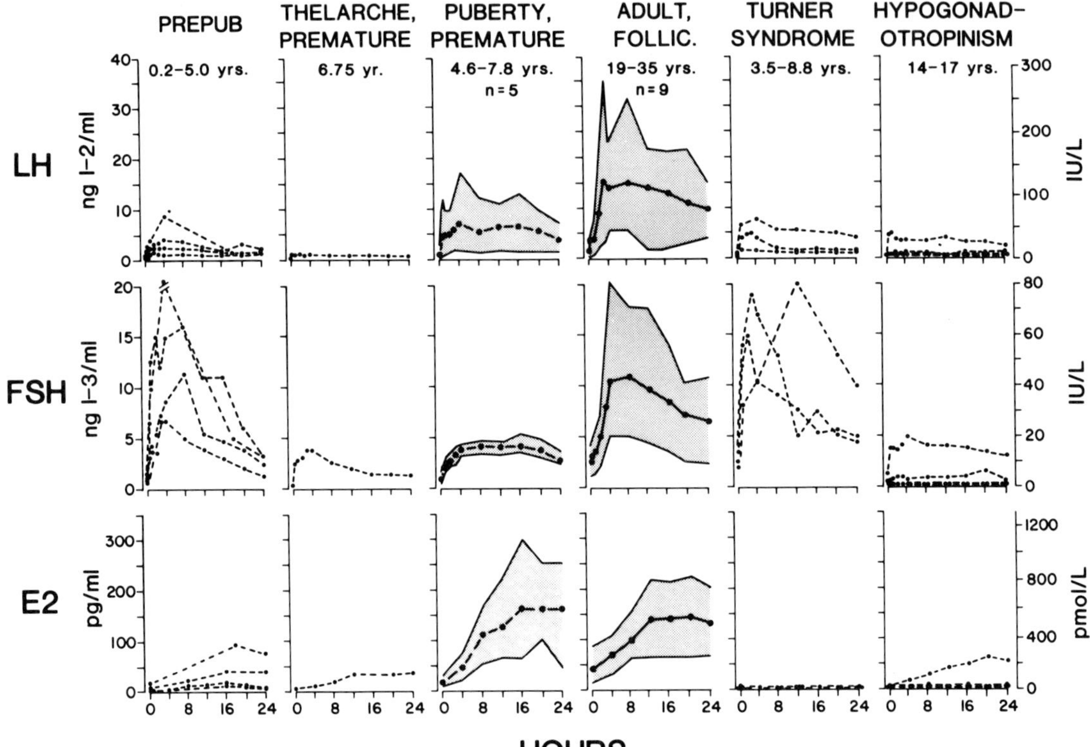

FIGURE 8–28. The pituitary-ovarian response to a test dose of GnRH agonist, FSH, and E2 responses to nafarelin 1 μg/kg (100 μg in adults) given subcutaneously at 0 hours. Mean and ranges or individual responses shown. Normal adult women in the first half of the follicular phase have greater LH and FSH responses than less mature girls. These preliminary data in prepubertal controls suggests a larger FSH reserve in young girls than in the 6.75-year-old with idiopathic premature thelarche. An E2 response is seen at all ages, but before puberty the peak is less than 50 pg/ml. Premenarcheal girls with idiopathic true sexual precocity have E2 responses as great as adults, in spite of their lower LH and FSH responses. Young girls with Turner syndrome have higher early (0.5 to 1.0 hour) FSH responses to the GnRH agonist than adults, yet there is no detectable E2 response. GnRH-deficient girls have heterogeneous responses: the sexually infantile have a flat response, the pubertally arrested girl has a pubertal response. (From Rosenfield R, Ehrmann D, Burstein S, Cuttler L, Cara JF, Levitsky LL: The use of Nafarelin for testing pituitary-ovarian function. In Proceedings of the XII World Congress of Gynecology & Obstetrics, Rio de Janeiro, October 1988. Fertil Steril, in press)

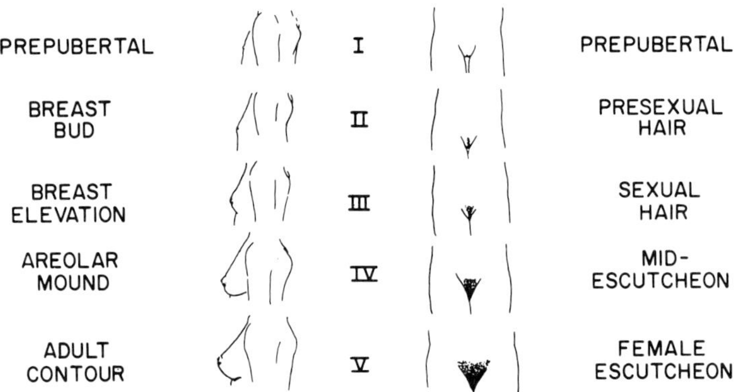

FIGURE 8–29. The stages of breast and pubic hair development, enumerated according to Marshall and Tanner.[243] (Redrawn from Ross and Vande Wiele.[244])

TABLE 8–5. AVERAGE AGE FOR ASCERTAINMENT OF PUBERTAL MILESTONES IN NORTH AMERICAN GIRLS[244,245]

	Years (mean ± SD)
Breast development	
Breast stage II	10.9 ± 1.0
Breast stage III	11.9 ± 1.0
Breast stage IV	12.9 ± 1.2
Pubic hair development	
Pubic hair stage II	11.2 ± 1.1
Pubic hair stage III	11.9 ± 1.1
Pubic hair stage IV	12.6 ± 1.1
Menarche	12.7 ± 1.0

escutcheon (inverted triangle pattern). Axillary hair usually appears about a year later than pubic hair and passes through similar stages.

The average age at which these pubertal milestones appear is given in Table 8–5. Tanner and Davies estimate that currently breast development (B II) begins at 10.9 ± 1.0 (SD) years of age and sexual pubic hair (PH II) begins to develop at 11.9 ± 1.1 years in North American children.[245] Menarche now occurs at 12.7 ± 1.0 years of age in the United States; it is about 0.1 year earlier than this in black children, 0.1 year later in Caucasians.[246]

The age at which puberty begins in normal children varies widely. For practical purposes, normal puberty is that which occurs within 3 SD of the average. Therefore, breast development is considered to be normal if it commences between 7.9 and 13.9 years, sexual pubic hair between 7.6 and 15.2 years, and menarche between 9.7 and 16.7 years of age. Another important normal variable is the span of time between the onset of breast development (B II) and menarche: since this is 2.3 ± 1.0 year regardless of the age at which B II occurs,[243] a girl whose breast development begins at 14 years may not experience the onset of menses before about 18.5 years of age! The earlier onset of puberty in girls than boys seems related to their having higher gonadotropin levels. Gonadotropins, especially FSH, tend to reach higher concentrations in girls than boys from infancy onward,[6,34,38] and their gonadotropin responses to GnRH tend to be greater during prepuberty too (Fig. 8–8).

The onset of puberty is more closely related to an individual's bone age than chronologic age. This is particularly important in the case of subjects who are later than average in entering puberty, as discussed previously. In the author's experience, puberty begins by the time the skeletal age reaches 12.5 years and menarche by the time skeletal age reaches 14 years in about 95 per cent of cases.

The pubertal growth spurt occurs during early adolescence. The peak of linear growth velocity corresponds most closely with stage B II and the increase in serum alkaline phosphatase levels with B III.[247] Fat accumulation increases and fat distribution tends to change as well,[248] in part because of the action of estrogen.[249] As a consequence of these pubertal changes occurring out of phase with chronologic age, girls begin to differ considerably in size and habitus during the nineth year of life. Consequently, examination of fourth to eighth graders reveals girls at all stages of puberty and phases of growth—short and tall, physically immature and mature.

Normal Variations in Development

Although the onset of breast development (stage B II) characteristically precedes the appearance of sexual pubic hair (PH II) and the onset of menses substantially (Table 8–5), there is normally considerable variation in the sequence of these events. Pubic hair may appear before breasts begin to develop, a situation arising from lack of direct linkage between adrenarche and gonadarche. Menarche may occur within months after the appearance of breasts; however, this is so unusual that its occurrence demands exclusion of an abnormal hyperestrogenic state.

A common normal variant is the unilateral onset of breast development. Unilateral breast development may exist up to 6 months before the other breast becomes palpable. This phenomenon seems related to an asymmetry that often normally persists into adulthood. Excisional biopsy of a normal unilateral breast papilla in search of a nonexistent tumor should be avoided, because such a procedure is equivalent to excision of the entire breast anlage.

Two extreme variations of normal are the most common causes of apparent premature sexual development. These are the isolated appearance of sexual hair (*premature pubarche*) and the isolated appearance of breast development (*premature thelarche*). Until recently it was thought by many that the cause of these situations was end-organ hypersensitivity to the trace amounts of sex hormones that normally circulate in small children. However, the vast majority of children with premature pubarche have responses to ACTH intermediate between those of normal young prepubertal children and adults, compatible with the diagnosis of premature adrenarche (Fig. 8–18).[151,250] That is, most children with this syndrome have undergone precocious maturation of adrenal androgen secretion. They typically have pubertal elevations of DHAS. Their testosterone levels are only marginally above the prepubertal range. In spite of the androgenic abnormality, the only other sign of increased androgen production may be minimal acne: clitoromegaly does not occur, there is no obvious growth spurt, the bone age typically does not advance abnormally, and there are no other signs of sexual maturation.

The cause of most cases of premature thelarche is not clear. However, it now appears that most idiopathic premature thelarche is usually due to slight secretion of estrogen by the ovary.[229,251–253] Intermittent or persistent low-grade estrogenization of the urogenital mucosa[49] and/or slight or intermittent elevation of the serum total or free E2 has sometimes been found. Ultrasound examination tends to show some ovarian follicular development.[254] Nevertheless, typically the breasts either do not progress or occasionally regress, a growth spurt does not occur, menses do not appear until the usual age, and the bone age does not advance abnormally. This phenomenon probably occurs because of early gonadarche in those individuals whose FSH and LH levels tend to be frequently—but not consistently—at the upper end of the prepubertal normal range (i.e., the lower end of the adult range) (Fig. 8–5). Thus, in infants the syndrome seems to be due to a failure to promptly inhibit the minipuberty of the neonate, and in older children it seems to be a form of unsustained or intermittent true sexual precocity. Therefore idiopathic premature thelarche seems to occur on a spectrum of neuroendocrine activation that includes true sexual precocity and may be the presenting feature of it. Follow-up is indicated to make the distinction with certainty. Our concept about the hormonal milieu in this syndrome is illustrated in Fig. 8–11.

By statistical definition, puberty can be delayed in 3 per cent of normal girls. This is termed "constitutional delay of growth and development" and is often familial. When puberty does ensue in such subjects it is perfectly normal in tempo. Endocrinologic status is normal for the stage of puberty.

There is considerable variation in the length of time it takes for a girl to establish a menstrual pattern that is normal by adult standards. The cycles in the early years tend to be a few days longer than in adults,[255] and Treloar has found that long phases of irregularity of menses may occur.[256] These variations seem to be due to the fact that about half of the menstrual cycles are anovulatory during the first two postmenarcheal (gynecologic) years.[257] By five gynecologic years the menstrual cycle is within normal limits for the sexually mature, with 80 per cent of cycles being ovulatory. Failure to establish a normal adult menstrual pattern by two postmenarcheal years or to sustain a normal pattern for 2 years after one has been established carries a greater than two-thirds risk of persistent oligoovulation (Fig. 8–30).[258] Thus, failure to establish regular cycles by this time is an indication to investigate for hypogonadism or dysfunctional ovulation (see later in this chapter).

There is considerable variation in the amount of acne, facial hair, adiposity, and muscularity among normal adolescent girls, most of which is related to familial factors. Virtually all adolescents experience some degree of acne. However, premature onset of acne, hirsutism at any age, or obesity in association with menstrual irregularity warrant investigation for hyperandrogenemia.

Profound psychological changes occur during adolescence. Sexually immature girls tend to be socially immature, and the onset of puberty is associated with increased independence and profound changes in outlook on life and intellectual capacities. The extent to which these developments occur in reaction to the physical changes of puberty and the extent to which they are direct effects of sex hormones are unknown. Masculine tomboyish traits usually have no clear hormonal basis, although there is some evidence that they may have prenatal hormonal determinants.[16] Social interactions have effects on these aspects of development, and these effects extend even to synchrony of the menstrual cycle.[259] The relative contribution of hormonal, pheromonal, psychological, and social factors to normal behavior is difficult to sort out.

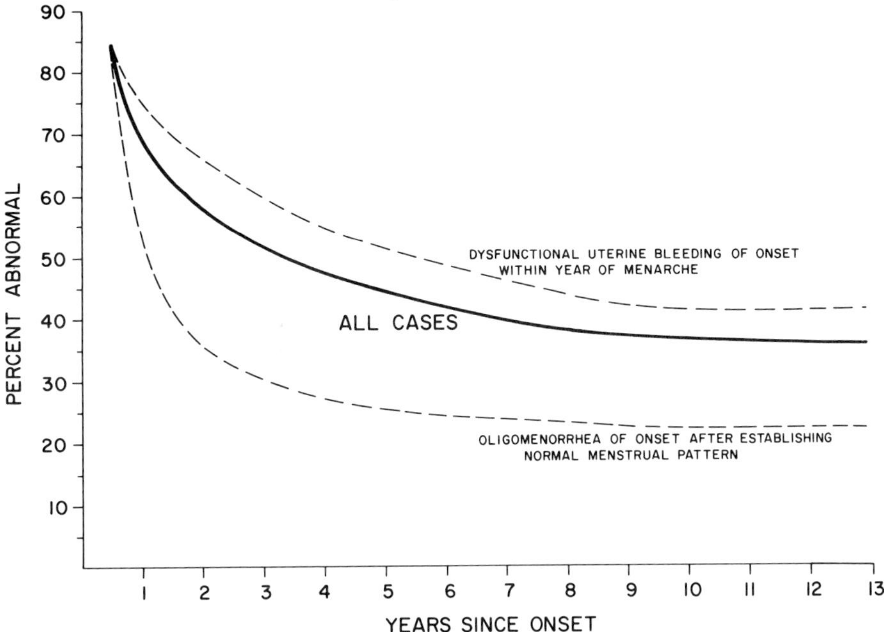

FIGURE 8–30. Probability that an adolescent with a menstrual abnormality severe enough to require gynecologic consultation will have continued menstrual abnormality. The lines show the cumulative rates at which subjects with menstrual abnormalities converted to normal patterns. The heavy curve shows the overall incidence of continued menstrual abnormality in adolescents when considering both types of anovulatory manifestation (dysfunctional uterine bleeding and oligoamenorrhea) regardless of time of onset. The dotted lines show those subgroups that differ most from the overall pattern; other subgroups fall within about 5 per cent of the mean for the entire group. Note that dysfunctional uterine bleeding of onset within 1 year of menarche carries the worst prognosis for continuing menstrual abnormality (upper dotted line). Note that oligomenorrhea of relatively short duration occurring after a normal menstrual pattern has been established carries the best overall prognosis. Nevertheless, it can be seen that if the menstrual abnormality persists for 2 years, there is a 67 per cent probability that the patient will not spontaneously evolve to normal cycles. That is, of the 60 per cent of patients with an abnormal menstrual pattern of 2 years' duration, two thirds (40 per cent of the total group) will continue to have abnormal periods. Similarly, if the problem persists for 5 years, there is an 80 per cent likelihood of persistence of the abnormality. (Redrawn from Southam and Richart.[258])

Normal Variation in Mature Cycles

The cyclic changes of LH, FSH, E2, and progesterone during the menstrual cycle are shown in Fig. 8–13. Some diurnal and episodic fluctuations are superimposed upon these, as noted in the related discussion.[80,83] Since testosterone and androstenedione have both adrenal and ovarian origins, their levels fluctuate to some extent in cyclic, diurnal, and episodic patterns. For example, testosterone levels tend to be 20 per cent greater in the morning than in the evening and to rise 50 to 100 per cent in midcycle.[78,260] The normal range for most of the important sex hormone levels of women during the early follicular phase of the menstrual cycle is given in Table 8–4. Progesterone levels are below 100 ng/dl until the periovulatory phase of the cycle and then peak to over 500 ng/dl in the midluteal

phase. Hormonal production rates for the midfollicular phase in women are given in Table 8–3.

Serum prolactin increases transiently in midcycle with maximum ovarian E2 secretion.[261] Prolactin levels are also transiently stimulated by mammary stimulation and psychological factors.[262]

The menstrual cycle of young adults averages 28 days in length (90 per cent confidence limits, 22 to 40 days by the fifth gynecologic year).[256] The variation in cycle length is almost entirely due to differences in the duration of the follicular phase. The luteal phase, the time between ovulation and the onset of menses, invariably lasts 14 ± 1 (SD) days.[79]

Behavioral symptoms frequently appear to be related to the menstrual cycle. Some dysmenorrhea is characteristic of ovulatory cycles, presumably as a result of prostaglandins released within the endometrium upon the withdrawal of progesterone. It becomes a source of morbidity in 14 per cent of adolescents and is ameliorated by antiprostaglandin therapy.[263,264] Mood changes confined to the second half of the menstrual cycle affect many women and are termed the premenstrual syndrome.[265] It is often disruptive of women's personal and professional lives. Neuropsychiatric symptoms are sometimes severe, ranging from mood disorders to epilepsy to quite bizarre behavior.[266-268] These represent aberrant responses to a normal endocrine milieu rather than a hormonal imbalance. Progestins have been the most widely used therapeutic agents, but why they should be beneficial when the hormonal environment is normal is unclear, and indeed their efficacy is limited. Reversible "medical ovariectomy" by GnRH agonist down-regulation of pituitary gonadotropin secretion has markedly attenuated premenstrual symptoms. Whether prolonged therapy would be safe and effective, or even necessary, remains to be determined.

ABNORMAL PUBERTY

Abnormal Development

Intersex

Patients with intersex syndromes—those whose genitalia are ambiguous or inappropriate for their gonadal sex as a result of endocrinopathy—may come to a physician's attention for the first time at puberty. One problem is primary amenorrhea in an otherwise normal adolescent on the basis of the testicular feminization syndrome. Another problem is the onset of inappropriate puberty. For example, a teenage girl came to us because she was becoming increasingly reclusive from her family and friends because her clitoris was growing to penile proportions while feminization was not occurring—she proved to have male pseudohermaphroditism on the basis of incomplete androgen resistance. Sometimes a delay in seeking medical help may occur because the clitoromegaly is modest. This can occur with true hermaphroditism or congenital adrenal hyperplasia. Both these situations are compatible with fertility.[16] Virilization beginning at puberty is sometimes the presenting complaint of girls with congenital adrenal hyperplasia (see "Hyper-

androgenism"). In about 5 per cent of females operated upon for inguinal hernia, a testicular gonad will be found.[269] The intersex syndromes are reviewed in Chapter 10.

Other Dysgenetic Disorders

Failure of the onset of menses can result from structural abnormalities of the genital tract that do not have an endocrinologic basis. The vagina may be aplastic or have an imperforate hymen; if the uterus is intact, hydrometrocolpos will occur. The uterus may be congenitally aplastic. Uterine synechiae develop as the consequence of endometritis, which may result from infection or irradiation. Congenital absence of the vagina may be associated with varying degrees of uterine aplasia; this is the Rokitansky-Küster-Hauser syndrome.[270] This syndrome seems to occur as a single gene defect or as an acquired teratogenic event involving mesodermal development and the mesonephric kidney, the latter resulting in abnormalities of the genital tract and sometimes the urinary tract.

Precocious Puberty

Causes

When breast development begins before the age of 7.5 years or menses before the age of 9.5, puberty is considered precocious, or premature. Puberty can occur prematurely as an extreme variation of normal, because of a disturbance in the hormonal axis normally involved in sexual maturation, or because of a disturbance outside that axis. Depending on which part of this hormonal axis is involved, different forms of precocious puberty are distinguished. A classification of the causes of premature puberty together with typical findings is given in Table 8–6.

It is important to distinguish between true precocious puberty and pseudoprecocious puberty. In true precocious puberty maturation is "complete." Both breasts and pubic hair develop as the result of activation of the pituitary to secrete both FSH and LH. Thus, *central* is a term sometimes applied to this type of precocity. Follicle-stimulating hormone brings about ovarian follicular development and estrogenization, and LH stimulates ovarian androgen production. Patients with true precocious puberty have "isosexual" precocity because the second-

TABLE 8–6. TYPICAL FINDINGS IN FEMALE SEXUAL PRECOCITY

Locus	Type	HA*	BA*	Estrogens†	Androgens†	LH/FSH†	Pathology	Characteristics
Complete precocity								
Neuroendocrine	Isosexual	+	+ +	+	+	+	Idiopathic Organic CNS	95% of female sexual precocity
Incomplete precocity								
Normal variant	Isosexual	–	–	±	–	±	None	Thelarche/gonadarche
	Isosexual	–	–	–	±	–	None	Pubarche/adrenarche
Neuroendrocrine	Heterosexual	+	+ +	–	+	+/+ + +	LH/hCG excess	Familial or tumor
	Isosexual	Low	Low	±	–	±	Hypothyroid	Growth arrest
Ovary	Iso/hetero	+	+ +	+/+ + +	+/+ + +	–	Tumor	
	Isosexual	+	+ +	+/+ + +	–	±	McCune-Albright	Bone lesions ± nevi ± ovarian cysts
Adrenal	Heterosexual	+	+ +	±	+ + +	–	CAH‡	Dexamethasone suppressible
	Hetero/iso	+	+ +	+/+ + +	+/+ + +	–	Tumor	
Exogenous	Iso/hetero	±	±	–	–	–	Steroid ingestion	
End organ	Iso/hetero	–	–	–	–	–	Tumor or vaginal foreign body	

* HA (height for age) and BA (bone age): –, normal; +, advanced; + +, markedly advanced.
† Hormone levels: –, normal prepubertal; +, pubertal level; + +, adult level; + + +, abnormally high.
‡ CAH, congenital adrenal hyperplasia.

ary sexual characteristics are appropriate for the sex of the child.

In pseudoprecocious puberty, maturation is *incomplete*, with only some of the sexual characteristics developing early. By contrast with true precocity, pseudoprecocious puberty suggests that the sexual development is not mediated by the pituitary gland (although breast development may be the sole manifestation of early complete precocity for as long as 6 months). In some patients with pseudoprecocity, pubertal development is isosexual—that is, it is appropriate for the sex of the child. In others it is "heterosexual," meaning that characteristics of the opposite sex are manifested.

The most common causes of sexual precocity in females are the extreme variants of normal mentioned previously—"premature thelarche" and "premature pubarche." These are incomplete forms of sexual precocity in which breast development (thelarche) *or* sexual hair development (pubarche) is of a degree appropriate for an early stage of adolescence and hence, isosexual. Typically, linear growth and skeletal maturation are not abnormally advanced and sexual development is virtually nonprogressive. Most cases of idiopathic premature thelarche have some evidence of gonadarche (Fig. 8–11), and most cases of premature pubarche have some evidence of premature adrenarche (Fig. 8–18). A related, but rare disorder is isolated prepubertal menses, which like premature thelarche has been attributed to transient ovarian activity.[271]

True isosexual precocity results from disturbance of the hypothalamic-pituitary axis.

About 95 per cent of true precocity in girls is idiopathic. Idiopathic true sexual precocity seems usually to be due to premature triggering of the normal pubertal mechanism. Pubertal development usually is qualitatively and quantitatively normal except for its early occurrence. Progressive puberty with a growth spurt ensues when activation of the pituitary-ovarian axis is sustained. However, puberty is not necessarily intense enough or sustained enough to cause the inexorable progression of normal puberty or to cause deterioration of height potential.[272] The predominance of the idiopathic syndrome in females, its usually sporadic occurrence, and its benign nature are compatible with the likelihood that this disorder is an extreme exaggeration of the normal tendency of girls to have relatively high gonadotropin levels. Although the majority of these patients are thought to go on to have normal menstrual cycles—and pregnancy has been documented to occur as early as 4 years of age—some patients with idiopathic true precocity prove to have anovulatory cycles. This is similar to the experimental model in which certain hypothalamic lesions in rats cause premature puberty followed by constant estrus.[1]

In true isosexual precocity, pubertal levels of estrogens and androgens are found and there is an associated pubertal growth spurt with advancement of bone age at variably increased rates. Random gonadotropin levels are in the pubertal range and are often indistinguishable by RIA from prepubertal or adult levels.

True sexual precocity sometimes results from noncentral disorders in which the bone age is advanced. Thus, we may see true puberty begin after correction of virilizing or feminizing disorders that have advanced the bone age to 10 to 12 years.[273]

True isosexual precocity can result from a variety of intracranial disturbances. These disorders apparently cause sexual precocity by interfering with tracts carrying inhibitory signals to the hypothalamus. It may be associated with congenital brain dysfunction, such as "cerebral palsy" or hydrocephalus. It may result from masses in the region of the hypothalamus. Such lesions may be as diverse as tuberculoma, astrocytoma, or neurofibromatosis. Neurofibromatosis type I (von Recklinghausen disease) tends to cause true sexual precocity in association with optic glioma, which is often relatively benign, or hamartoma.[274,275]

Hamartoma of the hypothalamus, unlike most brain lesions that produce sexual precocity by destruction of regions that normally suppress gonadotropin secretion, may act as an "accessory hypothalamus," which causes sexual precocity by releasing GnRH into the pituitary portal circulation.[276] Immunoreactive GnRH has been reported in the cerebrospinal fluid of some patients.

A small proportion of pineal tumors cause sexual precocity.[277,278] The incidence of sexual precocity is about 3.5 times as great in nonparenchymatous tumors (such as gliomas and teratomas) as in parenchymatous tumors. This suggests that in these tumors sexual precocity is due to absence of a normal pineal inhibitory factor rather than destructive effects on inhibitory tracts.[277] Although pineal tumors may cause paralysis of upward gaze by pressure on the corpora quadrigemina, this sign is present in only a minority of cases.

One of the most intriguing disorders causing true sexual precocity is the McCune-Albright syndrome.[279–283] This is a syndrome of precocious puberty, café-au-lait pigmentation occurring in nevi that have an irregular ("coast of Maine") border, and polyostotic fibrous dysplasia. Disorders that are occasionally associated include gigantism-acromegaly, hyperthyroidism, Cushing syndrome, and ovarian cysts. The syndrome occurs in incomplete and expanded forms. For example, precocious puberty and bony lesions may occur in the absence of cutaneous pigmentation; furthermore, not all patients with polyostotic fibrous dysplasia and cutaneous pigmentation have sexual precocity. The disorder has been recognized pre-dominantly in females. It was once postulated to result from hypersecretion of hypothalamic releasing hormones. Recently, the syndrome has been shown to occur independently of gonadotropin secretion.[284,285] A similarity of the Albright syndrome to the multiple endocrine adenomatosis syndromes has been pointed out. Pituitary adenomas capable of secreting LH and FSH and/or growth hormone have been reported, and the adrenal and thyroid glands in patients with Cushing syndrome and hyperthyroidism tend to show multinodular hyperplasia that seems to be independent of pituitary control. Luteinized follicular cysts within the ovaries function autonomously. Breast carcinoma has also been reported in this syndrome; it is unclear in this case whether it was related to the tendency for adenomatosis inherent in the syndrome, previous irradiation of the breast, or medroxyprogesterone acetate therapy.[286] The etiology of this syndrome is unknown. A unifying hypothesis would be that multiple receptor-related adenylate cyclase systems are turned on without trophic hormone stimulation. However, FSH has been reportedly detectable by bioassay in the absence of detectable immunoreactive FSH.[287]

The hypergonadotropinism of premature ovarian failure has once been reported to cause sexual precocity prior to premature menopause.[288]

An unusual disorder of functional isolated elevation of LH was recently reported.[289] Heterosexual precocious development occurred in the sister of a boy with true isosexual precocity. She developed stage III pubic hair and clitoral hypertrophy at 4 years, with slight to moderate advances in height and bone age in association with an adrenarchal level of DHAS and a moderately elevated testosterone level (91 ng/dl). The occurrence of virilization in this patient is unusual because girls with hCG-producing tumors have not been reported to have sexual precocity,[290] presumably because complete ovarian function cannot occur without FSH priming. It is possible that modest virilization would occur in patients with ectopic overproduction of hCG over prolonged periods of time.

One of the most intriguing pediatric complexes is the unusual syndrome of sexual precocity associated with juvenile hypothyroidism. A case is illustrated in Figure 8–31. This syndrome is often characterized by galactorrhea. This is often subtle, and the breasts must be carefully manipulated in order to express the few drops of milky fluid that may be present. Multicystic ovaries are often demonstrable by ultrasonography.[291] There is little, if any, sexual hair development. There is another clinically unique feature about the sexual precocity of hypothyroidism: it is the only form of sexual precocity in which growth is arrested rather than stimulated.

The prevailing concept of the mechanism by which juvenile hypothyroidism causes sexual precocity dates from the formulation of Van Wyk and Grumbach.[292] These workers postulated that this syndrome resulted from hormonal "overlap" in the negative feedback regulation of pituitary hormone secretion, with overproduction of gonadotropins as well as TSH in response to the thyroid deficiency. Although these workers realized that the seeming lack of specificity in the feedback control mechanism might have an explicit biologic basis, none was obvious at the time; consequently, many inferred that the overlap of the negative feedback effect of thyroxine was nonspecific. The nature of pituitary overlap has been considerably clarified in recent years. Overlap is now known not to apply to growth hormone secretion, which is subnormal in hypothyroidism. The increases in plasma TSH and prolactin that characterize the syndrome[293] could well be accounted for by common neurohumoral control systems, TRH stimulating, and dopamine inhibiting, both hormones. It has been speculated that gonadotropins are increased together with TSH, since all are glycoproteins and share a common subunit. However, gonadotropin excess seems unlikely to be the cause of the sexual precocity of hypothyroidism. A major argument against the prevailing concept is a clinical one: most children with prolonged hypothyroidism have delayed sexual maturation, as would be expected from the maturational retardation characteristic of states with delayed bone ages. In addition, although radioimmunoassayable gonadotropins are elevated, they are not significantly higher in hypothyroid patients with sexual precocity than in those without sexual precocity.[294] Furthermore, gonadotropins are not usually detectable by bioassay.[292,293,295]

Hyperprolactinemia may be the factor most closely related to the sexual precocity. Its causative role is by no means certain, however, because prolactin levels do not correlate with pubertal development in nor-

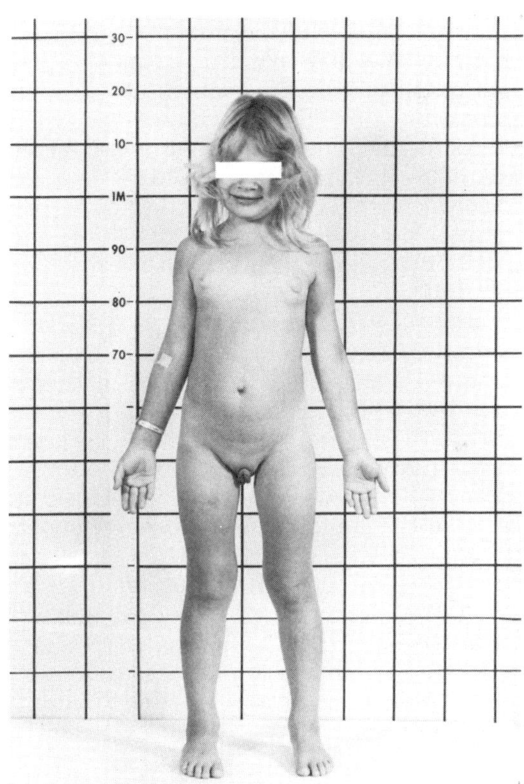

FIGURE 8–31. Sexual precocity due to hypothyroidism (#UC 133-33-55-4) in a 9.1-year-old with breast development since 7 years and menarche at 9.0 years. Growth failure had occurred and her height age was 6 years. In addition to breast enlargement and galactorrhea, the labia minora were noted to be enlarged and pigmented. There was no sexual hair or clitoromegaly. Rectal examination revealed an enlarged and palpable cervix without adnexal masses. There were typical physical findings of hypothyroidism. Bone age 6.2 years. Thyroxine less than 1 μg/100 ml, TSH 438 μu/ml, prolactin 66 ng/ml, and serum estrogens 72–182 pg/ml. Vaginal smear showed 45 per cent superficial cells and 55 per cent large intermediate cells. Immunoreactive LH and FSH were 300 and 174 ng LER-907/ml, respectively; however, bioactive LH was undetectable. Immunoreactive gonadotropins failed to suppress upon estrogen administration, their response to a 100-μg GnRH bolus was minimal, and they seemed responsive to TRH. All these hormonal findings were not obviously different from those of hypothyroid girls without sexual precocity except for the higher estrogens. Patient had withdrawal bleeding and evidence of regression of breast development within the first 3 months of thyroid hormone replacement treatment. After 6 months' treatment, normal puberty began; menarche occurred at 12.5 years of age.

mal or hypothyroid children. However, induced hyperprolactinemia causes sexual precocity in female rats.[135] Ovarian estrogen and progesterone responsiveness to hCG is increased, possibly by prolactin induction of ovarian LH receptors. Mean LH levels do not change, but an increase in episodic gonadotropin secretion has not been ruled out. This key role for prolactin is supported by the finding that suppression of hyperprolactinemia in experimental hypothyroidism blocks the ovarian cyst formation characteristic of hypothyroidism.[296] These data can be interpreted as indicating that hyperprolactinemia sensitizes the ovaries to the low circulating gonadotropin levels present prepubertally.

Primary ovarian disorders typically cause incomplete isosexual precocity. The most common tumor associated with isosexual feminization is the benign ovarian follicular cyst.[297,298] The cells lining these cysts are often luteinized. Estrogen production is modest to marked. Testosterone levels tend to be in the midadult female range (about 40 ng/dl). Some of these cysts may occur in the course of intermittent or unsustained true sexual precocity.[253] A case is shown in Figure 8–32.

The second most common ovarian feminizing neoplasm in girls is the granulosa cell tumor.[2,299] These often have some associated thecal tissue. Granulosa cell tumors are usually benign; when malignant, the granulosa cell component rather than the thecal component is generally the culprit. Characteristically tumors composed of granulosa-theca cells produce feminization. They are occasionally associated with mesodermal dysplasia syndromes[300] and may produce chorionic gonadotropin.[299]

Masculinizing tumors (characteristically Leydig-Sertoli cell tumors or arrhenoblastomas) are unusual before the teenage years. The abnormal differentiation that is essential to tumor formation often leads to an abnormal pattern of steroid secretion. Androstenedione secretion often predominates over testosterone secretion in interstitial cell tumors[301]; furthermore, masculinization on rare occasions occurs with granulosa-theca cell tumors and feminization with interstitial cell tumors. Thecomas (luteomas) are unusual in children and generally benign. Dysgerminomas virilize only if they have interstitial cell elements. Gonadoblastomas are virilizing tumors virtually confined to individuals with dysgenetic testes on the basis of XY pseudohermaphroditism. Adrenal rest and hilus cell tumors of the ovary are extremely rare causes of masculinization in childhood.[18,188] Lipid cell tumors must be considered in the differential diagnosis of late-onset congenital adrenal hyperplasia because they tend to produce

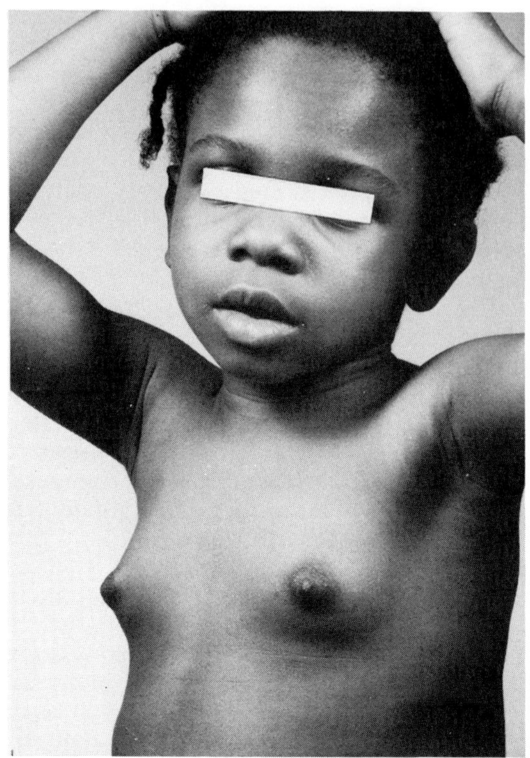

FIGURE 8–32. The appearance of a 5.2-year-old child (#UC 114-32-17-6) with complete isosexual precocity due to a luteinized follicular cyst. Her breast development is no different than that of other girls with idiopathic premature thelarche. She presented at 4.7 years with a 2-week history of breast development. Height and bone ages were 5 years. Over a 5-month follow-up period, breast development progressed, she developed sexual pubic hair and presexual axillary hair, and menstrual flow commenced at 3- to 5-week intervals. Four weekly determinations of plasma unconjugated estrogens (E2 and estrone) showed them to consistently range between 158 and 215 pg/ml. Luteinizing hormone averaged 50 and FSH 13 ng LER-907/ml by RIA. Testosterone was 37 ng/dl, DHAS 82 μg/dl. At the time of surgery, when she was 5.2 years old, her height age was 5.8 years and her bone age was 7.5. Exploratory laparotomy revealed a right ovarian cyst measuring about 5 cm in diameter, which was removed. Subsequently there was a rapid fall in plasma estrogens and testosterone to prepubertal levels. However, DHAS was unchanged. Menses ceased, but intermittent vaginal cornification (maturation index 90/10/0 to 0/90/10) was repeatedly found. Breast enlargement and sexual hair development resumed at 8.5 years with normal pubertal sex hormone levels; menarche occurred at 9.5 years.

17-hydroxyprogesterone and respond to ACTH as well as LH.[302]

Adrenal disorders cause pseudoprecocity, as discussed in Chapter 6. The hyperandrogenism of congenital adrenal hyperplasia can be so mild that there is no genital defect, and the presentation may resemble premature adrenarche. Adrenocortical tumors typically cause a rapid virilizing disorder characterized by very high DHAS production. A case discussion is given with Figure 8–33. On occasion adrenal tumors cause feminization. Androstenedione may be the predominant androgen. When feminization and virilization coexist from such a tumor, the clinical picture may resemble complete isosexual precocity.[303]

Exogenous steroids can cause sexual precocity. Estrogen-containing contraceptive pills and anabolic steroids are widely available. The administration of anabolic steroids can result in an expression of their androgenic effects. The ingestion of birth control pills can also result in breast development and vaginal withdrawal bleeding. Some cases of precocious thelarche may be caused by ingesting food contaminated with artificial estrogens.[304]

Common causes of genital bleeding and discharge are vaginal foreign bodies or sexual abuse. Occurence of vaginal bleeding (characteristically malodorous) without breast development is highly suggestive of foreign body. A hymenal opening of greater than 5 mm is compatible with vaginal penetration by a foreign object.[305] Tumors of the genital tract may present in this way as well. Neurofibromas have been reported to simulate breast development and clitoral hypertrophy.

Differential Diagnosis

A physician need not be experienced in endocrinology to handle most female patients presenting with early breast or pubic hair development. For the most part, these signs in girls are due to self-limited, natural processes occurring early for no reason more serious than premature thelarche/gonadarche or premature pubarche/adrenarche. In these cases, either early breast development or pubic hair growth occurs as an isolated unsustained phenomenon.

In the examination the physician should pay particular attention to symptoms and signs that might suggest intracranial, abdominal, or pelvic disease. The availability of steroid-containing hormones should be ascertained. The child's height and weight should be carefully recorded and the growth curve examined.

If no other abnormalities are found on physical examination, a limited workup, including bone age determination, should be done to check whether the symptom is indeed an isolated phenomenon or whether appreciable hormone excess exists. If the skeletal age is not abnormally advanced relative to chronologic age, it is likely that the presenting symptom is isolated and merely due to benign, subtle overactivity of some part of the hormonal axis. Therefore, it is no more than an extreme variant of normal. Confirmation of this impression is obtained if serum level of the relevant female or male hormones is low (E2 less than 10 pg/ml and testosterone less than 25 ng/dl).

To confirm the diagnosis of these benign nonprogressive disorders, the child must be similarly reevaluated after 6 months. The importance of this recheck is illustrated by the case shown in Figure 8–32. If the results are still negative, the family can be reassured that true puberty—including menses in girls—will not occur until the usual age.

If more than one sign of precocious puberty is present, if the growth is accelerated,

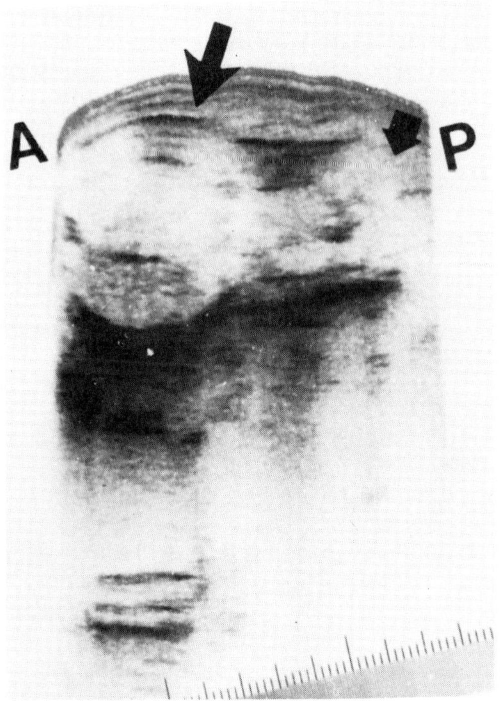

FIGURE 8–33. Abdominal ultrasound (decubitus view) showing a pedunculated, encapsulated 5-cm adrenal adenoma (large arrow) near upper pole of kidney (small arrow); the mass was not suspected from the intravenous pyelogram. A, anterior; P, posterior. This 1.3-year-old girl was virilized. Pubic hair had appeared 2 months previously, height had changed from the 10th to the 30th percentile, and clitoromegaly had occurred. Bone age was 2.3 years. Dehydroepiandrosterone sulfate was 3000 to 4271 μg/dl, testosterone 121 ng/dl, and urinary 17-ketosteroids 14 mg/day.

if there is evidence of excessive sex hormone levels or action, and/or if an additional sign of puberty appears, a more extensive investigation should be undertaken to rule out a discrete lesion affecting some part of the hormonal axis controlling puberty. For example, if a young girl with early breast development begins to grow pubic hair or show signs of a growth spurt (growth greater than 1 inch in 6 months), then something more than premature thelarche/gonadarche is possibly involved. The same is true if her bone age advances inordinately over the 6-month interval or if she begins menstruating. These additional signs indicate the need for more extensive studies.

The investigation of sexual precocity should be initiated with determinations of bone age, estrogenization indices, and androgen levels. Determination of serum thyroxine and prolactin is indicated if the sexual precocity is accompanied by growth arrest and/or galactorrhea. Advancement of bone age above height age suggests the presence of prolonged excess of sex hormones. Early in the course of sexual precocity the bone age may not reflect the disorder, but acceleration of the bone age observed over a period of several months is consistently found with a significant excess of sex hormone. Plasma E2 concentration is usually 10 pg/ml or more in true isosexual precocity. Because of the cyclic nature of sex hormone secretion, examination of a vaginal smear for E2 effect is often a more accurate indicator of the presence of modest E2 excess than is the E2 blood level because the vaginal cytology represents the integrated effect of estrogen over the preceding few weeks (Fig. 8–11). The finding of an E2 level at the upper end of the pubertal normal (over 75 pg/ml) is atypical and necessitates prompt workup to distinguish ovarian or adrenal tumor from true isosexual precocity[306]: Weekly determinations of E2 may be necessary to determine whether the level is fluctuating in a normal cyclic fashion or is persistently elevated.

Gonadotropin radioimmunoassay in a random sample is usually not diagnostically useful. However, the GnRH test is often useful in sorting out these disorders.[253,307] Patients with true isosexual precocity have a pubertal pattern of response to GnRH, whereas children with unsustained pseudopuberty as variants of normal or with estrogen/androgen secreting tumors will have a minimal gonadotropin response. Other

useful tests in specially equipped laboratories are the determination of the 24-hour patterns of LH and FSH[44] or determination of bioactive LH.[308] All of these approaches discriminate true precocious puberty from pseudoprecocity quite well.

Determination of the plasma androgen pattern is useful in discriminating among the causes of premature pubarche and virilization. We screen the androgen pattern by routinely determining plasma testosterone and DHAS for this purpose. Premature adrenarche is characterized by a pubertal level of DHEA and DHAS, but the other plasma androgens are, at most, marginally elevated above the prepubertal range. A greatly elevated level of DHAS is characteristic of adrenal tumors. Androstenedione is more obviously abnormal than testosterone or DHAS in congenital adrenal hyperplasia and many ovarian tumors.[302] Dexamethasone suppression testing and other means to determine the source of sex steroid excess are discussed in the section on "Hyperandrogenemia" and in Chapter 6.

Ancillary studies are often indicated. It has been customary in girls with true isosexual precocity that is neither rapidly progressive nor associated with alarming symptoms to settle for a simple set of skull films to rule out a serious cause of the disorder. However, if there are associated symptoms that are *at all* suggestive of intracranial disease, computed tomography (CT) of the hypothalamus and/or magnetic resonance imaging (MRI) is indicated. Ultrasonography is the method of choice to initiate investigation for abdominal or pelvic masses. Multiple small (less than 8 mm) ovarian follicles are typically detectable in the slightly enlarged ovaries of girls with true sexual precocity.[254] Occasionally, a larger cyst is seen, but these usually prove to be transient preovulatory follicles.

Isolated vaginal bleeding suggests sexual abuse, foreign body, tumor, or, rarely, isolated menses. Cytology, anaerobic culture, plasma E2, and in some cases pelvic ultrasound examinations are indicated.

Management*

The guidelines for management are to rule out an organic disorder that requires

---

* The use of GnRH agonists, Cyproterone acetate, Provera, Ketoconazole, and Testolactone has not been officially approved in the United States for treatment of sexual precocity. If these agents are to be used, proper informed consent must be obtained.

treatment in and of itself, and to ascertain whether sexual precocity is either rapidly compromising height potential or resulting in important secondary emotional disturbances in the child. The only permanent physical complication of true isosexual precocity, all else being normal, is short stature. The excessive sex hormone production in the first decade of life causes early maturation of the epiphyses, resulting in their premature closure. Thamdrup found that about half the females with this disorder reached an adult height of 53 to 59 inches and the remainder 60 to 65.6 inches.[2] Social withdrawal is common, but frank behavioral problems are unusual in girls.[309]

Intracranial lesions must be treated by appropriate measures, such as neurosurgery or irradiation. Granulosa cell tumors confined to the ovary have a good prognosis for cure by unilateral oophorectomy. Recurrence of tumor may occur 20 years after the initial operation, however. Biopsy of the opposite ovary is indicated in unilateral ovarian neoplasms.

When true sexual precocity is rapidly progressive to the point of significantly compromising height potential and its cause cannot be directly alleviated, we attempt to control the disorder medically.[173] Medroxyprogesterone acetate (Provera) has been administered intramuscularly in a dosage commencing at 50 mg/month. Doses as high as 400 mg/month have been used, although cushingoid side effects may be observed at this level.[310] Alternatively, the drug may sometimes be effective when given orally, commencing at doses of 5 mg twice daily and increasing to four times daily. Although Provera treatment reverses some of the physical changes of premature puberty, it does not necessarily reverse the inordinately rapid maturation of the skeleton, possibly because of its inherently weak androgenicity. Although medroxyprogesterone acetate has been implicated as an etiologic agent in experimentally produced mammary carcinoma, these findings seem to be unique to beagles, a species especially susceptible to such an effect by natural progestins. Progestational agents, however, are no longer considered appropriate for the therapy of sexual precocity. Danazol, a 19-nor-testosterone derivative, has been used in the treatment of sexual precocity because of its progestational and antiestrogenic effects. However, its androgenic effects are too predominant to make it a suitable form of treatment in girls.

Cyproterone acetate, a progestational and antiandrogenic steroid analog, has been widely used in Europe for the treatment of sexual precocity, but is not available in the United States. In a dosage of about 100 mg/m^2 orally in two to three divided doses daily, it inhibits the LH response to GnRH and causes a reduction in estrogen levels. Reduction in breast size and menstruation result. Although there has been a suggestion of a beneficial effect of this treatment on linear growth and bone maturation, statistical analysis does not indicate this effect to be significant.

The best treatment for idiopathic true sexual precocity appears to be with long-acting GnRH agonists.[173,311] Advantage has been taken of the down-regulating effects of such agents on pituitary gonadotropin release: daily use inhibits gonadotropin release and reduces plasma E2 to less than 9 pg/ml within 1 month. Potent agonists are capable of causing sex hormone secondary sexual characteristics to regress to early pubertal levels and height prediction to increase. Improvement in height prediction by approximately 5.5 cm after 4 years of therapy has been reported. No serious side effects have come to light, but long-term safety remains to be established. The use of GnRH agonists in the United States is currently investigational. Leuprolide, marketed for "medical orchiectomy" of metastatic prostatic cancer, is available by prescription, however. Therapy should be initiated with 2.0 mg/m^2 to avoid worsening the status by an agonist effect because large doses often are required to inhibit puberty. The dosage can be reduced later if tolerated. Other GnRH agonists such as nafarelin can be anticipated on the market soon.

The aromatase-inhibitor testolactone has been successfully used to treat the gonadotropin-independent McCune-Albright syndrome.[285] Gonadotropin-releasing hormone agonist treatment may be necessary for those in whom true puberty has been superimposed when the bone age has reached a pubertal level.[284]

Patients with premature thelarche or pubarche as variations of normal are counseled as follows. The child's early development is simply a matter of a normal stage of puberty occurring early. It is due either to an incomplete, slow kind of puberty (premature gonadarche or adrenarche) or to increased sensitivity to the trace levels of hormones that are normally present at her age (idiopathic thelarche or pubarche). Feminization with breast development and eventual menstruation can be expected to occur at an appropriate age. Because this is a normal type of development, no treatment is necessary. In order to ascertain that too much female hormone is not being made from time to time, we advise that such children be rechecked every 6 to 12 months.

Besides dealing with the physical consequences of true isosexual precocity, the physician must be ready to help the family and child cope with the psychological problems that come with early physical maturation. The doctor can help the family by explaining that even though their child looks older and more mature than other children of the same age, the child may not feel or act more maturely. Most children with these disorders tend to be withdrawn because they feel that they are different from their peers. The libido of these children is not increased. The family should be advised to take some precautions to downplay their child's development, for example, in the choice of clothing and swimsuits. Friendships with children a bit older will help shorten the time affected children spend in social limbo. This may be more easily said than done, however, since the intellectual and social maturity of these patients is not advanced. It is important to remind the family and child that in a few years the child will not be unique from the standpoint of sexual development. It is important to reassure parents and children with the usual idiopathic sexual precocity that the child is simply going through a normal process early because of a "mis-set timer." The following books may be helpful in explaining precocious puberty: for children, *What's Happening to Me?*, by Peter Mayle (Lyle Stuart, Inc., Secaucus, NJ, 1973); for parents, *Sex Errors of the Body*, by John Money (Johns Hopkins University Press, Baltimore, MD, 1969).

Hypogonadism

Causes

If hypogonadism is complete and present prepubertally, it causes sexual infantilism. If it is of lesser degree or of onset in the early teenage years, it interferes with the normal progression of feminization and prevents

TABLE 8–7. ANATOMIC AND FUNCTIONAL CLASSIFICATION OF OLIGOMENORRHEA AND AMENORRHEA

Abnormal genital structure
  Ambiguous genitalia
    Intersex
  Vaginal aplasia
  Normal introitus
    Uterus
      Intersex
      Aplasia
      Synechiae
    Vagina
      Imperforate hymen
Normal genital structure
  Hypoestrogenism—FSH high
    Primary ovarian failure*
      Gonadal dysgenesis
      Ovarian removal, x-ray, chemotherapy
      Oophoritis
      Adrenogenital syndrome affecting ovary
      Resistant ovaries
  Hypoestrogenism—FSH ≤ normal
    Ovarian insufficiency
    Hypogonadotropinism
      Delayed puberty
      Congenital
      Acquired: anorexia nervosa, brain tumors
      Hyperprolactinemia
    Primary ovarian failure*
    Virilization
  Normal estrogenization (follicular inadequacy)
    Lack of cyclic LH
      Psychogenic/athletic amenorrhea
      Post-pill
      Idiopathic
      Other: obesity, endocrine, pregnancy
    Hyperandrogenism
      Polycystic ovary syndrome
      Adrenogenital syndrome
      Idiopathic

* Patients with primary ovarian failure may not have clearly elevated gonadotropins until the bone age reaches about 10 to 12.5 years.

the onset of menses (primary amenorrhea). If the onset of hypoestrogenism is postmenarcheal, it causes secondary amenorrhea or oligomenorrhea (fewer than nine periods a year). Thus, disorders causing hypogonadism appear in the differential diagnosis of sexual infantilism, failure of pubertal progression, and oligomenorrhea, as well as of intersex. The causes of hypoestrogenism are listed in the differential diagnosis of amenorrhea in Table 8–7.

Primary ovarian failure is considered first; it is covered in Chapter 9 in greater detail. It is characterized by high levels of gonadotropins, particularly FSH. Two exceptions exist to the rule that FSH is elevated in this group of disorders. First, the gonadotropins may not be elevated until

CNS maturation has reached the stage at which bone age is 10 to 12.5 years. Secondly, patients with *partial* ovarian failure do not have high baseline gonadotropin levels, although FSH hyperresponds to GnRH administration.[312] It seems quite likely that there is a feedback relationship between FSH levels and gamete formation in women as there is in men. This hypothesis would explain why the presence of relatively few ovarian follicles—too few to permit a fully developed follicle to emerge—suffices to prevent a rise in FSH.

The most common cause of primary ovarian failure is gonadal dysgenesis due to deletions of an X chromosome. This diagnosis should be considered in all girls with primary hypogonadism or secondary amenorrhea whether or not they have the typical stigmata of Turner syndrome, as discussed elsewhere (see Chapter 9). A degree of ovarian dysgenesis occurs in autosomal trisomy 18 and 21, but the effect on ovarian function is not well described.[22]

The second most common cause of primary ovarian failure is physical and/or medical injury. Primary ovarian failure is becoming increasingly apparent now that irradiation and chemotherapy for childhood neoplasia are effectively prolonging life. The ovary is extremely radiosensitive, less than 1000 rads causing permanent ovarian failure in adults.[313] Shalet et al. studied 16 girls who had received abdominal irradiation for tumors in their prepubertal years. All had received 2500 to 3000 rads and all had evidence of gonadal failure.[313] In the majority of patients, such treatment therefore virtually assures subsequent sterility. The problem can be obviated by transposing the ovaries out of the irradiation field prior to such treatment if possible. About 75 per cent of mature women ingesting over 50 mg/day of cyclophosphamide will develop permanent ovarian failure.[314] The incidence of ovarian failure seems to increase with duration of treatment beyond about a year. Busulfan treatment for chronic myelogenous leukemia in postmenarcheal subjects causes ovarian failure. The 6-mercaptopurine-methotrexate-vincristine-corticosteroid protocols used for childhood leukemia carry perhaps only a 5 per cent risk of causing permanent ovarian failure.[315]

Autoimmune oophoritis tends to occur in association with hypoadrenalism, autoimmune thyroiditis, diabetes, hypoparathyroidism, vitiligo, pernicious anemia, and a variety of other autoimmune disorders.[316,317] Adrenal failure nearly always accompanies ovarian failure, and both organ systems tend to fail within a short time of each other. The strong association between these two disorders probably reflects sharing of antigens between the steroid-producing cells of the gonads and adrenal cortex. A family of autoantibodies is found in the sera of these patients that react with a spectrum of antigens in steroid-producing cells: some sera react with luteal, others with theca, and others with granulosa cells. Steroid cell antibodies can generally, but not necessarily, be absorbed out by extracts of adrenal cortex. The antibodies to granulosa cells are generally cytotoxic. Current evidence suggests that the basic defect in the autoimmune endocrine deficiency syndromes is deficient T cell suppressor function. The histologic picture of the ovaries in affected patients is sometimes that of lymphocytic infiltration; yet sometimes there is only selective loss of primordial follicles, and in other cases nothing is left of the ovary but streaks. Gonadotropin elevation may be only intermittent while puberty progresses, and it has been postulated that treatment with replacement doses of glucocorticoids slows the course of the oophoritis.[318]

Functional ovarian failure has been most often described to result from certain hereditary defects in the biosynthesis of androgens and estrogens, the congenital adrenogenital syndromes. Desmolase deficiency (A in Fig. 8–23), 17α-hydroxylase deficiency (B'), and C_{17-20}-lyase deficiency (G) cause hypogonadism in phenotypic females.

Resistance to gonadotropin action is a rare cause of functional hypogonadism. These patients' gonadotropins are elevated and evidence an exaggerated response to GnRH. In addition, the histologic appearance of the ovary shows a normal number of ova but no growing follicles. We found gonadotropin resistance to be the cause of secondary amenorrhea in a patient with pseudohypoparathyroidism.[319] This patient is now known to have the generalized defect in the guanine nucleotide regulatory unit, which is characteristic of most patients with the Albright osteodystrophy form of the syndrome.[320] Functional ovarian failure has also been described in galactosemia.[321]

The *hypogonadotropic hypogonadism* syndromes present the most difficult diagnostic problems. This type of hypoestrogenism does not have elevated gonadotropins. These disorders are particularly difficult to distinguish from delayed puberty. Extreme delay in puberty as a variant of normal is a relatively unusual presenting complaint in girls. Delayed puberty can result from endocrine or metabolic disorders that arrest or delay growth.[322] Attenuation of growth is caused by growth hormone deficiency, hypothyroidism, hypercortisolism, acidemia, alkalosis, liver or renal disease, severe chronic illness, or cachexia. A delayed growth pattern can result from chronic illness, prolonged undernutrition, hypophosphatemia, or the tissue hypoxia of chronic anemia or congenital heart disease (see Chapter 1).

Congenital gonadotropin deficiency can occur as an isolated pituitary defect—sometimes inherited in association with anosmia (Kallmann syndrome)—or in association with congenital errors of hypophysis formation, which are often signaled by a midline facial defect. It may occur in association with other neurologic or endocrine dysfunction, such as in the Prader-Willi syndrome (congenital benign hypotonia, hypothalamic obesity with or without diabetes insipidus) or the Laurence-Moon-Biedl syndrome (retinitis pigmentosa, obesity, mental deficiency). Gonadotropin deficiency can also be acquired, as a consequence of tumors, accidents, autoimmune hypophysitis,[323] degenerative disorders involving the hypothalamus and pituitary,[324] or irradiation.[325] Pituitary adenoma, craniopharyngioma, and dysgerminoma are the most common neuroendocrine neoplasms responsible in children. A case of hypothalamic tumor is presented with Figure 8–34. The most common disturbance of sexual development in girls with pinealomas is delayed adolescence. This has led to the suggestion that these tumors may act by secreting a pineal inhibitory substance such as melatonin, rather than by compression of areas of the brain.[277]

The most common cause of hypogonadotropic hypogonadism in pediatric practice is anorexia nervosa. This is a syndrome of amenorrhea, undernutrition due to voluntary starvation, and a particular psychological dysfunction.[326,327] Some are bulimic.[328] The onset tends to be at 12 years of age or later. Earlier onset is associated with growth arrest and delay of puberty.[329] The symptom complex consistently includes a distorted body image; these patients uniformly con-

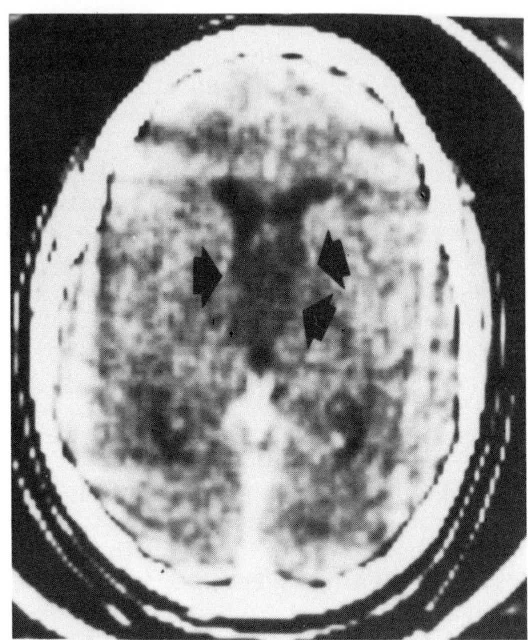

FIGURE 8–34. Computed tomography of the brain of a 16-year-old girl with hypothalamic astrocytoma. The low-density tumor mass (arrows) extends superiorly from the hypothalamus, obliterates the third ventricle, and partially compresses the frontal horns of the lateral ventricles, particularly the right. This patient presented with secondary amenorrhea. Menarche had occurred at age 13, and menses were normal until 15.3 years. The patient then became amenorrheic in association with lethargy, episodic headaches, polyuria, and weight gain, despite little change in appetite. Physical examination was negative. The skull x-ray, electroencephalogram, visual fields, and serum prolactin and thyroxine levels were normal, and urine specific gravity was 1.016. After biopsy of the cyst wall, studies revealed her to have gonadotropin, growth hormone, and partial antidiuretic hormone deficiencies.

sider themselves too fat in the face of objective evidence that they are not. Their physical activity level tends to be high, too. These patients tend to be highly intelligent with a strong ability to rationalize with "pseudologic" their fundamental misconception about food and fatness.

Anorexia nervosa patients have poor self-esteem and tend to be depressed. They are reserved and do not date at the usual age. They tend to have a very poor self-image, which is sometimes obvious in the area of physical attractiveness, but sometimes a less obvious problem is in not being able to live up to their own standards. These patients are quite anxious about their feelings of social inadequacy. More deep-seated is the tendency to feel insufficient in self-control over resentments and frustrations. In contrast to other depressive individuals, they are characterized by a greater degree of intellectual achievement and high regard for educational and vocational goals; they are generally content with themselves in this sphere. They adjust well in most ethical areas. The basic psychological conflicts seem to arise over the implications of maturational changes: increasing concern about bodily changes may make the patients aware of their long-standing self-dissatisfaction, which includes a problem disengaging from their parents. It is as if these teenagers seize upon dieting as a means of differentiating themselves and establishing their identity. Dieting not only meets a need for approval, which is easily forthcoming in our culture with its diet fads, and demonstrates self-control, but the emaciation is the girl's means of making herself unattractive so as to avoid sexual relationships with the opposite sex. These emotional problems are difficult to discern in the initial disagreements over the need for eating.

The cause of the disorder is unclear. Normal nutrition is critical for recovery of gonadal function.[330] These cases almost always have fat stores at or below the 10th percentile, and those who recover to the point of resuming menstruation do so after achieving body fat stores above this level (Fig. 8–35). The weight changes leading to cessation or restoration of menstrual cycles are in the range of 10 to 15 per cent of body weight and seem to represent mainly changes in fat. There is an inverse relationship between body weight and the maturity of gonadotropin release in these patients. The 24-hour pattern of gonadotropin release tends to be comparable to that of prepubertal or pubertal children, and the diurnal LH pattern has been reported to revert from a pubertal to a mature pattern with recovery from malnutrition.[331] The gonadotropin response to GnRH is blunted in the malnourished state and becomes normal with weight gain to 70 to 94 per cent of ideal.[332,333] Ovulation generally occurs in response to clomiphene after body weight has returned to 80 per cent or more of normal.[334,335]

However, weight is not the only consideration. A primary psychological disturbance or hypothalamic disturbance[326,336] is necessary to explain why some cases give a history of becoming amenorrheic before weight loss, and about half of the cases remain amenorrheic after treatment. The author favors the concept that these psychological problems lead to amenorrhea only in certain women who are predisposed to amenorrhea by some unique preexisting anatomic or functional feature of their neuroendocrine system.

A number of features attributed to hypothalamic dysfunction, such as cold intolerance, may be due to the subtle hypothyroid state that is secondary to the malnutrition: serum triiodothyronine levels are consistently low, serum thyroxine levels tend to be lower than average (although usually within normal limits), the pattern of TSH release indicates TRH deficiency, and the state of deep tendon reflexes and metabolism is consistent with hypothyroidism.[337]

Mild hypercortisolism is typical.[338] Afternoon ACTH and cortisol levels are high and the response to CRH is blunted. Anorexia nervosa bears some similarity to other psychogenic causes of amenorrhea, such as depression[339] and to athletic amenorrhea,[119,340] and the distinction may be difficult. These similarities are both clinical and biochemical. Luteinizing hormone pulse frequency may be restored by opiate antagonists in anorexic patients[54] as in other forms of hypothalamic amenorrhea.[339]

Not only must brain tumor be excluded in anorexic amennorrheic patients, but partial bowel obstruction as well. The superior mesenteric artery syndrome may produce symptoms suggestive of anorexia nervosa.[341]

Hyperprolactinemia can cause functional gonadotropin deficiency.[342] Galactorrhea is present in about half the cases, particularly those with residual estrogen production. Luteinizing hormone pulses tend to be infrequent and LH secretion variable in response to GnRH.[343] Hirsutism and seborrhea are common because of the multiple effects of prolactin on androgen metabolism.[138] About one third of hyperprolactinemic women have an identifiable pituitary adenoma. Prolactinomas may be so small as to cause no problems due to local extension (microadenomas). Elevated serum prolactin levels also occur with a variety of tumors that cause functional or anatomic pituitary stalk section, thereby preventing inhibitory pituitary control. Many cases have a functional abnormality: decrease in hypothalamic dopaminergic tone or in production of prolactin inhibitory factor may underlie such cases.[344] In about a quarter of adult cases, the malfunction is due to phenothiazine ingestion or associated with oral contraceptive use. Selective secretion of exces-

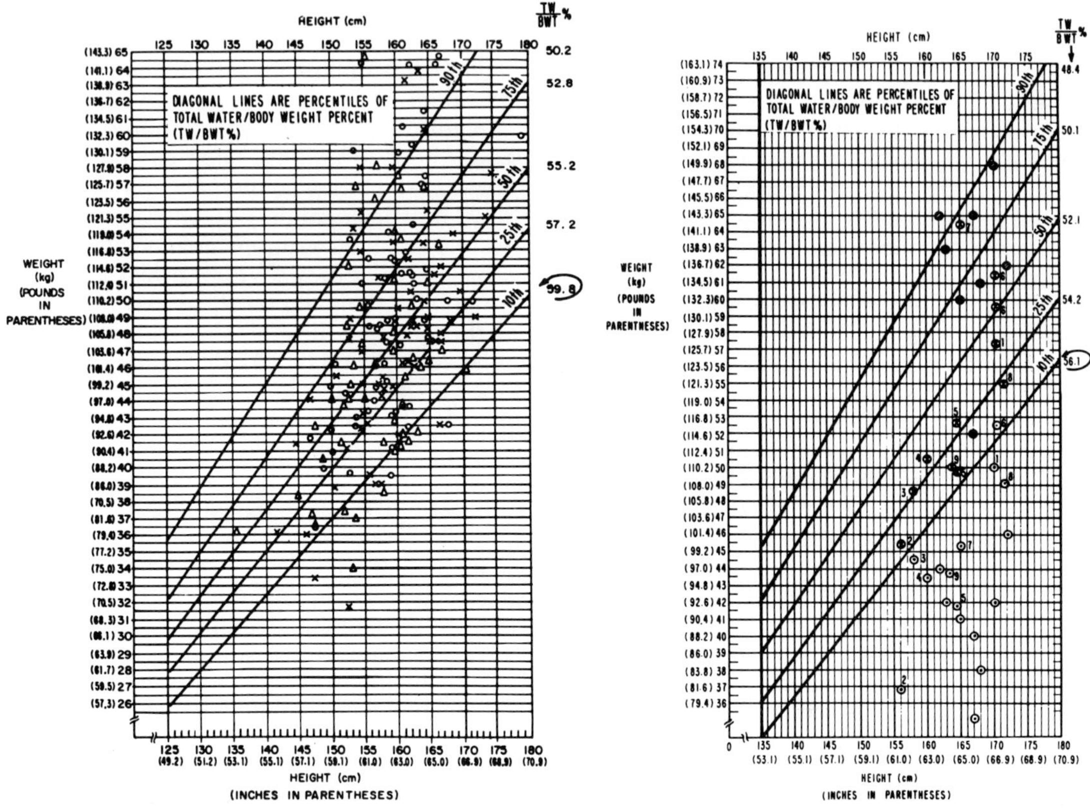

FIGURE 8–35. Percentiles of fatness (diagonal lines) for Caucasian girls at menarche (left) and after menarche (right) equated with computed percentiles of total water as a percentage of total body weight. The minimal weight necessary at a particular height for the onset or maintenance of menses is very close to the 10th percentile of fatness on these respective charts. Data for anorexia nervosa cases are shown on the right chart: ⊙, at presentation, ⊗ = at resumption of menses. (From Frisch RE, McArthur JW: Menstrual cycles: Fatness as a determinant of minimum weight for height necessary for their maintenance or onset. Science 185:949, 1974. Copyright© by the American Association for the Advancement of Science.)

sive prolactin may cause not frank gonadotropin deficiency, but more subtle ovarian dysfunction (see "Follicular Inadequacy" section).

Frank virilization as a result of very high androgen levels causes defeminization. However, the modestly hyperandrogenic disorders, which are more common, are associated with normal estrogenization.

Differential Diagnosis

The differential diagnosis of amenorrhea is outlined in Table 8–8. Investigation should be undertaken for hypogonadism when the onset of puberty has not occurred by the chronologic or bone age of 13 years, if puberty has not progressed as indicated by failure of menses to occur within 4.5 years of the onset of puberty or by a chron-

ologic or bone age of 14 years, or if secondary oligo- or amenorrhea has persisted for 2 years (see Table 8–5 and Fig. 8–30 and related discussion). Delayed puberty in the female usually has an organic basis. A family history of delayed puberty may suggest that the delay is inherited and not due to organic

TABLE 8–8. INITIAL DIAGNOSTIC WORKUP FOR OLIGOMENORRHEA OR AMENORRHEA

1. Systemic history and physical exam
2. Gynecologic exam
3. Bone age
4. Estrogenization assessment
   a. Estrogen level
   b. Vaginal smear, spinnbarkeit, and/or ferning
   c. Progestin ± estrogen trial
5. Androgen measurement
6. LH, FSH measurement
7. Prolactin measurement

causes. The evaluation should include taking a careful history of previous medical problems and possible intracranial, visual, olfactory, emotional, abdominal, or pelvic symptoms. It should be kept in mind that chronic systemic disease of almost any kind can lead to delayed puberty—pulmonary, renal, gastrointestinal, hematologic, immunologic, or collagen diseases, for example. Upon examining the patient, the height should be carefully measured for determination of growth rate, and assessment should be made of the appropriateness of weight (Fig. 8–35). The physician should pay particular attention to measurement of blood pressure, eye movements, visual fields, and optic fundi. The patient should be tested for loss of sense of smell and other neurologic deficits. One should be on the lookout for evidence of other endocrinopathies. On examination of the breasts an attempt should be made to express milk from the ducts to the nipple. Careful examination of the introitus, hymen, and clitoris and categorization of the stage of sexual development are essential. The finding of a structural abnormality upon gynecologic examination may indicate that amenorrhea is due to abnormal development of the genital tract.

The initial diagnostic workup of amenorrheic patients proceeds as outlined in Table 8–8. Bone age determination is necessary to assess the expected state of neuroendocrine maturation. The initial tests must include an assessment of estrogen and gonadotropin levels. A single plasma E2 measurement is of limited value without a biologic assessment of overall estrogenization. In pediatric practice, this is best ascertained by performing a vaginal smear for the determination of hormonal effects on cytology (Fig. 8–19). A useful clinical tool for the assessment of degree of estrogenization in an adolescent who is well feminized is to ascertain the response to progestin therapy. Following administration of medroxyprogesterone acetate, 10 mg nightly for 5 to 7 days or a single intramuscular injection of 200 mg progesterone in oil, withdrawal bleeding will occur in individuals who are well estrogenized (average plasma E2 approximately 40 pg/ml or more). If bleeding does not occur in response to this maneuver, the integrity of the uterus can be tested by the response to a 3-week course of estrogen-progestin; these hormones are most conveniently administered in the form of birth-control pills.

Plasma total testosterone and DHAS should be measured if virilization is suspected. For the detection of more subtle hyperandrogenism that may cause anovulation without hypogonadism, assay of plasma free testosterone is necessary.

The direction of study of a hypoestrogenic patient takes one course if the gonadotropins are high and another if they are not (Table 8–7).

Finding elevated gonadotropins suggests primary ovarian failure. Therefore, the workup should include determination of serum electrolytes and chromosomes. If these studies are normal and there is no obvious explanation for the hypogonadism, an ACTH test may be indicated for the assay of 17-hydroxyprogesterone and progesterone in addition to cortisol in order to assess adrenal reserve and the possibility of a defect in a steroidogenic step common to the adrenal and ovary. Biopsy of the ovary with histologic examination is indicated if the diagnosis remains in doubt. This can be adequately done in most instances via laparoscopy.

If gonadotropins are not elevated, a different course should be taken. Complete blood count, erythrocyte sedimentation rate, urinalysis, and assessment of liver and renal function should be taken as the first step to rule out various types of chronic illness. If prolactin excess is discovered, the best endocrinologic indicator of tumor as the cause is a prolactin level over 100 ng/ml.[342] The height of the prolactin level correlates with the size of the tumor. Very high blood or cerebrospinal fluid[345] prolactin levels indicate invasiveness of the tumor. The workup should include formal testing of visual fields (Goldman perimetry or evoked response) and CT or MRI of the sella turcica (Fig. 8–34). The patient should also be studied for the possibility of deficiency of other pituitary hormones, starting with thyroid function tests and somatomedin-C.

Arrangements for psychiatric evaluation for possible anorexia nervosa should be considered at the same time that plans are laid for the other diagnostic studies. Diet faddism may be difficult to distinguish from anorexia nervosa.

Gonadotropin-releasing hormone testing may permit the differentiation between hypogonadotropic hypogonadism and delayed puberty relatively early. The GnRH test as usually performed, measuring the gonadotropin response to a 50- to 100-μg bolus, has limitations because some normal teenagers have minimal responses and because one third of hypogonadotropic subjects have a normal response. The major utility of the GnRH test in the premenarchial teenager is that a brisk response strongly suggests that the delayed puberty is a variation of normal. It is presently unclear whether GnRH agonist testing will discriminate better (Fig. 8–28). Gonadotropin profiles during sleep have not proven useful to distinguish hypothalamic dysfunction from constitutional delay of puberty.[346]

Management

Underlying disorders must be treated appropriately. For example, most tumors require surgery, although a deeply situated hypothalamic location may preclude this approach in favor of irradiation therapy. The medical treatment of choice for hypogonadism in patients with hyperprolactinemia is bromergocriptine.[342] Small doses are used initially to minimize nausea. Treatment is initiated with a dose of 1.25 mg (1/2 tablet) at bedtime and gradually increased to a full dosage of 2.5 mg twice or three times a day. If menses occur, they will do so within 4 to 6 weeks of achievement of the maximal dose.

In anorexia nervosa, rehydration and reversal of starvation are the first priorities, and management of the psychiatric problem is the next. In selected patients with anorexia nervosa in whom menses do not return in spite of normal weight gain, ovulatory cycles may be induced with clomiphene. Initial psychiatric management of mild cases of anorexia nervosa, and psychogenic and athletic amenorrhea (see "Lack of Normal Cyclic Gonadotropin Surges") can be undertaken on an outpatient basis. It must be emphasized that menses cannot be expected to resume until the amount of body fat is restored to normal for the patient's height (see Fig. 8–35). The long-term prognosis is variable. Anorexia nervosa "by proxy" has been described in the offspring of former patients.[347]

There are two aspects of therapy that are uniformly involved in managing hypogonadism—psychological support and hormone administration. Patients with delayed development that is a variation of normal should be reassured that there is nothing wrong, only a delay in timing of onset of menses. The wide normal variation in the pattern and time of the pubertal growth spurt should be explained in detail and the girl should be informed of her predicted eventual height. It is of interest that the majority of children with delayed puberty do not have overt psychological symptoms. Complex compensations and sublimations obviously occur. However, peer group pressures may make adjustment to sexual infantilism especially difficult when the age of 13 is approached,[348] and a poor self-image may lead to social withdrawal and feelings of hopelessness. Physical immaturity may prolong psychological immaturity. A short course of physiologic sex hormone therapy at this time may help alleviate these anxieties. The physician should discuss the fact, when the evidence favors it, that the odds are overwhelmingly in favor of the "timer" in the "subconscious area of the brain" eventually turning on. When this will happen can be roughly estimated from the skeletal age. One should not hesitate to advise more intensive psychological counseling if it becomes apparent that the concern about puberty is but one aspect of a more general maladjustment. Ultimately the decision as to whether to undertake treatment for delayed puberty is up to the patient and her family.

It is important to assure the teenager with an organic basis for hypoestrogenism that feminization will occur, although in response to appropriate hormone treatment. It should be kept in mind that normal breast development in the girl with panhypopituitarism requires replacement of growth hormone and cortisol deficits. The only patient in whom the author has not succeeded in producing normal feminization was a child with refractory systemic lupus erythematosus who could not be weaned from doses of glucocorticoids that produced Cushing syndrome.

Estrogen replacement therapy is best begun with a physiologic form of treatment because the use of inappropriately large estrogen doses results in failure to achieve children's genetic growth potential. We recommend that the initial course of therapy consist of monthly intramuscular injections of 0.5 mg of a depot form of estradiol. The growth, development, and predicted height should be carefully evaluated prior to treatment. Menses may not occur within the first year of therapy on this regimen. However, closely approximating midpubertal sex hormone production by increasing the dose to 1.5 mg/month will bring on menses within 3 to 12 months.[121] When this form of estrogen treatment is given to hypogonadal girls whose bone ages are 11 or more years, the patients achieve their genetic height potential. If intramuscular therapy is not acceptable, a reasonable alternative is to commence with 5 μg ethinyl estradiol given in a cyclic fashion, daily for 3 weeks out of four.[349] The suggestion that this regimen improves height potential has been disputed. However, it is clearly wise to commence therapy with very low dosage estrogen. The use of low doses of androgens or androgen derivatives for improvement of growth rate is seldom indicated in patients with hypogonadal disorders other than Turner syndrome variants. Either 30 mg/m^2 depot-testosterone monthly[350] or about 0.0625 mg/kg/day oxandrolone (2-oxo-17α-methyldihydrotestosterone [Anavar])[351] on a 6 months on, 6 months off cycle does not seem to interfere with the realization of normal height potential and may be useful in the hypogonadal child who wishes to commence estrogen therapy, yet whose bone age is only 10 years.

Eventually progestin must be added to estrogenic regimens when bleeding begins to occur at unpredictable times. This is the first sign of endometrial hyperplasia. In those patients in whom achievement of full genetic height potential is important, we prefer adding medroxyprogesterone acetate, 10 mg at bedtime, coincident with the third week of estrogen. This will uniformly bring about normal menstruation during the week preceding resumption of estogen therapy. Once optimal height is achieved, most patients prefer to switch to birth control pills as a convenient form of estrogen-progestin therapy. The pills containing the lowest dose of estrogen that will result in normal-appearing menstrual cycles are advisable. The lowest estrogen dosages currently available in combination contraceptive pills in the United States contain 20 μg (Loestrin 1⁄20) to 30 μg (Lo-Ovral, Loestrin 1.5⁄30) ethinyl estradiol (see also Chapter 9).

Hypogonadotropic patients can achieve ovulation with gonadotropin therapy. Hyperprolactinemic patients are relatively resistant to clomiphene or gonadotropin therapy, however.[352] There has recently been considerable interest in treatment of those patients whose hypogonadotropinism is based on hypothalamic GnRH deficiency with pulsatile GnRH.[54,346] Fertility has been achieved by this means. For detailed discussions of induction of ovulation for purposes of promoting conception, the reader is referred elsewhere.

Follicular Inadequacy Syndromes

The disorders to be discussed in this section are those that cause amenorrhea or menstrual disturbances in sexually mature, well-estrogenized women. In these disorders the neuroendocrine system stimulates ovarian estrogen secretion to a level normal for an early- or midfollicular phase female, but follicular development is incomplete and a normal dominant follicle does not emerge. Therefore, ovulation does not occur or an inadequate corpus luteum is formed. Such disorders result either from subtle alterations of hypothalamic-pituitary function such that normal FSH or LH surges do not occur or from impaired follicular maturation in association with ovarian hyperandrogenism. Dysfunctional uterine bleeding (menstrual bleeding at irregular, abnormally frequent intervals) is a manifestation of anovulatory cycles in which follicular maturation is apparently arrested at a late enough stage to result in overall excessive estrogen production.[353]

Lack of Normal Cyclic Gonadotropin Surges

Causes. Patients with hypothalamic hypogonadism as the cause of secondary amenorrhea have reduced LH pulse frequency.[354] The causes include emotional stress, physical stress, exercise amenorrhea, and "post-pill" amenorrhea. Many cases are unexplained. Amenorrhea from severe psychic stress has long been known to cause anovulation (e.g., "boarding-school amenorrhea").[355] The onset of psychogenic amenorrhea may be identified as being associated with a discrete event, but the ovarian dysfunction tends to be long lasting.

Exercise amenorrhea may be difficult to distinguish from anorexia nervosa, partly because of the obsession with weight control.[119,340] Protracted strenuous physical activity coupled with a dietary regimen that leads to leanness is related to delayed menarche and oligomenorrhea. Because menarche may occur when the female athlete's activity level suddenly decreases and before weight gain occurs, it has been postulated that energy reserve is more important than body fat per se for the maintenance of the menstrual cycle.

Mild hypercortisolism is now known to exist in both psychological and athletic stress states.[139,338,339] Endogenous overproduction of corticotropin-releasing hormone (CRH) may serve to raise afternoon cortisol concentrations to morning levels. Then further ACTH response to CRH is blunted by the negative feedback of this cortisol excess. The anovulation apparently results from the inhibitory effect of CRH on gonadotrope responsiveness to GnRH.

An extremely rare form of psychogenic amenorrhea is that due to persistence of the corpus luteum (pseudocyesis). This syndrome tends to occur in infertile women with an overwhelming desire for pregnancy and conversion hysteria. Prolactin and LH excess appear to mediate this syndrome.[356]

Hyperprolactinemia occasionally causes secondary amenorrhea without frank hypoestrogenism.[357] Presumably this situation results from a diminution in FSH secretion that is so marginal as to only inhibit the emergence of a dominant follicle. An even more subtle change of a similar type would seem to account for the occasional presentation of hyperprolactinemia as luteal insufficiency.[358]

The cause of oligoovulation is usually unexplained, but seems to result from excessive endorphinergic tone[359] interfering with the feedback effects of estrogens on LH release. Prolonged negative feedback suppression after E2 administration,[360] failure of estrogenic enhancement of LH responsiveness to GnRH,[361] and failure of a positive feedback effect of estrogen on LH[353,362] have been reported. Opiate antagonists may restore ovulation.

Birth control medications have been suspected of causing amenorrhea. About one third of patients with secondary amenorrhea after discontinuation of estrogen and progestin-containing pills have a history of previous menstrual disturbance and ongoing menstrual problems.[363] Another third can expect spontaneous remission of the amenorrhea. About half of the remainder of cases will have resolution of their menstrual disturbance after induced pregnancy. The most common cause of post-pill amenorrhea is probably hyperprolactinemia because over 20 per cent of such cases have galactorrhea.

How often this antedates ingestion of the contraceptive pill is unknown. Menses may be restored in normoprolactinemic cases by bromergocryptine treatment, which suggests that their cessation is related to excessive pituitary prolactin secretion that is sometimes too subtle to be detected by measurement of plasma levels.[364] The anovulation resulting from depot-medroxyprogesterone acetate contraception is related to the extremely slow rate of absorption and metabolism of this steroid; menses return when the blood levels of this progestin fall below the threshold for suppression of the LH surge,[365] and only rarely has it been associated with disturbed prolactin secretion.[366]

Luteal phase defects may be the cause of short or infertile ovulatory cycles. The immediate cause of an inadequate luteal phase is failure of the serum progesterone to rise to a normal level of 500 ng/dl or more.[367,368] This situation seems to arise from relative deficiency of FSH during the follicular phase, with subsequent diminished follicular development; this may be associated with hirsutism, obesity, or hyperprolactinemia.

Nonhypothalamic endocrine, metabolic, or systemic disorders may cause hypothalamic dysfunction; these include obesity, glucocorticoid excess, disturbed thyroid function, marihuana, chronic illness, and pregnancy. Over-production of estrogen from plasma precursors in adipose tissue is thought to mediate the effect of obesity.[203] Glucocorticoids interfere with the gonadotropin response to GnRH[369,370] and perhaps act at a higher CNS level as well.[371] Thyroid hormone deficiency interferes with gonadotropin action on the ovary.[372] Blood concentrations of tetrahydrocannabinol similar to those found in heavy marihuana users cause anovulatory cycles in the rhesus monkey.[373] The effects of chronic illness may well be mediated by undernutrition.

It must be remembered that pregnancy must be excluded in all sexually mature women with amenorrhea. An elevation of the plasma hCG level, as determined by β-hCG assay, is the earliest laboratory sign.[374] Constant overproduction of estrogens and progestins successively by the hCG-driven corpus luteum of pregnancy and the fetoplacental unit leads to suppression of endogenous pituitary gonadotropin release.

Differential Diagnosis. The medical evaluation should be performed as discussed in the preceding section, with particular attention to the possibilities of emotional disturbances, excessive exercise, the use of birth control pills or other drugs, and state of health. The physical examination should be particularly directed to the state of nutrition, the possibilities of intracranial or systemic disease, galactorrhea, thyroid dysfunction, glucocorticoid excess, hirsutism, and obesity.

Unusually frequent vaginal bleeding requires first and foremost consideration of genital tract tumors. These characteristically cause bleeding that cannot be controlled with cyclic progestin or estrogen-progestin therapy. Endocrine causes include dysfunctional uterine bleeding resulting from anovulation or a short luteal phase. The latter situation tends to cause a relatively regular 3-week cycle. Measurement of plasma androgens and estrogens or weekly determinations of progesterone will make the distinction.

Hypothalamic secondary amenorrhea is characterized by subnormal LH pulse frequency. Gonadotropin-releasing hormone testing may help in the differential diagnosis by demonstrating an immature response. The induction of an ovulatory cycle by clomiphene citrate may be of value in predicting the potential for ovulation.

Management. Many cases falling in this category will benefit from nutritional counseling. Diet faddists and athletes should be advised about the necessity of optimal body energy reserves for the maintenance of normal menstrual cycles (see Fig. 8–35). The teleological significance of this should be pointed out, namely, that inherent in the evolutionary process is the inhibition of pregnancy in times of inadequate food supplies. Ongoing psychological counseling is advisable for patients who cannot change their dietary patterns because of an abnormal body image. Obese girls should be advised that there is a substantial possibility that reduction to a normal weight will result in restoration of menses and improved chances of fertility.

Mature teenagers whose amenorrhea is unexplained should be so informed. They should be assured that they have a high likelihood of fertility with appropriate endocrinologic treatment. However, such treatment is unlikely to be of any benefit to them until such time as they desire to become pregnant.

In the meanwhile, the main objective of therapy is to normalize the endometrial cycle by periodic progestin administration. For this purpose, medroxyprogesterone acetate, 10 mg at bedtime for 5 to 7 consecutive days once every 2 months, usually is effective and is the treatment least likely to produce undesirable side-effects. This will prevent endometrial hyperplasia and theoretically, therefore, endometrial carcinoma.

Induction of an ovulatory cycle sometimes leads to resumption of spontaneous normal menses.[363] An ovulatory cycle can normally be induced by the administration of 50 to 150 mg of clomiphene citrate once nightly for five doses. If treatment is successful, bleeding generally occurs about 1 month from commencement of the treatment. One should start with the 50-mg dose because larger doses may cause hyperstimulation of the ovaries with the development of ovarian cysts; for this reason, too, one should either wait 2 months before starting with the next higher dose or perform an examination to rule out cystic ovaries before going to the next higher dose. Bromergocriptine has been reported to be successful in causing the resumption of ovulation in post-pill amenorrhea, the amenorrhea resulting from modest undernutrition, and other unexplained cases of secondary amenorrhea. Otherwise, induction of ovulation is best left to the endocrinologic gynecologist to supervise at such time as the woman wishes to conceive. The vast majority of patients with no obvious cause for their secondary amenorrhea will become pregnant after appropriate treatment with clomiphene, bromergocriptine, estrogen, human menopausal gonadotropins, or pulsatile GnRH therapy.

Hyperandrogenism

Causes. Polycystic ovary syndrome (PCOS) is the most common cause of hyperandrogenemia presenting at or after the onset of puberty. The common denominator in PCOS seems to be functional, gonadotropin-dependent ovarian hyperandrogenism.[375,376] The disorder is functional rather than anatomic; the classic histologic abnormalities (multiple atretic follicles, stromal hyperplasia, thickened ovarian capsule) of the Stein-Leventhal syndrome are not necessarily present. It is gonadotropin dependent: ovarian hyperandrogenism does not occur in hypogonadotropic amenorrhea, and suppression of gonadotropins reverses the hyperandrogenemia. Finally, the ovarian response to gonadotropins is masculinized.

Polycystic ovary syndrome arises from heterogeneous disturbances. How these cause the syndrome has been intensely controversial. The most popular theory has been that PCOS results from a complex cycle of events in which secretion of androstenedione, in part by the adrenals, and its peripheral conversion to estrone is essential.[377] According to this concept, increased estrone concentrations sensitize the pituitary to secrete excessive LH. However, this theory is not universally accepted because estrone is a weak estrogen, not all cases of PCOS have elevated estrone or LH levels, and our data suggest that androstenedione and estrone are secreted in excess by the ovaries.

We have proposed an alternate theory in which ovarian overproduction of androgen is central. We postulate that PCOS arises from disorders that directly increase one of three variables: the ratio of the serum concentration of LH to FSH, the ratio of the intraovarian concentrations of androgen to estrogen, or follicular atresia. An increase in one of these can then induce successive abnormalities in the others in a reciprocal manner. This concept is diagrammed in Figure 8–36. The common denominator in most PCOS seems to be hyperandrogenic regulation of ovarian P450c17 activities. In classic PCOS (type I), a masculine-type, high LH:FSH ratio is probably the initiating factor. This leads to a masculinized ovarian response. In other cases of PCOS, the gonadotropin abnormalities are mild or absent (Type II PCOS). These latter cases of PCOS are probably initiated by primary abnormalities of androgen production, particularly those arising within the ovaries, or by disorders directly causing follicular atresia. Such cases usually appear to have excessive theca-interstitial cell 17-hydroxylase/C_{17-20}-lyase activity, possibly because of intrinsic defect(s) in the desensitization of the response to LH. This intraovarian androgen excess leads to follicular atresia.[71,100] Conversely, disturbances causing follicular atresia in partially matured follicles would seem to cause intraovarian androgen excess (Fig. 8–15).

The causes of the perturbations underlying PCOS are usually not known. It has been reported to follow idiopathic true sexual precocity.[378] This suggests tonic overproduction of LH, analogous to the situation wherein certain hypothalamic lesions result in sexual precocity that is followed by constant estrus. Most PCOS patients, however, have symptoms dating from an apparently normal menarche. Inefficient E2 biosynthesis from androgenic precursors as a result of deficient activity of ovarian 3β-hydroxysteroid dehydrogenase, C_{17-20}-lyase, or aromatase may cause PCOS. However, such causes appear to be the exception rather than the rule, and whatever aromatase deficiency is present appears to be secondary to the FSH deficit.[89] Disorders characterized by insulin resistance or hyperinsulinism would appear to respectively interfere directly with granulosa cell maturation or promote thecal androgen secretion by interfering with desensitization of the LH re-

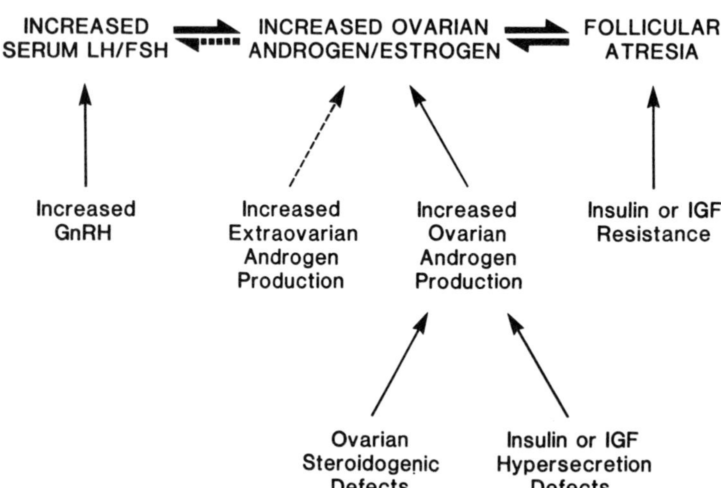

FIGURE 8–36. Model of the etiology of polycystic ovary syndrome (PCOS). Broad arrows show the interrelationships among the key variables that are the proximate causes of PCOS. Perturbation of one of these variables causes a disturbance in the others, as indicated. Narrow arrows show where six pathophysiologic states impinge to cause PCOS. Dotted lines show relationships for which evidence is inconsistent. (From Barnes R, Rosenfield RL: Polycystic ovary syndrome: Pathogenesis and treatment. Ann Int Med 110:368, 1989.[376])

ceptor.[379,380] In Type A insulin resistance, PCOS is due to a congenital disorder of ovarian function first expressed at adolescence.

Hyperandrogenemia has been reported in cases with gonadotropin-resistant ovarian follicles.[381] It seems possible that such rare cases represent defects in the FSH receptor, which in turn result in overproduction of gonadotropins and overstimulation of the LH-sensitive ovarian compartments.

Adrenal hyperandrogenemia is sometimes clearly due to late-onset adrenogenital syndrome. These are mild forms of congenital virilizing adrenal hyperplasia. Late-onset hirsutism has been well documented for 21-hydroxylase, 11β-hydroxylase, and 3β-ol deficiencies.[206] However, most hirsute women with dexamethasone-suppressible hyperandrogenemia cannot be proven to have an adrenogenital syndrome if rigorous criteria are applied regarding the response of plasma steroid intermediates to ACTH. Most of these patients have a pattern of response to ACTH that suggests an exaggeration of adrenarche.[233] Although frankly virilizing levels of androgens inhibit the neuroendocrine axis, we believe that modest elevations of plasma androgens do not in and of themselves interfere with ovulation or menstruation. Therefore, we doubt that very mild excesses of adrenal androgens necessarily cause menstrual disturbances.

Hyperprolactinemia often presents with mild hyperandrogenic symptoms.[138] In rare cases, anomalous presence of adrenal enzymes in the ovaries, perhaps in the form of "adrenal rests" that are under bihormonal control, has been postulated.[302]

Differential Diagnosis. Hirsutism must be differentiated from hypertrichosis, the situation in which vellus hair predominates on "nonsexual" areas of the body. Hypertrichosis is not caused by sex hormone imbalance but appears with heredity, glucocorticoid excess, starvation, and certain medications.

The pilosebaceous response to modest hyperandrogenemia is variable. An increase in the plasma free testosterone concentration underlies half of the cases of mild hirsutism and a third of the cases of persistent mild acne. Hyperandrogenemia should also be suspected if substantial acne appears before feminization at puberty. Many cases are cryptic. Therefore, hyperandrogenemia should also be suspected in the oligomenorrheic female if there is obesity or insulin resistance, even without hirsutism. The distribution of fat to the upper waist and upper limbs may suggest an androgenic basis.[382]

A history of sudden onset and rapid progression of androgenization is very suggestive of virilizing tumor. The presence of ovulatory menstrual cycles in the presence of modest hyperandrogenemia tends to suggest an adrenal source of androgen overproduction. In performing the examination, a search should be made for the stigmata of Cushing syndrome. Upon gynecologic examination, clitoromegaly and the possibility of posterior labial fusion should be ruled out. Bimanual pelvic examination for evaluation of size and configuration of the ovaries is indicated in sexually active teenagers, although it is not now critical in the initial evaluation of virgins.

The first step in diagnosis is to document excessive plasma androgen levels. This may require persistence. The best initial test is a plasma testosterone level, but often one or more other plasma androgen assays are necessary. A normal total plasma testosterone level does not rule out an important, reversible virilizing process, because a depressed TEBG level may lead to an abnormally great fraction of the total testosterone being free and bioavailable. If the plasma concentrations of total or free testosterone as well as DHAS are normal, *virilizing states* are ruled out. However, repeated measurement of plasma free testosterone or other androgens may be necessary to document subtle hyperandrogenemia because in some cases testosterone secretion is episodic or cyclic.

The next step in the differential diagnosis is to determine the source of androgen excess in those patients with elevated androgens. We feel that the dexamethasone suppression test is the method of choice if properly interpreted. Dexamethasone is given for 5 days (or longer in patients who are very obese or have relatively high DHAS levels) in a "low" dose of 1.0 mg/m² daily by mouth in three to four divided doses. The pattern of response of plasma free testosterone, DHAS, and cortisol segregates patients diagnostically (Fig. 8–37). The adequacy of adrenal suppression is judged from the response of cortisol and DHAS to the test: if they do not fall normally, the patient either has Cushing syndrome, has failed to comply with taking the dexamethasone properly, or is under stress. The criterion for

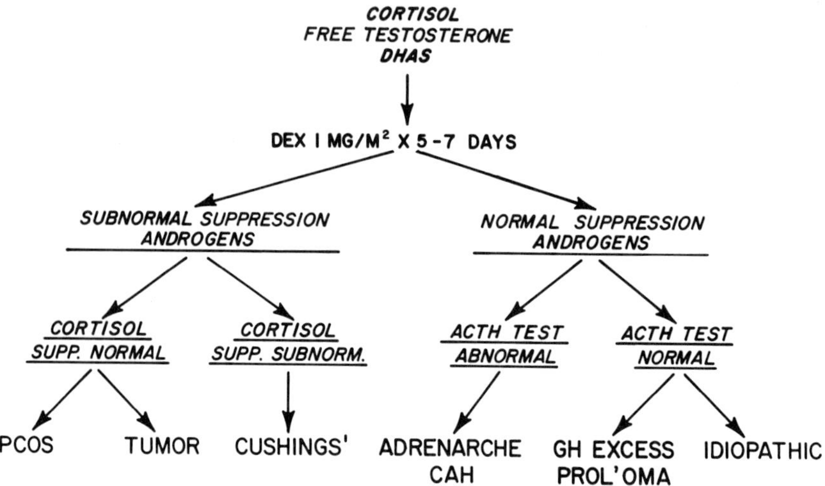

FIGURE 8–37.   Algorithm for the differential diagnosis of hyperandrogenemia. The response of the plasma free testosterone, DHAS, and cortisol to dexamethasone (DEX) 1.0 mg/m² for 5 days or more is evaluated. Subnormal suppression of androgens by dexamethasone points toward PCOS (if both DHAS and cortisol suppress normally), tumor (if only cortisol suppresses normally), or Cushing syndrome (if cortisol does not suppress normally). Normal suppression of androgens by dexamethasone indicates an abnormality of adrenal function: an ACTH test elicits characteristic patterns of adrenal steroid secretion in congenital adrenal hyperplasia (CAH) and exaggerated adrenarche. GH, growth hormone; PROL'OMA prolactinoma, See text for more details.

determining whether a patient has an ovarian source of androgens is whether the plasma free androgens fail to fall into the *normal range for dexamethasone-suppressed nonhirsute women* in the presence of normal adrenocortical suppression.[206] Specifically, in our laboratory, dexamethasone suppressibility is considered normal in a postmenarchial female if the free plasma testosterone is 8 pg/ml or less (plasma total testosterone should be 58 ng/dl or less, but this criterion is not adequate in women with abnormally low testosterone binding). Adequate adrenal suppression is indicated by the DHAS decreasing at least 50 per cent (ordinarily over 75 per cent) with both DHAS and cortisol coming to fall below the normal adult control range. Adrenal virilizing tumors have been reported that suppress with low-dose dexamethasone, although it is not clear whether the suppression was ever truly normal.

Subnormal suppressibility of androgens by dexamethasone indicates that the excess androgen arises at least in part from the ovary or by autonomous adrenal production. Polycystic ovary syndrome is present in the majority of hyperandrogenic patients with menstrual abnormalities and is much more common than tumor or Cushing syndrome.[383] Serum LH measurement is a useful ancillary test. However, it is not elevated in most cases. In part, the lack of LH increase may be an artifact of clinical testing because the elevation of serum LH may be missed if the abnormal diurnal rhythm (midday zenith) or pulsatility are not taken into account. A pelvic ultrasound examination that shows 10 or more microcysts (8 mm diameter or smaller) with increased amounts of ovarian stroma is a supportive but seldom diagnostic test.[254,384] A serum 17-hydroxyprogesterone level over 220 ng/dl in response to a 100 μg test dose of the GnRH agonist nafarelin seems to be useful in confirming the diagnosis.[376] Further extensive diagnostic studies are not indicated unless there is reason to suspect a virilizing tumor. Tumor is suggested by a testosterone level over 200 ng/dl. A DHAS level of over 800 μg/dl suggests the tumor is in the adrenal. Ultrasound, CT, or MRI scan will usually demonstrate the mass in such cases.

If androgens are suppressed to normal concentrations, the patient either has a functional adrenal source for the hyperandrogenemia or a type of androgen imbalance of an obscure nature. In the former group would be late-onset congenital adrenogenital syndrome or exaggerated adrenarche. Hyperprolactinemia or acromegaly are other causes of adrenal androgenic hyperfunction.[138]

Management.   Cyclic oral progestins are

the method of choice for initiating treatment of the menstrual irregularities of anovulatory cycles. Medroxyprogesterone acetate (Provera), 10 mg at bedtime daily for 5 to 7 days, is prescribed, commencing at 3-week to 3-month intervals. The more frequent intervals are chosen for patients with intractable dysfunctional uterine bleeding and the less frequent intervals for patients with amenorrhea, the wide spacing permitting one to ascertain the possibility of occurrence of spontaneous menses. The only indication for the use of estrogen-progestin–containing contraceptive pills in the management of menstrual irregularity alone is in those patients whose problem cannot be controlled with progestin. Relatively high-dose estrogen pills should be used in these situations; if starting with 50 μg ethinyl estradiol, one should double the dose on each day that breakthrough bleeding occurs to a maximum dose of 200 μg daily for 3 weeks. In unusual cases in which extreme blood loss results from dysfunctional uterine bleeding, high-dose estrogen (e.g., 10 mg conjugated estrogen intravenously every 6 hours) is given until bleeding stops, followed by an oral regimen. We then use conjugated estrogens, 10 mg/day orally for 2 to 3 weeks. If breakthrough bleeding occurs, the estrogen is increased in 5-mg increments up to 20 mg/day. During the last 5 days of the regimen, medroxyprogesterone acetate is added so that withdrawal bleeding will result in "medical curettage." Thereafter, periodic progestin withdrawal treatment is usually a satisfactory form of treatment. Over the long term, appreciable weight reduction may result in normalization of the menstrual cycle in obese patients. In resistant cases on rare occasions, suction curettage or dilation and curettage may be needed to control hemorrhage.

The first line of management of hirsutism in functional ovarian hyperandrogenism is to take cosmetic measures. The most effective of these, if properly done, is electrolysis, the electrolytic destruction of individual hair roots. In some cases, after the patient's menstrual pattern is well established, estrogen-progestin–combination (contraceptive) pills can be prescribed in conjunction with the electrolysis in order to control the rate of hair growth enough to reduce the frequency of electrolysis. The least androgenic of the progestins should be used; this is ethynodiol diacetate, which is contained in Demulin. Before undertaking treatment

with these agents, the risk-benefit ratio must be considered in view of the uncommon side effects of these agents, such as amenorrhea, galactorrhea, ovarian cysts, and thrombotic phenomena.

Antiandrogens are effective in reversing hirsutism in about 70 per cent of cases. The most potent, cyproterone acetate, is not available for treatment in the United States. Spironolactone has been found to be antiandrogenic at the high doses that are also progestational.[170] We give 100 to 200 mg daily concomitantly with ethinyl estradiol 20 μg daily cyclically. The effect on hirsutism is not ascertainable for 6 months and the maximum effect takes 9 to 12 months. A preliminary report suggests that flutamide will be efficacious.

Although infertility is a major cause for concern in PCOS cases, it is not invariable. In some adolescents, contraceptive regimens are indicated. These patients can be reassured that they will probably ultimately be able to bear children with endocrinologic help. Ovulation can usually be induced with clomiphene, glucocorticoid, FSH, or pulsatile GnRH therapy. Ovarian wedge resection is a last resort, used only when pregnancy cannot be achieved by medical management.

Corticoid therapy normalizes menses and reduces hirsutism and acne in virilizing adrenogenital syndromes. It is only occasionally effective in PCOS.[383] The lowest glucocorticoid dose for congenital adrenal hyperplasia is that which normalizes androgen and progestin levels. Control of androgens may not suffice to normalize the menstrual cycle unless progestin levels are also controlled.[385] Progesterone excess appears to blunt pulsatile gonadotropin release.[386] Prednisone 5 to 10 mg twice daily or dexamethasone about 0.25 mg orally at bedtime may be useful in blunting the abnormal steroidogenesis in adolescents who are recalcitrant in taking hydrocortisone thrice daily.

ACKNOWLEDGMENTS: This work was supported in part by USPHS grant HD-06308.

REFERENCES

1. Donovan BT, van der Werff ten Bosch JJ: Physiology of Puberty. London, Edward Arnold Ltd, 1965.
2. Wilkins L: The Diagnosis and Treatment of En-

docrine Disorders in Childhood and Adolescence. Springfield, Illinois, CC Thomas, 1968.

3. Ramirez DV, McCann SM: Comparison of the regulation of luteinizing hormone (LH) secretion in immature and adult rats. Endocrinology 72:452, 1963.

4. Mills IH, Brooks RV, Prunty FTG: The relationship between the production of cortisol and androgen by the human adrenal. *In* Currie AR, Symington T, Grant JK (eds): The Human Adrenal Cortex. Baltimore, Williams & Wilkins, 1962.

5. Grumbach MM, Roth JC, Kaplan SL, et al: Hypothalamic-pituitary regulation of puberty in man: Evidence and concepts derived from clinical research. *In* Grumbach MM, Grave GD, Mayer FE (eds): The Control of the Onset of Puberty. New York, John Wiley & Sons, 1974.

6. Winter JSD, Hughes IA, Reyes FI, et al: Pituitary-gonadal relations in infancy: 2. Patterns of serum gonadal steroid concentrations in man from birth to two years of age. J Clin Endocrinol Metab 42:679, 1976.

7. Arey LB: Development of the Female Reproductive System. *In* Developmental Anatomy. 6th ed. Philadelphia, WB Saunders Company, 1974.

8. Clements JA, Reyes FI, Winter JSD, et al: Ontogenesis of gonadotropin-releasing hormone in the human fetal hypothalamus. Proc Soc Exp Biol Med 163:437, 1980.

9. Kaplan SL, Grumbach MM, Aubert ML: The ontogenesis of pituitary hormones and hypothalamic factors in the human fetus. Recent Prog Horm Res 32:161, 1976.

10. Siler-Khodr TM, Khodr GS: Studies in human fetal endocrinology. I. Luteinizing hormone-releasing factor content of the hypothalamus. Am J Obstet Gynecol 130:795, 1978.

11. Ojeda SR, Andrews WW, Advis JP, et al: Recent advances in the endocrinology of puberty. Endocr Rev 1:228, 1980.

12. Tapanainen J, Koivisto M, Vihko R, et al: Enhanced activity of the pituitary-gonadal axis in premature human infants. J Clin Endocrinol Metab 52:235, 1981.

13. King JC, Gerall AA: Localization of luteinizing hormone-releasing hormone. J Histochem Cytochem 24:829, 1976.

14. Raisman G, Field PM: Sexual dimorphism in the neuropil of the preoptic area of the rat and its dependence on neonatal androgen. Brain Res 54:1, 1973.

15. Gorski RA, Gordon JH, Shryne JE, et al: Evidence for a morphological sex difference within the medial preoptic area of the rat brain. Brain Res 148:333, 1978.

16. Rosenfield RL, Lucky AW, Allen TD: The diagnosis and management of intersex. Curr Probl Pediatr 10 (May), 1980.

17. Gulyas BJ, Hodgen GD, Tullner WW, et al: Effects of fetal or maternal hypophysectomy on endocrine organs and body weight in infant rhesus monkeys (*Macaca mulatta*): With particular emphasis on oogenesis. Biol Reprod 16:216, 1977.

18. Merrill JA: Ovarian hilus cells. Am J Obstet Gynecol 78:1258, 1959.

19. van Wagenen G, Simpson ME: Embryology of the Ovary and Testis. *Homo sapiens* and *Macaca mulatta*. New Haven, Yale University Press, 1965.

20. Peters H: Migration of gonocytes into the mammalian gonad and their differentiation. Philos Trans R Soc Lond [Biol] 259:91, 1970.

21. Baker TG: A quantitative and cytological study of germ cells in human ovaries. Proc Roy Soc [Biol] 158:417, 1963.

22. Peters H, Byskov AG, Grinsted J: Follicular growth in fetal and prepubertal ovaries of humans and other primates. Clin Endocrinol Metab 7:469, 1978.

23. Block E: A quantitative morphological investigation of the follicular system in newborn female infants. Acta Anat 17:201, 1953.

24. Richardson SJ, Senikas V, Nelson JF: Follicular depletion during the menopausal transition: Evidence for accelerated loss and ultimate exhaustion. J Clin Endocrinol Metab 65:1231, 1987.

25. Ross GT, Schreiber JR: The ovary. *In* Yen SSC. Jaffe R (eds): Reproductive Endocrinology. Philadelphia, WB Saunders Company 1978, p 63.

26. Peters H: The human ovary in childhood and early maturity. Eur J Obstet Gynecol Reprod Biol 9/3:137, 1979.

27. Page DC: Sex reversal: Deletion mapping the male-determining function of the human Y chromosome. Cold Spring Harbor Symp Quant Biol 51:229, 1986.

28. Ohno S, Smith JB: Role of fetal follicular cells in meiosis of mammalian oocytes. Cytogenetics 3:324, 1964.

29. Gartler SM, Andina R, Gant N: Ontogeny of X-chromosome inactivation in the female germ line. Exp Cell Res 91:454, 1975.

30. Carr DH, Haggar RA, Hart AG: Germ cells in the ovaries of XO female infants. Am J Clin Pathol 19:521, 1968.

31. Byskov AG: The role of the rete ovarii in meiosis and follicle formation in the cat, mink and ferret. J Reprod Fert 45:201, 1975.

32. Besedovsky HO, Sorkin E: Thymus involvement in female sexual maturation. Nature 249:356, 1974.

33. Winter JSD, Faiman C: Pituitary-gonadal relations in female children and adolescents. Pediatr Res 7:948, 1973.

34. Winter JSD, Faiman C, Hobson WC, Prasad AV, Reyes FI: Pituitary-gonadal relations in infancy. I. Patterns of serum gonadotropin concentrations from birth to four years of age in man and chimpanzee. J Clin Endocrinol Metab 40:545, 1975.

35. Conte FA, Grumbach MM, Kaplan SL, et al: Correlation of luteinizing hormone-releasing factor-induced luteinizing hormone and follicle-stimulating hormone release from infancy to 19 years with the changing pattern of gonadotropin secretion in agonadal patients: Relation to the restraint of puberty. J Clin Endocrinol Metab 50:163, 1980.

36. Rosenfield RL: Hormonal events and disorders of puberty. *In* Gynecologic Endocrinology. Chicago, Year Book Medical Publishers, 1977.

37. Attardi B, Ohno S: Androgen and estrogen receptors in the developing mouse brain. Endocrinology 99:1279, 1976.

38. Penny R, Olambiwonnu NO, Frasier SD: Serum gonadotropin concentrations during the first four years of life. J Clin Endocrinol Metab 38:320, 1974.

39. Bourginon J-P, Hoyoux C, Reuter A, et al: Urinary excretion of immunoreactive luteinizing

hormone-releasing hormone-like material and gonadotropins at different stages of life. J Clin Endocrinol Metab 48:78, 1979.

40. Kulin HE, Reiter EO: Gonadotropins during childhood and adolescence: A review. Pediatrics 51:(2)260, 1973.

41. Rifkind AB, Kulin HE, Ross GT: Follicle stimulating hormone (FSH) and luteinizing hormone (LH) in the urine of prepubertal children. J Clin Invest 46:1925, 1967.

42. Penny R, Olambiowonnu NO, Frasier SD: Episodic fluctuations of serum gonadotropins in pre- and post-pubertal girls and boys. J Clin Endocrinol Metab 45:307, 1977.

43. Kulin HE, Moore RG Jr, Santner SJ: Circadian rhythms in gonadotropin excretion in prepubertal and pubertal children. J Clin Endocrinol Metab 42:770, 1976.

44. Chipman JJ, Moore RJ, Marks JF, et al: Interrelationship of plasma and urinary gonadotropins: Correlations for 24 hours, for sleep/wake periods, and for 3 hours after luteinizing hormone-releasing hormone stimulation. J Clin Endocrinol Metab 52:225, 1981.

45. Ross GT: Gonadotropins and preantral follicular maturation in women. Fertil Steril 25:522, 1974.

46. Funkenstein B, Nimrod A. Lindner HR: The development of steroidogenic capability and responsiveness to gonadotropins in cultured neonatal rat ovaries. Endocrinology 106:98, 1980.

47. Stanhope R, Adams J, Jacobs HS, Brook CGD: Ovarian ultrasound assessment in normal children, idiopathic precocious puberty, and during low dose pulsatile gonadotrophin releasing hormone treatment of hypogonadotrophic hypogonadism. Arch Dis Child 60:116, 1985.

48. Bidlingmaier F, Knorr D: Oestrogens: Physiological and clinical aspects. Pediatr Adolesc Endocrinol 4:43, 1978.

49. Collette-Sollberg PR, Grumbach MM: A simplified procedure for evaluating estrogenic effects and the sex chromatin pattern in exfoliated cells in urine: Studies in premature thelarche and gynecomastia of adolescence. J Pediatr 66:883, 1965.

50. Dickerman Z, Prager-Lewin R. Laron Z: Response of plasma LH and FSH to synthetic LH-RH in children at various pubertal stages. Am J Dis Child 130:634, 1974.

51. Rettig K, Duckett GE, Sweetland M, et al: Urinary excretion of immunoreactive luteinizing hormone-releasing hormone-like material in children: Correlation with pubertal development. J Clin Endocrinol Metab 52:1150, 1981.

52. Barnea A, Cho G. Porter JC: A role for the ovaries in maturational processes of hypothalamic neurons containing luteinizing hormone-releasing hormone. Endocrinology 105:1303, 1979.

53. Knobil E: The neuroendocrine control of the menstrual cycle. Recent Prog Hor Res 36:53, 1980.

54. Marshall JC, Kelch RP: Gonadotropin-releasing hormone: Role of pulsatile secretion in the regulation of reproduction. N Engl J Med 315:1459, 1986.

55. Boyar R, Finkelstein J, Roffwarg H, et al: Synchronization of augmented luteinizing hormone secretion with sleep during puberty. N Engl J Med 287:582, 1972.

56. Weitzman ED, Perlow M, Boyar R, et al: Light and luteinizing hormone. N Engl J Med 286:932, 1972.

57. Boyar RM, Wu RHK, Roffwarg H, et al: Human puberty: 24-Hour estradiol patterns in pubertal girls. J Clin Endocrinol Metab 43:1418, 1976.

58. Hansen JW, Hoffman HJ, Ross GT: Monthly gonadotropin cycles in premenarcheal girls. Science 190:161, 1975.

59. Lucky AW, Rich BH, Rosenfield RL, et al: LH bioactivity increases more than immunoreactivity during puberty. J Pediatr 97:205, 1980.

60. Solano AR, Garcia-Vela A, Catt KJ, et al: Modulation of serum and pituitary luteinizing hormone bioactivity by androgen in the rat. Endocrinology 106:1941, 1980.

61. Burstein S, Schaff-Blass E, Blass J, Rosenfield RL: The changing ratio of bioactive to immunoreactive luteinizing hormone (LH) through puberty principally reflects changing LH radioimmunoassay dose-response characteristics. J Clin Endocrinol Metab 61:508, 1985.

62. Eklind-Hirsch K, Ravnikar V, Schiff I, Tulchinsky D, Ryan KJ: Determinations of endogenous immunoreactive luteinizing hormone-releasing hormone in human plasma. J Clin Endocrinol Metab 54:602, 1982.

63. Norman RL, Gliessman P, Lindstrom SA, Hill J, Spies HG: Reinitiation of ovulatory cycles in pituitary stalk-sectioned rhesus monkeys: Evidence for a specific hypothalamic message for the preovulatory release of luteinizing hormone. Endocrinology 111:1874, 1982.

64. Lin WW, Ramirez VD: Effect of pulsatile infusion of progesterone on the in vivo activity of the luteinizing hormone-releasing hormone neural apparatus of awake unrestrained female and male rabbits. Endocrinology 122:868, 1988.

65. Gasc J-M, Baulieu E-E: Regulation by estradiol of the progesterone receptor in the hypothalamus and pituitary: An immunohistochemical study in the chicken. Endocrinology 122:1357, 1988.

66. Moll GW Jr, Rosenfield RL: Direct inhibitory effect of estradiol on pituitary luteinizing hormone responsiveness to luteinizing hormone releasing hormone is specific and of rapid onset. Biol Reprod 30:59, 1984.

67. Young JR, Jaffe RB: Strength-duration characteristics of estrogen effects on gonadotropin response to gonadotropin-releasing hormone in women. II. J Clin Endocrinol Metab 42:432, 1976.

68. March CM, Goebelsmann U, Nakamura RM, et al: Roles of estradiol and progesterone in eliciting the midcycle luteinizing hormone and follicle-stimulating hormone surges. J Clin Endocrinol Metab 49:507, 1979.

69. Chang RJ, Jaffe RB: Progesterone effects on gonadotropin release in women pretreated with estradiol. J Clin Endocrinol Metab 47:119, 1978.

70. Advis JP, Krause JE, McKelvy JF: Evidence that endopeptidase-catalyzed luteinizing hormone releasing hormone cleavage contributes to the regulation of median eminence LHRH levels during positive steroid feedback. Endocrinology 112:1147, 1983.

71. Harlow CR, Shaw HJ, Hillier SG, Hodges JK: Factors influencing follicle-stimulating hormone-responsive steroidogenesis in marmoset granulosa cells: Effects of androgens and the

stage of follicular maturity. Endocrinology 122:2780, 1988.

72. Richards JS, Bogovich K: Effects of human chorionic gonadotropin and progesterone on follicular development in the immature rat. Endocrinology 111:1429, 1982.

73. Jia X-C, Kessel B, Welsh TH, Jr, Hsueh AJW: Androgen inhibition of follicle-stimulating hormone-stimulated luteinizing hormone receptor formation in cultured rat granulosa cells. Endocrinology 117:13, 1985.

74. Richards JS, Hedin L: Molecular aspects of hormone action in ovarian follicular development, ovulation, and luteinization. Ann Rev Physiol 50:441, 1988.

75. Hsueh AJW, Adashi EY, Jones PBC, Welsh TH Jr: Hormonal regulation of the differentiation of cultured ovarian granulosa cells. Endocrinol Rev 5:76, 1984.

76. White SS, Ojeda SR: Changes in ovarian LHRH receptor content during the onset of puberty in the female rat. Endocrinology 108:347, 1981.

77. Eckstein B, Shani J, Ravid R, et al: Effect of androstanediol sulfates on luteinizing hormone release in ovariectomized rats. Endocrinology 108:500, 1981.

78. Abraham GE: Ovarian and adrenal contributions to peripheral androgens during the menstrual cycle. J Clin Endocrinol Metab 39:340, 1974.

79. Ross GT, Cargille CM, Lipsett MB, et al: Pituitary and gonadal hormones in women during spontaneous and individual ovulatory cycles. Recent Prog Horm Res 26:1, 1970.

80. Soules MR, Steiner RA, Cohen NL, Bremner WJ, Clifton DK: Nocturnal slowing of pulsatile luteinizing hormone secretion in women during the follicular phase of the menstrual cycle. J Clin Endocrinal Metab 61:43, 1985.

81. Johnson DC, Naqvi RH: A positive feedback action of androgen on pituitary follicle stimulating hormone: induction of a cyclic phenomenon. Endocrinology 85:881, 1969.

82. Melrose P, Gross R: Steroid effects on the secretory modalities of gonadotropin-releasing hormone release. Endocrinology 121:190, 1987.

83. Soules MR, Steiner RA, Clifton DK, Cohen NL, Aksel S, Bremner WJ: Progesterone modulation of pulsatile luteinizing hormone secretion in normal women. J Clin Endocrinol Metab 58:378, 1984.

84. Erickson GF, Magoffin DA, Dyer CA, Hofeditz C: The ovarian androgen producing cells: A review of structure/function relationships. Endocrin Rev 6:371, 1985.

85. Voutilainen R, Tapanainen J, Chung B-C, Matteson KJ, Miller WL: Hormonal regulation of P450scc (20,22-desmolase) and P450c17 (17α-hydroxylase/17,20-lyase) in cultured human granulosa cells. J Clin Endocrinol Metab 63:202, 1986.

86. McNatty KP, Makris A, Reinhold VN: Metabolism of androstenedione by human ovarian tissues in vitro with particular reference to reductase and aromatase activity. Steroids 34:429, 1979.

87. McNatty KP, Smith DM, Makris A, et al: The microenvironment of the human antral follicle: Interrelationships among the steroid levels in antral fluid, the population of granulosa cells, and the status of the oocyte in vivo and in vitro. J Clin Endocrinol Metab 49:851, 1979.

88. Tsang BK, Armstrong DT, Whitfield JF: Steroid biosynthesis by isolated human ovarian follicular cells in vitro. J Clin Endocrinol Metab 51:1407, 1980.

89. Erickson GF, Hsueh AJW, Quigley ME, et al: Functional studies of aromatase activity in human granulosa cells from normal and polycystic ovaries. J Clin Endocrinol Metab 49:514, 1979.

90. Hild-Petito S, Stouffer RL, Brenner RM: Immunocytochemical localization of estradiol and progesterone receptors in the monkey ovary throughout the menstrual cycle. Endocrinology 123:2896, 1988.

91. McNatty KP, Hunter WM, McNeilly AS, et al: Changes in the concentration of pituitary and steroid hormones in the follicular fluid of human Graafian follicles throughout the menstrual cycle. J Endocrinol 64:555, 1975.

92. McNatty KP, Makris A, DeGrazia C, et al: The production of progesterone, androgens, and estrogens by granulosa cells, thecal tissue, and stromal tissue from human ovaries in vitro. J Clin Endocrinol Metab 49:687, 1979.

93. McNatty KP, Makris A, DeGrazia C, et al: Steroidogenesis by recombined follicular cells from the human ovary in vitro. J Clin Endocrinol Metab 51:1286, 1980.

94. DiZerega GS, Hodgen GD: Folliculogenesis in the primate ovarian cycle. Endocrinol Rev 2:27, 1981.

95. Jonassen JA, Bose K, Richards JS: Enhancement and desensitization of hormone-responsive adenylate cyclase in granulosa cells of preantral and antral ovarian follicles: Effects of estradiol and follicle-stimulating hormone. Endocrinology 111:74, 1982.

96. Brailley S, Gougeon A, Milgrom E, Bomsel-Helmreich O, Papiernik E: Androgens and progestin in the human ovarian follicle: Differences in the evolution of preovulatory, healthy nonovulatory, and atretic follicles. J Clin Endocrinol Metab 53:128, 1981.

97. Schreiber JR, Nakamura K, Truscella AM, Erickson GF: Progestins inhibit FSH-induced functional LH receptors in cultured rat granulosa cells. Molec Cell Endocrinol 25:113, 1982.

98. Bellin ME, Ax RL: Chondroitin sulfate: An indicator of atresia in bovine follicles. Endocrinology 114:428, 1984.

99. Lindner HR, Tsafriri A, Lieberman ME, et al: Gonadotropin action on cultured Graafian follicles: Induction of maturation division of the mammalian oocyte and differentiation of the luteal cell. Recent Prog Horm Res 30:79, 1974.

100. Hillier S, Ross GT: Effects of exogenous testosterone on ovarian weight, follicular morphology and intraovarian progesterone concentration in estrogen-primed hypophysectomized immature female rats. Biol Reprod 20:261, 1979.

101. Polan ML, Seu D, Tarlatzis B: Human chorionic gonadotropin stimulation of estradiol production and androgen antagonism of gonadotropin-stimulated responses in cultured human granulosa-luteal cells. J Clin Endocrinol Metab 62:628, 1986.

102. Ying S-Y: Inhibins, activins, and follistatins: Gonadal proteins modulating the secretion of

follicle-stimulating hormone. Endocr Rev 9:267, 1988.

103. Tsonis CG, Messinis IE, Templeton AA, McNeilly AS, Baird DT: Gonadotropic stimulation of inhibin secretion by the human ovary during the follicular and early luteal phase of the cycle. J Clin Endocrinol Metab 66:915, 1988.

104. Lumpkin M, Negro-Vilar A, Franchimont P, et al: Evidence for a hypothalamic site of action of inhibin to suppress FSH release. Endocrinology 108:1101, 1981.

105. Shander D, Anderson LD, Barraclough CA: Follicle-stimulating hormone and luteinizing hormone affect the endogenous release of pituitary follicle-stimulating hormone and the ovarian secretion of inhibin in rats. Endocrinology 106:1047, 1980.

106. Auletta FJ, Flint APF: Mechanisms controlling corpus luteum function in sheep, cows, nonhuman primates, and women especially in relation to the time of luteolysis. Endocr Rev 9:88, 1988.

107. Vande Wiele RL, Bogumil J, Dyenfurth I, et al: Mechanisms regulating the menstrual cycle in women. Recent Prog Horm Res 26:63, 1970.

108. Stouffer RL, Hodgen GD, Ottobre AC, Christina CD: Follicular fluid treatment during the follicular versus luteal phase of the menstrual cycle: Effects on corpus luteum function. J Clin Endocrinol Metab 58:1027, 1984.

109. Terasawa E, Noonan JJ, Nass TE, Loose MD: Posterior hypothalamic lesions advance the onset of puberty in the female rhesus monkey. Endocrinology 115:2241, 1984.

110. Marshall WA: Interrelationships of skeletal maturation, sexual development and somatic growth in man. Ann Human Biol 1:29, 1974.

111. Simmons K, Greulich W: Menarcheal age and the height, weight, and skeletal age of girls age 7 to 17 years. J Pediatr 22:518, 1943.

112. Boyar RM, Finkelstein JW, David R, et al: Twenty-four hour patterns of plasma luteinizing hormone and follicle-stimulating hormone in sexual precocity. N Engl J Med 289:282, 1973.

113. Tanner JM, Whitehouse RH: A note on the bone age at which patients with true isolated growth hormone deficiency enter puberty. J Clin Endocrinol Metab 41:788, 1975.

114. Frisch RE: Critical weight at menarche, initiation of the adolescent growth spurt, and control of puberty. *In* Grumbach MM, Grave GD, Mayer FE (eds): The Control of the Onset of Puberty. New York, John Wiley & Sons, 1974.

115. Crawford JD, Osler DC: Body composition at menarche: The Frisch-Revelle hypothesis revisited. Pediatrics 56:449, 1975.

116. Plant TM: Puberty in primates. *In* Knobil W, Neill J, et al (eds); Physiology of Reproduction. New York, Raven Press, 1988, pp 1763–1788.

117. Frisch RE, Hegsted DM, Yoshinaga K: Carcass components at first estrus of rats on high-fat and low-fat diets: Body water, protein, and fat. Proc Natl Acad Sci (USA) 74:379, 1977.

118. Wilen R, Naftolin F: Pubertal food intake and body length, weight, and composition in the feed-restricted female rat: Comparison with well fed animals. Pediatr Res 12:263, 1978.

119. Warren MP: The effects of exercise on pubertal progression and reproductive function in girls. J Clin Endocrinol Metab 51:1150, 1980.

120. Arslan M, Pohl CR, Plant TM: DL-2-amino-5-phosphonopentanoic acid, a specific N-methyl-D-aspartic acid receptor antagonist, suppresses pulsatile LH release in the rat. Neuroendocrinology 47:465, 1988.

121. Rosenfield RL, Fang VS: The effects of prolonged physiologic estradiol therapy on the maturation of hypogonadal teenagers. J Pediatr 85:830, 1974.

122. Reiter EO, Kulin HE, Hamwood SM: The absence of positive feedback between estrogen and luteinizing hormone in sexually immature girls. Pediatr Res 8:740, 1974.

123. Reiter RJ: The pineal and its hormones in the control of reproduction in mammals. Endocrinology 1:109, 1980.

124. Waldhauser F, Weiszenbacher G, Tatzer E, Gisinger B, Waldhauser M, Schemper M, Frisch H: Alterations in nocturnal serum melatonin levels in humans with growth and aging. J Clin Endocrinol Metab 66:648, 1988.

125. Bogumil RT, Ferlin M, Rootenberg J, et al: Mathematical studies of the human menstrual cycle. I. Formation of a mathematical model. J Clin Endocrinol Metab 35:126, 1972.

126. Kalra SP, Kalra PS: Neural regulation of LH secretion in the rat. Endocr Rev 4:311, 1983.

127. Krey JC, Butler WR, Knobil E: Surgical disconnection of the medial basal hypothalamus and pituitary function in the rhesus monkey. I. Gonadotropin secretion. Endocrinology 96:1073, 1975.

128. Wildt L, Hutchison JS, Marshall G, et al: On the site of action of progesterone in the blockade of the estradiol-induced gonadotropin discharge in the rhesus monkey. Endocrinology 109:1293, 1981.

129. Bourguignon J-P, Gerard A, Debougnoux G, Rose J, Franchimont P: Pulsatile release of gonadotropin-releasing hormone (GnRH) from the rat hypothalamus in vitro: Calcium and glucose dependency and inhibition by superactive GnRH analogs. Endocrinology 121:993, 1987.

130. Clayton RN, Catt KJ: Gonadotropin-releasing hormone receptors: Characterization, physiological regulation, and relationship to reproductive function. Endocrinol Rev 2:186, 1981.

131. Turgeon JL, Waring DW: Acute progesterone and 17β-estradiol modulation of luteinizing hormone secretion by pituitaries of cycling rats superfused in vitro. Endocrinology 108:413, 1981.

132. Drouin J, Labrie F: Interactions between 17β-estradiol and progesterone in the control of luteinizing hormone and follicle-stimulating hormone release in rat anterior pituitary cells in culture. Endocrinology 108:52, 1981.

133. Hirono M, Igarashi M, Matsumoto S: Short- and auto-feedback mechanism of LH. Endocrinology 18:175, 1971.

134. Patritti-Laborde N, Wolfsen AR, Odell WD: Short loop feedback system for the control of follicle-stimulating hormone in the rabbit. Endocrinology 108:72, 1981.

135. Advis JP, Richards JS, Ojeda, SR.: Hyperprolactinemia-induced precocious puberty: Studies on the intraovarian mechanism(s) by which PRL enhances ovarian responsiveness to gonadotropins in prepubertal rats. J Clin Endocrinol Metab 108:1333, 1981.

136. Garcia A, Herbon L, Barkan A, Papavasiliou S, Marshall JC: Hyperprolactinemia inhibits go-

nadotropin-releasing hormone (GnRH) stimulation of the number of pituitary GnRH receptors. Endocrinology 117:954, 1985.

137. Demura R, Ono M, Demura H, Shizume K, Oouch H: Prolactin directly inhibits basal as well as gonadotropin-stimulated secretion of progesterone and 17β-estradiol in the human ovary. J Clin Endocrinol Metab 54:1246, 1982.

138. Glickman SP, Rosenfield RL, Bergenstal RM, Helke J: Multiple androgenic abnormalities, including elevated free testosterone, in hyperprolactinemic women. J Clin Endocrinol Metab 55:251, 1982.

139. Suh BY, Liu JH, Berga SL, Quigley ME, Laughlin GA, Yen SS: Hypercortisolism in patients with functional hypothalamic-amenorrhea. J Clin Endocrinol Metab 66:733, 1988.

140. Hwan J-C, Freeman ME: A physiological role for luteinizing hormone release-inhibiting factor of hypothalamic origin. Endocrinology 121:1099, 1987.

141. Reid RL, Ling N, Yen SSC: Gonadotropin-releasing activity of α-melanocyte-stimulating hormone in normal subjects and in subjects with hypothalamic-pituitary dysfunction. J Clin Endocrinol Metab 58:773, 1984.

142. Sutton SW, Toyama TT, Otto S, Plotsky PM: Evidence that neuropeptide Y (NPY) released into the hypophysial-portal circulation participates in priming gonadotropes to the effects of gonadotropin releasing hormone (GnRH). Endocrinology 123:1208, 1988.

143. Dahl KD, Bicxak TA, Hsueh AJW: Naturally occurring antihormones: Secretion of FSH antagonists by women treated with a GnRH analog. Science 239:72, 1988.

144. Feng P, Catt KJ, Knecht M: Transforming growth factor-β stimulates meiotic maturation of the rat oocyte. Endocrinology 122:181, 1988.

145. Kudlow JE, Kobrin MS, Purchio AF, Twardzik DR, Hernandez ER, Asa SL, Adashi EY: Ovarian transforming growth factor-α gene expression: Immunohistochemical localization to the theca-interstitial cells. Endocrinology 121:1577, 1987.

146. Fukuoka M, Mori T, Taii S, Yasuda K: Interleukin-a inhibits luteinization of porcine granulosa cells in culture. Endocrinology 122:367, 1988.

147. Wiebe JP, Wood PH: Selective suppression of follicle-stimulating hormone by 3 α-hydroxy-4-pregnen-20-one, a steroid found in Sertoli cells. Endocrinology 120:2259, 1987.

148. Aten RF, Polan ML, Bayless R, Behrman HR: A gonadotropin-releasing hormone (GnRH)-like protein in human ovaries: Similarity to the GnRH-like ovarian protein of the rat. J Clin Endocrinol Metab 64:1288, 1987.

149. Barnes RB, Scommegna A, Schreiber JR: Decreased ovarian response to human menopausal gonadotropin caused by subcutaneously administered gonadotropin-releasing hormone agonist. Fertil Steril 47:512, 1987.

150. Bramley TA, Menzies GS, Baird DT: Specific binding of gonadotrophin-releasing hormone and an agonist to human corpus luteum homogenates: Characterization, properties, and luteal phase levels. J Clin Endocrinol Metab 61:834, 1985.

151. Rich BH, Rosenfield RL, Lucky AW, et al: Adrenarche: Changing adrenal response to ACTH. J Clin Endocrinol Metab 52:1129, 1981.

152. Korth-Shutz S, Levine LS, New MI: Dehydroepiandrosterone sulfate (DS) levels, a rapid test of abnormal adrenal androgen secretion. J Clin Endocrinol Metab 42:1005, 1976.

153. Grumbach MM, Richards GE, Conte FA, et al: Clinical disorders of adrenal function and puberty: An assessment of the role of the adrenal cortex in normal and abnormal puberty in man and evidence for an ACTH-like pituitary adrenal androgen stimulating hormone. In James VHT, Serio M, Giusti G, Martini L (eds): The Endocrine Function of the Human Adrenal Cortex. London, Academic Press, 1978, p 583.

154. Kennerson AR, McDonald DA, Adams JB: Dehydroepiandrosterone sulfotransferase localization in human adrenal glands: A light and electron microscopic study. J Clin Endocrinol Metab 56:786, 1983.

155. Dickerman Z, Grant DR, Faiman C, Winter JSD: Intraadrenal steroid concentrations in man: Zonal differences and developmental changes. J Clin Endocrinol Metab 59:1031, 1984.

156. Schiebinger RJ, Albertson BD, Cassorla FG, et al: The developmental changes in plasma adrenal androgens during infancy and adrenarche are associated with changing activities of adrenal microsomal 17-hydroxylase and 17.20-desmolase. J Clin Invest 67:1177, 1981.

157. Byrne GC, Perry YS, Winter JSD: Kinetic analysis of adrenal 3 β-hydroxysteroid dehydrogenase activity during human development. J Clin Endocrinol Metab 60:934, 1985.

158. Miller WL: Molecular biology of steroid hormone synthesis. Endocr Rev 9:295, 1988.

159. Cutler GB Jr, Davis SE, Johnsonbaugh RE, Loriaux DL: Dissociation of cortisol and adrenal androgen secretion in patients with secondary adrenal insufficiency. J Clin Endocrinol Metab 49:604, 1979.

160. Sklar CA, Kaplan SL, Grumbach MM: Evidence for dissociation between adrenarche and gonadarche: Studies in patients with idiopathic precocious puberty, gonadal dysgenesis, isolated gonadotropin deficiency, and constitutionally delayed growth and adolescence. J Clin Endocrinol Metab 51:548, 1980.

161. Cumming DC, Rebar RW, Hopper BR, Yen SSC: Evidence for an influence of the ovary on circulating dehydroepiandrosteone sulfate levels. J Clin Endocrinol Metab 54:1069, 1982.

162. Puche RC, Roman MC: Effect of dehydroepiandrosterone sulfate on the mineral accretion of chick embryo frontal bones cultivated in vitro. Calcif Tissue Res 4:39, 1969.

163. Miller RW: DES daughters: Further studies of pregnancy wastage. Childhood Cancer Etiology Newsletter 65, March 25, 1980.

164. Schumacher GFB: Soluble proteins in cervical mucus. In Blandau RJ, Moghissi K (eds): The Biology of the Cervix. Chicago, University of Chicago Press, 1973.

165. Wied GL, Bibbo M: Evaluation of endocrinologic condition by exfoliative cytology. In Gold JJ (ed): Gynecologic Endocrinology. 2nd ed. New York, Harper & Row, 1975.

166. Rosenfield RL, Fang VS, Dupon C, et al: The effects of low doses of depot estradiol and testosterone in teenagers with ovarian failure and Turner's syndrome. J Clin Endocrinol Metab 574, 1973.

167. Robbins SL, Cotran RS: Pathologic Basis of Disease. The Breast. Philadelphia, WB Saunders Company, 1979, p 1305.
168. Topper YJ: Multiple hormone interactions in the development of mammary gland in vitro. Recent Prog Horm Res 26:287, 1970.
169. Lyons WR: Hormonal synergism in mammary growth. Proc Roy Soc Lond [Biol] 149:303, 1958.
170. Rosenfield RL: Pilosebaceous physiology in relation to hirsutism and acne. Clin Endocrinol Metab 15:341, 1986.
171. Catt KJ, Harwood JP, Clayton RN, et al: Regulation of peptide hormone receptors and gonadal steroidogenesis. Recent Prog Horm Res 36:557, 1980.
172. Veldhuis JD, Klase PA: Mechanisms by which calcium ions regulate the steroidogenic actions of luteinizing hormone in isolated ovarian cells *in vitro*. Endocrinology 111:i, 1982.
173. Boepple PA, Mansfield MJ, Wierman ME, Rudlin CR, Bode HH, Crigler JF Jr, Crawford JD, Crowley WF Jr: Use of a potent, long acting agonist of gonadotropin-releasing hormone in the treatment of precocious puberty. Endocr Rev 7:24, 1986.
174. Adelman JP, Mason AJ, Hayflick JS, Seeburg PH: Isolation of the gene and hypothalamic cDNA for the common precursor of gonadotropin-releasing hormone and prolactin release-inhibiting factor in human and rat. Proc Natl Acad Sci (USA) 83:179, 1986.
175. Redding TW, Schally AV, Arimura A, et al: Stimulation of release and synthesis of luteinizing hormone (LH) and follicle stimulating hormone (FSH) in tissue cultures of rat pituitaries in response to natural and synthetic LH and FSH releasing hormone. Endocrinology 90:764, 1972.
176. Hall JE, Brodie TDD, Badger TM, Rivier J, Vale W, Conn PM, Schoenfeld D, Crowley WF Jr: Evidence of differential control of FSH and LH secretion by gonadotropin-releasing hormone (GnRH) from the use of a GnRH antagonist. J Clin Endocrinol Metab 67:524, 1988.
177. Farland L, Marchetti B, Seguin C, et al: Dissociated changes of pituitary luteinizing hormone releasing hormone (LHRH) receptors and responsiveness to the neuro-hormone induced by 17β-estradiol and LHRH in vivo in the rat. Endocrinology 109:87, 1981.
178. Shome B, Parlow AF: Human follicle stimulating hormone: first proposal for the amino acid sequence of the hormone-specific, β-subunit (hFSHβ). J Clin Endocrinol Metab 39:203, 1974.
179. Chin WW: Hormonal regulation of thyrotropin and gonadotropin gene expression. Clin Res 36:484, 1988.
180. Phifer RF, Midgley AR, Spicer SS: Immunohistologic and histologic evidence that follicle-stimulating hormone and luteinizing hormone are present in the same cell type in the human pars distalis. J Clin Endocrinol Metab 36:125, 1973.
181. Suginami H, Robertson DM, Diczfalusy E: Influence of the purity of the iodinated tracer on the specificity of the radioimmunoassay of human luteinizing hormone. Acta Endocrinol 89:506, 1978.
182. Bangham DR, Berryman I, Burger H, et al: An international collaborative study of 69/104, a reference preparation of human pituitary FSH and LH. J Clin Endocrinol Metab 36:647, 1973.
183. Chappel SC, Ulloz-Agiuirre A, Cotifaris C: Biosynthesis of follicle-stimulating hormone. Endocr Rev 4:179, 1983.
184. Wang C: Bioassays of follicle stimulating hormone. Endocr Rev 9:374, 1988.
185. Padmanabhan V, Chappel SC, Beitins IZ: An improved in vitro bioassay for follicle-stimulating hormone (FSH): Suitable for measurement of FSH in unextracted human serum. Endocrinology 121:1089, 1987.
186. Kohler PO, Ross GT, Odell WD: Metabolic clearance and production rates of human luteinizing hormone in pre- and postmenopausal women. J Clin Invest 47:38, 1968.
187. Coble YD, Kohler PO, Cargille CM, et al: Production rates and metabolic clearance rates of human follicle-stimulating hormone in premenopausal and postmenopausal women. J Clin Invest 48:359, 1969.
188. Rosenfield RL: Role of androgens in growth and development of the fetus, child, and adolescent. Adv Pediatr 19:171, 1972.
189. Baulieu EE, Corpechot C, Dray F, et al: An adrenal-secreted "androgen": Dehydroisoandrosterone sulfate. Recent Prog Horm Res 21:411, 1965.
190. Sandberg E, Gurpide E, Lieberman S: Quantitative studies on the metabolism of dehydroisoandrosterone sulfate. Biochemistry 3:1256, 1964.
191. Longcope C, Pratt JH: Blood production rates of estrogens in women with differing ratios of urinary estrogen conjugates. Steroids 29:483, 1977.
192. Little B, Billiar RB: Progesterone production. *In* Gual C (ed): Progress in Endocrinology. Amsterdam, Excerpta Medica Foundation, 1969, p 871.
193. Strott CA, Yoshimi T, Lipsett MB: Plasma progesterone and 17-hydroxyprogesterone in normal men and children with congenital adrenal hyperplasia. J Clin Invest 48:930, 1969.
194. Yen SSC, Llerena O, Little B, et al: Disappearance rates of endogenous luteinizing hormone and chorionic gonadotropin in man. J Clin Endocrinol Metab 28:1763, 1968.
195. Yen SSC, Llerena LA, Pearson OH, et al: Disappearance rates of endogenous follicle-stimulating hormone in serum following surgical hypophysectomy in man. J Clin Endocrinol Metab 30:325, 1970.
196. Veldhuis JD, Johnson ML: In vivo dynamics of luteinizing hormone secretion and clearance in man: Assessment by deconvolution mechanics. J Clin Endocrinol Metab 66:1291, 1988.
197. Raiti S, Foley TP Jr, Penny R, et al: Measurement of the production rate of human luteinizing hormone using the urinary excretion technique. Metabolism 24:937, 1975.
198. Prentice LG, Ryan RJ: LH and its subunits in human pituitary, serum and urine. J Clin Endocrinol Metab 40:303, 1975.
199. Foreman MM, Porter JC: Prolactin augmentation of dopamine and norepinephrine release from superfused medial basal hypothalamic fragments. Endocrinology 108:800, 1981.
200. Rosenfield RL, Miller WL: Congenital adrenal hyperplasia. *In* Mahesh VG, Greenblatt RB

(eds): Hirsutism and Virilism. Boston, John Wright-PSG, Inc, 1983, pp 87–119.

201. Siiteri PK, MacDonald PC: Role of extraglandular estrogen in human endocrinology. *In* Greep RO, Astwood EB (eds): Handbook of Physiology, Endocrinology II, Part I, Chap. 28. Washington, D.C., American Physiology Society, 1973, p 615.

202. Rivarola MA, Singleton RT, Migeon CJ: Splanchnic extraction and interconversion of testosterone and androstenedione in man. J Clin Invest 46:2095, 1967.

203. Edman CD. MacDonald PC: Effect of obesity on conversion of plasma androstenedione to estrone in ovulatory and anovulatory young women. Am J Obstet Gynecol 130:456, 1978.

204. Morimoto I, Edmiston A, Hawks D, et al: Studies of the origin of androstanediol and androstanediol glucuronide in young and elderly men. J Clin Endocrinol Metab 52:772, 1981.

205. Gurpide E. MacDonald PC, Chapdelaine A, et al: Studies on the secretion and interconversion of the androgens. II. Methods for estimation of rates of secretion and of metabolism from specific activities of urinary metabolites. J Clin Endocrinol 25:1537, 1965.

206. Hatch R, Rosenfield RL, Kim MH, et al: Hirsutism: Implications, etiology, and management. Am J Obstet Gynecol 140:815, 1981.

207. Moll GW Jr, Rosenfield RL, Helke JH: Estradiol-testosterone binding interactions and free plasma estradiol under physiological conditions. J Clin Endocrinol Metab 52:868. 1981.

208. Rosenfield RL: Studies of the relation of plasma androgen levels to androgen action in women. J Steroid Biochem 6:695, 1975.

209. Moll GW Jr, Rosenfield RL: Estradiol inhibition of pituitary luteinizing hormone release is antagonized by serum proteins. J Steroid Biochem 25:308, 1986.

210. Pardridge WM: Transport of protein-bound hormones into tissues in vivo. Endocr Rev 2:103, 1981.

211. Giorgi EP, Stein WD: The transport of steroids into animal cells in culture. Endocrinology 108:688, 1981.

212. Nimrod A. Rosenfield RL, Otto P: Relationship of androgen action to androgen metabolism in isolated rat granulosa cells. J Steroid Biochem 13:1015, 1980.

213. Gurpide E: Metabolic influences on the action of estrogens: Therapeutic implications. Pediatrics 62:1114, 1978.

214. Paul SM, Axelrod J: Catechol estrogens: Presence in brain and endocrine tissues. Science 19:657, 1977.

215. Naess O, Hansson V, Djoeseland O, et al: Characterization of the androgen receptor in the anterior pituitary of the rat. Endocrinology 97:1355, 1975.

216. Lieberburg I, McEwen BS: Brain cell nuclear retention of testosterone metabolites, 5α-dihydrotestosterone and estradiol-17β, in adult rats. Endocrinology 100:588, 1977.

217. Flores F, Naftolin F, Ryan KJ: Aromatization of androstenedione and testosterone by rhesus monkey hypothalamus and limbic system. Neuroendocrinology 11:177, 1973.

218. Gladue BA, Clemens LG: Flutamide inhibits testosterone-induced masculine sexual behavior in male and female rats. Endocrinology 106:1917, 1980.

219. Chan L, O'Malley BW: Mechanism of action of the steroid hormones. N Engl J Med 294:1322, 1976.

220. Muldoon TG: Regulation of steroid hormone receptor activity. Endocr Rev 1:339, 1980.

221. Chang C, Kokontis J, Liao S: Molecular cloning of human and rat complementary DNA encoding androgen receptors. Science 240:324, 1988.

222. Lubahn DB, Joseph DR, Sullivan PM, Willard HF, French FS, Wilson EM: Cloning of human androgen receptor complementary DNA and localization to the X chromosome. Science 240:327, 1988.

223. MacLusky NJ, McEwen BS: Progestin receptors in rat brain: Distribution and properties of cytoplasmic progestin-binding sites. Endocrinology 106:192, 1980.

224. Attardi B: Facilitation and inhibition of the estrogen-induced luteinizing hormone surge in the rat by progesterone: Effects on cytoplasmic and nuclear estrogen receptors in the hypothalamic-preoptic area, pituitary, and uterus. Endocrinology 108:1487, 1981.

225. Korenman SG: Radio-ligand binding assay of specific estrogens using a soluble uterine macromolecule. J Clin Endocrinol Metab 28:127, 1968.

226. Brown TR, Bullock L, Bardin CW: In vitro and in vivo binding of progestins to the androgen receptor of mouse kidney: Correlation with biological activities. Endocrinology 105:1281, 1979.

227. Cyproterone acetate (editorial). Lancet 1:1003, 1976.

228. Winter JSD, Faiman C, Reyes FI, et al: Gonadotrophins and steroid hormones in the blood and urine of prepubertal girls and other primates. Clin Endocrinol Metab 7:513, 1978.

229. Radfar N, Ansusingha K, Kenny FM: Circulating bound and free estradiol and estrone during normal growth and development and in premature thelarche and iso-sexual precocity. J Pediatr 89:719, 1976.

230. Forest MG, Cathiard AM: Pattern of plasma testosterone and Δ^4-androstenedione in normal newborns: Evidence for testicular activity at birth. J Clin Endocrinol Metab 41:977, 1975.

231. Schnakenberg K, Bidlingmaier F, Knorr D: 17-Hydroxyprogesterone, androstenedione, and testosterone in normal children and in prepubertal patients with congenital adrenal hyperplasia. Eur J Pediatr 133:259, 1980.

232. Reiter EO, Root AW: Hormonal changes of adolescence. Med Clin North Am 59:1289, 1975.

233. Lucky AW, Rosenfield RL, McGuire J, Rudy S, Helke J: Adrenal androgen hyperresponsiveness to adrenocorticotropin in women with acne and/or hirsutism: Adrenal enzyme defects and exaggerated adrenarche. J Clin Endocrinol Metab 62:840, 1986.

234. Forest MG: Function of the ovary in the neonate and infant. Eur J Obstet Gynecol Reprod Biol 9:145, 1979.

235. Solomon LM, Esterly NB: Neonatal dermatology. I. The newborn skin. J Pediatr 77:888, 1970.

236. Betend B, Claustrat B, Bizollon CA, Ehre G, Francois R: Étude de la fonction gonadotrope hypophysaire par le test à la LH-RH pendant la

premiere année de la vie. Ann Endocrinol (Paris) 36:325, 1975.

237. Kulin HE, Santner SJ: Timed urinary gonadotropin measurements in normal infants, children and adults, and in patients with disorders of sexual maturation. J Pediatr 90:760, 1977.

238. Penny R. Goldstein IP, Frasier SD: Overnight gonadotropin excretion in normal females. J Clin Endocrinol Metab 44:780, 1977.

239. Beitins IZ, O'Loughlin K, Ostrea T, et al: Gonadotropin determinations in timed 3-hour urine collections during the menstrual cycle and LHRH testing. J Clin Endocrinol Metab 43:46, 1976.

240. Reiter EO, Root AW, Duckett GE: LH and FSH levels in urine and serum of prepubertal and pubertal children receiving a 3-hour infusion of LH-RH. J Clin Endocrinol Metab 44:56, 1977.

241. Rosenfield RL, Burstein S, Cuttler L, Cara JF, Levitsky LL, Barnes RB, Ehrmann DA: The use of Nafarelin for testing pituitary-ovarian function. In Proceedings of the XII World Congress of Gynecology & Obstetrics, Rio de Janeiro, October 1988. Fertil Steril, in press.

242. Ehara Y, Yen SSC, Siler TM: Serum prolactin levels during puberty. Am J Obstet Gynecol 121:995, 1975.

243. Marshall WA, Tanner JM: Variations in pattern of pubertal changes in girls. Arch Dis Child 44:291, 1969.

244. Ross GT, Vande Wiele R: The ovary. In Williams RH (ed): Textbook of Endocrinology. 5th ed. Philadelphia, WB Saunders Company, 1974.

245. Tanner JW, Davies PWS: Clinical longitudinal standards for height and height velocity for North American children. J Pediatr 107:317, 1985.

246. MacMahon B: Age at Menarche. In Vital Health Stat [11], No. 133.

247. Bennett DL, Ward MS, Daniel WA Jr: The relationship of serum alkaline phosphatase concentrations to sex maturity ratings in adolescents. J Pediatr 88:633, 1976.

248. Tanner JM, Whitehouse RH: Revised standards for triceps and subscapular skinfolds in British children. Arch Dis Child 50:142, 1975.

249. Wade GN: Some effects of ovarian hormones on food intake and body weight in female rats. J Comp Psychol 88:183, 1975.

250. Rosenfield RL, Helke J, Lucky AW: Dexamethasone preparation does not alter corticoid and androgen responses to adrenocorticotropin. J Clin Endocrinol Metab 60:585, 1985.

251. Pescovitz OH, Hench KD, Barnes KM, Loriaux DL, Cutler GB Jr: Premature thelarche and central precocious puberty: The relationship between clinical presentation and the gonadotropin response to luteinizing hormone-releasing hormone. J Clin Endocrinol Metab 67:474, 1988.

252. Escobar ME, Rivarola MA, Bergada C: Plasma concentration of oestradiol-17-β in premature thelarche and in different types of sexual precocity. Acta Endocrinol 31:351, 1976.

253. Zipf WB, Kelch RP, Hopwood NJ, et al: Suppressed responsiveness to gonadotropin-releasing hormone in girls with unsustained isosexual precocity. J Pediatr 95:38, 1979.

254. Salardi S, Orsini LF, Cacciari E, Partesotti S, Brondelli L, Cicognani A, Frejaville E, Pluchinotta V, Tonioli S, Bovicelli L: Pelvic ultrasonography in girls with precocious puberty, congenital adrenal hyperplasia, obesity, or hirsutism. J Pediatr 112:880, 1988.

255. Vollman RF: Patterns of menstrual performance in adolescent girls. In Proceedings of 2nd World Congress on Fertility and Sterility, Naples, 1956, p 27.

256. Yen SSC: The human menstrual cycle. In Yen SSC, Jaffe RB (eds): Reproductive Endocrinology. Philadelphia, WB Saunders Company, 1978, p 126.

257. Apter D, Vihko R: Serum pregnenolone, progesterone, 17-hydroxyprogesterone, testosterone, and 5-α-dihydrotestosterone during female puberty. J Clin Endocrinol Metab 45:1039, 1977.

258. Southam AL, Richart RM: The prognosis for adolescents with menstrual abnormalities. Am J Obstet Gynecol 94:637, 1966.

259. McClintock MK: Menstrual synchrony and suppression. Nature 229:244, 1971.

260. Rosenfield RL: Plasma free androgen patterns in hirsute women and their diagnostic implications. Am J Med 66:417, 1979.

261. Vekemans M, Delvoye P, L'Hermite M, et al: Serum prolactin levels during the menstrual cycle. J Clin Endocrinol Metab 44:989, 1977.

262. Kolodny RC, Jacobs LS, Daughaday WH: Mammary stimulation causes prolactin secretion in non-lactating women. Nature 238:284, 1972.

263. Rosenwaks Z, Jones GS, Henzl MR, et al: Naproxin sodium, aspirin, and placebo in primary dysmenorrhea. Am J Obstet Gynecol 140:592, 1981.

264. Klein JR, Litt IF, Cushey R: The effect of aspirin on dysmenorrhea in adolescents. J Pediatr 98:987, 1981.

265. Muse KN, Cetel NS, Futterman LA, Yen SSC: The premenstrual syndrome. Effects of "medical ovariectomy". N Engl J Med 311:1345, 1984.

266. Rubinow DR, Hoban MC, Grover GN, Galloway DS, Roy-Byrne R, Andersen R, Merriam GR: Changes in plasma hormones across the menstrual cycle in patients with menstrually related mood disorder and in control subjects. Am J Obstet Gynecol 158:5, 1988.

267. Zimmerman AW, Holden KR. Reiter EO, et al: Medroxyprogesterone acetate in the treatment of seizures associated with menstruation. J Pediatr 83:959, 1973.

268. Dalton K: Cyclical criminal acts in premenstrual syndrome. Lancet 2:1070, 1980.

269. Nielsen DF, Bulow S: The incidence of male hermaphroditism in girls with inguinal hernia. Surg Gynecol Obstet 142:875, 1976.

270. Griffin JE, Edwards C, Madden JD, et al: Congenital absence of the vagina: The Mayer-Rokitansky-Kuster-Hauser syndrome. Ann Intern Med 85:224, 1976.

271. Blanco-Garcia M, Evain-Brion D, Roger M, Job MC: Isolated menses in prepubertal girls. Pediatrics 76:43, 1985.

272. Kreiter, ML, Rosenfield RL, Burstein SR, Cara JF, Cuttler L, Levitsky LL: Preserved height potential in untreated true precocious puberty. Clin Res 36:901A, 1988.

273. Pescovitz OH, Comite F, Cassorla F, et al: True precocious puberty complicating congenital adrenal hyperplasia: Treatment with a luteinizing hormone-releasing hormone analog. J Clin Endocrinol Metab 58:857, 1984.

274. Martuza RL, Eldridge R: Neurofibromatosis 2 (bilateral acoustic neurofibromatosis). N Engl J Med 318:684, 1988.

275. Laue L, Comite F, Hench K, Loriaux DL, Cutler GB Jr, Pescovitz OH: Precocious puberty associated with neurofibromatosis and optic gliomas. Am J Dis Child 139:1097, 1985.

276. Hochman HI. Judge DM, Reichlin S: Precocious puberty and hypothalamic hamartoma. Pediatrics 67:236, 1981.

277. Kitay JI. Altschule MD: The Pineal Gland. Cambridge, MA, Harvard University Press, 1954.

278. Cohen RA. Wurtman RJ. Axelrod J, et al: Some clinical. biochemical, and physiological actions of the pineal gland. Ann Intern Med 61:1144, 1964.

279. DiGeorge AM: Albright's syndrome: Is it coming of age? J Pediatr 87:1018, 1975.

280. Cuttler L, Jackson J, Uzzafar S, Levitsky L, Mellinger RC, Frohman L: Hypersecretion of growth hormone and prolactin in McCune-Albright syndrome. J Clin Endocrinol Metab 68:1148, 1989.

281. Danon M, Robboy SJ, Kim S, et al: Cushing syndrome, sexual precocity, and polyostotic fibrous dysplasia (Albright syndrome) in infancy. J Pediatr 87:917, 1975.

282. Lightner ES, Penny R, Frasier SD: Pituitary adenoma in McCune-Albright syndrome: Follow-up information. J Pediatr 89:159, 1976.

283. Joishy SK. Morrow LB: McCune-Albright syndrome associated with a functioning pituitary chromophobe adenoma. J Pediatr 89:73, 1976.

284. Foster CM, Comite F, Pescovitz OH, Ross JL, Loriaux DL, Cutler GB Jr: Variable response to a long-acting agonist of luteinizing hormone-releasine hormone in girls with McCune-Albright syndrome. J Clin Endocrinol Metab 59:801, 1984.

285. Feuillan PP, Foster CM, Pescovitz OH, Hench KD, Shawker T, Dwyer A, Malley JD, Barnes K, Loriaux DL, Cutler GB Jr: Treatment of precocious puberty in the McCune-Albright syndrome with the aromatase inhibityor testolactone. N Engl J Med 315:1115, 1986.

286. Scanlon EF, Burkett FE, Sener SF, et al: Breast carcinoma in an 11-year-old girl with Albright's syndrome. Breast 6:5, 1974.

287. Foster CM, Feuillan P, Padmanabhan V, Pescovitz OH, Beitins IZ, Comite F, Shawker TH, Loriaux DL, Cutler GB Jr: Ovarian function in girls with McCune-Albright syndrome. Pediatr Res 20:859, 1986.

288. Baer KA: Premature ovarian failure and precocious puberty. Obstet Gynecol 49:15s, 1977.

289. Rosenfeld RG, Reitz RE, King AB, et al: Familial precocious puberty associated with isolated elevation of luteinizing hormone. N Engl J Med 303:859, 1980.

290. Scully RE, Galdabini JJ, McNeely BU (eds): Case Records of the Massachusetts General Hospital. N Engl J Med 293:653, 1975.

291. Lindsay AN, Voorhess ML, MacGillivray MH: Multicystic ovaries detected by sonography in children with hypothyroidism. Am J Dis Child 134:588, 1980.

292. Van Wyk JJ, Grumbach MM: Syndrome of precocious menstruation and galactorrhea in juvenile hypothyroidism: An example of hormonal overlap in pituitary feedback. J Pediatr 57:416, 1960.

293. Costin G, Kershnar AK, Kogut MD, et al: Prolactin activity in juvenile hypothyroidism and precocious puberty. Pediatrics 50:881, 1962.

294. Lee PA, Blizzard RM: Serum gonadotropins in hypothyroid girls with and without sexual precocity. Johns Hopkins Med J 135:55, 1974.

295. Beitins IZ, Bode HH: Hypothyroidism with elevated gonadotropin secretion. Pediatr Res 14:475, 1980.

296. Copmann TL, Adams WC: Relationship of polycystic ovary induction to prolactin secretion: Prevention of cyst formation by bromocriptine in the rat. Endocrinology 108:1095, 1981.

297. Towne BH, Mahour GH, Woolley MM, et al: Ovarian cysts and tumors in infancy and childhood. J Pediatr Surg 10:311, 1975.

298. Wieland RG, Bendezu R, Hallberg MC, et al: Hormonal evaluation of premature menarche produced by a follicular cyst. Am J Obstet Gynecol 126:731, 1976.

299. Gallion HH, van Nagell JR, Donaldson ES, Powell DE: Ovarian dysgerminoma: Report of seven cases and review of the literature. Am J Obstet Gynecol 158:591, 1988.

300. Vaz RM, Turner C: Ollier disease (enchondromatosis) associated with ovarian juvenile granulosa cell tumor and precocious pseudopuberty. J Pediatr 108:945, 1986.

301. Mandel FP, Voet RL, Weiland AJ, et al: Steroid secretion by masculinizing and "feminizing" hilus cell tumors. J Clin Endocrinol Metab 52:779, 1981.

302. Rosenfield RL, Cohen RM, Talerman A: Lipid cell tumor of the ovary in reference to adult-onset congenital adrenal hyperplasia and polycystic ovary syndrome. J Reprod Med 32:363, 1987.

303. Scully RE, Galdabini JJ, McNeely BU: Case Records of the Massachusetts General Hospital. N Engl J Med 300:1322, 1979.

304. Saenz de Rodriguez CA, Bongiovanni AM, Conde de Borrego L: An epidemic of precocious development in Puerto Rican children. J Pediatr 107:393, 1985.

305. Herman-Giddens ME, Frothingham TE: Prepubertal female genitalia: Examination for evidence of sexual abuse. Pediatrics 80:203, 1987.

306. Bidlingmaier F, Butenandt O, Knorr D: Plasma gonadotropins and estrogens in girls with idiopathic precocious puberty. Pediatr Res 11:91, 1977.

307. Reiter EO, Kaplan SL, Conte FA, et al: Responsivity of pituitary gonadotropes to luteinizing hormone-releasing factor in idiopathic precocious puberty, precocious thelarche, precocious adrenarche, and in patients treated with medroxyprogesterone acetate. Pediatr Res 9:111, 1975.

308. Lucky AW, Rich BH, Rosenfield RL et al: Bioactive LH: A useful test to discriminate true precocious puberty from premature thelarche and adrenarche. J Pediatr 97:214, 1980.

309. Sonis WA, Comite F, Blue J, Pescovitz OH, Rahn CW, Hench KD, Cutler GB Jr, Loriaux DL, Klein RP: Behaviour problems and social competence in girls with true precocious puberty. J Pediatr 106:156, 1985.

310. Richman RA, Underwood LE, French FS, et al: Adverse effects of large doses of medroxyprogesterone (MPA) in idiopathic isosexual precocity. J Pediatr 79:963, 1971.

311. Comite F, Cassorla F, Barnes KM, Hench KD, Dwyer AD, Skerda MC, Loriaux DL, Cutler GB Jr, Pescovitz OH: Luteinizing hormone releasing hormone analogue therapy for central precious puberty. JAMA 255:2613, 1986.

312. Razdan AK, Rosenfield RL, Kim MH: Endocrinologic characteristics of partial ovarian failure. J Clin Endocrinol Metab 43:449, 1976.

313. Shalet SM, Beardwell CG, Morris Jones PH, et al: Ovarian failure following abdominal irradiation in childhood. Br J Cancer 33:655, 1976.

314. Warne GL, Fairley KF, Hobbs JB, et al: Cyclophosphamide-induced ovarian failure. N Engl J Med 289:1159, 1973.

315. Siris ES, Leventhal BG, Vaitukaitis JL: Effects of childhood leukemia and chemotherapy on puberty and reproductive function in girls. N Engl J Med 294:1143, 1976.

316. Irvine WJ: Autoimmunity in endocrine disease. Recent Prog Horm Res 36:509, 1980.

317. Vazquez AM, Kenny FM: Ovarian failure and antiovarian antibodies in association with hypoparathyroidism, moniliasis, and Addison's and Hashimoto's disease. Obstet Gynecol 41:414, 1973.

318. Lucky AW, Rebar RW, Blizzard RM, et al: Pubertal progression in the presence of elevated serum gonadotropins in girls with multiple endocrine deficiencies. J Clin Endocrinol Metab 45:673, 1977.

319. Wolfsdorf JI, Rosenfield RL. Fang VS, et al: Partial gonadotrophin-resistance in pseudohypoparathyroidism. Acta Endocrinol 88:321, 1978.

320. Levine MA, Downs RW Jr, Moses AM, et al: Resistance to multiple hormones in patients with pseudohypoparathyroidism association with deficient activity of guanine nucleotide regulatory protein. Am J Med 74:545, 1983.

321. Kaufman FR, Xu YK, Ng WG, Donnell GN: Correlation of ovarian function with galactose-1-phosphate uridyl transferase levels in galactosemia. J Pediatr 112:754, 1988.

322. Schaff-Blass E, Burstein S, Rosenfield RL: Advances in diagnosis and treatment of short stature, with special reference to the role of growth hormone. J Pediatr 104:801, 1984.

323. Barkan AL, Kelch RP, Marshall JC: Isolated gonadotrope failure in the polyglandular autoimmune syndrome. N Engl J Med 312:1535, 1985.

324. Hendricks SA, Lippe BM, Kaplan SA, et al: Hypothalamic atrophy with progressive hypopituitarism in an adolescent girl. J Clin Endocrinol Metab 52:562, 1981.

325. Rappaport R, Brauner R, Czernichow P, Thibaud E, Renier D, Zucker JM, Lemerle J: Effect of hypothalamic and pituitary irradiation on pubertal development in children with cranial tumors. J Clin Endocrinol Metab 54:1164, 1982.

326. Warren MP, Vande Wiele RL: Clinical and metabolic features of anorexia nervosa. Am J Obstet Gynecol 117:435, 1973.

327. Casper RC, Offer D, Ostrov E: The self-image of adolescents with acute anorexia nervosa. J Pediatr 98:656, 1981.

328. Herzog DB, Copeland PM: Bulimia nervosa—psyche and satiety. N Engl J Med 319:716, 1988.

329. Pugliese MT, Lifshitz F, Grad G, Fort P, Marks-Katz M: Fear of obesity. A cause of short stature and delayed puberty. N Engl J Med 309:513, 1983.

330. Frisch RE, McArthur JW: Menstrual cycles: Fatness as a determinant of minimum weight for height necessary for their maintenance or onset. Science 185:949. 1974.

331. Boyar RM, Katz J, Finkelstein JW, et al: Anorexia nervosa: Immaturity of the 24-hour luteinizing hormone secretory pattern. N Engl J Med 291:861, 1974.

332. Sherman BM, Halmi KA, Zamudio R: LH and FSH response to gonadotropin-releasing hormone in anorexia nervosa: Effects of nutritional rehabilitation. J Clin Endocrinol Metab 41:135, 1975.

333. Beumont PJV, George GCW, Pimstone BL, et al: Body weight and the pituitary response to hypothalamic releasing hormones in patients with anorexia nervosa. J Clin Endocrinol Metab 43:487, 1976.

334. Beumont PJV, Carr PJ, Gelder MG: Plasma levels of luteinizing hormone and of immunoreactive oestrogens (oestradiol) in anorexia nervosa: Response to clomiphene citrate. Psycholog Med 3:495, 1973.

335. Marshall JC, Fraser TR: Amenorrhoea in anorexia nervosa: Assessment and treatment with clomiphene citrate. Br Med J 4:590, 1971.

336. Mecklenburg RS, Loriaux DL, Thompson RH, et al: Hypothalamic dysfunction in patients with anorexia nervosa. Medicine 53:147, 1974.

337. Croxson MS, Ibbertson HK: Low serum triiodothyronine (T_3) and hypothyroidism in anorexia nervosa. J Clin Endocrinol Metab 44:167, 1977.

338. Luger A, Deuster PA, Kyle SB, Gallucci WT, Montgomery LC, Gold PW, Loriaux DL, Chrousos GP: Acute hypothalamic-pituitary-adrenal responses to the stress of treadmill exercise. N Engl J Med 316:1309, 1987.

339. Gold PW, Goodwin FK, Chrousos GP: Clinical and biochemical manifestations of depression. Relation to the neurobiology of stress. N Engl J Med 319:413, 1988.

340. Frisch RE, Wyshak G, Vincent L: Delayed menarche and amenorrhea in ballet dancers. N Engl J Med 303:17, 1980.

341. Burrington JD, Wayne ER: Obstruction of the duodenum by the superior mesenteric artery—does it exist in children? J Pediatr Surg 9:733, 1974.

342. Sakiyama R, Quan M: Galactorrhea and hyperprolactinemia. Obstet Gynecol Surv 38:689, 1983.

343. Sauder SE, Frager M, Case GD, Kelch RP, Marshall JC: Abnormal patterns of pulsatile luteinizing hormone secretion in women with hyperprolactinemia and amenorrhea: Responses to bromocriptine. J Clin Endocrinol Metab 59:941, 1984.

344. Tallo D, Malarkey WB: Physiologic concentrations of dopamine fail to suppress prolactin secretion in patients with idiopathic hyperprolactinemia or prolactinomas. Am J Obstet Gynecol 151:651, 1985.

345. Schroeder LL, Johnson JC, Malarkey WB: Cerebrospinal fluid prolactin: A reflection of abnormal prolactin secretion in patients with pituitary tumors. J Clin Endocrinol Metab 43:1255, 1976.

346. Stanhope R, Pringle PJ, Brook CGD, Adams J, Jacobs HS: Induction of puberty by pulsatile go-

nadotropin releasing hormone. Lancet 2:552, 1987.

347. Katz RL, Mazer C, Litt IF: Anorexia nervosa by proxy. J Pediatr 107:247, 1985.

348. Rothchild E, Owens RP: Adolescent girls who lack functioning ovaries. J Am Acad Child Psychiatry 11:88, 1972.

349. Ross JL, Long LM, Skerda M, et al: The effect of low dose ethinyl estradiol on six monthly growth rates and predicted height in patients with Turner syndrome. J Pediatr 109:950, 1986.

350. Rosenfield RL: Low-dose testosterone effect on somatic growth. Pediatrics 77:853, 1986.

351. Rosenfeld RG, Hintz RL, Johanson AJ, Sherman B, Brasel JA, Burstein S, Chernausek S, Compton P, Frane J, Gotlin RW, Kuntze J, Lippe BM, Mahoney PC, Moore WV, New MI, Saenger P, Sybert V: Three-year results of a randomized prospective trial of methionyl human growth hormone and oxandrolone in Turner syndrome. J Pediatr 113:393, 1988.

352. Mroueh AM, Siler-Khodr TM: Ovarian refractoriness to gonadotropins in cases of inappropriate lactation: Restoration of ovarian function with bromocryptine. J Clin Endocrinol Metab 43:1398, 1976.

353. Van Look PFA, Hunter WM, Fraser IS, et al: Impaired estrogen-induced luteinizing hormone release in young women with anovulatory dysfunctional uterine bleeding. J Clin Endocrinol Metab 46:816, 1978.

354. Reame NE, Sauder SE, Case GD, Kelch RP, Marshall JC: Pulsatile gonadotropin secretion in women with hypothalamic amenorrhea: Evidence that reduced frequency of gonadotropin-releasing hormone secretion is the mechanism of persistent anovulation. J Clin Endocrinol Metab 61:851, 1985.

355. Rakoff AE: Psychogenic factors in anovulatory women. Fertil Steril 13:1, 1962.

356. Yen SSC: Chronic anovulation due to CNS-hypothalamicpituitary dysfunction. *In* Yen Y, Jaffe R (eds): Reproductive Endocrinology. Philadelphia, WB Saunders Company, 1978.

357. Boyar RM, Kapen S, Weitzman ED, et al: Pituitary microadenoma and hyperprolactinemia. N Engl J Med 294:263, 1976.

358. Seppälä M, Hirvonen E, Ranta T: Hyperprolactinaemia and luteal insufficiency. Lancet 1:229, 1976.

359. Wildt L, Leyendecker G: Induction of ovulation by the chronic administration of naltrexone in hypothalamic amenorrhea. J Clin Endocrinol Metab 64:1334, 1987.

360. Santen RJ, Friend JN, Trojanowski D, et al: Prolonged negative feedback suppression after estradiol administration: Proposed mechanism of eugonadal secondary amenorrhea. J Clin Endocrinol Metab 47:1220, 1978.

361. Shaw RW: Differential response to LHRH following oestrogen therapy in women with amenorrhoea. Br J Obstet Gynaecol 86:69, 1979.

362. Weiss G, Nachtigall LE, Ganguly M: Induction of an LH surge with estradiol benzoate. Obstet Gynecol 47:415, 1976.

363. Shearman RP: Secondary amenorrhoea after oral contraceptives—treatment and follow-up. Contraception 11:123, 1974.

364. van der Steeg HJ, Bennink HJT: Bromocriptine for induction of ovulation in normoprolactinaemic post-pill anovulation. Lancet 1:502, 1977.

365. Ortiz A, Hiroi M, Stanczyk FZ, et al: Serum medroxy-progesterone acetate (MPA) concentrations and ovarian function following intramuscular injection of depo-MPA. J Clin Endocrinol Metab 44:32, 1977.

366. Bolognese RJ, Piver S, Feldman JD: Galactorrhea and abnormal menses associated with a long-acting progesterone. JAMA 199:100, 1967.

367. Strott CA, Cargille CM, Ross GT, et al: The short luteal phase. J Clin Endocrinol Metab 30:246, 1970.

368. Sherman BM, Korenman SG: Measurement of plasma LH, FSH, estradiol and progesterone in disorders of the human menstrual cycle: the short luteal phase. J Clin Endocrinol Metab 38:89, 1974.

369. Boccuzzi G, Angeli A, Bisbocci D, et al: Effect of synthetic luteinizing hormone releasing hormone (LH-RH) on the release of gonadotropins in Cushing's disease. J Clin Endocrinol Metab 40:892, 1975.

370. Sakakura M, Takebe K, Nakagawa S: Inhibition of luteinizing hormone secretion induced by synthetic LRH by long-term treatment with glucocorticoids in human subjects. J Clin Endocrinol Metab 40:774, 1975.

371. Baldwin DM: The effect of glucocorticoids on estrogen-dependent luteinizing hormone release in the ovariectomized rat and on gonadotropin secretion in the intact female rat. Endocrinol 105:120, 1979.

372. Maruo T, Hayashi M, Matsuo H, Yamamoto T, Okada H, Mochizuki M: The role of thyroid hormone as a biological amplifier of the actions of follicle-stimulating hormone in the functional differentiation of cultured porcine granulosa cells. Endocrinology 121:1233, 1987.

373. Asch RH, Smith CG, Siler-Khodr TM, et al: Effects of Δ^9-tetrahydrocannabinol during the follicular phase of the rhesus monkey (*Macaca mulatta*). J Clin Endocrinol Metab 52:50, 1981.

374. Mishell DR Jr, Nakamura RM, Barberia JM et al: Initial detection of human chorionic gonadotropin in serum in normal human gestation. Am J Obstet Gynecol 118:990, 1974.

375. Barnes R, Rosenfield RL: Polycystic ovary syndrome: Pathogenesis and treatment. Ann Intern Med 110:386, 1989.

376. Barnes RB, Rosenfield RL, Burstein S, Ehrmann D: Pituitary-ovarian responses to nafarelin testing in polycystic ovary syndrome. New Engl J Med 320:559, 1989.

377. McKenna TJ: Pathogenesis and treatment of polycystic ovary syndrome. N Engl J Med 318:558, 1988.

378. Root AW, Moshang T Jr: Evolution of the hyperandrogenism-polycystic ovarian syndrome from isosexual precocious puberty: Report of two cases. Am J Obstet Gynecol 149:763, 1984.

379. Cara JF, Rosenfield RL: Insulin-like growth factor I and insulin potentiate luteinizing hormone-induced androgen synthesis by rat ovarian thecal-interstitial cells. Endocrinology 123:733, 1988.

380. Cara JF, Rosenfield RL: Somatomedin-C/Insulin-like growth factor-I (IGF-I) enhances LH binding to rat ovarian theca-interstitial cells. Clin Res 36:901A, 1988 (abstract).

381. Meldrum DR, Frumar AM, Shamonki IM, et al: Ovarian and adrenal steroidogenesis in a virilized patient with gonadotropin-resistant ovaries and hilus cell hyperplasia. Obstet Gynecol 56:216, 1980.
382. The shape of fatness (editorial): Lancet 1:889, 1984.
383. Emans SJ, Grace E, Woods ER, Mansfield J, Crigler JF Jr: Treatment with dexamethasone of androgen excess in adolescent patients. J Pediatr 112:821, 1988.
384. Polson EW, Wadsworth J, Adams J, Franks S: Polycystic ovaries—a common finding in normal women. Lancet 1:870, 1988.
385. Rosenfield RL, Bickel S, Razdan AK: Amenorrhea related to progestin excess in congenital adrenal hyperplasia. Obstet Gynecol 56:208, 1980.
386. Burstein S, Turkington E, Rosenfield RL: Elevated progesterone (P) in congenital adrenal hyperplasia (CAH) alters LH secretory dynamics. Proceedings 7th International Congress of Endocrinology, Quebec. Princeton, NJ, Excerpta Medica, 1984, Abstract #336.

9

PRIMARY OVARIAN FAILURE

Barbara M. Lippe

FEMALE SEXUAL DIFFERENTIATION AND OVARIAN DEVELOPMENT

Sexual development and differentiation is a complex process involving events at several genetic and embryologic levels. At the first level, fertilization, and during the immediate postfertilization cell cleavages, the sex chromosome constitution is established in the zygote. This may be normal, 46,XX or 46,XY, or may consist of some abnormality in all cells (such as all being 45,X or 47,XXY) or abnormalities in a mosaic pattern (such as 46,XX/45,X or 45,X/47,XXY). At the second level, the differentiation of the paired genital ridges into gonads, between the fifth and sixth postfertilization week, changes occur independently on each side of the embryo.[1] These changes depend on a series of events initiated by the Y chromosome.

The presence of a Y chromosome is associated with the induction of a testis. The mechanisms of testis induction are complicated, however; the presence of a Y chromosome does not invariably result in testicular differentiation, and the absence, using classic cytogenetics, of a demonstrable Y chromosome does not guarantee ovarian development. Until recently, it was thought that the factor responsible for the induction of the testis was the Y chromosome—encoded minor histocompatibility antigen called H-Y antigen. However, new evidence suggests that this plasma membrane protein is coded for by a region of the Y chromosome that does not appear to be directly associated with the presence or absence of a testis. If the H-Y antigen has a role in testicular development it may be in tissue organization since the protein's structure is suggestive of a cell adhesion type of molecule (so-called CAM protein). Further complicating interpretation of the data on the role of H-Y antigen in sexual differentiation are the differing methods used to detect it. Graft rejection and cell-mediated cytotoxicity methods are used to detect the Y-encoded cell membrane protein. However, serologic methods appear to detect a totally unrelated protein, coded for by a gene on chromosome 6, and expressed in both males and females, albeit in different quantities. The role for this "serologic" H-Y antigen remains to be identified and the search for the sex-determining factor remains active.[2]

Recently, molecular genetic techniques that can probe for the presence of specific DNA sequences too small to be detected by cytogenetics, appear to have localized a Y chromosome "testis-determining factor" or TDF. This region of DNA is a small fraction of the Y chromosome located in the distal part of the short arm adjacent to the terminal pseudoautosomal region (the tip of the Y that participates in crossing over with the X chromosome during meiosis). When this small region of the Y is absent, the individual fails to develop testes; when present, regardless of how little else of the Y is present, the testes develop. Using molecular genetic techniques, including cloning a segment of this TDF region, Page and coworkers have made observations suggesting that this gene encodes a protein with multiple "fingers" that bind to nucleic acids in a sequence-specific manner, thereby regulating the transcription of other genes downstream in the process from TDF.[3] This model for the role of TDF that invokes the action and products of several genes, including genes located on the X chromosome as well as on autosomes, is important since a single TDF gene alone cannot explain all examples of genetic disorders of sexual differentiation. While TDF can be detected in the genome of most cytogenetic XX males and is absent from the genome of some phenotypic XY females bearing deletions of the Y chromosome including the TDF, there are several exceptions where the TDF model is insufficient to explain gonadal differentiation. The most notable examples are the XX hermaphrodites, who uniformly do not appear to have TDF, and those phenotypic female XY familial gonadal dysgenesis patients who inherit their defect (failure of a testis to develop) as an X-linked recessive trait independent of TDF (which is present). The explosion in number of molecular techniques that can be applied to the study of gonadal differentiation will yield additional data to expand and clarify these mechanisms. What is likely to remain valid, however, is that neither abnormalities of this or other TDFs are responsible for the gonadal failure in Turner syndrome. Instead, it appears that the genetic dosage effect of a complete or partial monosomic X chromosome in the germ cells that enter the developing gonadal structure may be responsible for the gonadal dysgenesis.

The germ cells originate in the wall of the yolk sac at the caudal end of the embryo and migrate to the genital ridges by the fourth week postconception. In the case of the XX-containing cells, after reaching the genital ridge they undergo successive mitotic divisions to reach their maximum number (7,000,000) by about 5 fetal months, although many germ cells are also lost during oogonial division.[4] As the oogonia cease mitosis, they initiate nuclear changes characteristic of the prophase of the first meiotic division (primary oocyte). Concomitantly, the primary oocyte becomes closely associated with a single layer of spindle-shaped cells that are the precursors of the granulosa cells. This complex of oocyte and spindle-shaped cells, and the basal lamina enclosing it, is a "primary follicle." Shortly after the granulosa cells proliferate into the primary follicle, the cortical stromal cells change in shape and begin to acquire organelles characteristic of the steroid hormone–secreting cells of the theca interna. The size of the maturing follicle increases and antral fluid accumulates among the granulosa cells at the junction of the cortex and medulla. This results in the transformation of the primary follicle into a graafian follicle.[5] At the same time that primary follicles are developing, the degenerative process of follicular atresia also begins.[6] It is this atretic process that is responsible for the decline in the number of follicles from a maximum of 7,000,000 to about 2,000,000 at birth and to only 300,000

to 400,000 at the time of menarche.[4] In ovaries that contain cells bearing abnormal sex chromosome constitutions, the process of oogonial division may begin normally but then exhibit accelerated loss of oogonia and an accelerated rate of follicular atresia. This mechanism may be responsible for the stromal fibrosis of the ovary in the female with the 45,X karyotype[7] as well as the decreased fertility or early menopause reported in women with X chromosome mosaicism or structural abnormalities of the X, as well as in those with extra X chromosome karyotypes such as the 47,XXX, 48,XXXX and 49,XXXX.

Events at the third level, embryogenesis of the internal genital ducts, occur subsequently (weeks 6 to 8) and depend on influences arising ipsilaterally from the developing gonad. Normally, there are two sets of ducts present in close proximity to each gonad at the 6- to 8-week stage (the paramesonephric or müllerian ducts and the mesonephric or wolffian ducts). If an ovary is present, whether it is destined to be normal or not, or if no gonad is present at all, the wolffian duct regresses and the müllerian duct differentiates into a fallopian tube, a uterine horn, and part of the upper one third of the vagina. When this occurs bilaterally, as in the case of normal females or those with Turner syndrome, the structures fuse to form a normal uterus and upper vagina. If a normal testis is present, however, active secretion of a protein called müllerian regression substance or müllerian inhibitory factor results in regression of the paramesonephric duct. Simultaneously, the wolffian duct persists, and if testosterone is secreted by the testis, the ductal structure on the side with the testis is further organized into the accessory male reproductive structures (the epididymis and vas deferens).

During the development of the external genitalia, there is also an undifferentiated stage. The final anatomy is dependent on both embryologic mechanisms of cloacal division and hormonal effects on genital fold fusion and genital tubercle elongation. Normal synthesis and secretion of testosterone by the fetal testis, its enzymatic conversion to dihydrotestosterone (DHT), and the local action of DHT on genital anlage are necessary for the virilization of the external genitalia and the apparent male phenotype. This process of fusion is a late embryologic phenomenon, occurring at the 12th to 14th week. If the gonads do not secrete testosterone and there are no abnormal extragonadal sources of androgen, the genitalia will retain the unfused anatomy of the female phenotype.[8]

THE X CHROMOSOME AND THE CHROMOSOMAL KARYOTYPE

Over the last 40 years numerous advances have occurred that have contributed significantly to our ability to identify and study the human X chromosome. The classical cytologic demonstration by Barr that an intranuclear body was present in a large majority of cells from females, but not males, was a significant breakthrough.[9] Subsequent demonstration that this represented an inactivated X chromosome added to the importance of the observation. However, the quantitative estimation of the presence of the Barr body in cells such as are obtained from a smear of the buccal mucosa is an imprecise clinical test. The Barr body can be identified only in a small percentage of female cells, the number varying with the tissue studied (buccal mucosa, hair root sheath, or leukocyte). Additionally, in the neonate, the Barr body, or so-called sex chromatin body, is somewhat more difficult to detect. Mosaicism is difficult or impossible to detect, as are structural abnormalities of the X chromosome. Finally, positive cells are sometimes reported when normal male tissue is examined. Therefore, as cytogenetic techniques that enabled direct visualization of individual chromosomes became available, the value of the buccal smear for Barr body determination declined. Thus obtaining such a study is no longer considered to be sufficient, even as a screening technique, if an X chromosome abnormality is suspected. Instead, a chromosomal karyotype, prepared from either peripheral leukocytes, skin fibroblasts, bone marrow elements, or tissue samples, should always be utilized.

The normal karyotype consists of 22 pairs of homologous autosomes and one pair of sex chromosomes. The chromosomes were classified originally into seven groups, A through G, according to the length of the chromosome and the position of the centromere. By convention, the short arms were designated by lower case "p" (petit), while the long arms were assigned the next letter in the alphabet, lower case "q." The X chromosome has the characteristic of a C group chromosome; it is similar in size and has a metacentric centromere. The Y chromosome, on the other hand, is a small structure, similar in configuration to the G group chromosomes. Thus, the older literature will describe a patient with Turner syndrome, who is missing an X chromosome, as having a 45 chromosome count and missing a C group, which is consistent with 45,X. Similarly, a male with Down trisomy would have been described as having 47 chromosomes with an extra G group chromosome (now recognized as chromosome 21). More recently, newer cytogenetic techniques have been developed to visualize individual chromosomal architecture and specific biologic properties. Differential staining of various regions of the chromosome with Giemsa or acridine orange, or differential fluorescence with quinacrine, has permitted recognition of unique patterns of bands in each pair of autosomes and the X and Y. Within each group from A to G the chromosome pairs are now numbered specifically from 1 to 22. The X chromosome is separated from chromosomes 6 to 12 in the C group, and the Y, from 21 and 22 in the G group.[10]

A typical normal female karyotype, prepared with the trypsin-Giemsa banding technique, is shown in Figure 9–1. If a part of the short arm were missing, the banding pattern would reflect this deletion, and the chromosomal karyotype report might now read 46,XXp –. Similarly, if part of the long arm were deleted, this would be designated as 46,XXq –. Should a ring (r) chromosome be identified, composed of material with X-like staining patterns of both the short and long arms, it would be designated 46,X,r(X). Another recognized rearrangement is when the entire X chromosome appears to consist of almost two complete long arms with little short arm material, or two short arms with little or no long arm material. These structurally abnormal chromosomes are called isochromosomes. A schematic representation of the X isochromosome for the long arm, X,i(Xq), which occurs more frequently than the X,i(xp) is shown in the right panel of Figure 9–2; a normal X chromosome is shown on the left.

Finally, X chromosome material may be translocated to an autosome, or additional chromosomal material (autosomal, X, or Y) may be translocated to the X chromosome. Both of these abnormalities have been recognized with the newer staining tech-

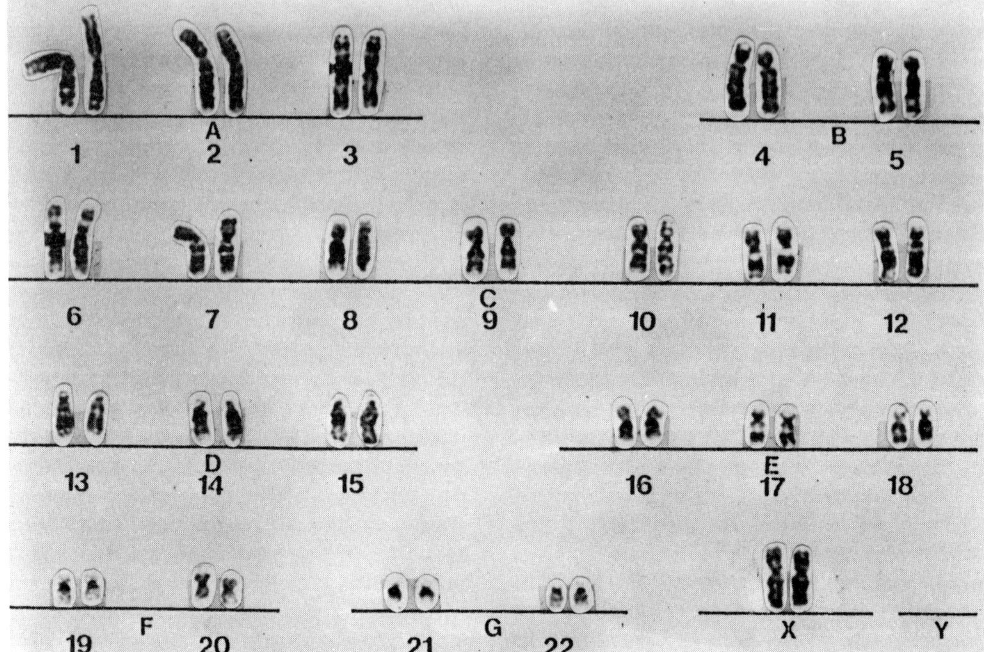

FIGURE 9–1. Complete 46,XX chromosomal karyotype. Trypsin-Giemsa technique demonstrates characteristic banding of each chromosomal pair.

niques. Therefore, banding studies are indicated whenever an X chromosome disorder is suspected, and may be omitted only if a 45,X karyotype is demonstrated for all cells studied.

Concurrent with the development of the techniques for chromosome identification, cytogenetic, clinical, and experimental investigations were carried out to attempt to localize specific genes to the X chromosome and to attempt to characterize which regions of the chromosome are responsible for the

genotypic and phenotypic abnormalities that occur in women with X chromosome disorders. It is beyond the scope of this discussion to review the data localizing the genes for such factors as the Xg_a blood group antigens and the genes for enzymes such as phosphoglycerate kinase and α-galactosidase to the X chromosome,[10] save to mention that genetic studies of families often employ the measurement of these gene products in linkage analysis studies. Similarly, while a complete review of X-linked disorders, such as hemophilia A,[11] red-green color blindness, ocular albinism, muscular dystrophy, and ichthyosis is not feasible here, it is noteworthy that full expression of these disorders has been reported in females with Turner syndrome. Genetic determinants for thyroxine-binding globulin (TBG) appear to be X-linked as well, and TBG deficiency has been reported in a 45,X member of an affected kindred.[12]

More pertinent to this discussion are those studies that examine the relationship between the chromosomal karyotype and the phenotypic characteristics that appear in Turner syndrome. In a classic paper by Ferguson-Smith,[13] the karyotypes of 307 patients with various forms of gonadal dysgenesis were correlated with their clinical

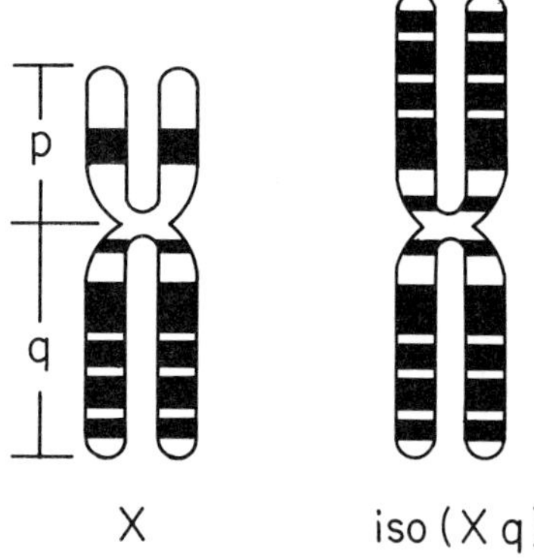

FIGURE 9–2. Schematized illustrations of a normal X chromosome (*left*) and an iso-X chromosome with duplicated long arms (*right*).

findings. He noted that short stature was the only clinical finding invariably associated with the 45,X karyotype. Complete gonadal insufficiency was not always present, since seven 45,X patients had had some evidence of spontaneous puberty. He also noted that as a whole, patients with mosaic karyotypes, including one normal XX line (i.e., 45,X/ 46,XX), tended to have fewer pheotypic abnormalities. However, save for a very few mosaic patients who were not short, on physical examination individual patients with mosaicism could not be readily distinguished from patients with the monosomic karyotype. Finally, he proposed that the area of the X chromosome responsible for the disturbance in growth was localized to the short arm of the X chromosome. Although banding studies were not yet available at the time of this study, the majority of these observations are still valid. A subsequent study of a large group of patients, which included banding,[14] confirmed that short stature is the only characteristic present in virtually 100 per cent of the patients.

Although the data tended to confirm the primacy of the short arm as the location of the determinant of stature, no cases of nonmosaic long arm deletions were detected in that series. Over the last few years, we, as well as others, have reported individual patients in whom nonmosaic deletions of the long arm have been associated with both short stature and gonadal dysgenesis.[15] However, patients who manifested normal stature have also been described with long arm deletions and long arm autosomal translocations. Thus, the functional integrity of only part of the long arm may be necessary for the attainment of normal stature. Conversely, to date, clinical and cytogenetic data suggest that almost the entire short arm is necessary for normal growth.[16] This is especially interesting, since evidence suggests that during X chromosome inactivation not all of the short arm is inactivated.[17] Thus, true monosomy for the entire short arm may never occur normally, and when it is present, owing to either complete absence of an X or significant short arm loss, somatic growth may be impaired.

TURNER SYNDROME

Definition

Recent advances in our understanding of the factors that affect ovarian development have made it possible to place the extensive literature describing patients with phenotypic and ovarian abnormalities into perspective. While there are many descriptions of women with short stature, childlessness, hypoplastic female genitalia and absent ovaries, the report of Henry Turner in 1938 of seven cases of rather uniform appearance led to general recognition of the phenotype that bears his name.[18] These women had short stature in association with sexual infantilism, webbing of the neck, low posterior hairline, and increased carrying angle of the elbows (cubitus valgus). An earlier report by Ullrich in 1930 of an 8-year-old female with short stature, lymphedema of the neck, hands, and feet, and subsequent neck webbing, cubitus valgus, and other phenotypic abnormalities (including a high arched palate, ptosis, low-set auricles, and small upwardly curved nails), described several other features that are now associated with Turner syndrome, hence the less common but more appropriate eponym, Ullrich-Turner syndrome. Ullrich himself later recognized that his patients and those of Turner appeared to have the same condition.[19] He also called attention to the work of Kristin Bonnevie, who described a group of congenital anomalies in mice, consisting of distention of the neck and malformations of the ears, face, and limb buds, all secondary to dissection of the subcutaneous tissues by fluid. This "bleb" mechanism for producing multiple anomalies was suggested by Ullrich as being responsible for the cervical lymphangiectasia noted in some human female abortuses, which appeared to produce a scarred, webbed neck (pterygium colli). Ullrich proposed the eponym Status Bonnevie-Ullrich to describe the set of specific anomalies arising from a single mechanism (lymphangiectasia) and resulting in the phenotype of Turner syndrome.

The links between these phenotypic descriptions, the pathologic evidence of streak ovaries, and the X chromosome came with the introduction of the technique for sex chromatin identification by Barr and the demonstration that most patients with Turner syndrome had absence of the sex chromatin material. Initially, this absence of sex chromatin, or lack of a Barr body, was associated with "maleness," since a similar pattern was found in normal phenotypic males. Only after it was demonstrated that it was the second X chromosome that, in the inactivated state, constituted the Barr body, was it clear that the 45,X karyotype would result in a chromatin pattern similar to the normal 46,XY karyotype. Thus, Turner syndrome patients were in fact not XY males, but in most cases, 45,X females. In fact, one of the original seven patients Turner described was reinvestigated and found to have a 45,X chromosomal karyotype.[20]

Expansion of the use of leukocytes and fibroblasts for chromosomal karyotyping has led to the discovery of many other X chromosome abnormalities, including mosaicism, rings, deletions, and rearrangements, all of which can be associated with one or more of the features of Turner syndrome and ovarian dysgenesis. However, other groups of patients were recognized after chromosomal karyotypes were used to characterize patients with phenotypic similarities and/or ovarian dysgenesis. One source of confusion is the group of patients in whom the phenotype of webbed neck and short stature is associated with normal chromosomes in both XX females and XY males. A group of these patients was described by Noonan,[21] who noted the frequent occurrence of pulmonic valvular heart disease. The eponym Noonan syndrome is applied to these patients. This syndrome is often confused with Turner syndrome, and when it occurs in males, has been referred to as the male Turner syndrome phenotype. However, the chromosomes are normal in the 46,XX females and 46,XY males who bear this phenotype. The gonads of the females do not show the early follicular loss or fibrosis characteristic of X chromosome abnormalities, nor is there a chromosomal abnormality in those males in whom cryptorchidism occurs. Therefore, Noonan syndrome both in males and females should be clearly separated from Turner syndrome. The nomenclature, evaluation, genetic counseling, and endocrine management that are appropriate to the female with Turner syndrome do not apply to patients with Noonan syndrome.

Another area of confusion arises from the demonstration of gonadal dysgenesis or aplasia in females without demonstrable chromosomal abnormalities. Most, but not all, of these patients tend to have normal phenotypes and normal stature, and some have similarly affected siblings, which is consistent with an autosomal recessive pattern of inheritance. Finally, there is a group of phenotypic female patients with gonadal dysgenesis and a 46,XY karyotype. These patients (not to be confused with those with testicular feminization) also have a genetic disorder affecting testicular induction, so that gonads do not form. Thus, the concept of "gonadal dysgenesis," so elegantly reviewed by Opitz and Pallister,[22] includes a large number of disorders. For the purpose of this chapter, Turner syndrome will be used to describe the patient with an abnormality of the chromosomal karyotype involving the X chromosome associated with phenotypic abnormalities that include short stature and the potential for or the presence of ovarian failure.

Incidence and Etiology

The incidence of abnormalities in the sex chromosomal karyotype resulting in the loss of all or part of an X chromosome has been variously reported as 1:2000 to 1:5000 in live-born phenotypic females.[23,24] Population screenings by Barr body assessment are likely to have underestimated the incidence because mosaic or structural X abnormalities may have been missed. Studies using lymphocyte chromosomal analysis would have detected some mosaic karyotypes such as 45,X/46,XX as well as some nonmosaic karyotypes such as 46,X,r(X), but may have missed deletions and rearrangements. Finally, studies using banding techniques applied to the lymphocyte karyotype analysis would tend to detect minor changes in the architecture of the X chromosome such as partial deletions or an X isochromosome and should yield the highest incidence. However, these latter methods have not been applied to large population screening programs. Thus, the true incidence of X chromosomal abnormalities and the distribution of types is still unknown. However, when large series of patients with previously diagnosed Turner syndrome are examined with these newer techniques and categorized according to chromosomal karyotype, the relative frequencies of the different karyotypes suggest that the 45,X karyotype may represent only 50 to 60 per cent of all cases.[10] Our own data for a group of 141 patients are shown in Table 9–1. The percentage of 45,X patients is 56.7, which is almost identical to the percentages quoted in the literature. This would suggest that the frequency of X chromosomal abnormalities in live-born females may indeed be as high as 1:2000.

The number of affected live births actually reflects only a small fraction of total

TABLE 9–1   SUMMARY OF THE CYTOGENETIC FINDINGS IN 141 TURNER SYNDROME PATIENTS

N	Per cent	Karotype		
80	56.7	45,X		
24	17.0	46,X,i(Xq)	(thirteen	:45,X/46,X,i(Xq))
			(ten	:46,X,i(Xq))
			(one	:45,X/46,X,i(Xq)/46,XXp-)
12	8.5	45, X/46,XX		
8	5.7	46, X,r(X)	(all	:45,X/46,X,r(X)
7	5.0	45,X/46, XY		
4	2.8	46,XXq-	(two	:45,X/46,XXq-)
			(two	:46,XXq-)
4	2.8	46,XXp-	(two	:46,XXp-)
			(one	:45,X/46,XXp-)
			(one	:45,X/46,XXp-/46,X + mar)
2	1.4	45,X/47,XXX		

conceptuses with X chromosome abnormalities. It is estimated that 99.9 per cent of XO conceptuses do not survive beyond 28 weeks' gestation, and that the XO karyotype occurs in 1 of 15 spontaneous abortions.[25,26] Associated with the very high incidence of this abnormality in abortuses appears to be an inverse correlation between increasing frequency and advancing maternal age.[27] This negative correlation has not been noted for the mosaic or structural X chromosomal abnormalitics, nor has it been noted in the case of 45,X infants that are born after gestations resulting in viable infants. Thus, young women do not have an increased risk for having a term infant with Turner syndrome, only for having the abnormality in a fetus spontaneously aborted. There are no data to support a positive or negative correlation between the 45,X karyotype in aborted or term pregnancies and paternal age. However, there is a suggestion that the mechanism responsible for the 45,X conceptus may be different from that responsible for structural X chromosome rearrangements. There is evidence, for example, that the X,i(Xq) karyotype may have an association with advanced paternal age.[28] More than one dose of certain loci on the long arm of the X chromosome delivered to the fetus will enhance its chance of survival. Therefore live-born infants with the X,i(Xq) karyotype constitute an unusually large percentage of Turner syndrome individuals.[24]

The association of a seasonal incidence with a birth abnormality such as Turner syndrome would implicate either an environmental cause or, conversely, an environmental effect on preservation of prenatal viability. When such associations are sought in Turner syndrome, the results are somewhat conflicting; but when all the series are reviewed, significant peaks do not appear to emerge. We examined our own group of 141 patients according to month and year of birth, and utilizing birth date, rather than conception date, found no systematic variation in incidence with seasons of the year.

Other etiologic factors examined previously include birth order and sibling sex (for which there were no apparent associations)[28] and twinning. In the latter there does appear to be a slightly higher occurrence rate for both the XO[9] and the (X,i,(Xq) karyotypes, although not at a level of statistical significance. At least three cases of Turner syndrome resulting from artificial insemination have been reported.[30] In two, studies of blood group antigens suggest the lost chromosome was of paternal origin. In our own series, we have one patient who was the offspring from pregnancy by artificial insemination.

The issue of the relationship between autoimmune disorders and chromosomal defects is unresolved. It has been well documented that autoimmune phenomena occur with increased frequency, not only in Turner syndrome, but also in trisomy 21 and Klinefelter syndrome.[31] It has also been suggested that autoimmune disorders occur with increased frequency in first-degree relatives of affected individuals. However, preliminary studies of the human leukocyte antigens (HLAs) of Turner patients and their families failed to show any preponderance of those specific types most commonly associated with autoimmune disorders (HLA B8 and BW15).[32]

The role of environmental factors, such as

maternal or paternal drug abuse or ethanol consumption, therapeutic medications, cigarette smoking, and so on, in the pathogenesis of Turner syndrome has not been systematically investigated or reported.

The lack of evidence for any etiologic mechanisms responsible for the occurrence of Turner syndrome applies equally to the occurrence of the "Turner-Down polysomy" or "double aneuploidy syndrome" as well. In this condition trisomy 21 is associated with either a 45,X karyotype or with mosaic cell lines for the X chromosome. While this is a rare occurrence, its frequency is estimated to be greater than that due to chance alone.[33] Similarly, the double aneuploidy for Down syndrome and Klinefelter syndrome also occurs with a frequency greater than that expected from chance alone.

There does not appear to be an increased risk for the recurrence of the 45,X karyotype in families, but X chromosome structural malformations may have an increased risk of recurrence, since some deletions, for example, may be transmitted by the carrier of a balanced translocation.[34] There are also reports in the literature of trisomy 21 and Turner syndrome occurring in the same sibship.[35] We have two such sibships in our series. Taken in conjunction with the evidence that there appears to be an increased risk of a second defect occurring in most other chromosomal disorders, one would have to counsel parents accordingly. In the absence of significantly increased parental age, assignment of a risk figure of 1 per cent may be reasonable.

Clinical Findings

Since the original description of Turner, it has been recognized that there are a multiplicity of findings in patients with Turner syndrome, occurring with varying frequencies. More significantly, it has been recognized that the multiple findings may reflect a smaller number of fundamental events. In Table 9–2 and in the following discussion, the common features illustrated by the patients in our series will be described, and, when possible, categorized according to the developmental defects proposed to be fundamentally responsible. What cannot be illustrated are the multiple combinations of findings that occur in any one patient. Thus, it is difficult to appreciate from Table 9–2

that, in fact, one patient may have only one of the many features described while others may have multiple features.

Physical Features

Skeletal Growth Disturbances. The single most common physical abnormality is short stature. Although the entire problem of the growth disturbance in Turner syndrome is discussed in a subsequent section, the impairment is most pronounced along the longitudinal body axis.[36] This gives affected individuals the visual appearance of being stocky or squarely shaped and accounts for the predominantly illusory finding of widely spaced nipples[37] and shield-like chest. In fact, when chest width and internipple distances are measured and ratios calculated, the majority of patients do not differ from normal subjects of the same age. What differs is their overall height, and the relative width to height of the thorax. Thus, the impaired longitudinal osseous growth is the primary defect. Conversely, the short neck is not illusory, but secondary, in many cases, to hypoplasia of one or more of the cervical vertebrae.[38] The osseous abnormalities responsible for the short stature are not limited to the cervical vertebrae. Our own data, and those of others, confirm that long bone growth may be impaired even to a greater degree than vertebral growth. Thus there is disproportion in the axial segmental measurements, resulting in short-leggedness and an abnormal upper-to-lower segment ratio.[39] However, the limbs themselves do not have the radiologic or histologic appearance of a true skeletal dysplasia. The low hairline, on the other hand, is secondary both to the short neck and to the intrauterine mechanism responsible for the neck webbing (see "Lymphatic Obstruction").

Individual bones appear to be affected to varying degrees. For example, cubitus valgus is commonly appreciated. What this reflects is an increase in the so-called carrying angle. Clinically, this can be measured as the angle of intersection of the long axis of the upper arm with the long axis of the supinated forearm when the elbow is fully extended. In x-rays it is measured as the acute angle formed between the humerus and the ulna. Normally, in adult women this angle is about 12° while in adult men it is about 6°.[40] The major determinant of the angle is

TABLE 9–2. CLINICAL FINDINGS COMMONLY DESCRIBED IN PATIENTS WITH TURNER SYNDROME

Primary Defects	Secondary Features	Incidence (Per cent)
Physical features		
Skeletal growth disturbances	Short stature	100
	Short neck	40
	Abnormal upper-to-low segment ratio	97
	Cubitus valgus	47
	Short metacarpals	37
	Madelung deformity	7.5
	Scoliosis	12.5
	Genu valgum	35
	Characteristic facies with micrognathia	60
	High arched palate	36
Lymphatic obstruction	Webbed neck	25
	Low posterior hairline	42
	Rotated ears	Common
	Edema of hands/feet	22
	Severe nail dysplasia	13
	Characteristic dermatoglyphics	35
Unknown factors	Strabismus	17.5
	Ptosis	11
	Multiple pigmented nevi	26
Physiologic features		
Skeletal growth disturbances	Growth failure	100
	Otitis media	73
Germ cell	Gonadal failure	96
chromosomal	Infertility	99.9
defects	Gonadoblastoma	4.0
Unknown factors—embryogenic	Cardiovascular anomalies	55
	Hypertension	7
	Renal and renovascular anomalies	39
Unknown factors— metabolic	Hashimoto's thyroiditis	34
	Hypothyroidism	10
	Alopecia	2
	Vitiligo	2
	Gastrointestinal disorders	2.5
	Carbohydrate intolerance	40

the depth of the inner lip of the trochlea relative to the outer lip. When this relationship is disturbed, abnormalities occur. In many patients with Turner syndrome, the angle will be between 15° and 30° (Fig. 9–3) as a consequence of developmental abnormalities of the trochlear head. Thus, again, it is a skeletal abnormality that is responsible for a physical finding. That the development of the head of the ulna appears to be regulated by the sex chromosomes (and not, as has been previously inferred, primarily by sex hormones during puberty) is suggested by the abnormalities in Turner syndrome as well as by those in other disorders. It has been noted that the carrying angle is most pronounced with the 45,X karyotype and that the angle decreases progressively in association with XX and XY karyotypes. The angle decreases further, approaching cubi-

tus rectus, in patients with an extra X or Y, and frank radioulnar synostosis and radial head dislocation occur in many patients with multiple extra sex chromosomes.[41]

The knuckle sign, a depression due to diminished prominence of the head of the fourth metacarpal, so that a straight edge can be placed between the third and fifth metacarpals, is another physical finding that occurs in a large number of patients. It, as well as the so-called knuckle, knuckle, dimple, dimple sign, reflecting a depression of both the fourth and fifth knuckles, is a consequence of abnormally small metacarpals. These signs may be seen on a bone age x-ray and are often clues to the possible diagnosis (Fig. 9–4A). Short toes, due to shortening of the metatarsals, may also be found.

Other deformities of the hand and wrist occur commonly. The carpal bones of the

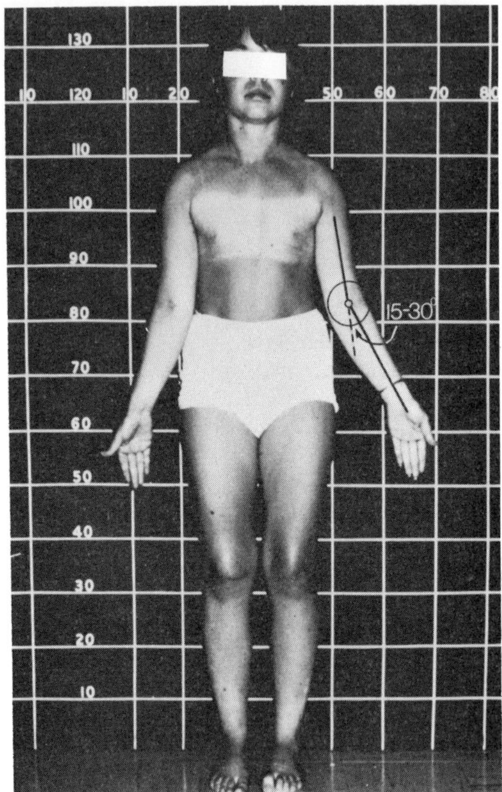

FIGURE 9–3. A 16-year-old girl with Turner syndrome and absence of puberty. Note absence of most characteristic stigmata save short stature and an increased carrying angle.

first line are frequently arched together abnormally. Superimposed on this, a further deformity, originally described by Madelung in 1898, has been described in Turner syndrome and occurred in 7.5 per cent of our patients. This so-called "bayonet deformity" is due to lateral and dorsal bowing of the radius, coupled with the carpal crowding and dorsal dislocation or subluxation of the distal ulna[42] (Fig. 9–5). It also occurs as part of the autosomal dominant mesomelic chondrodystrophy, dysoschondrosis, or Leri-Weil syndrome. Because these patients are also short, the differential diagnosis in the girl may be difficult. Although gonadal dysgenesis is not a feature of Leri-Weil syndrome, chromosomal analysis may be necessary to distinguish the two, especially in the prepubertal girl without an obviously affected parent.

Scoliosis is reported in a significant number of patients. In our own series 12.5 per cent had a deformity. The etiology was demonstrated radiologically to be secondary to obvious hemivertebrae in three patients and secondary to documented leg length inequality, with a functional scoliosis occurring secondarily, in two patients. In the remaining patients, no obvious bony deformities were noted, and the scoliosis was classified as idiopathic. That severity sufficient to warrant surgical correction has not been reported may be related to the lack of a pubertal growth spurt. As we begin to use more aggressive programs of hormonal treatment for growth acceleration we may find an increase in clinically significant scoliosis, and appropriate measures should be taken to ensure its early detection.

The knock-kneed appearance of many patients described in the literature is due to abnormalities in the medial tibial and femoral condyles. The medial tibial condyles are enlarged and project medially; the medial femoral condyles are enlarged and project downward below the levels of the lateral condyles; and the epiphyseal plates are deformed and displaced.[43]

The development of the face is also affected by a number of osseous malformations, contributing in part to the so-called characteristic facies. The high incidence of micrognathia, antimongoloid palpebral fissures, downward droop of the outer corners of the eyes, and epicanthal folds are also consequences of defective facial morphogenesis. The palate is frequently abnormally arched and, when examined using maxillary casts, exhibits deformities that differ from the more typical gothic or inverted V shape of other syndromes. Instead, both an inverted U shape form and a form with a narrow vault and bulges of the lateral alveolar ridges have been described.[44]

Not manifest clinically, but present radiologically, is the so-called osteoporotic appearance of the bones. This is observed in childhood and may therefore be independent of estrogen deficiency. Examination of the hand and wrist for bone age, a procedure frequently performed even before the diagnosis of Turner syndrome is established, often reveals this osteoporotic appearance. In some patients the carpal bones may be so characteristically affected that the appearance, which we describe as fishnet, has been reported as a clue to the diagnosis.[45] Others find that ballooning of the tips of the terminal phalanges is a most consistent finding.[46] Both findings are illustrated in Figure 9–4B.

Lymphatic Obstruction. The appear-

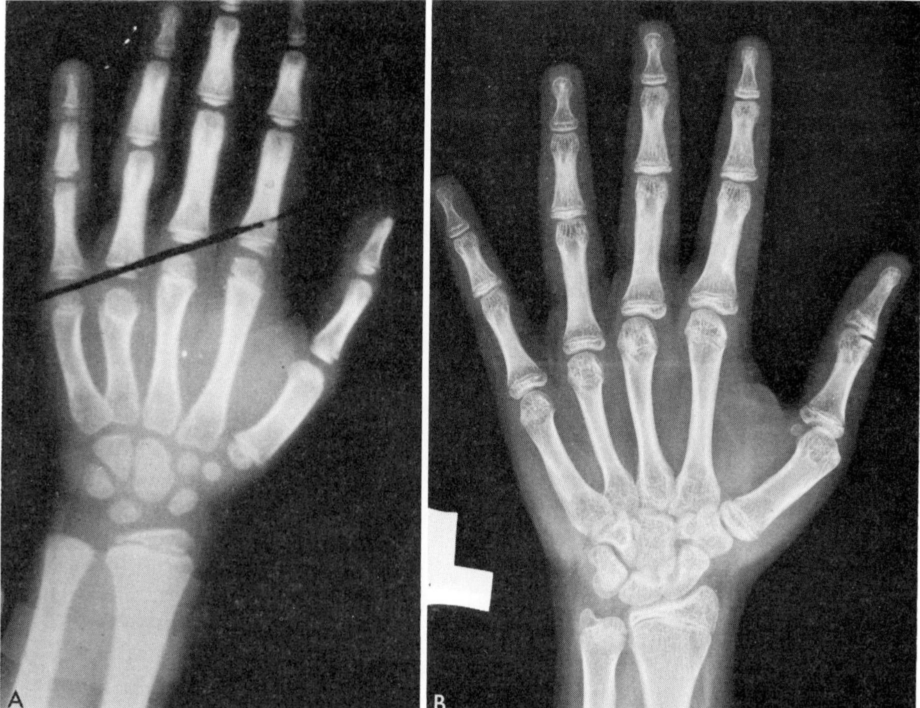

FIGURE 9–4. Two characteristic hand radiographs. *A*, Demonstrates a short fourth metacarpal, the tip falling below a straight line drawn between the third and fifth metacarpals. *B*, Demonstrates a generalized lacy ("fishnet") appearance of the carpals and tufting of the distal phalanges, characteristic of the so-called osteoporotic appearance of the bones of patients with Turner syndrome.

ance of the 45,X fetus illustrated in Figure 9–6 dramatically illustrates the fetal edema that occurs in many conceptuses with Turner syndrome. The edema appears to result from lymphatic malformations and obstruction.[47] This type of obstruction may result from a lag in the formation of a communication between the developing jugular lymph sac and the internal jugular vein. This communication normally develops between the fifth and sixth weeks of gestation, and failure to establish it appropriately results in lymphatic distention.[48] This occurs most often in the nuchal region, with the dilatation of at least two cavities separated by the nuchal ligament. In many cases, each cavity is subdivided by incomplete septa. The cavities extend from the upper part of the occipital bone caudally to the scapular region and medially to beneath the sternocleidomastoid muscle. If the blockage persists, the increased pressure within the lymphatics may alter their development and result in the more generalized malformations of peripheral lymphatics. Peripheral lymphatic hypoplasia or aplasia has also been demonstrated using lymphangiogra-

phy in adult patients with Turner syndrome.[49] Thus, as in the case of the mice with subcutaneous blebs described by Bonnevie, a single process may be responsible for a host of the apparently varied physical findings in this syndrome.

Webbed neck, or pterygium colli, is, perhaps, the most obvious consequence of lymphatic obstruction. It results from a scarring process that affects the distended loose skin over the large cystic hygromas that were present in the nuchal region. Some patients may, therefore, have a severe anomaly. Others, however, who never had significant distention or in whom the obstruction was minimal or in whom rupture and decompression occurred early do not have a webbed neck. In fact, in some patients in whom neither webbing nor abnormalities of the cervical vertebrae exist, the neck will appear long in proportion to the stature (Fig. 9–3). Thus webbing per se is not a primary anomaly. In our series, only 25 per cent of patients had any webbing at all.

The dilatation of the nuchal region is also thought to be responsible for mechanical effects on the pattern of hair direction, re-

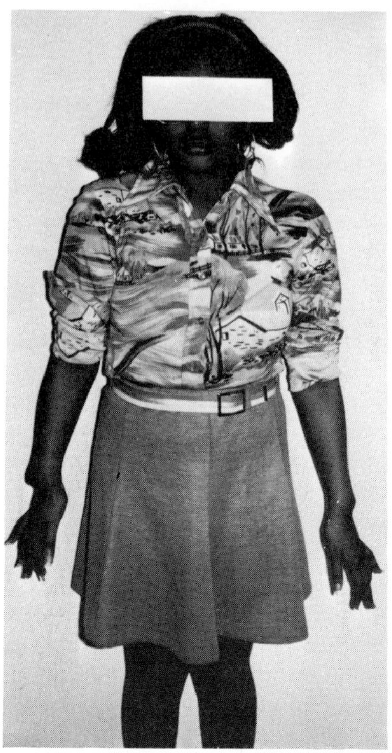

FIGURE 9–5. A 19-year-old patient with Turner syndrome and bilateral "bayonet-like" Madelung deformities of the wrists.

mal ridge whorl patterning, a characteristic dermatoglyphic feature.[51] That a compressive or restrictive effect on the developing ossification centers may have occurred also, resulting in some of what has been categorized as skeletal defects, is also possible.

Unknown Factors. The factors that are responsible for several other common physical features are less clear. Strabismus and ptosis occur more commonly than normal, contributing other features to the characteristic facies. Seventeen and one-half per cent of our patients had strabismus, and two thirds of these children required surgical correction. Eleven per cent had ptosis. Most were bilateral but in several cases it was unilateral (Fig. 9–8). We also noted a 2.5 per cent incidence of horizontal nystagmus. These findings indicate that cranial nerve dysfunction occurs frequently. Again, however, it is unclear if this represents intrinsic neurologic dysfunction or acquired neuropathy, perhaps secondary to the compressive lymphedema of the face. Multiple pigmented nevi, in excess of what is expected from familial patterns, occur frequently and were noted in 26 per cent of our patients.

sulting in the lower position of the posterior hairline (Fig. 9–7). This may also be responsible for the heavy, extended growth of the eyebrow. Similarly, the dilatation may result in rotation of the axis of the auricle posteriorly and elevation of the lower pinna, resulting in the prominent and low-set appearance of the ears.[50]

Edema of the dorsum of the hands and feet at birth is an obvious consequence of the incompletely resolved process if it involved peripheral lymphatics. Postnatally, the lymphedema usually resolves, although some patients demonstrate residual involvement. Others may complain of intermittent or recurrent edema, often following institution of estrogen replacement therapy. Less obvious are the mechanical effects that the lymphedema may have had on the developing extremities. It is probable that the abnormalities in the nails described in many patients (deeply set into the nail bed with lateral hyperconvexity) are secondary to mechanical distortion of the developing nail bed.[48] Severely dysplastic or even absent nails are noted at birth in some patients as a more obvious consequence. The result on the fingertip pads is a predominance of der-

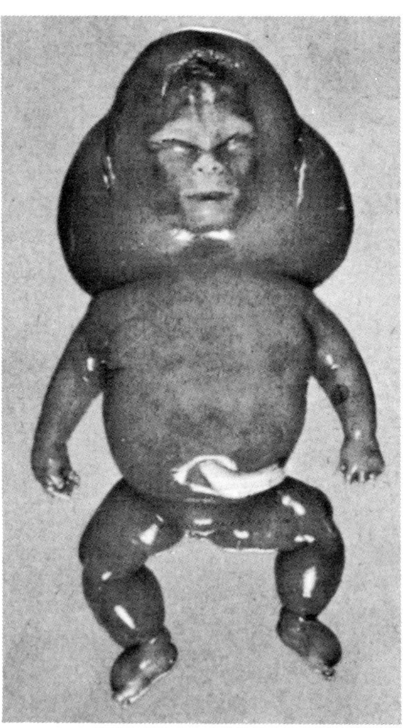

FIGURE 9–6. A 45,X abortus demonstrating generalized lymphedema. Note the distended cervical region. With resolution of the edema the redundant skin may cicatrize, resulting in a webbed neck. The edema of the hands and feet may persist and be present at birth. (From Gellis SS, Feingold M: Picture of the month. Am J Dis Child 132:417, 1978. Copyright 1978, American Medical Association.)

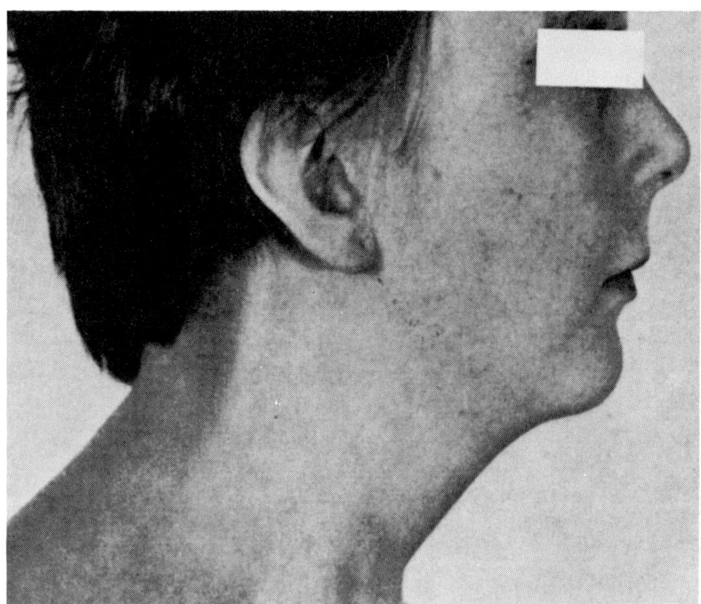

FIGURE 9–7.   Lateral picture of face of a girl with Turner syndrome, demonstrating low posterior hair line, residual neck webbing, and micrognathia.

Several had surgical excisions of one or more lesions that had been subjected to trauma, and histologic examination did not show evidence of malignant degeneration. The mechanism responsible for the excessive presence of these lesions, especially on the face and arms, is unknown. Since migration of melanocytes into the skin begins at a relatively early stage (10 weeks), it is unlikely that this process is affected by the lymphedema.

Physiologic Features

Skeletal Growth Disturbances

Growth Failure.   Adult short stature appears to be the most common phenotypic feature in women with Turner syndrome. The mean adult heights from numerous series are remarkably similar, and in a recent compilation of data from 366 patients the average height was found to be 143.1 cm.[52] Patterns of growth are illustrated in Figure 9–9, which shows cross-sectional height and velocity data from a series of 150 Turner children who had not received therapy for growth promotion.[53] The pattern described by Ranke et al. is distinguished by four components: (1) intrauterine growth retardation, with mean birth length 1 SD below the mean or an average reduction of 2.8 cm, and mean birth weight (not shown in the figure) of 2.18 kg, which is also 1 SD below the mean; (2) a period of normal or near-normal growth velocity for 2 to 3 years; (3) after age 3, a more rapid than normal growth deceleration so that between ages 3 and 13 years the Turner girls fall farther and farther away from the normal height curves; and (4) if untreated, failure to experience a pubertal growth spurt, but continued growth at a slow rate for several more years. A positive correlation is found between ultimate height

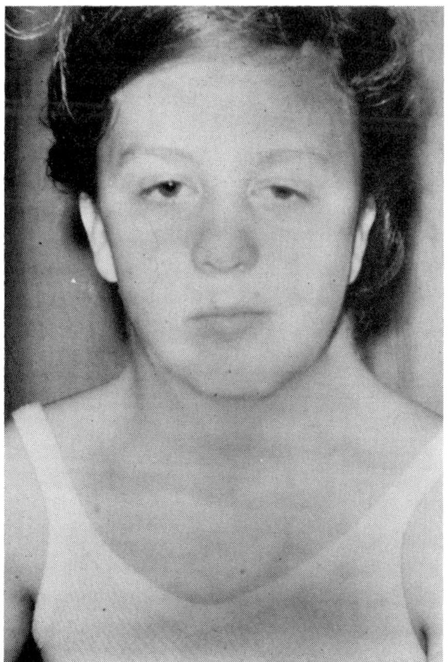

FIGURE 9–8.   Unilateral ptosis in a girl with Turner syndrome. Note also significant webbing of the neck.

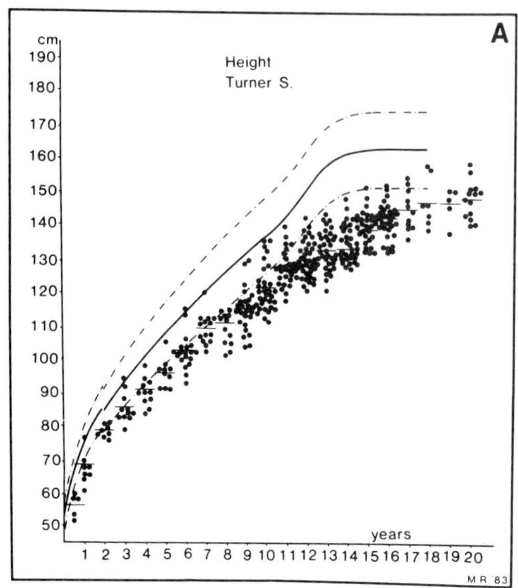

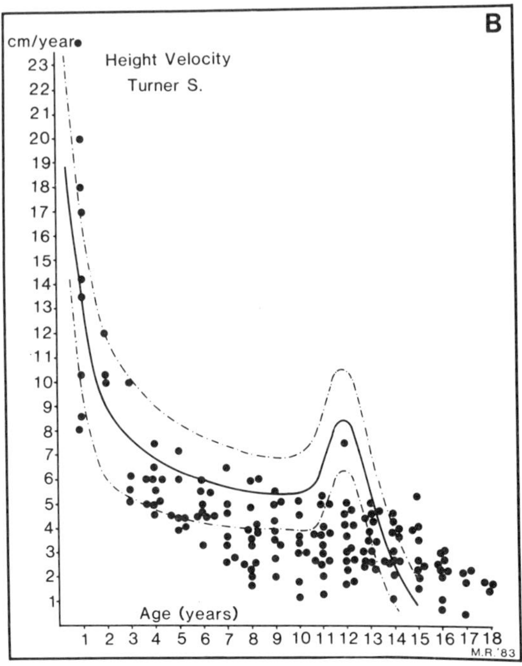

FIGURE 9–9.   Height and height velocity in Turner syndrome. *A,* 384 single measurements of height for 150 children with Turner syndrome. *B,* Height velocity from a total of 159 measurements. The normal ranges shown by the heavy and dashed lines were taken by the authors from Tanner JM, Whitehouse RH, Takaishi M: Arch Dis Child 41:454, 613, 1966. (From Ranke MB, Pfluger H, Rosendahl W, et al: Turner syndrome: Spontaneous growth in 150 cases and review of the literature. Eur J Paediatr 141:81, 1983.)

achieved and midparental height.[54] These authors concluded that the short stature was primarily the result of a generalized abnormality in the growth response of the skeleton but other genetic factors also play a role. Whether this abnormal growth response is due to a prolongation of cell generation time associated with the chromosomal disturbance per se[55] or is an intrinsic disturbance of the skeleton is not known. We have shown that another factor, disproportionate growth of the lower extremities, appears to contribute, in some degree, to the short stature in Turner syndrome.[39] In a group of 16 adult Turner patients, the mean height ± SD was 144.1 ± 2.0 cm, the sitting height 79.9 ± 1.6 cm, and the sitting height–to–height ratio 0.553. This observation of a short lower segment has been confirmed by some[56] but not all[57] observers. Additionally, we found a significant negative correlation between the ratio of sitting height to lower segment and height, indicating that the patients with the greatest proportional reduction in the length of their legs were the shortest. However, this finding, alone does not account entirely for the short stature of these women.

In the last few years there has been a re-surgence in the investigation of the role of growth-promoting hormones in Turner syndrome. Early studies failed to demonstrate that abnormalities of thyroid hormone or growth hormone (GH) could account for the growth failure. Although the incidence of Hashimoto thyroiditis and thyroid failure is high in Turner syndrome (see section on "Autoimmune Disorders"), until hypothyroidism supervenes thyroid hormone replacement is not helpful in promoting growth. The status of GH is less clear. Growth hormone responses to pharmacologic stimuli were reported to be normal[58] or paradoxically increased,[59] although at least one patient with Turner syndrome and true GH deficiency has been reported.[60] However, it is now recognized that responses to pharmacologic stimuli may not reflect endogenous spontaneous GH secretion. When the issue of GH secretory dynamics was addressed by measuring pulsatile GH release over 24 hours, the data suggested that girls with Turner syndrome are not different from normal girls until they reach their early adolescent years.[61] Then, in the absence of the hormonal changes of puberty, they do not experience the normal increases in total integrated concentration of

GH, nor the increased GH pulse amplitude or frequency. This finding is to be expected, since estrogen increases GH secretion, but its role in contributing to the short stature of Turner syndrome is questionable[62] since the major loss of height in Turner syndrome occurs prior to the adolescent years. Nevertheless, the availability of increased supplies of biosynthetic human GH has brought about a resurgence of interest in investigating its use to augment the growth velocity and final height of girls with Turner syndrome. These investigations include the use of GH alone and in combination with anabolic (androgen) and estrogen treatment.

The use of anabolic steroids in Turner syndrome began over 25 years ago,[63] but their efficacy in increasing final adult height is still being debated. Some studies indicate that augmented growth velocity may not be accompanied by a concomitant bone age increase and suggest that ultimate height is increased.[64–66] Others either found no differences in adult height between androgen and estrogen–treated girls[67] or pointed out that changes in stature, over time, could make the results difficult to interpret if treated patients were compared to untreated controls of previous years.[68] Of the more recent studies, two conclude that androgens, alone, do have a positive effect on final height[69,70] and one concludes that they do not.[71] Our own retrospective analysis of growth data failed to demonstrate that anabolic steroids promoted a statistically significant increase in final adult height. However, we and others[72,73] have confirmed that they do promote marked growth acceleration in the first year or more of therapy, which is usually perceived as highly beneficial by the patients and their families. Thus, many pediatric endocrinologists have used and continue to use low-dose androgen therapy for one or more years before the introduction of estrogen therapy.

The use of GH dates back to the early 1960s. However, the ensuing years have not clarified its role, because the studies comprehensively reviewed by Wilton[74] have yielded conflicting and inconclusive results. Some studies were very short term; others did not use comparable doses of GH, and little is known about final adult height. The most recent studies, using biosynthetic human GH, involve larger numbers of patients and hold promise of clarifying the role of GH therapy, either alone or in conjunction with androgens or estrogens, in pro-moting an increase in adult height. The use of a combination of androgen and GH was first reported in 1980,[75] and it was suggested that in the short term combination therapy might promote more rapid growth than either agent alone. These data formed the basis for a large multicenter study that has now completed its third year.[76] Seventy girls with Turner syndrome, ranging in age from 4 to 12 years, were initially enrolled. Sixty-seven completed the first year and 65 the first 3 years. The first year of the study included a control group (no therapy), as well as the three treatment groups [methionyl human GH (met-hGH), oxandrolone, and a combination of met-hGH and oxandrolone]. The patients were randomized according to chronologic age, bone age, karyotype, and pretreatment growth rate, so that study groups would be comparable. Oxandrolone was administered daily at a dose of 0.125 mg/kg/day (although it was soon recognized that this dose may have been unnecessarily high, and a 0.0625 mg/kg dose was used for the subsequent years of the study). Met-hGH was administered three times a week at a dose of 0.125 mg/kg/injection (or 0.25 units/kg/injection). No patient was dropped from the study because of an adverse reaction to either medication. In the second and third years of the study the control and oxandrolone treatment groups began to receive combination therapy, while the treatment of the original combination group and GH treatment groups were unchanged. The pretreatment growth velocity and the treatment responses for each patient in each group are shown in Figure 9–10. The numbers in the upper right-hand corner of each box represent mean Z scores ± 1 SD for each group. The growth grids used in the figure were adapted by the authors from the data of Ranke et al.,[53] as illustrated in Figure 9–9. The pretreatment velocities of all four groups were similar to those of the Ranke et al. data (a mean of 4.2 ± 1.1 cm). In year 1, the control patients continued to experience growth velocities within the range of those expected for untreated Turner patients, and the expected deceleration with age that Ranke et al. described, with the mean growth rate being 3.8 ± 1 cm over the year. The met-hGH–treated patients and the oxandrolone-treated patients showed marked increases in growth velocity, to 7.6 ± 1.5 and 6.6 ± 1.2 cm, respectively. While not unexpected for oxandrolone therapy, these data unequivo-

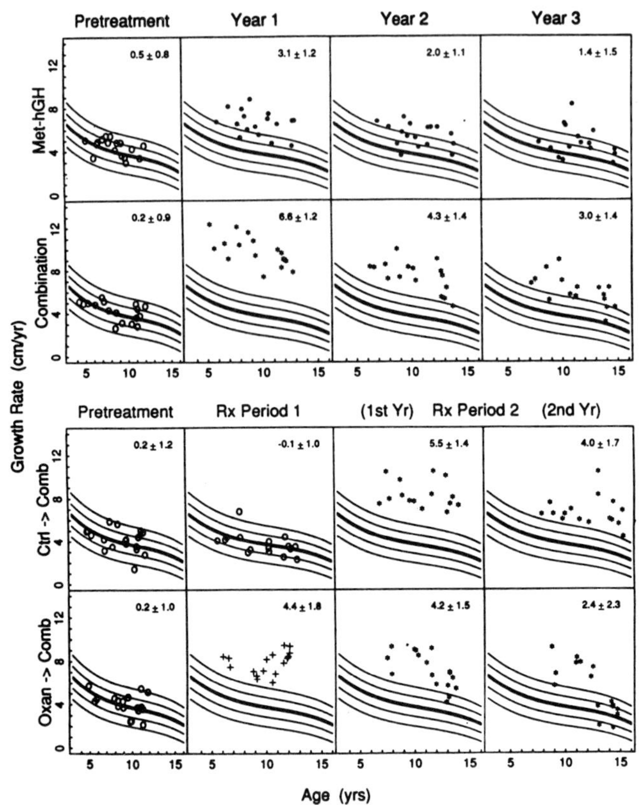

FIGURE 9–10. The effect of treatment with growth hormone (met-hGH) and oxandrolone on growth velocity in Turner syndrome. Growth velocity for individual patients is plotted in centimeters per year. Numbers in the upper right-hand corner of each box represent mean Z score ± 1 SD for each group. The top set of panels refer to the patients who received met-hGH for 3 years (closed circles) following the pretreatment period (open circles) The second set of panels shows the responses of the patients who received combination met-hGH and oxandrolone (stars). The third set (Ctrl→ Comb) refers to those patients who began as controls for treatment (Rx) Period 1 (open circles) and then were switched to combination therapy for Rx Period 2 (stars). The lowest set of panels (Oxan→Comb) refers to those patients who received oxandrolone for Rx period 1 (crosses) and then were switched to combination therapy for Rx Period 2 (stars). The growth velocity lines show the mean (heavy line) and 2 SD (light lines) for Turner girls as derived from the data of Ranke et al. shown in Figure 9–9. (From Rosenfeld RG, Hintz RL, Johanson AJ, et al: Three-year results of a randomized prospective trial of methionyl human growth hormone and oxandrolone in Turner syndrome. J Pediatr 113:393, 1988.)

cally demonstrated that GH therapy resulted in short-term growth acceleration. The synergistic effect of the combination of drugs was most impressive, with the growth velocity over the year being 9.8 ± 1.4 cm. In the second and third years of treatment the growth velocities of the original met-hGH and combination groups declined somewhat (5.4 ± 1.1 cm and 4.6 ± 1.4 cm for met-hGH and 7.4 ± 1.4 cm and 6.1 ± 1.5 cm for combination therapy), although the growth of the combination group remained significantly accelerated even in the third year. The control group responded to the change to combination therapy (8.2 ± 1.7 cm and 6.7 ± 1.4 cm) as did the group that was changed from oxandrolone to combination therapy (7.1 ± 1.6 cm and 5.3 ± 2.4 cm). The Bayley-Pinneau method of height prediction was used by the authors to calculate a prediction for final height increment in each of the four groups. The mean increases in predicted height for the met-hGH group was 4.5 ± 0.9 cm and that for the group treated with the combination of drugs from the beginning of the study was 8.2 ± 1.4 cm. The original control group, which received 2 years of combination therapy with the lower oxandrolone dose, had a 7.2 ± 1.5 cm increase in predicted height while the group that started on the higher dose of oxandrolone and then switched to the lower dose in combination with met-hGH had a 6.6 ± 1.0 cm increase. The authors point out that it is premature to assess the effects of treatment on ultimate adult height, although their data, and those of others, do support the conclusion that linear growth in Turner syndrome can be successfully accelerated by these regimens without compromising adult stature.

Otitis Media. Perhaps the most common medical problem reported by patients with Turner syndrome is bilateral otitis media. In a series of 76 patients, Anderson and coworkers[77] recorded medically significant middle ear infection in 68 per cent, with more than one half of these patients reporting not only recurrent episodes but also spontaneous perforations or the need for surgical treatment, or both. In our own series, complete system reviews were recorded for over 80 per cent of patients. Of these almost 75 per cent had either undergone tonsillectomy and adenoidectomy because of recurrent otitis or had had polyethylene tubes placed for the drainage of serous otitis media, or both. Of these, 4 patients had also undergone mastoid surgery.

The etiology of otitis does not appear to be related to a specific or generalized immunologic dysfunction. Other infections, as well as other disorders of the mucous membranes, are not reported to occur with increased frequency in Turner syndrome. Although levels of secretory immunoglobulins have not been reported, serum concentrations are not abnormal. Immunoglobulin (Ig) G and IgA concentrations, however, appear to be in the adult male range, which is significantly lower than the adult female range.[78] Instead, frequent occurrence of otitis may be the consequence of abnormalities in growth of the cranial base in Turner syndrome. Cephalometry[77,79] has demonstrated that both structural growth of the temporal bone and growth of the condylar cartilage and spheno-occipital synchondrosis are abnormal. The result is that the final development of the facial skeleton only reaches a level corresponding to that of an 11-year-old girl, while that of the posterior portion of the cranial base is even less advanced. As a consequence, not only is the position of the external auditory meatus abnormal, giving the appearance of low-set ears, but the relationship of the middle ear to the eustachian tube is disturbed. These factors, coupled with abnormalities in the shape of the palate, create a predisposition to fluid collection and secondary infection. Marked hypocellularity of the mastoid air cells may also be found, further predisposing the individual to both acute and chronic suppurative disease.[80]

The relationship of chronic otitis media to hearing deficit was also explored by Anderson et al.[77] Their data suggest that a component of the hearing loss reported to be a common occurrence in Turner syndrome is, in fact, conductive in nature. However, true sensorineural hearing impairment was also documented in a high percentage (64 per cent) of patients. This was generally bilateral and characterized by symmetric dips in the audiogram in the midfrequency range. Audiologic manipulations tended to identify the defect as one of recruitment and specifically localized the defect to the outer hair cells of the organ of Corti. When older patients were compared to children under the age of 10, conductive losses were more frequently found in the children, and sensorineural losses in the adults. Thus, the sensorineural losses appear to develop with age, and represent a degenerative rather than a congenital abnormality. No relationship between the type of hearing defect and the specific chromosomal karyotype has been recorded.

Germ Cell Chromosomal Defects

Gonadal Failure. Histologic evidence suggests that the ovary of the fetus with a 45,X karyotype (and presumably the ovary of the fetus with karyotypes with X chromosome deletions, rings, or mosaicism) undergoes an initial phase of differentiation that is the same as that in the 46,XX fetus. If the ovary is examined at 14 to 18 weeks of gestation, no abnormalities are seen. Subsequently, however, when there is a chromosomal defect in the germ cells, the process of oocyte loss appears to be accelerated, with a concomitant acceleration of stromal fibrosis. Thus, what is considered to be the normal process of oocyte loss, beginning prenatally and continuing over 30 to 50 years of postnatal life in normal females, occurs either entirely prenatally or in the first few months or years of postnatal life in most females with Turner syndrome.[7] The processes of oocyte loss and fibrosis are, however, neither absolute nor inevitable. Therefore, some patients with Turner syndrome may demonstrate evidence of ovarian function at puberty.[81]

In as many as 5 to 10 per cent of patients the degree of estrogen secretion is sufficient to initiate breast development at puberty, and in a small percentage of this small group it is sufficient to initiate menses. In our own series, six patients have menstruated without the benefit of treatment (two with a 45,X, one with a 45,X/46,XX, one with a 45,X/46,X,i(Xq), and one with 45,X/46,X,r(X) karyotype). A very few (probably less than 1 per cent of all affected patients) will maintain normal ovarian function, so that ovulatory menses occur and pregnancy may result.[82,83] While maintenance of some ovarian function is more often reported in patients with mosaic karyotypes, it may occur in the 45,X individual as well.[84] Although these latter cases remain rare enough to continue to merit individual reports, they illustrate the spectrum of ovarian function in this condition. Counseling about the expectations and future management of the patient with Turner syndrome who is diagnosed before puberty needs to include the very high possibility of gonadal failure and infertility but not its inevitable occurrence. However, even in those instances in which fertility does occur, reproductive failure is high and the risk of an abnormal offspring,[85] notably trisomy 21, appears significant.[86]

Physiologic evidence for gonadal failure in Turner syndrome is provided by the response of the hypothalamic-pituitary (H-P) axis to functional agonadism. It has long been recognized that the negative feedback loop between the gonad and the H-P axis is operative in the fetus and demonstrable at birth. In normal infants, both follicle-stimulating hormone (FSH) and luteinizing hormone (LH) rise after birth. In the male, the gonadotropin rise is accompanied by a significant surge in plasma testosterone in the first months of life. Both gonadotropin and testosterone then gradually decline to prepubertal concentrations by the end of the first year. In the female, although the gonadotropin rise does not appear to be accompanied by as striking a response in estradiol secretion from the ovary, the plasma FSH remains slightly elevated for a period of several years.

In Turner syndrome, a markedly exaggerated rise in both plasma gonadotropins, but especially in FSH, has been demonstrated as early as 5 days of age.[87] These abnormally elevated gonadotropin levels decline again after the first 2 years, although to mean concentrations significantly higher than those in gonadally competent female children. Between ages 4 and 10 to 11 years, a trough is noted, which is followed by the gradual rise of gonadotropins in normal children, and a more rapid and exaggerated rise in most children with Turner syndrome. This diphasic pattern for FSH, determined on a large number of patients with gonadal dysgenesis, is illustrated in Figure 9–11A. In Figure 9–11B, serial determinations graphically demonstrate the fall that occurs in the first years of life and the abrupt rise that occurs in early adolescence. The range of values considered normal for a female are:

> FSH (mIU/ml): prepubertal less than 2 to 8; pubertal 5 to 40
> LH (mIU/ml): prepubertal less than 2 to 10; pubertal 5 to 35

Save for the transient midcycle preovulatory surge, FSH concentrations in excess of 50 mIU/ml and LH concentrations in excess of 40 mIU/ml are considered suggestive of gonadal failure. Although it is believed that under most circumstances gonadotropin-releasing hormone (GnRH) releases both FSH and LH, the metabolic clearance of these gonadotropins is different, so that simultaneous FSH concentrations exceed those of LH.

The mechanisms that are responsible for the feedback suppression of gonadotropin secretion in the normal child and the similar pattern, although at a higher set-point, in the child with gonadal dysgenesis are unclear. It has been presumed that increased sensitivity to circulating steroids of gonadal and adrenal origin results in decreased hypothalamic GnRH release in the prepubertal subject. Recently, studies in primate species suggest that one component of the feedback inhibition may be at the level of the pituitary and that another may be at the hypothalamic level. There may also be significant central neuronal inhibition that is not affected by gonadal steroids.

Increased FSH and LH would most likely be detectable in infancy and again in adolescence. The development of sensitive radioimmunoassays for FSH and LH in plasma has resulted in the virtual elimination of the need for the 24-hour urine collections for gonadotropin determination. Plasma gonadotropin concentrations can be assessed at the time of diagnosis and again in early adolescence prior to the institution of steroid hormone therapy and counseling about ultimate fertility. When GnRH is administered to assess the function of the H-P axis the responses of patients with Turner syndrome with gonadal failure are exaggerated as compared with normal subjects.[88] This procedure may be used to provide a second test for gonadal integrity in some patients. However, in most patients a single determination of plasma FSH and LH is sufficient to document gonadal failure. In the absence of estrogen replacement therapy, gonadotropin secretion will continue unabated and unmodulated. While no systemic manifestations are known to result from these excessive concentrations of FSH and LH, reactive pituitary abnormalities have been reported in some patients.[89] Skull x-rays may show enlargement of the pituitary fossa, which is suggestive of pituitary hyperplasia or microadenoma formation. Although enlargement sufficient to result in organic dysfunction has not yet been reported, the recognition of this phenomenon is important so that the gonadal dysgenesis is not misdiagnosed as being secondary to a pituitary tumor. The potential for progres-

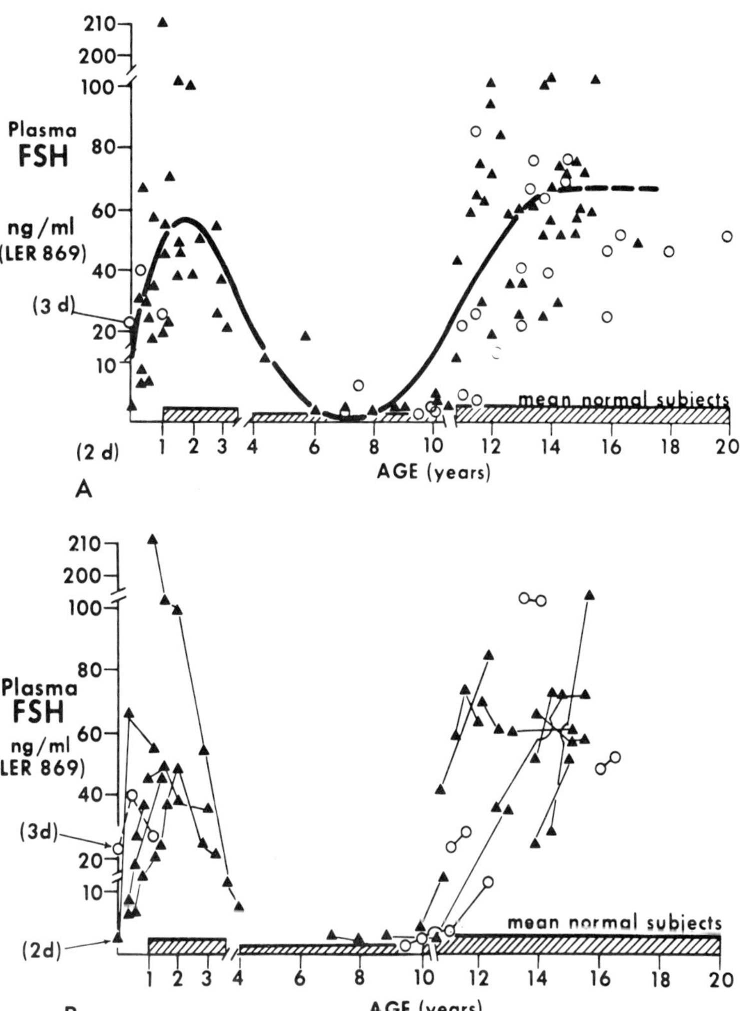

FIGURE 9–11. *A,* Plasma FSH values in patients with Turner syndrome. Triangles (▲) indicate patients with 45,X karyotype and circles (○) denote those with X chromosome mosaicism or structural abnormalities of the X. The curve is a polynomial regression plot; the hatched lines indicate mean plasma FSH values in normal females. Note the very high levels in infancy and adolescence, with lower levels in the mid first decade. FSH is expressed as ng/ml of standard LER-869. To convert these values to mIU/ml of the second IRP, multiply by 3.5. *B,* Symbols indicating serial plasma FSH values in several individuals are connected by straight lines. Note the rise and fall in infancy and the dramatic and abrupt rises in adolescence. (From Conte FA, Grumbach MM, Kaplan SL: A diphasic pattern of gonadotropin secretion in patients with the syndrome of gonadal dysgenesis. J Clin Endocrinol Metab 40:670, 1975. Reprinted with permission of the publisher.)

sive pituitary enlargement is an additional reason for instituting estrogen replacement therapy.

Gonadoblastoma. Gonadoblastomas are distinctive tumors composed of at least two different cell types. The large cells have the appearance and ultrastructure of oogonial germ cells, and the small cells are ovarian stromal cells that are not clearly differentiated.[90] They most closely resemble primitive sex-cord mesenchymal cells and are termed granulosa-Sertoli cells. The tumor arises in a gonad that is dysgenetic, that is, a gonad that has not completely differentiated into a normal ovary or normal testis or that does not behave like a normal ovary or testis. The dysgenesis that leads to gonadoblastoma formation almost invariably occurs in patients with Y chromosome material in their karyotype. In the case of

Turner syndrome most karyotypes do not contain a Y. The ovary is induced normally and then usually rapidly degenerates into fibrous streaks with loss of oogonial germ cells. These ovaries are not believed to be at risk for gonadoblastoma formation.

There is a small percentage of patients (between 2 and 5 per cent in most series, and 5 per cent in our own), however, who fit all the criteria for Turner syndrome, in whom the karyotype contains a Y chromosome. Most commonly the karyotype is the mosaic 45X/46,XY. More complex karyotypes, including 46,XX/45,X/46,XY and even 46,XY, however, have been associated with Turner syndrome. Thus the karyotype, per se, does not determine the phenotype. What defines these patients as having Turner syndrome, rather than being hermaphrodites or having mixed gonadal dysgenesis, is their short stature, their symmetric female external genitalia, and their normal female internal genitalia (bilateral fallopian tubes, uterus, and vagina). The only expression of the Y may be its effect on gonadal ridge induction, with the result that some number of cells no longer resemble differentiated ovarian stroma. In this case, all the oogonial germ cells that develop in these dysgenetic ridges do not necessarily undergo atresia as rapidly as they do in typical Turner syndrome. Instead, some may persist, continue to divide, and develop into a gonadoblastoma.

In some, but not all, patients with a Y in their karyotype, the granulosa-Sertoli cell stroma more closely resembles a testis and produces some androgen. This may occur whether or not a gonadoblastoma will eventually develop. These patients, while still having the Turner phenotype, may show some evidence of virilization, including clitoromegaly or partial fusion of the posterior labia. However, since many patients bearing the Y will not virilize, these findings are not necessarily helpful in deciding which Turner patient may be at risk for gonadoblastoma. For this reason it is essential to obtain a complete chromosomal karyotype even in the most obvious of Turner syndrome patients. If a marker or fragment chromosome is detected, which cannot be assigned to a specific chromosome, then more specific studies can be performed, including preparing DNA from the patient's leukocytes and probing it with Y-specific probes.

The risk for the development of the tumor, either unilaterally or bilaterally, in the patient with the Y-bearing dysgenetic gonad is estimated to be as high as 15 to 25 per cent.[91] In our own series, 4 of the 7 patients with a Y in the karyotype have had gonadoblastomas removed. This represents almost 4 per cent of our patients. Although the tumor usually does not metastasize, local invasion of the surrounding stroma to form microscopic or gross germinomas is seen in about one half the cases.[92] Gonadoblastomas may also be found in conjunction with malignant germinomas, although these latter tumors tend to occur in conditions other than Turner syndrome. The age at which these tumors are detected varies, but a number have now been reported in early childhood.[92,93] In some patients, calcification is present, which assists in detection, and in others a tumor mass may be demonstrated

with ultrasound, magnetic resonance imaging (MRI) or computed tomography (CT) scan. In many the disease is microscopic, however. Recommendations for dealing with the problem vary from prophylactic removal of the gonadal ridge streaks in all Turner syndrome patients with a Y in their karyotype to prospective monitoring of the patient at risk with some visualization technique such as ultrasonography. Examples of ultrasonographic studies in a normal pubertal female, a girl with Turner syndrome, and a girl with Turner syndrome and a gonadoblastoma are shown in Figure 9–12A, B, and C, respectively.

Unknown Factors—Embryogenic

Embryogenic Cardiovascular Abnormalities. The association of cardiovascular abnormalities, notably coarctation of the aorta, with Turner syndrome has been well documented.[13,94–96] However, the determination of its frequency, as well as the clarification of the conflicting reports of occurrence of other major structural cardiovascular anomalies, was impaired by the lack of chromosomal karyotyping in early series. One of the major sources of confusion was the inclusion of patients with normal chromosomes but phenotypic abnormalities, of whom a large number may have had Noonan syndrome.[97,98] Now that these so-called chromatin-positive patients, noted to have a high incidence of right-sided heart defects, are no longer categorized as having Turner syndrome, it is evident that left-sided heart defects are, in fact, the most typically reported structural lesions.

Coarctation appears to occur in about 15 to 20 per cent of patients, somewhat less frequently than previously suggested. The reason may be that in the past the diagnosis of Turner syndrome was made more often in patients with 45,X karyotypes and typical physical stigmata, and these patients do indeed appear to have a higher incidence of this abnormality. Engle and Forbes suggested that coarctation was only found in patients with the 45,X karyotype and in association with webbed neck.[96] While other series have subsequently shown that this is not necessarily the case, coarctation does, in fact, occur most frequently in the 45,X group and does not yet appear to have been noted in association with the 46,X,i(Xq), 45,X, or 46,X, r(X) variants.[14] In our own series (Table 9–3), of patients who had cardiac examinations 14, or 10.4 per cent, were diag-

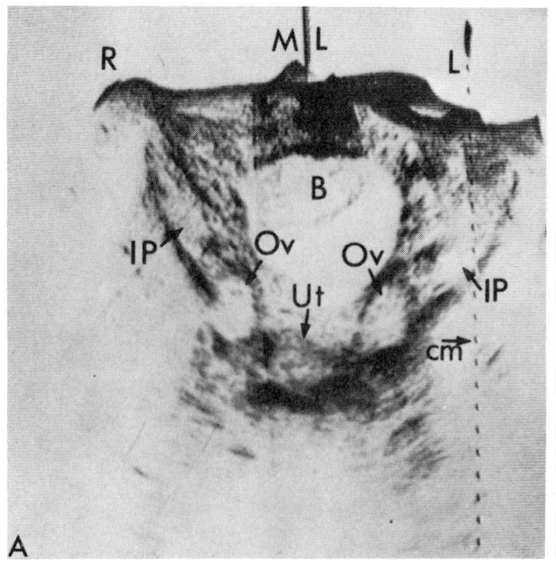

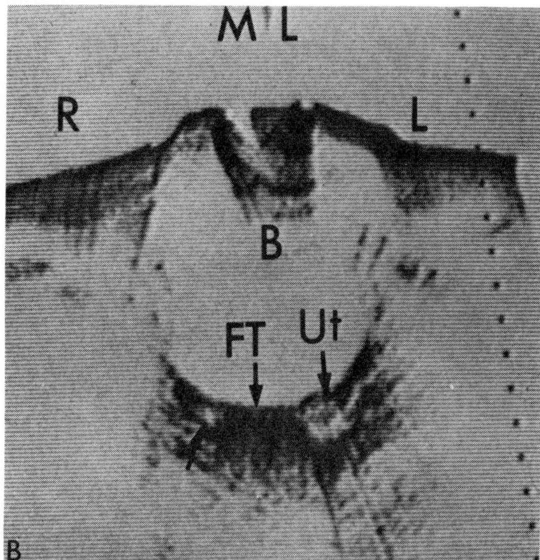

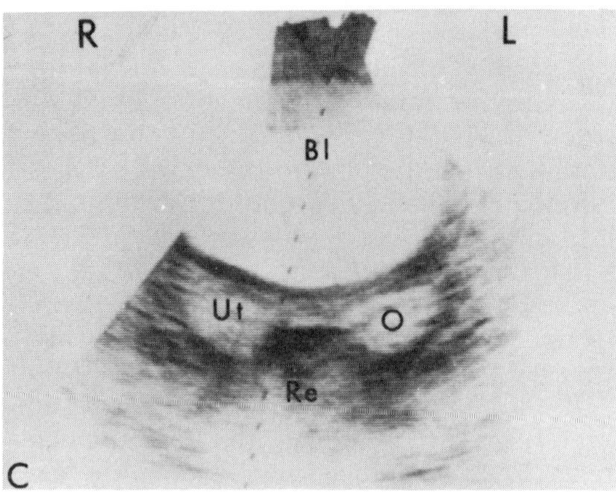

FIGURE 9–12. Examples of pelvic ultrasound studies. The images are transverse, oriented right (R) and left (L) of the midline (ML). The dotted scales are in centimeters. BL = bladder, Ov = ovary, Ut = uterus, IP = ileopsosas, Re = rectum, FT = fallopian tube, O = gonadoblastoma. *A*, Normal pubertal female demonstrating ovaries of adult size. *B*, Patient with Turner syndrome. The corpus of the uterus is seen slightly to the left of the midline. The fallopian tube can be followed into the right adnexa and observed to terminate in a small structure (arrow) believed to be the fimbriated end of the tube. No ovaries are identified. *C*, Patient with XO/XY Turner syndrome previously treated with estrogen. The corpus of the uterus is enlarged to adult size. In the left adnexa a large, gonadal mass (O) is seen. Histologically this was identified as a gonadoblastoma.

nosed as having coarctation, and all but one of these had a 45,X karyotype. We also noted that the webbed neck phenotype was more common in this group. Eleven of the 14 patients with coarctation had an obvious webbing deformity, whereas of the remaining 122 patients examined for cardiac defects only 22 were described as having an obvious webbed neck. The relationship of coarctation to karyotype and phenotype and to the actual defect in embryogenesis is unknown. Since it appears that the defect in the lymphatic system and its connection to the jugular venous system that is responsible for lymphedema is a very frequent primary structural malformation in 45,X Turner syndrome, it is interesting to speculate upon a relationship between coarctation and lymphatic obstruction.

Coarctation per se, especially the preductal, adult-type coarctation most characteristic of this condition, is not likely to result from the same mechanisms as other congenital heart defects. While the final structure of the four chambers of the heart and the orientation of the great vessels are established by 6 to 7 weeks after fertilization, the preductal area of the aorta subject to coarctation may be affected at any time. Moreover, coarctation occurring in this so-called isthmus region has been considered in some cases to be a result of the differential flows through the two fetal circulatory systems that interface at this point (the ductal-placental flow and the systemic-cardiac-pulmonary flow). In a recent report Clark[99] elegantly reviewed the embryology of lymphatic sac drainage into the venous system, and noted that in the chick disordered drainage implicates a mechanism that distends the cardiac lymphatics. He proposed that this would encoach upon the ascending aorta and alter intracardiac blood flow. A more recent pathologic examination of 12 fe-

TABLE 9–3. CARDIOVASCULAR ABNORMALITIES OBSERVED IN TURNER SYNDROME: THE RELATIONSHIP TO KARYOTYPE AND PHENOTYPE

Abnormality	Positive/ Examined*	Per Cent	45,X	Webbed Neck
Coarctation	14/134	10.4	13/14	11†/14
Dilated aorta	6/67	8.9	6/6	5/6
"Bicuspid" aortic valve without coarctation	20/67	29.9	12/20	6‡/20
Mitral valve prolapse	6/67	8.9	4/6	3/6
Hypertension	9/80	11.2	5/9	3/5

* Initially by chest X-rays; recently, patients have routine echocardiography (n = 67).
† All 45,X.
‡ Four were 45,X.

tuses with Turner phenotype of nuchal cystic hygromas found that 75 per cent had left-sided flow defects and aberrations of the lymphatics at the base of the heart.[100] If the lymphatic defect is a consequence of the loss of a gene that requires the deletion of a major portion of the X chromosome for its expression, then the relationship between webbing, coarctation, and karyotype would be established.

It may be inferred, both from reports of a high incidence of unclassified murmurs and from small patient series,[101] that the incidence of aortic valvular abnormalities may also be increased in Turner syndrome. With the introduction of echocardiography, we have been able to undertake a study of the frequency of this association.[102] Of 67 patients without coarctation studied to date with two-dimensional or M-mode echocardiography (or both), 20 (almost 30 per cent) have findings characteristic of bicuspid aortic valve. Some of these valves are anatomically tricuspid but have eccentric closure and are functionally "bicuspid," whereas the majority are actually bicuspid. Our data currently suggest that the percentage distribution of patients with isolated bicuspid valve does not appear to be confined to any karyotype, nor does there appear to be a preponderance of the webbed neck phenotype. Thus, bicuspid aortic valve may not only be more common than coarctation, but may also represent a more fundamental manifestation of a small X chromosome defect in Turner syndrome. We also diagnosed six patients as having mitral valve prolapse (Barlow syndrome). This frequency, 8.9 per cent, may be in excess of that believed to be the occurrence rate in the population at large.[103]

Another cardiovascular abnormality that occurs in Turner syndrome is dissecting aortic aneurysm. We recently reported our experience with two patients who had aortic dissection and rupture and summarized the reports of 18 other cases.[104] Subsequently, a third patient we had previously followed has had a fatal aortic dissection. With the introduction of echocardiography and then cardiac MRI we are also finding dilation of the aortic root in an unexpectedly large number of girls with Turner syndrome. Figure 9–13 demonstrates the utility of echocardiography in assessment of the aortic root, as well as of MRI in the imaging of the entire aorta. Risk factors that appear to be associated with dissection include prior coarctation or "pseudo"-coarctation, bicuspid aortic valve, and systemic hypertension, although one or more need not be present. That aortic root diameters are greater in 45,X patients than in matched controls[105] suggests a degree of intrinsic primary abnormality. Pathologic evidence of cystic medial necrosis is reported in some cases of dissection and suggests that the intrinsic disorder might represent an example of a mesenchymal defect in Turner syndrome. This may explain the increased incidence of mitral valve prolapse as well. Alternatively, the tendency toward significant aortic root dilation may be related to intrauterine hemodynamic events that are a consequence of the lymphatic disorder. The report that death from aortic dissection was greatly in excess of that expected in a large prospective study of Turner syndrome patients registered with a karyotype registry[106] has prompted us to adopt an aggressive approach to diagnosis, follow-up, and risk factor management in these patients. This is discussed in the section on "Consultative Studies."

Hypertension, per se, without coarctation, has been described as occurring in increased frequency in Turner syndrome. While a renovascular abnormality is considered to be the most likely mechanism for development of hypertension in most cases, obvious structural renal lesions are not always present. Similarly, a history of infectious nephritis or even urinary tract infection is usually absent. Thus, in the majority of patients the cause of the hypertension is unknown. In our own series, nine patients

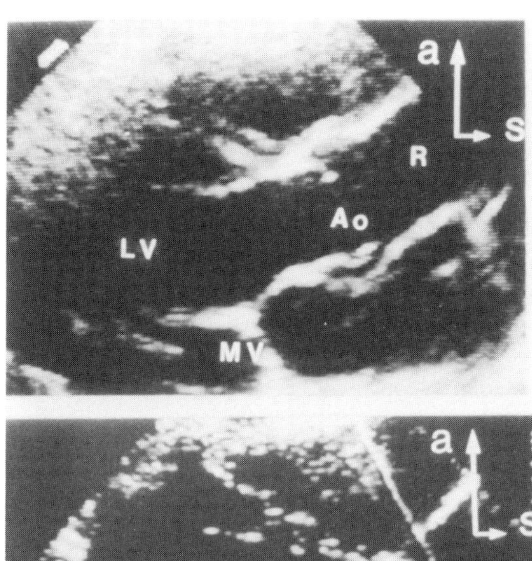

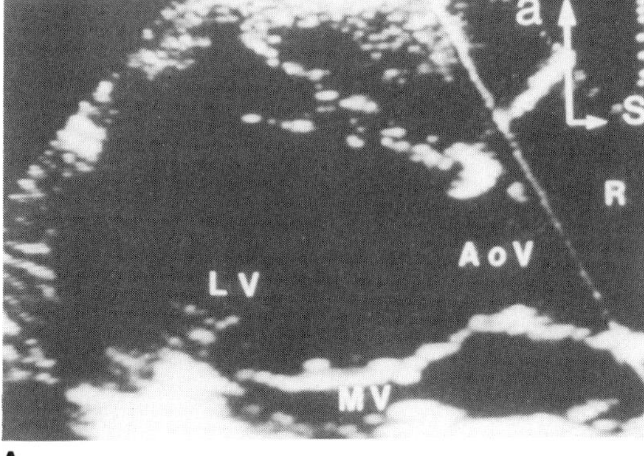

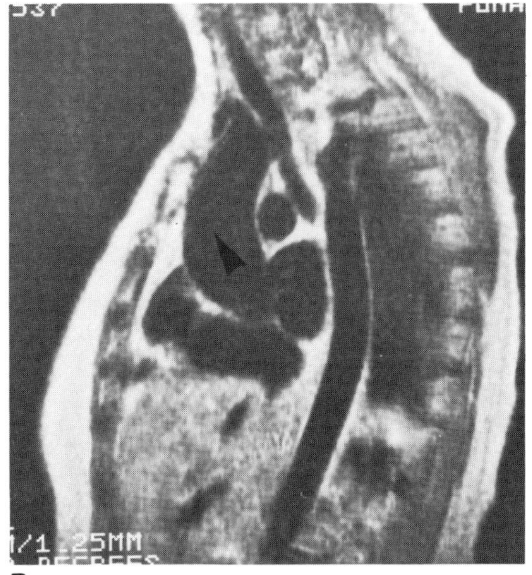

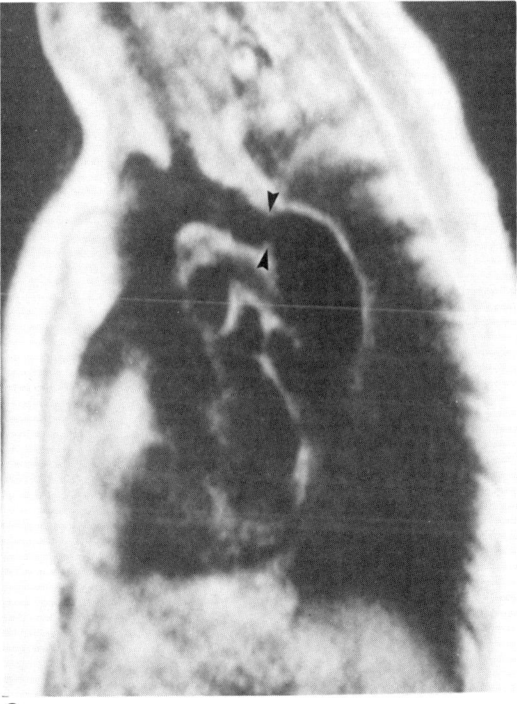

FIGURE 9–13. Cardiac imaging in Turner syndrome. *A*, Ultrasonographic parasternal long axis views of the left ventricle outflow tract and the ascending aorta in two patients with Turner syndrome. The top image is normal. The bottom image shows a dilated proximal aortic root and dilated left ventricle. LV = left ventricle, Ao = aorta, R = aortic root, MV = mitral valve. *B*, Sagittal MRI scan of the thoracic aorta in a patient with Turner syndrome and a dilated aortic root. The arrow lies in the dilated aortic root. *C*, Sagittal MRI scan of the thoracic aorta in a patient with Turner syndrome who had undergone surgery for aortic coarctation 10 years previously. The arrows show a stenotic area at the site of surgery. The aorta distal to the stenosis shows mild poststenotic dilation.

with hypertension were identified, and in only one did it appear to be of renovascular origin. There was no apparent relationship with any particular karyotype or phenotype.

Finally, only one patient with atrial septal defect and one with ventral septal defect were found in our series and no other more complex cyanotic heart lesions were detected or suspected.

In summary, therefore, the most common primary cardiovascular abnormality may be bicuspid aortic valve, and the most common secondary defect may be coarctation of the aorta.

Renal and Renovascular Abnormalities. Renal and renovascular abnormalities occur in Turner syndrome with greatly increased frequency. While the incidence varies from 35 to 70 per cent among different series reported,[107–109] the abnormalities tend to be of three specific types: those that primarily involve the pelvocalyceal collecting system, such as complete or partial duplication; those that are associated with the position and alignment of the organ, such as horseshoe kidney and retrocaval ureter; and those that are associated with abnormal vascular supply.

The development of the collecting system begins with the formation of the ureteric bud, its dorsocranial migration, and its penetration of the metanephric blastema. At about 5 weeks of gestation it dilates into a primitive pelvis and simultaneously splits into cranial and caudal portions, forming the future major calyces. Thus, duplications of the collecting system are due to abnormal or early splitting of the ureteric bud, at or before 5 fetal weeks, and are therefore primary malformations of organogenesis. Conversely, the upward migration of the already preformed kidney from its position in the pelvis to the lumbar region is a somewhat later event. The kidney must pass through the arterial fork formed by the umbilical arteries and if there are disturbances in either the anatomy of these vessels or the path of migration, secondary positional malformations occur. If one kidney fails to traverse the arterial fork, it will remain ectopically in the pelvis. If there is a partial mechanical effect on the kidney during migration, then rotational abnormalities may result.

The vascular supply of the kidneys may be anomalous (Fig. 9–14B), secondary to the multiple budding segments of the kidney, the final positioning, or the presence of an aberrant vessel crossing the upper renal

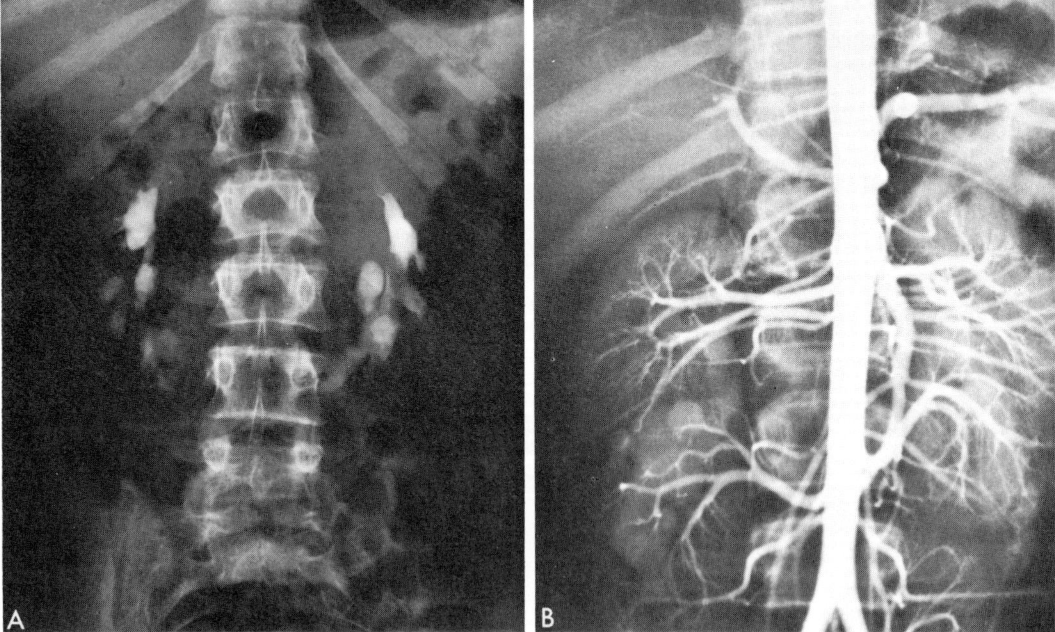

FIGURE 9–14.   *A,* Radiography from an intravenous pyelogram demonstrating a horseshoe kidney deformity. *B,* Radiograph following an aortic injection, illustrating multiple renal arteries in a patient with Turner syndrome and hypertension.

pole. Finally, the horseshoe kidney, which occurs with increased frequency (Fig. 9–14A), may represent either a primary defect in embryogenesis resulting in the union of the two metanephric blastemae or a secondary defect due to malposition of the umbilical arteries.

In our own experience in 141 patients (Fig. 9–15), studied either by intravenous pyelography (IVP), with contrast enhancement at the time of cardiac catherterization, or, more recently, with ultrasonography, we found that 47 patients (33 per cent) had some structural abnormality. The lesions we detected covered the spectrum of defects described previously except that we did not have a case of retrocaval ureter.[110] Ultrasound, which we have used as the initial screening method in recent years, was effective in demonstrating all the anomalies previously seen with IVP except for mild, clinically insignificant, rotational abnormalities. While the overall morbidity of the renal lesions is relatively low, with only four patients requiring surgery, one requiring long-term antibiotic therapy, and four having an absent kidney, the potential for calyceal obstruction, parenchymal infection, and secondary renal impairment is real and we therefore suggest that all patients should undergo an ultrasound imaging study. The high percentage of horseshoe kidneys in our series (7 per cent) and in those of others merits further comment since there may be an increased incidence of Wilms tumor in the horseshoe kidney.[111] If the increased incidence of Wilms tumor results from an abnormal proliferation of the metanephric blastema and if that were the mechanism in Turner syndrome, these patients would be at the same risk as other patients with a horseshoe kidney and the incidence of Wilms tumor in Turner syndrome should be high. Alternatively, if the mechanism in Turner syndrome is vascular, these patients should be at no greater risk for Wilms tumor than the general population. At present, only one patient with both Wilms tumor and Turner syndrome has been reported, suggesting that the latter hypothesis is correct. Therefore, at this time we do not recommend repeat ultrasound or MRI examination of the horseshoe kidney of a Turner patient if the first study is adequate and otherwise normal.

Unknown Factors—Metabolic

Autoimmune Disorders. An apparent increased frequency of autoimmune disorders has been noted in patients with Turner syndrome. The reason for this increase is unknown, but it has been theorized that families with a high frequency of autoimmune diseases may be prone to nondisjunctional events. This hypothesis is based on the observations that (1) there is also an increased

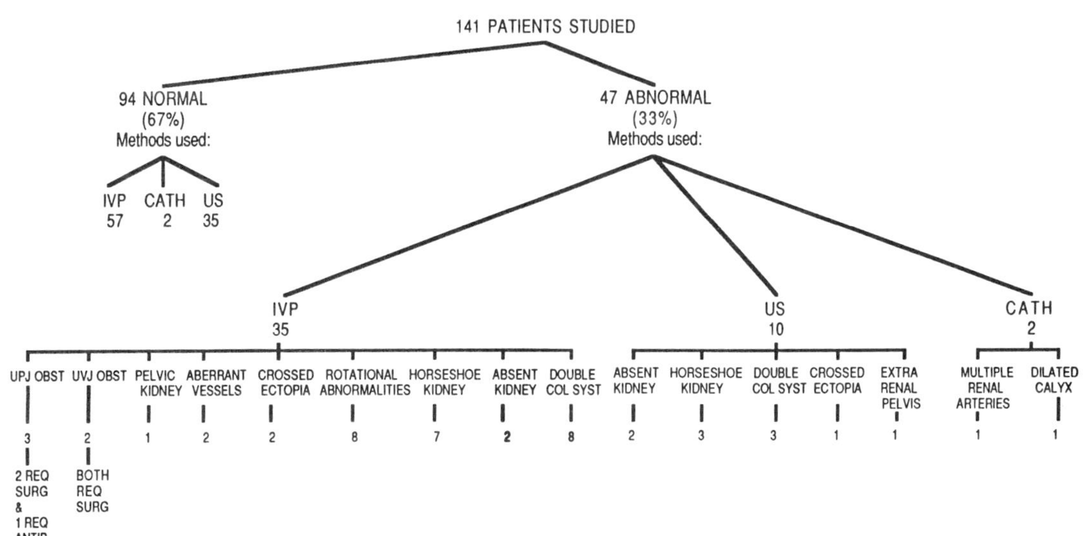

FIGURE 9–15.   Renal abnormalities detected in 141 patients with Turner syndrome. Abbreviations: Cath, catheterization; US, ultrasonography, UPJ OBST, ureteropelvic junction obstruction; UVJ OBST, ureterovesical junction obstruction; REQ, required; Surg, surgery; ANTIB, antibiotics. (From Lippe BM, Geffner ME, Dietrich RB, et al: Renal malformations in patients with Turner syndrome: Imaging in 141 patients. Pediatrics 82:852, 1988.)

frequency of autoimmune disorders in other nondisjunctional chromosomal disorders such as Down and Klinefelter syndromes and (2) that when the families of patients with Turner and Down syndromes are investigated, autoimmune disease appears to be reported or diagnosed frequently. A second theory—that autoimmune diseases might result from, or be associated with, genes or gene mutations on the X chromosome—is supported by the increased incidence of these disorders in X chromosomal disorders as well as by their increased incidence in women. A third theory, that familial (maternal) autoimmunity may lead to the preferential survival of a fetus with chromosomal aneuploidy, remains to be investigated.

The most prevalent autoimmune disorder in Turner syndrome appears to be Hashimoto lymphocytic thyroiditis. Depending on the series reported and on the methods utilized to measure the antibodies, the prevalence of significant titers may be as high as 50 per cent. While originally described in association with structurally abnormal X chromosomes, notably the isoX,[112] increased titers of antithyroid antibodies with or without thyroid failure has been reported in 45,X individuals as well as in patients with mosaic karyotypes without a structurally abnormal X (i.e., 45,X/46,XX).[113,114] In our own series, approximately 30 per cent of patients have positive antithyroid antibodies at the time of first testing. However, of six patients who were overtly hypothyroid two did not have abnormal antibody titers at the time of diagnosis. This is not unexpected, since it is well known that children with biopsy-proven Hashimoto thyroiditis often do not have abnormal titers of circulating antithyroid antibodies.[115]

There are reports now to indicate that Graves hyperthyroidism[116] may also occur more commonly than previously recognized in girls with Turner syndrome, and we have one affected girl in our series. We also have two patients with vitiligo and three with alopecia. However, other forms of polyglandular autoimmunity, such as Addison disease, hypoparathyroidism, and pernicious anemia, have not yet been noted to be increased in frequency in Turner patients.

Gastrointestinal Disorders. A number of reports have called attention to gastrointestinal bleeding, often massive, occurring in patients with Turner syndrome.[117,118] The bleeding has been ascribed to intestinal te-

langiectasias, hemangiomatoses, phlebectasia, or dilated veins and venules. These vascular malformations occur without evidence of mesenteric, portal, or hepatic vascular abnormalities, and this suggests a developmental rather than an acquired etiology. However, they do not appear to be associated with cutaneous hemangiomata or other obvious vascular malformations. It is not known which patients may be at risk for development of vascular bleeding. Whether or not these vascular abnormalities are a consequence of the same obstructive processes that result in the lymphedema is not known. Since large segments of bowel may be involved we recommend conservative management, when possible, to avoid massive resections.

A second cause of gastrointestinal bleeding and dysfunction appears to be inflammatory bowel disease. Several reports suggest an increased incidence of both Crohn disease and ulcerative colitis in infants and children with Turner syndrome.[119–121] Whether this increase in Crohn disease may represent another autoimmune phenomenon, or is perhaps associated with a particular genetic haplotype (HLA type) that may also prove to be increased in Turner syndrome, remains to be established. Similarly, there is as yet no conclusive evidence for a genetic or familial predisposition to ulcerative colitis in these patients. Since growth retardation and delayed sexual maturation are characteristic manifestations of both inflammatory bowel disease and Turner syndrome, careful attention must be paid to the review of systems of patients with Turner. Conversely, girls with inflammatory bowel disease and growth and pubertal delay may need assessment of gonadal function before their sexual delay is ascribed to their bowel disease alone.

Carbohydrate Intolerance. A high incidence of carbohydrate intolerance in Turner syndrome has been reported.[122,123] In our own series 40 per cent of patients tested with oral glucose tests have abnormal responses. The clinical features are those of what is now termed type II or non-ketosis-prone, non-insulin-dependent diabetes.[124] The abnormality may be reflected only in a hyperglycemic response to oral glucose or a meal, or it may progress to fasting hyperglycemia and polyuria. Insulin levels in the serum may be high, in the normal range, or low. Typical type I insulin-dependent diabetes has also been noted in Turner syndrome patients, but not clearly with a frequency in excess of that in the general population.

There is some evidence to suggest that the carbohydrate intolerance in Turner syndrome may be the genetic type II disorder, since abnormal or borderline glucose tolerance tests have been demonstrated in 51 per cent of parents of patients.[125] However, in that same series, only one parent had clinical diabetes, far less than the usual clinical expression in type II families of similar ages. Thus, the questions of both the genetics of the diabetes as well as the potential relationship between diabetes in parents and Turner syndrome in the offspring remain unresolved.

A number of physiologic factors are known to be associated with this form of diabetes. They include obesity, estrogen therapy, GH hypersecretion, hyperglucagonemia, and insulin receptor defects resulting in insulin resistance. Obesity per se is frequently characterized by an insulin-resistant form of carbohydrate intolerance. Although many patients with Turner syndrome appear obese, when assessed by measurement of skinfold thickness they are not significantly obese.[126] Similarly, when this method is used in conjunction with standards for ideal body weight appropriate for their age and height, their degree of fatness or percentage of ideal body weight does not correlate with their carbohydrate intolerance.[127]

Estrogen/progesterone replacement therapy is known to be associated with changes in carbohydrate tolerance. However, many patients with Turner syndrome manifest the abnormality prior to institution of replacement therapy. Thus, while replacement therapy may be an aggravating factor in some patients, it is probably not an important factor in the pathogenesis of diabetes.[128]

The use of GH alone or in combination with anabolic steroids has prompted the reassessment of the carbohydrate status of girls with Turner syndrome with specific focus on the effects of these agents. In a recently reported study[129] of the 71 girls enrolled in the previously discussed growth hormone/oxandrolone protocol of Rosenfeld et al.,[76] glucose tolerance was evaluated before and after acute (5 days) and chronic (2 months and 12 months) administration of GH, oxandrolone, or combination therapy. Pretreatment fasting glucose concentrations were normal in the Turner syndrome patients but their glucose responses to an oral glucose challenge were higher than in normal controls, with 15 per cent classified as having impaired glucose tolerance. Insulin responses were so varied as to be impossible to distinguish from normal. Following either acute or chronic hormone therapy, carbohydrate tolerance, as measured by integrated glucose or insulin responses, did not change in the GH-treated group. This was contrary to the expectation that GH treatment might induce a deterioration in carbohydrate tolerance, especially in what was considered a high-risk group. However, higher glucose and insulin responses were noted in the oxandrolone alone and the combination oxandrolone-GH group. The clinical significance of what appears to be an effect due to the oxandrolone remains to be determined.

Hyperglucagonemia is usually associated with relative or absolute hypoinsulinemia, and it contributes to hyperglycemia and the development of ketoacidosis in insulin-deficient diabetics. However, a primary abnormality in glucagon secretion, which may precede or be fundamental to the pathogenesis of diabetes, does not appear to occur in most Turner syndrome patients. In our own studies of a group of unselected patients, glucagon hypersecretion was not present in the fasting state and its concentration in the plasma was normally suppressed by hyperglycemia.[127]

Although there is a high incidence of autoimmune disease in Turner syndrome, it is unlikely that the diabetes is of the autoimmune type commonly described in other autoimmune polyendocrinopathies. This type of diabetes is usually ketosis prone and insulin dependent, and the type in Turner syndrome is not. The type in Turner syndrome also contrasts with the diabetes that occurs in Down syndrome, which does tend to have an explosive onset, as often occurs in the insulin-dependent type, and may well have an autoimmune basis.

We and others have recently raised the question of whether or not a defect in the insulin receptor is responsible for a component of the peripheral insulin resistance described in Turner syndrome. However, the variables affecting insulin receptor binding studies in these patients have precluded a definitive answer, and further investigations are needed. Finally, there does not appear to be a relationship with a specific chromosomal karyotype. Thus, the etiology of the carbohydrate intolerance in Turner syndrome remains obscure.

Psychologic Features

The weight of the currently available evidence is that the intelligence of persons with Turner syndrome is normal. There does not appear to be an increased incidence of either moderate or severe mental retardation, nor do the individuals differ from their siblings in overall intelligence.[130] There also does not appear to be a specific chromosomal karyotype or a single somatic malformation that is associated with either lowered general intelligence or a specific deficit in intellectual performance. This is in contrast to both the initial general impression of increased prevalence of mental retardation and the specific impression that it is more common among persons with a 45,X karyotype or those with a webbed neck.[13] Of note is a report of two severely retarded institutionalized patients with the Turner syndrome phenotype. In these patients, in addition to the 45,X karyotype, extra chromosomal material, apparently of chromosome 21 in origin, was noted.[131] Thus, some of the earlier reports of mental retardation may be the result of unrecognized coexistent autosomal aneuploidy, a condition recognized to occur in association with Turner syndrome.

In specific areas such as spatiotemporal processing,[132] perceptual stability,[133] or visual-motor coordination and motor learning,[134] however, it has been demonstrated that Turner syndrome patients have a deficiency in performance. While almost all investigators concur that specific cognitive deficits are present, the areas of presumed cognitive dysfunction differ in different reports and the interpretation of the results depends on numerous variables related to the testing instrument and data analysis. Nevertheless, the most commonly observed pattern is one of diminished nonverbal processing. The spatial deficit affects space form perception and, in testing situations, is most clearly demonstrable in mental rotation tasks.[135] In actual performance in school it is most often reflected by difficulties with mathematics and constructional tasks. Socially it is reflected by a poor directional sense and difficulty in driving an automobile. However, while this is a statistically significant finding among patients with Turner's syndrome as a group, not all individuals demonstrate impairment.

Personality trait assessment has also been carried out in patients with Turner syndrome. Most significant is the conclusion that sexual attitudes are feminine.[136] This normal finding allows the physician to reassure the patient and family that this aspect of future psychosocial adaptation should not differ from the female population at large. However, the psychosocial function of girls and adult women with Turner syndrome may not be entirely normal. In school, they are described as being immature, having fewer friends, and needing more structure to socialize and complete tasks as compared to short-stature controls.[137] They have more difficulties understanding social and nonverbal cues, so that, as a younger sibling of an adolescent Turner patient recently commented about her sister, "she just doesn't get the point and that isolates her." As adult women, they tend to begin dating later than their peers, leave home later, and have more limited heterosexual contact, and a subgroup may have a considerably impaired sense of self-esteem.[138] Whether delayed sexual maturation, infertility, short stature, or other more basic psychodynamic factors, including selective cognitive dysfunctions, are responsible is unknown. Nevertheless, as more aggressive and innovative endocrine therapies begin to alter the outlook for stature, timing of feminization, and fertility, attention should still be paid to assessment of psychosocial adaptation.

There have been a number of reports describing the occurrence of anorexia nervosa in patients with Turner syndrome[139] but it is unclear if anorexia is increased in Turner syndrome in comparison with normal girls. Kron and coworkers have pointed out the danger of overlooking an X chromosomal disorder in a patient in whom growth arrest and pubertal delay are attributed to excessive weight loss alone. This is especially relevant since gonadotropins may revert to prepubertal levels.[140]

Evaluation

The clinical aspects of which child should be evaluated for Turner syndrome and at what age have been addressed, in part, in the chapters of this text dealing with growth disorders (Chapter 1) and with amenorrhea (Chapter 8) and are implicit in the previous discussion of the salient features of the syndrome presented in this chapter. Nevertheless, certain clinical aspects warrant review. It is obvious that the female neonate with a webbed neck or edema of the hands and feet merits further investigation. Similarly, the girl with multiple physical stigmata, the girl with coarctation of the aorta, or the girl with radiologic evidence of abnormalities in the urinary collecting system or a horseshoe kidney should also be considered for evaluation. What is less obvious is which girl without obvious stigmata or highly suggestive organic defects should be evaluated.

Many girls with Turner syndrome do not have obvious physical stigmata, and it is necessary to recognize that the diagnosis may be difficult in such cases. We reviewed the records of 144 of our patients and found that only 41 had been diagnosed as neonates or toddlers because of obvious physical stigmata. The remaining 103 (71 per cent) presented with short stature or short stature and pubertal delay.[141] Therefore, presence of short stature alone must be sufficient to consider the diagnosis. The incidence of Turner syndrome is about 1:2000 live female births, but the statistics change as one considers stature. For example, among 2000 girls, only 60 are at or below the 3rd centile. Therefore, the group at risk, even if no stigmata at all are present, is much smaller. Given other genetic causes for short stature among this group, as well as other acquired causes, and the possible presence of one or more clinical features, the number of girls who might need evaluation becomes less than 1 in 60. Thus, the rationale for considering performing a complete chromosomal karyotype on a girl with short stature becomes more obvious.

Once the diagnosis of Turner syndrome has been established and a chromosome analysis has been carried out several additional diagnostic procedures are required.

Initial and Follow-up Studies

Since the clinical manifestations of gradually developing thyroid failure can be subtle, and easily overlooked in a short child, routine serum thyroid function tests, including thyroxine (T_4), thyroid-stimulating hormone (TSH), and antithyroid antibodies, are indicated. Subsequently T_4 and TSH levels should be determined at yearly intervals in all patients whether or not significant titers of antithyroid antibodies were detected initially. Once estrogen therapy has been initiated, even in low doses, the serum T_4 may be elevated consequent to the estrogen-mediated increase in serum thyroid-binding globulin (TBG). Therefore, use of a corrected T_4 [T_4 index or T_4 and triiodothyronine (T_3) resin uptake] is helpful. If GH is being used thyroid function should be checked at frequent intervals since it may unmask latent primary hypothyroidism or provoke temporary tertiary hypothyroidism. Routine testing for other autoimmune glandular failures does not appear necessary unless other evidence of autoimmune disease such as alopecia, vitiligo, or a glandular failure develops.

A routine renal ultrasound may detect structural abnormalities in renal architecture or collecting system anatomy (Fig. 9–14). If no abnormalities are present, follow-up studies are not routinely indicated. Bone age determinations are indicated in all pediatric patients prior to hormone replacement therapy and subsequently to monitor the effects of such therapy. If skeletal age is severely retarded, this may serve as an indication that other conditions resulting in short stature, such as hypothyroidism or inflammatory bowel disease, may also be present. Plasma FSH and LH concentrations at the time of diagnosis may or may not be elevated, but could serve as an indication of future gonadal function. However, we have observed two girls with significantly elevated FSH levels in early childhood who went on to the spontaneous onset of puberty. Therefore, predictions of gonadal failure may be given, but with care.

Although insulin-dependent diabetes is rare in Turner syndrome, significant carbohydrate intolerance does occur. This develops as the patient's age increases and may be exaggerated by increased weight or hormonal replacement therapy.

Although the osseous abnormalities of Turner syndrome may be multiple, unless they cause significant morbidity, radiologic survey of the entire skeleton is not routinely recommended. Once a skeletal deformity is noted, however, orthopedic consultation may be indicated. In our experience, scoliosis does not progress rapidly and is usually managed conservatively. However, if growth-promoting regimens are used, careful attention should be paid to detecting progressive scoliosis. If noted, its etiology should be determined radiographically, since we have observed two patients in whom it was due to leg length inequality.

Madelung deformity requires recognition so as to exclude other causes of this bony malposition, but it does not require orthopedic correction.

Pelvic visualization techniques, including ultrasound or MRI, appear to be initially indicated only in those clinical situations in which there is a question of gonadal anatomy or function. The most potentially serious of these occurs in the patient with a Y chromosome in the karyotype, since she is at risk for the development of gonadoblastoma. Imaging studies in a patient with uncomplicated 45,X karyotype generally do not demonstrate gonadal structures, but the ultrasound may demonstrate an adnexal mass in the patient with the Y chromosome in comparison with the normal female (Fig. 9–12). Surgical removal of the bilateral adnexal structures is then indicated.

The recommendation for a concomitant hysterectomy as a prophylactic measure against endometrial carcinoma in an agonadal individual who will be on long-term estrogen replacement therapy is controversial. Some physicians believe that since it lends little extra morbidity to the indicated pelvic surgery it is a warranted consideration. Others believe that the psychological benefit of monthly menstruation, independent of the artificiality of its method of production and its irrelevance to fertility, precludes the procedure unless there is evidence of local spread of the gonadoblastoma. Finally, oocyte donation, in vitro fertilization, and embryo transfer are being performed successfully in agonadal women who have an intact uterus.[142] Thus the issue bears complete discussion with the individual patient and physicians involved. A more difficult management decision concerns the method of follow-up of the patient with a Y in the karyotype in whom the initial radiographic studies are normal. The question of whether prophylactic removal of the adnexal streaks should be performed electively, or delayed until the ultrasound or MRI suggests a mass, has not been entirely resolved. However, the data indicating that tumor formation may be present microscopically at a very young age are a strong argument for elective surgery even in the absence of a demonstrable mass.[92]

Pelvic visualization techniques may also be useful in patients with evidence of some gonadal function at puberty. In such patients either unilateral or bilateral gonadal structures may be demonstrable. The anatomic findings would lend supportive evidence to the clinical or gonadotropin data, and might deter the physician from the institution of hormonal replacement therapy.

Renal arteriography or selective venous catheterization, or both, may be indicated in some patients with hypertension. While the evidence of multiple arterial and venous abnormalities in Turner syndrome suggests that gross or segmental renal vascular disease may be responsible for the hypertension, the disordered anatomy may also render detection of treatable lesions difficult. An example of a study performed in an 11-year-old patient with significant hypertension is shown in Figure 9–13A. Multiple renal arteries and veins were noted, and selective catheterization was virtually impossible. Nevertheless, in some patients surgically treatable lesions may be apparent.

The high prevalence of hearing loss, either primary or secondary to residual serous otitis media, suggests that otorhinolaryngologic evaluation with audiometry may be indicated in a large number of patients. In infancy, feeding techniques such as those used for cleft palate patients may also be indicated. We have the clinical impression that mild abnormalities in phonation, independent of hearing impairment, are present in a number of our older patients. Because these abnormalities in speech may be a consequence of a palatal deformity, speech evaluation may also be indicated. While myringotomy and polyethylene tube placement are considered the primary modes of therapy for serous otitis media, tonsillectomy or adenoidectomy, or both, are often performed as well. However, in those patients in whom a palatal abnormality is pronounced, removal of the tonsils and adenoids may not be advisable because of its dubious value for the treatment of serous otitis media, and because the pharyngeal tissue often serves as an anatomic prosthesis for pharyngeal competence.

Consultative Studies

Since the detection of cardiovascular abnormalities requires specialized diagnostic and clinical evaluation, and their presence may indicate the need for cardiac surgery or lifelong antibiotic therapy for subacute bacterial endocarditis (SBE) prophylaxis, a cardiologic consultation should be obtained for all patients. If no abnormalities are detected, follow-up evaluation is suggested at

2- to 3-year intervals, since aortic dilation may occur without any other risk factors. If bicuspid aortic valve or mitral valve prolapse is detected, SBE prophylaxis is recommended and follow-up should be more frequent. If aortic root dilation is found follow-up should probably be yearly. If unexplained chest pain occurs, even with initially normal studies, the diagnosis of aneurysm or dissection must always be considered. Coarctation of the aorta is treated surgically in most cases. Although the postoperative risk of the development of mesenteric arteritis is higher in males than females,[143] the author has observed this syndrome in a patient with Turner syndrome. Long-term prognosis is generally good, with few reports of recurrence or complications. However, asymptomatic poststenotic aneurysmal dilation of the aorta may be detectable on screening chest x-ray or cardiac MRI (Fig. 9–13C) and should be followed.

The decision to seek consultation for plastic surgery to correct the webbed neck deformity or the forwardly displaced ears is an individual decision. It must be pointed out to the patient and family that in addition to the webbing, the neck may also be short. Therefore, cosmetic surgery may be somewhat disappointing. In some cases, however, satisfactory results are achieved. The apparent predisposition toward the development of keloids in these patients must also be taken into account. There is some evidence to suggest that early surgery may have a better cosmetic result.[144] This author has noted an increased frequency in development of keloids following ear piercing in adolescence, and suggests that this procedure be performed with great care.

If, or when, to suggest psychometric testing, should be individualized. A preschool evaluation to rule out major areas of cognitive dysfunction might be advisable. School performance should be monitored and specific problems attended to in light of the previous discussion.

Endocrinologic Management

The many and varied protocols for growth promotion currently being tested in Turner syndrome patients make it difficult to give uniform guidelines for endocrinologic management. It behooves the practitioner to recognize that there are several different approaches to this problem and to explore the options that are available, not only in the community in which the patient lives but also in the major regional referral centers.

Prior to the recognition that there might be methods to increase the final height of Turner patients, this author believed that the psychologic benefit of increased growth during early adolescence as well as the need for the development of secondary sexual characteristics at a relatively normal age could best be met by a management strategy that utilized androgenic steroids prior to estrogen therapy. I considered those girls between the ages of 10 and 12 years who were more than 2 SD below the mean in height and growing less than 5.0 cm year (which, as shown in Figure 9–9, is characteristic of most but not all Turner individuals) and who were not showing signs of spontaneous onset of puberty to be candidates for therapy. The potential side effects of androgen therapy, including deepening of the voice, acne, increased body hair, and clitoromegaly, were discussed. Additionally, the potential risks of hepatotoxicity and hepatic neoplasia were also discussed, although at the doses used the side effects are minimal and no cases of hepatic dysfunction are known to the author from androgens used in this manner. I began either fluoxymesterone (Halotestin) or oxandrolone (Anavar) at doses of 0.05 to 0.1 mg/kg/day and monitored growth rate and the physical examination at 3-month intervals. Bone age determinations were made at 3- to 6-month intervals. The goal of therapy was an increase in growth velocity without noticeable side effects and without advancement of bone age in excess of the incremental height increase that was achieved. Most commonly, a significant increase in growth velocity was maintained for 6 to 12 months. As deceleration began a small increase in dose would often promote reacceleration. In the absence of side effects, this latter dose was maintained until either the growth rate again declined or the patient expressed a desire to initiate estrogen therapy. At this time, usually a 12 to 24 month interval, androgen was discontinued, the patient was reassessed for the presence of spontaneous gonadal function, and, if not previously started, estrogen therapy was begun. Were a GH therapy program not available or otherwise contraindicated this is the program I would still recommend.

Protocols for estrogen replacement therapy are also based on a risk-benefit assessment. The physiologic and psychological needs for estrogen are incontrovertible, but the compounds employed and the dosage schedules used are changing.[145] Diethylstilbestrol, which was used as the primary source of estrogen for many years, has now been recognized as a potential carcinogen. Thus, it is no longer recommended for replacement therapy, and may have contributed to the apparent increase in endometrial carcinoma reported in women with gonadal dysgenesis who had received this compound for 5 or more years.[146] Only two cases of adenocarcinoma have been reported in untreated women with Turner syndrome,[147,148] and few cases have been reported in patients receiving both an estrogen and a progesterone regimen.[149,150] Conjugated equine estrogen (Premarin) does not appear to have the same structural carcinogenic potential as diethylstilbestrol. Whether this preparation, or a synthetic oral or transdermal estrogen is used, after an initial priming phase, it is recommended that the estrogen be administered in a cyclic fashion in conjunction with progesterone. There is an accumulating body of evidence that unopposed estrogen is associated with an increased risk of estrogen-related neoplasms, especially uterine carcinoma. Data on steroid receptors in hormone-dependent target tissues suggest that progesterone down-regulates or blocks the estrogen receptors[151] and when given in conjunction with estrogen may be protective against estrogen-induced neoplasia. Progestins also act to attenuate the action of estrogen by increasing the activities of enzymes that convert estrogen into biologically less active estrone and inactive estrogen sulfate. When endometrial responses were prospectively evaluated in Turner syndrome patients receiving long-term replacement therapy, hyperplastic changes were noted in only a small percentage of those receiving combined therapy as compared with those receiving cyclic estrogen alone.[152] Thus, therapy with progesterone appears to have a protective effect.[153] While the precise amount of estrogen that is necessary for both feminization and long-term protection from osteoporosis has yet to be determined, most investigators believe it is less than that present in most oral contraceptive preparations. Similarly, the amount of progesterone needed for protection may also be less than that in contraceptive preparations, although most authorities recognize that it must be administered for 12 or 13 days per month. The goal is the complete conversion of the endometrium from a proliferative to a whole or predominantly secretory state.[153] For these reasons, the most commonly used protocols for the long-term treatment of Turner syndrome women are slightly more cumbersome than the single pill of a contraceptive package.

Our current protocol usually consists of the administration of 0.3 to 0.625 mg of Premarin per day for 3 to 6 months. If the lower dose is used initially, it is then raised to 0.625 mg for 3 months and then cyclic therapy is begun. If the higher dose is used it is not increased unless there is very poor estrinization of the breasts, and then a higher dose (a 0.9-mg tablet is now available) may be tried. The Premarin is taken from day 1 through day 23 of the calendar month and the progestin (Provera, 5 to 10 mg) is taken from day 10 through day 23. No medication is ingested for the remainder of the calendar month, when withdrawal menses usually ensue. Estrogen is then restarted on day 1 of the next calendar month, and progesterone again added subsequently. If bleeding occurs earlier than day 21 of the month, especially on the lower dose of Provera, the dose should be increased since a predominantly proliferative endometrium characteristically bleeds before 10 days of progestin therapy.[154] If no menses occur after several cycles, especially on the higher dose of Provera, it can be lowered. While plasma FSH and LH concentrations may not be suppressed to normal concentrations, hot flushes are rare, as are other symptoms of hypoestrinization. Follow-up includes monthly breast self-examination and yearly pelvic examination and Papanicolaou smears commencing 3 to 4 years after cyclic therapy or earlier if the patient is sexually active.

Other preparations of estrogen and progesterone are currently being assessed for long-term use as replacement therapy. These include oral synthetic ethinyl estradiol and micronized estradiol-17β, transdermal estradiol-17β, and transvaginal suppositories of estrogen and progesterone. The issues that need to be considered are the route of administration and effects of different preparations on systems such as the hepatic enzymes that contribute to the potential adverse affects of estrogen on blood pressure, clotting, and gallstone formation. Transdermal estrogen, for example, unlike oral estrogens, avoids the so-called first-pass effect on the liver and may therefore obviate adverse effects on hepatic proteins.[155] We have had some experience with transdermal estradiol (Estraderm) in a Turner patient who had recurrence of pedal lymphedema with the institution of oral estrogen replacement. She has experienced less swelling with the transdermal preparation and has continued to use it. Subsequently, we have tried it in several other older patients, who find it quite acceptable. We use the 50-μg patch, which appears to be similar in potency to 0.625 mg of Premarin, and the patient changes the patch after 3 1/2 days (2 per week) for the first 21 days (3 weeks) of the calendar month. Provera, 10 mg, is taken from days 10 through 21 and no patch or Provera are used after day 21 until the next month. Follow-up is the same as for oral estrogen therapy.

An additional comment should be made about breast development in response to estrogen replacement in Turner syndrome. The author has observed that the final size of the breast is more consistent with genetic predisposition of the family than with the dose of estrogen or the time it was initiated. The only clear exception appears to be in the girl in whom there are marked clinical signs of extensive fetal edema of the upper body. This includes severe webbing and/or marked nipple hypoplasia at birth. It is my impression that some of these girls develop very little breast tissue in response to estrogen and that this may be due to mechanical damage to the breast primordium in utero. In such patients I would encourage breast augmentation in late adolescence if the patient is so inclined and if she has not had a problem with keloid formation.

Additional Management Notes

There are some unusual clinical problems that must be recognized by the physician. These have been called to the attention of the author by her own patients ("I can't swim backstroke and I can't play the bass violin because my elbows are funny"), by the patient's parents ("I can't find clothes that are proportionate because my child is broad shouldered and short legged"), and by the patient's siblings ("My sister is smarter than she looks"). They call to our attention that patients with Turner syndrome may require social or psychosocial support. Turner syndrome societies have taken an active role in this regard in Canada and in Scandinavia and currently efforts are underway to link local United States groups into a National Society. It must also be recognized that repeated discussion must take place between family, patient, and clinician. After years of follow-up one tends to overlook the fact that the patient is no longer a child, and reeducation and new lines of communication may need to be established. It must also be reemphasized that the classical textbook stigmata and descriptions of Turner syndrome are antiquated at best and should not serve as a source of information for patient and physician. A most common source of anxiety in our own experience is the patient or family who reads of stigmata or complications that they do not have, but that they anticipate could befall them. Finally, the self-image any person develops is in part a product of the image others have of them. Girls and women with Turner syndrome have the potential to live normal, healthy, productive lives but may need the guidance of understanding physicians to enable them to achieve their potential.

PURE GONADAL DYSGENESIS

In the early and middle 1950s several other forms of gonadal dysgenesis were described. A group of phenotypically normal women, usually of normal stature, were noted to demonstrate so-called "pure" gonadal dysgenesis.[156] A form with positive sex chromatin, subsequently shown to have a normal 46,XX karyotype was noted to occur in sisters, suggesting a recessive pattern of inheritance.[157] Since there is no evidence that in this condition the gonad was ever genetically determined to be anything other than an ovary, the term *pure ovarian dysgenesis* seems appropriate for this condition.[22] Although most affected women have no other systemic abnormalities, a subgroup with severe sensorineural deafness was identified by Perrault et al. in 1951 and has more recently reviewed.[158] The genetic defect responsible for the ovarian failure in both conditions appears to be inherited as an autosomal recessive.

The diagnosis is suspected when pubertal failure is associated with high levels of gonadotropins (increase of both FSH and LH), a normal 46,XX karyotype, normal stature, and normal female internal genitalia. However, in some patients the external genitalia may show some degree of virilization (clitoromegaly), and hirsutism may develop.[159] In these patients the virilization is associated with hilus cell hyperplasia and luteinized gonadal stromal cells. Gonadoblastoma does not appear to occur, however, since germ cells containing Y chromosomes are not present. Therefore, surgical removal of the streaks may not be indicated in the patient with pure gonadal dysgenesis unless virilization is a problem. The differential diagnosis between pure ovarian dysgenesis and a form of acquired ovarian dysfunction (see page 360) may be difficult in the absence of either a similarly affected sibling in the former case or evidence of a process responsible for acquired ovarian failure in the latter. Pelvic ultrasound may be helpful, since the streak ovaries present in pure gonadal dysgenesis may be too small to be adequately visualized, while in gradually acquired postnatal ovarian dysfunction the ovaries can often be clearly imaged. Since it is possible that some viable ovarian follicles may exist in some forms of acquired ovarian failure, if family planning is contemplated laparoscopy with gonadal biopsy may be necessary at that time.

The term *pure gonadal dysgenesis* was also applied to phenotypic females with streak gonads who were demonstrated to be sex chromatin negative. Subsequently, these patients were identified as having 46,XY karyotypes. This entity, now more appropriately termed *XY testicular dysgenesis*, may also occur in siblings.[160] The pedigrees of several families suggest that the defect can be transmitted as an X-linked mutant gene.[161,162] In other families it follows an autosomal pattern. This fits current thinking that the testis-determining gene on the Y chromosome acts in conjunction with both Y and autosomal genes for complete testicular development. If incomplete development occurs, XY germ cells do not survive well and the gonad gradually loses ovarian architecture and is replaced by fibrous stroma (Swyer syndrome).

Clinically, XY testicular dysgenesis is differentiated from XY testicular feminization syndrome in that the internal genitalia are female in the former, with uterus and full vagina. The patients are also peripherally sensitive to androgen, so that they develop normal pubic and axillary hair. Finally, rather than having testes that have developed sufficiently, so that they may be located anywhere along the path of testicular descent, including herniae in the labia, the gonadal streaks of XY testicular dysgenesis are located in the normal pelvic position of ovaries. Hypergonadotrophic hypogonadism is present at puberty and the response to estrogen administration is normal feminization. However, these gonads may not be completely inert, and may actually produce some androgen at the time of puberty or thereafter, resulting in clitoromegaly or hirsutism. So-called lutein-Leydig cells may be seen on histologic examination.[163] In these XY patients the risk for gonadoblastoma formation is significant whether virilization occurs or not since the germ cells carry the Y chromosome.[164] Therefore, prophylactic surgical removal of the streaks is usually recommended.

Finally, there are several syndromes of XY phenotypic females associated with major malformations, anomalies, or mesenchymal dysplasias. Campomelic dysplasia is frequently associated with XY sex reversal.[165] These phenotypic female infants have a severe bony dysplasia and rarely live beyond infancy. However, it is possible that some affected individuals will eventually survive to become adults and if so should undergo prophylactic gonadectomy. Although the condition is usually sporadic, in occurrence there is a report of sibling pairs, supporting the likelihood of a recessive form of inheritance. The Drash syndrome[166] was described as the association of XY pseudohermaphroditism and Wilms tumor. However, it is now recognized that the ambiguity is due to testicular dysgenesis or damage and may be sufficiently severe that the genitalia are not ambiguous but instead phenotypically female.[167] The renal lesions are also varied and the symptoms and signs may be those of nephrosis, or a glomerulopathy. Since these children are at risk not only for Wilms tumor but also for malignant transformation of the dysgenetic gonads, nephrectomy and gonadectomy are often both indicated. The Smith-Lemli-Opitz (SLO) syndrome is an autosomal recessive disorder with a heterogeneous spectrum of congenital anomalies. Several infants have been reported with SLO and phenotypic female external and internal genitalia but with an XY karyotype and intra-abdominal testes.[168] It is therefore recommended that a karyotype be obtained when SLO is diagnosed in any phenotypic female.

OVARIAN FUNCTION AND OTHER CHROMOSOME ABNORMALITIES

Multiple X Chromosomes

When there are an excessive rather than deficient number of X chromosomes, ovarian function may also be impaired. The incidence of the 47,XXX (Triplo-X) karyotype in newborn phenotypic female infants is approximately 1:1000.[169] The majority of these patients do not have obvious phenotypic or developmental abnormalities and would be unrecognized save for the research-based chromosome screening programs that identified them. However, when prospective studies are performed on women with the 47,XXX karyotype, infertility and gonadal failure are noted more frequently than in the normal population.[170] Gonadotropins are increased in the plasma, indicating that the hypogonadism is due to primary gonadal failure. Histologic data are scanty, but the mechanism of ovarian failure is presumed to be accelerated follicular atresia. Therefore, the manner in which this diagnosis is established is somewhat similar to that of the phenotypically normal patient with Turner syndrome. Primary gonadal failure, per se, whether short stature is present or not, necessitates a complete chromosomal karyotype. However, should the Triplo-X karyotype be identified in a girl prior to pubertal development, assurance may be given that the majority of the patients are fertile. There is also a low incidence of chromosomal aneuploidy among their offspring,[171] and although amniocentesis might be performed during pregnancy, the value of this procedure in prenatal counseling is debatable.

The 48,XXXX karyotype is exceedingly rare[172] with less than 50 cases reported. These patients are also phenotypic females, but they tend to have more phenotypic abnormalities, including skeletal dysplasias, intellectual impairment, and speech dysfunctions.[173] The skeletal abnormalities, including those of carrying angle varus disturbances and radioulnar synostosis, are similar to those in Klinefelter syndrome. Thus, in contrast to the increased carrying angle of the 45,X patient or the normal angle of the 46,XX patient, the angle of the 48,XXXX patient may be decreased to an extent indistinguishable from that of the 47,XXY or 48,XXXY male. In these so called

Tetra-X women fertility appears to be decreased to an extent even greater than in the Triplo-X patients. Again primary gonadal failure is responsible. Plasma gonadotropin concentrations in adolescence are helpful in predicting whether ovarian function and fertility will be normal. We reported one such patient in whom ovarian development was virtually absent. This case represents one extreme within the spectrum of the abnormality.[172]

The Penta-X karyotype, 49,XXXXX, has also been reported.[174] It is extremely rare, and the principal phenotypic features are those associated with microcephaly, postnatal growth failure, and skeletal dysplasia, including radioulnar synostosis. The frequency with which gonadal function is impaired, however, is less well documented, since the oldest patient was only 16 years old when reported. However, this patient was still not fully pubertal, and this suggests that she had ovarian dysfunction.

Thus, the evidence confirms that ovarian function may be adversely affected by the presence of multiple X chromosomes. The mechanism is unknown, since the precise effect of aneuploidy, be it autosomal or X chromosomal in nature, is unclear. The presence of an additional X chromosome, or multiple X chromosomes, however, appears to accelerate the rate of follicular atresia in most patients. In some patients, such as our patient with apparent ovarian agenesis, normal induction of the ovaries may be impaired in the fetus. A possible mechanism for the ovarian failure could be impaired migration of the abnormally constituted germ cells. In no cases without demonstrable or presumptive Y chromosomal material has ovarian neoplasia been documented, and surgical intervention is therefore not indicated.

Autosomal Abnormalities

As more information becomes available in patients with autosomal abnormalities, increased associations are seen with ovarian dysfunction.[175] Trisomy 21, the most commonly described autosomal trisomy to result in survival into adult life, is clearly associated with some degree of ovarian dysfunction. Gonadotropins are often elevated and delayed menarche, anovulatory menstrual cycles, or true gonadal failure may occur.[176] The majority of female patients with Downs syndrome are unaffected and fertile, however.

Phenotypic females with trisomy 18 (Edwards syndrome) and trisomy 13 (Patau syndrome) have also been reported to have ovarian dysgenesis. In these infants, however, the incidence of ovarian failure appears to be extraordinarily high.[177] A number of theoretical mechanisms have been proposed to explain this observation, including (1) the potential difficulty of coupling of unbalanced chromosomal sets, (2) specific gene-expressed dysfunction, (3) failure of stromal-oogonial interactions, and (4) possible autoimmune or immunologic phenomena. When genetic counseling is offered to the parents of children with these trisomic syndromes it should be remembered that gonadal dysgenesis may be part of, rather than separate from, the other findings of the syndrome.

ACQUIRED OVARIAN FAILURE

In the absence of an X chromosome abnormality or a familial pattern of ovarian dysgenesis, the finding of hypergonadotropic hypogonadism in a phenotypically normal 46,XX female suggests acquired ovarian failure.

We currently recognize at least four forms of this type of hypogonadism: (1) autoimmune ovarian failure, (2) gonadal damage from therapeutic irradiation or systemic chemotherapy, (3) gonadal failure associated with systemic diseases, and (4) gonadal insensitivity to pituitary trophic hormone stimulation.

Autoimmune Ovarian Failure

The association of autoimmune ovarian failure with other systemic autoimmune disorders, including Addison disease, Hashimoto thyroiditis, and moniliasis, is well recognized.[178,179] In an appropriate assay system, antiovarian antibodies can be demonstrated,[179,180] and histologic investigation of ovarian tissue obtained at laparoscopy has shown lymphocytic infiltration of developing ovarian follicles (oophoritis) analogous to the changes in Hashimoto thyroiditis.[181] However, as in some autoimmune disorders, such as myasthenia gravis, in which circulating antibodies are directed against receptors, the premature ovarian failure may be antibody mediated though an antibody

that blocks the LH receptor.[182] Thus both cellular and humoral autoimmune processes may affect the ovary. When the ovarian failure is manifested as secondary amenorrhea in a patient who has another autoimmune disorder (with Addison disease being most common), it rarely represents a diagnostic dilemma. However, autoimmune oophoritis may lead to pubertal failure in early adolescence, or to premature menopause, and even if no other evidence of autoimmune disease is present, this condition must be considered in the differential diagnosis of hypergonadotropic hypogonadism.[183] Signs of autoimmune disease such as vitiligo and alopecia may be present, and serologic evidence for other glandular involvements should be sought. Unfortunately, assays for antiovarian antibodies are not as generally available as they are for antithyroid antibodies or antiadrenal antibodies, and in the absence of other manifestations of autoimmune disease the diagnosis of oophoritis may be difficult. Pelvic ultrasound will show a normal uterus, and may show the presence of gonadal structures. Since there is no risk for gonadoblastoma, surgical intervention is not indicated. Estrogen replacement therapy may be initiated at the expected time of puberty, because there is no evidence that this will adversely affect the remote possibility of any future therapeutic intervention aimed at trying to activate potentially residual ovarian function. The possibility exists that in the future specific therapy may be available to arrest the progression of the autoimmune disease at a stage at which some viable follicles may still be present. Thus, we are currently recommending that laparoscopic biopsy be postponed until such time as family planning is contemplated, and then be performed only if there is a possibility of therapeutic intervention.

Irradiation or Chemotherapy

Progress in the therapy of many forms of childhood cancer, as well as aplastic anemia and lethal immunologic disorders, has led to the development of complications, among which is gonadal damage. Many female survivors of the specific high-dose local radiation for Wilms tumor and Hodgkin disease are now well into their reproductive years, and hypergonadotropic hypogonadism is a well-recognized complication. Bone marrow transplantation following total body irradiation and chemotherapy may also lead to hypergonadotropic hypogonadism in many patients.[184] Intracranial tumors may be treated with chemotherapy and craniospinal irradiation, and this combination has also been associated with gonadal damage.[185] Chemotherapy alone may also be associated with gonadal failure, but this association varies with the regimen used and may vary with the age of the patient.

In pubertal women treated for Hodgkin disease, the incidence of gonadal failure is high, although it does not occur in all.[186] On the other hand, long-term female survivors of aggressively treated childhood leukemia have an excellent prognosis for normal gonadal function, especially if they were prepubertal at the onset of disease.[187] Since these protocols may involve irradiation of the central nervous system as well as systemic chemotherapy, if gonadal function is not normal determination of gonadotropins will identify whether the dysfunction is central (hypogonadotropic) or gonadal (hypergonadotropic). In the former exogenous gonadal stimulation with gonadotropins could induce fertility, whereas in the latter such therapy is less likely to be effective. Less aggressive chemotherapeutic protocols, such as the use of cyclophosphamide for nephrotic syndrome, appear to affect females to a lesser degree than males, and in some series no evidence has been obtained that primary ovarian failure occured.[188]

In all cases, replacement estrogen therapy is indicated if ovarian failure is present. However, careful gynecologic follow-up is essential since there is both an increased risk of a second neoplasm developing in any patient with a first cancer and a risk of tumorogenesis in someone treated with chemotherapy, radiotherapy, or both.

Association with Systemic Disease

Apart from the aforementioned association with autoimmune glandular diseases, ovarian failure has been sporadically reported in a variety of other systemic disorders. These include two diseases with associated immunologic disturbances, ataxia-telangectasia and Di George syndrome,[177] albeit the mechanisms do not appear to be based on acquired autoimmune tissue destruction. Hypergonadotropic hypogonadism has been reported in females with galactosemia, who may have either primary or secondary amenorrhea or oligomenor-

rhea,[189] and in both females and males with a form of cerebellar ataxia.[190]

Insensitivity to Pituitary Trophic Hormones

A defect in ovarian function that results in the picture of hypergonadotropic ovarian failure may be the result of either an isolated or a more generalized defect in end-organ sensitivity to hormonal stimulation. In the case of the so-called isolated defect, gonadotropin-resistant ovary syndrome or "Savage" syndrome, the gonadal failure is usually secondary.[191] Histologically, numerous primordial follicles are usually present and stromal hyperplasia may also be found. The nature of the defect is unknown. Current theories include insensitivity to FSH, an abnormal FSH or abnormal FSH receptor, or an abnormal response of the ovary to dysrhythmic gonadotropin stimulation.[192,193]

A more generalized end-organ insensitivity disorder may be present in some patients who have the syndrome of pseudohypoparathyroidism. In these patients, target organ insensitivity to parathyroid hormone has been recognized as the most common manifestation. The defect in one form of this disorder appears to be a failure of activity of a protein that couples receptor occupancy with generation of the second message, cyclic AMP.[194] It has been noted that parathormone is clearly not the only hormone whose interaction with its target tissue is abnormal. Hypothyroidism due to apparent TSH insensitivity appears to occur commonly, and ovarian dysfunction characteristic of ovarian insensitivity is now recognized as a part of the syndrome.[195]

REFERENCES

1. Langman J: The Urogenital System. *In* Medical Embryology. 2nd ed. Baltimore, Williams & Wilkins, 1969, p 149.
2. Wiberg UH: Facts and considerations about sex-specific antigens. Hum Genet 76:207, 1987.
3. Page DC, Mosher R, Simpson EM, et al: The sex-determining region of the human Y chromosome encodes a finger protein. Cell 51:1091, 1987.
4. Baker TG: Quantitative and cytological study of germ cells in human ovaries. Proc Roy Soc 158:417, 1963.
5. Richardson GS: Ovarian physiology. New England Journal of Medicine Progress Series. Boston, Little, Brown, & Co., 1967, p 1.
6. Ross GT, Schreiber JR: The ovary. *In* Yen SSC, Jaffe RB (eds.): Reproductive Endocrinology:

Physiology, Pathophysiology and Clinical Management. Philadelphia, WB Saunders Company, 1978, p. 63.

7. Weiss L: Additional evidence of gradual loss of germ cells in the pathogenesis of streak ovaries in Turner's syndrome. J Med Genet 8:540, 1971.

8. Lippe BM: Ambiguous genitalia and pseudohermaphroditism. Pediatr Clin North Am 26:91, 1979.

9. Barr ML, Bertram EG: A morphological distinction between neurones of the male and female, and the behavior of the nucleolar satellite during accelerated nucleo-protein synthesis. Nature 163:676, 1949.

10. deGrouchy J, Turleau C: Clinical Atlas of Human Chromosomes. New York, John Wiley & Sons, 1977, p 222.

11. Gilchrist GS, Hammond D, Melnyk J: Hemophilia A in a phenotypically normal female with XX/XO mosaicism, N Engl J Med 273:1403, 1965.

12. Refetoff S, Selenkow HA: Familial thyroxine-binding globulin deficiency in a patient with Turner's syndrome (XO): Genetic study of a kindred. N Engl J Med 278:1081, 1968.

13. Ferguson-Smith MA: Karyotype-phenotype correlations in gonadal dysgenesis and their bearing on the pathogenesis of malformations. J Med Genet 2:142, 1965.

14. Palmer CG, Reichman A: Chromosomal and clinical findings in 110 females with Turner syndrome, Hum Genet 35:35, 1976.

15. Lippe BM, Crandall BF: Turner syndrome with partial deletion of the X chromosome long arm. Am J Dis Child 126:222, 1973.

16. Hoo JJ: Clinical consequence of Xp-. Hum Genet 46:349, 1979.

17. Mohandas T, Sparkes RS, Shapiro LJ: Reactivation of an inactive human X chromosome: evidence for X inactivation by DNA methylation. Science 211:393, 1981.

18. Turner HH: A syndrome of infantilism, congenital webbed neck and cubitus valgus. Endocrinology 23:566, 1938.

19. Ullrich O: Turner's syndrome and status Bonnevie-Ullrich. Am J Hum Genet 1:179, 1949.

20. Males JL, Seely JR: Turner's syndrome: Index case after 44 years (A Tribute to Dr. Henry H. Turner). J Clin Endocrinol Metab 46:163, 1978.

21. Noonan JA: Hypertelorism with Turner phenotype: A new syndrome with associated congenital heart disease. Am J Dis Child 116:373, 1968.

22. Opitz JM, Pallister PD: Brief historical note: The concept of "gonadal dysgenesis." Am J Med Genet 4:333, 1979.

23. Hook EB, Hamerton JL: The frequency of chromosome abnormalities detected in consecutive newborn studies—differences between studies. Results by sex and severity of phenotypic involvement. In Hooke B, Porter IH (eds): Population Cytogenetics. New York, Academic Press, 1977, pp 63–79.

24. Hook EB, Warburton D: The distribution of chromosomal genotypes associated with Turner's syndrome: Livebirth prevalence rates and evidence for diminished fetal mortality and severity in genotypes associated with structural X abnormalities or mosaicism. Hum Genet 64:24, 1983.

25. Carr DH, Gedeon M: Population cytogenetics in human abortuses. In Hook EB, Porter IH (eds): Population Cytogenetics. New York, Academic Press, 1977, pp 1–9.

26. Warburton D, Kline J, Stein I, et al: Monosomy X: A chromosomal anomaly associated with young maternal age. Lancet 1:167, 1980.

27. Kajii T, Ohama K: Inverse maternal age effect in monosomy X. Hum Genet 51:147, 1979.

28. Carothers AD, Frackiewicz A, DeMey R, et al: A collaborative study of the aetiology of Turner syndrome. Ann Hum Genet 43:355, 1980.

29. Pescia G, Ferrier PE, Wyss-Hutin D, et al.: 45,X Turner's syndrome in monozygotic twin sisters. J Med Genet 12:390, 1975.

30. King CR, Magenis E: Turner syndrome in the offspring of artificially inseminated pregnancies. Fertil Steril 30:604, 1978.

31. Salmon MA, Ashworth M: Association of autoimmune disorders and sex chromosome anomalies. Lancet 2:1085, 1970.

32. Cassidy SB, Niblack GD, Lorber CA, et al: HLA frequencies, diabetes mellitus and autoimmunity in Turner's patients and their relatives. Ann Genet 21:203, 1978.

33. Villaverde MM, DaSilva JA: Turner-mongolism polysyndrome: Review of the first eight known cases. JAMA 234:844, 1975.

34. Leichtman DA, Schmickel RD, Gelehrter TD, et al: Familial Turner syndrome. Ann Intern Med 89:473, 1978.

35. Casteels-Van Daele M, Proesmans W, Van den Berghe H, et al: Down's anomaly (21 trisomy) and Turner's syndrome (46,XXqi) in the same sibship. Helv Paediatr Acta 25:412, 1970.

36. Park E: Body shape in Turner's syndrome. Hum Biol 49:215, 1977.

37. Collins E: The illusion of widely spaced nipples in the Noonan and the Turner syndromes. J Pediatr 83:557, 1973.

38. Felix A, Capek V, Pashayan M: The neck in the XO and XX/XO mosaic Turner's syndrome. Clin Genet 5:77, 1974.

39. Neufeld ND, Lippe BM, Kaplan SA: Disproportionate growth of the lower extremities: A major determinant of short stature in Turner's syndrome. Am J Dis Child 132:296, 1978.

40. Beals RK: Orthopedic aspects of the XO (Turner's) syndrome. Clin Orthop 97:19, 1973.

41. Baughman FA, Higgins JV, Wadsworth TG, et al: The carrying angle in sex chromosome anomalies. JAMA 230:718, 1974.

42. Kaitila II, Leisti JT, Rimoin DL: Mesomelic skeletal dysplasias. Clin Orthop 114:94, 1976.

43. Levin B: Gonadal dysgenesis: Clinical and roentgenologic manifestations. Am J Roentgenol Rad Ther Nucl Med 87:1116, 1962.

44. Horowitz SL, Morishima A: Palatal abnormalities in the syndrome of gonadal dysgenesis and its variants and in Noonan's syndrome. Oral Surg 38:839, 1974.

45. Bercu BB, Kramer SS, Bode HH: A useful radiologic sign for the diagnosis of Turner's syndrome. Pediatrics 48:737, 1976.

46. Necic S, Grant DB: Diagnostic value of hand x-rays in Turner's syndrome. Acta Paediatr Scand 67:309, 1978.

47. van der Putte SCJ: Lymphatic malformation in human fetuses: A study of fetuses with Turner's syndrome or status Bonnevie-Ullrich. Virchows Arch Hum Pathol Anat Histol 376:233, 1977.

48. Smith DW: Recognizable Patterns of Human De-

formation. Philadelphia, WB Saunders Company, 1981, pp 119–120.

49. Vittay P, Bosze, P, Gaal M, et al: Lymph vessel defects in patients with ovarian dysgenesis. Clin Genet 18:387, 1980.

50. Horowitz SL, Morishima A, Vinkk A: The position of the external ear in Turner's syndrome. Clin Genet 9:333, 1976.

51. Reed T, Reichmann A, Palmer, CG: Dermatoglyphic differences between 45,X and other chromosomal abnormalities of Turner syndrome. Hum Genet. 36:13, 1977.

52. Lyon AJ, Preece MA, Grant DB: Growth curve for girls with Turner syndrome. Arch Dis Child 60:932, 1985.

53. Ranke MB, Pfluger H, Rosendahl W, et al: Turner syndrome: Spontaneous growth in 150 cases and review of the literature. Eur J Paediatr 141:81, 1983.

54. Brook CGD, Murset G, Zachmann M, et al: Growth in children with 45,XO Turner's syndrome. Arch Dis Child 49:789, 1974.

55. Verp MS, Rosinsky B, Le Beau MM, et al: Growth disadvantage of 45,X and 46,X, del (X)(p11) fibroblasts. Clin Genet 33:277, 1988.

56. Ikeda Y, Higurashi M, Egi S, et al: An anthropometric study of girls with Ullrich-Turner syndrome. Am J Med Genet 12:271, 1982.

57. Varrela J, Vinkka H, Alvesalo L: The phenotype of 45,X females: An anthropometric quantification. Ann Hum Biol 11:53, 1984.

58. Kaplan SL, Abrams CAL, Bell JJ, et al: Growth and growth hormone: I. Changes in serum levels of growth hormone following hypoglycemia in 134 children with growth retardation. Pediatr Res 2:43, 1968.

59. Lindsten J, Cerasi E, Luft R, Hultquist G: The occurrence of abnormal insulin and growth hormone (HGH) responses to sustained hyperglycaemia in a disease with sex chromosome aberrations (Turner's syndrome). Acta Endocrinol 56:107, 1967.

60. Brook CGD: Growth hormone deficiency in Turner's syndrome. N Engl J Med 298:1203, 1978.

61. Ross JL, Long LM, Loriaux DL, Cutler GB: Growth hormone secretory dynamics in Turner syndrome. J Pediatr 106:202, 1985.

62. Ranke MB, Blum WF, Haug F, et al: Growth hormone, somatomedin levels and growth regulation in Turner's syndrome. Acta Endocrinol 116:305, 1987.

63. Whitelaw MJ, Thomas SF, Graham W, et al: Growth response in gonadal dysgenesis to the anabolic steroid norethandrolone. Am J Obstet Gynecol 84:501, 1962.

64. Johanson AJ, Brasel JA, Blizzard RM: Growth in patients with gonadal dysgenesis receiving fluoxymesterone. J Pediatr 75:1015, 1969.

65. Rosenbloom AL, Frias JL: Oxandrolone for growth promotion in Turner syndrome. Am J Dis Child 125:385, 1973.

66. Urban MD, Lee PA, Dorst JP, et al: Oxandrolone therapy in patients with Turner syndrome. J Pediatr 94:823, 1979.

67. Lev Ran A: Androgens, estrogens, and the ultimate height in XO gonadal dysgenesis. Am J Dis Child 131:648, 1977.

68. Snider ME, Solomon IL: Ultimate height in chromosomal gonadal dysgenesis without androgen therapy. Am J Dis Child 127:673, 1974.

69. Joss E, Zuppinger K: Oxandrolone in girls with Turner's syndrome: A pair-matched controlled study up to final height. Acta Paediatr Scand 73:674, 1984.

70. Stahnke N, Lingstaedt K, Willig RP: Oxandrolone increased final height in Turner's syndrome. Pediatr Res 19:620, 1985.

71. Sybert VP: Adult height in Turner syndrome with and without androgen therapy. J Pediatr 104:365, 1984.

72. Moore DC, Tattoni DS, Ruvalcaba RHA, et al: Studies of anabolic steroids. VI: Effect of prolonged administration of oxandrolone on growth in children and adolescents with gonadal dysgenesis. J Pediatr 90:462, 1977.

73. Lenko HL, Perheentupa J, Soderholm A: Growth in Turner's syndrome: Spontaneous and fluoxymesterone stimulated. Acta Paediatr Scand Suppl 277:57, 1979.

74. Wilton P: Growth hormone treatment in girls with Turner's syndrome: A review of the literature. Acta Paediatr Scand 76:193, 1987.

75. Rudman D, Goldsmith M, Kutner M, et al: Effect of growth hormone and oxandrolone singly and together on growth rate in girls with X chromosome abnormalities. J Pediatr 96:132, 1980.

76. Rosenfeld RG, Hintz RL, Johanson AJ, et al: Three-year results of a randomized prospective trial of methionyl human growth hormone and oxandrolone in Turner syndrome. J Pediatr 113:393, 1988.

77. Anderson H, Filipsson R, Fluur E, et al: Hearing impairment in Turner's syndrome. Acta Otolaryngol Suppl 247:1, 1969.

78. Jensen K, Petersen PH, Nielsen EL, et al: Serum immunoglobin M, G, and A concentration levels in Turner's syndrome compared with normal women and men. Hum Genet 31:329, 1976.

79. Filipsson R, Lindsten J, Almquist S: Time of eruption of the permanent teeth, cephalomotric and tooth measurement and sulphation factor activity in 45 patients with Turner's syndrome with different types of X chromosome aberrations. Acta Endocrinol 48:91, 1965.

80. Szpunar J: Middle ear disease in Turner's syndrome. Arch Otolaryngol 87:34, 1968.

81. McDonough PG, Byrd RJ, Tho PT, et al: Phenotypic and cytogenetic findings in eighty-two patients with ovarian failure—changing trends. Fertil Steril 28:638, 1977.

82. King CR, Magenis E, Bennett S: Pregnancy and the Turner syndrome. Obstet Gynecol 52:617, 1978.

83. Reyes FI, Koh KS, Faiman C: Fertility in women with gonadal dysgenesis. Am J Obstet Gynecol 126:668, 1976.

84. Philip J, Sele V: 45,XO Turner's syndrome without evidence of mosaicism in a patient with two pregnancies. Acta Obstet Gynecol Scand 55:283, 1976.

85. Dewhurst J: Fertility in 47,XXX and 45,X patients. J Med Genet 15:132, 1978.

86. King CR, Magenis E: Fetal wastage and chromosome anomalies in offspring of patients with Turner syndrome. Lancet 2:928, 1977.

87. Conte FA, Grumbach MM, Kaplan SL: A diphasic pattern of gonadotropin secretion in pa-

tients with the syndrome of gonadal dysgenesis. J Clin Endocrinol Metab 40:670, 1975.

88. Illig R, Tolksdorf M, Murset G, et al: LH and FSH response to synthetic LH-RH in children and adolescents with Turner's and Klinefelter's syndrome. Helv Paediatr Acta 30:221, 1975.

89. Samaan NA, Stepanas AV, Danziger J, et al: Reactive pituitary abnormalities in patients with Klinefelter's and Turner's syndrome. Arch Intern Med 139:198, 1979.

90. Hou-Jensen K, Kempson RL: The ultrastructure of gonadoblastoma and dysgerminoma. Hum Pathol 5:79, 1974.

91. Mulvihill JJ, Wade WM, Miller RW: Gonadoblastoma in dysgenetic gonads with a Y chromosome. Lancet 1:863, 1975.

92. Scully RE: Gonadoblastoma: A review of 74 cases. Cancer 25:1340, 1970.

92. Cuseen LJ, MacMahon RA: Germ cells and ova in dysgenetic gonads of a 46-XY female dizygotic twin. Am J Dis Child 133:373, 1979.

93. Khodr GS, Cadena GD, Ong TC, et al: Y-autosome translocation, gonadal dysgenesis, and gonadoblastoma. Am J Dis Child 133:277, 1979.

94. Haddad HM, Wilkins L: Congenital anomalies associated with gonadal aplasia: Review of 55 cases. Pediatrics 23:885, 1959.

95. Goldberg MB, Scully AL, Solomon IL, et al: Gonadal dysgenesis in phenotypic female subjects. A review of eighty-seven cases, with cytogenetic studies in fifty-three. Am J Med 45:529, 1968.

96. Engel E, Forbes AP: Cytogenetic and clinical findings in 48 patients with congenitally defective or absent ovaries. Medicine 44:135, 1965.

97. Nora JJ, Torres FG, Sinha AK, et al: Characteristic cardiovascular anomalies of XO Turner syndrome, XX and XY phenotype and XO/XX Turner mosaic. Am J Cardiol 25:639, 1970.

98. Rainier-Pope CR, Cunningham RD, Nadas AS, et al: Cardiovascular malformations in Turner's syndrome. Pediatrics 33:919, 1964.

99. Clark EB: Neck web and congenital heart defects: A pathogenic asociation in 45 X-O Turner syndrome? Teratology 29:355, 1984.

100. Larco RV, Jones KL, Bernirschke K: Coarctation of the aorta in Turner syndrome: A pathologic study of fetuses with nuchal cystic hygromas, hydrops fetalis, and female genitalia. Pediatrics 81:445, 1988.

101. Gunning JF, Oakley CM: Aortic-valve disease in Turner's syndrome. Lancet 1:389, 1970.

102. Miller MJ, Geffner ME, Lippe BM, et al: Echocardiography reveals a high incidence of bicuspid aortic valve in Turner syndrome. J Pediatr 102:47, 1983.

103. Bisset GS, Schwartz DC, Meyer RA, et al: Clinical spectrum and long-term follow-up of isolated mitral valve prolapse in 119 children. Circulation 62:423, 1980.

104. Lin AE, Lippe BM, Geffner ME, et al: Aortic dilation, dissection, and rupture in patients with Turner syndrome. J Pediatr 109:820, 1986.

105. Allen DB, Hendricks SA, Levy JM: Aortic dilation in Turner syndrome. J Pediatr 109:302, 1986.

106. Price WH, Clayton JF, Collyer S, et al: Mortality ratios, life expectancy, and causes of death in patients with Turner's syndrome. J Epidemiol Commun Health 40:97, 1986.

107. Reveno JS, Palubinskas AJ: Congenital renal abnormalities in gonadal dysgenesis. Radiology 86:49, 1966.

108. Matthies F, Macdiarmid WD, Rallison M, et al: Renal anomalies in Turner's syndrome: Types and suggested embryogenesis. Clin Pediatr 10:561, 1971.

109. Litvak AS, Rousseau TG, Wrede LD, et al: The association of significant renal anomalies with Turner's syndrome. J Urol 120:671, 1978.

110. Uson AC, Braham SB, Abrams CAL, et al: Retrocaval ureter in a child with Turner's syndrome. Am J Dis Child 119:267, 1970.

111. Mesrobian H-GJ, Kelalis PP, Hrabovsky E, et al: Wilms tumor in horseshoe kidneys: A report from the National Wilms Tumor Study. J Urol 133:1002, 1985.

112. Sparkes RS, Motulsky AB: Hashimoto's disease in Turner's syndrome with isochromosome X. Lancet 1:947, 1963.

113. Pai GS, Leach DC, Weiss L, et al: Thyroid abnormalities in 20 children with Turner's syndrome. J Pediatr 91:267, 1977.

114. Germain EL, Plotnick LP: Age-related anti-thyroid antibodies and thyroid abnormalities in Turner syndrome. Acta Paediatr Scand 75:750, 1986.

115. Ling SM, Kaplan SA, Weitzmann JJ, et al: Euthyroid goiters in children: Correlation of needle biopsy with other clinical and laboratory findings in chronic lymphocytic thyroiditis and simple goiter. Pediatrics 44:695, 1969.

116. Brooks WH, Meek JC, Schimke RN: Gonadal dysgenesis with Grave's disease. J Med Genet 14:128, 1977.

117. Rosen KM, Sirota DK, Marinoff SC: Gastrointestinal bleeding in Turner's syndrome. Ann Intern Med 67:145, 1967.

118. Salomonowitz E, Staffen A, Potzi R, et al: Angiographic demonstration of phlebectasia in a case of Turner's syndrome. Gastrointest Radiol 8:279, 1983.

119. Arulanantham K, Kramer MS, Gryboski JD: The association of inflammatory bowel disease and X chromosomal abnormality. Pediatrics 66:63, 1980.

120. Price WH: A high incidence of chronic inflammatory bowel disease in patients with Turner's syndrome. J Med Genet 16:263, 1979.

121. Knudtzon J, Svane S: Turner's syndrome associated with chronic inflammatory bowel disease: A case report and review of the literature. Acta Med Scand 223:375, 1988.

122. Forbes AP, Engel E: The high incidence of diabetes mellitus in 41 patients with gonadal dysgenesis, and their close relatives. Metabolism 12:428, 1963.

123. Nielsen J, Johansen K, Yde H: The frequency of diabetes mellitus in patients with Turner's syndrome and pure gonadal dysgenesis. Acta Endocrinol 62:251, 1969.

124. National Diabetes Data Group: Classification and diagnosis of diabetes mellitus and other categories of glucose intolerance. Diabetes 28:1039, 1979.

125. Rimoin DL, Harder E, Whitehead B, et al: Abnormal glucose tolerance in patients with gonadal dysgenesis and their parents. Clin Res 18:395, 1970.

126. Karp M, Snir A, Doron M, et al: Glucose tolerance tests and insulin response in juvenile pa-

tients with gonadal dysgenesis. Mod Probl Paediatr 12:251, 1975.

127. Neufeld ND, Lippe B, Sperling MA: Carbohydrate (CHO) intolerance in gonadal dysgenesis: A new model of insulin resistance. Diabetes 25(Suppl):379, 1980.

128. Polychronakos C, Letarte J, Collu R, et al: Carbohydrate intolerance in children and adolescents with Turner syndrome. J Pediatr 96:1009, 1980.

129. Wilson DM, Frane JW, Sherman B, et al: Carbohydrate and lipid metabolism in Turner syndrome: Effect of therapy with growth hormone, oxandrolone, and a combination of both. J Pediatr 112:210, 1988.

130. Garron DC: Intelligence among persons with Turner's syndrome. Behav Genet 7:105, 1977.

131. Nielsen J, Fischer M, Friedrich U: Mental retardation in Turner's syndrome. J Ment Defic Res 17:227, 1973.

132. Silbert A, Wolff PH, Lilienthal J: Spatial and temporal processing in patients with Turner's syndrome. Behav Genet 7:11, 1977.

133. Nyborg H, Nielsen J: Sex chromosome abnormalities and cognitive performance: III. Field dependence, frame dependence, and failing development of perceptual stability in girls with Turner's syndrome. J Psychol 96:205, 1977.

134. Waber DP: Neuropsychological aspects of Turner's syndrome. Dev Med Child Neurol 21:58, 1979.

135. Rovet J, Netley C: Processing deficits in Turner's syndrome. Dev Psychol 18:77, 1982.

136. Garron DC, Van der Stoep LP: Personality and intelligence in Turner's syndrome. Arch Gen Psychiatry 21:339, 1969.

137. McCauley E, Ito J, Kay T: Psychosocial functioning in girls with Turner's syndrome and short stature: Social skills, behavior problems, and self-concept. J Am Acad Child Psychiatry 25:105, 1986.

138. McCauley E, Sybert V, Ehrhardt AA: Psychosocial adjustment of adult women with Turner syndrome. Clin Genet 29:284, 1986.

139. Kron L, Katz JL, Gorzynski G, et al: Anorexia nervosa and gonadal dysgenesis: Further evidence of a relationship. Arch Gen Psychiatry 34:332, 1977.

140. Kauli R, Gurewitz R, Galazer A, et al: Effect of anorexia nervosa on gonadotropin secretion in a patient with gonadal dysgenesis. Acta Endocrinol 100:363, 1982.

141. Gottschalk M, Lippe BM, Frane JW: Turner syndrome: Delayed diagnosis when short stature is the predominant finding. Clin Res 37:184A, 1989.

142. Navot D, Laufer N, Kopolovic J, et al: Artificially induced endometrial cycles and establishment of pregnancies in the absence of ovaries. N Engl J Med 314:806, 1986.

143. Ho ECK, Moss AJ: The syndrome of "mesenteric arteritis" following surgical repair of aortic coarctation: Report of nine cases and review of the literature. Pediatrics 49:40, 1972.

144. Crawford JD: Management of children with Turner's syndrome. *In* The Management of Genetic Disorders. New York, Alan R. Liss, 1979, pp 97–109.

145. Levine LS: Treatment of Turner's syndrome with estrogen. Pediatrics 62:1178, 1978.

146. Cutler BS, Forbes AP, Ingersol FM, et al: Endometrial carcinoma after stilbestrol therapy in gonadal dysgenesis. N Engl J Med 287:628, 1972.

147. Gray PH, Anderson T, Munnell EW: Endometrial adenocarcinoma and ovarian agenesis: Report of a case. Obstet Gynecol 35:513, 1970.

148. Ostor AG, Fortune DW, Evans JH, et al: Endometrial carcinoma in gonadal dysgenesis with and without estrogen therapy. Gynecol Oncol 6:316, 1978.

149. Krishnamurthy S, Adcock LL, Okagaki T: Endometrial carcinoma following estrogen-progestogen therapy in Turner's syndrome: A case report and review of the literature. Gynecol Oncol 5:291, 1977

150. Louka MH, Ross RD, Lee JH, et al: Endometrial carcinoma in Turner's syndrome. Gynecol Oncol 6:294, 1978.

151. Chan L, O'Malley BW: Mechanism of action of the sex steroid hormones. N Engl J Med 294:1430, 1976.

152. Benjamin I, Block RE: Endometrial response to estrogen and progesterone therapy in patients with gonadal dysgenesis. Obstet Gynecol 50:137, 1977.

153. Dewhurst CJ, DeKoos EB, Haines RM: Replacement hormone therapy in gonadal dysgenesis. Br J Obstet Gynaecol 82:412, 1975.

154. Padwick ML, Pryse-Davies J, Whitehead MI: A simple method for determining the optimal dosage of progestin in postmenopausal women receiving estrogens. N Engl J Med 315:930, 1986.

155. Chetkowski RJ, Meldrum DR, Steingold KA, et al: Biologic effects of transdermal estradiol. N Engl J Med 314:1615, 1986.

156. Harnden DG, Stewart JSS: The chromosomes in a case of pure gonadal dysgenesis. Br Med J 2:1285, 1959.

157. Nazareth HR de S, Farah, LMS, Cunha AJB, et al: Pure gonadal dysgenesis (Type XX): Report on a family with four affected sibs. Hum Genet 37:117, 1977.

158. Pallister PD, Opitz JM: The Perrault syndrome: Autosomal recessive ovarian dysgenesis with facultative, non-sex-limited sensorineural deafness. Am J Med Genet 4:239, 1979.

159. Judd HL, Scully RE, Atkins L, et al: Pure gonadal dysgenesis with progressive hirsutism: Demonstration of testosterone production by gonadal streaks. N Engl J Med 282:881, 1970.

160. Sternberg WH, Barclay DL, Kloepfer HW: Familial XY gonadal dysgenesis. N Engl J Med 278:695, 1968.

161. German J, Simpson JL, Chaganti RSK, et al: Genetically determined sex-reversal in 46,XY humans. Science 202:53, 1978.

162. Wachtel SS: The dysgenetic gonad: Aberrant testicular differentiation. Biol Reprod 22:1, 1980.

163. Rose LI, Underwood RH, Williams GH, et al: Pure gonadal dysgenesis: Studies of in vitro androgen metabolism. Am J Med 57:957, 1974.

164. Amarose AP, Kyriazis AA, Dorus E, Azizi F: Clinical, pathologic, and genetic findings in a case of 46, XY pure gonadal dysgenesis (Swyer's syndrome). I. Dysgerminoma and gonadoblastoma. Am J Obstet Gynecol 127:824, 1977.

165. Hall BD, Spranger JW: Campomelic dysplasia: Further elucidation of a distinct entity. Am J Dis Child 134:285, 1980.

166. Drash A, Sherman F, Hartman WH, Blizzard RM: A syndrome of pseudohermaphroditism, Wilms' tumor, hypertension, and degenerative renal disease. J Pediatr 76:585, 1970.

167. Eddy AA, Mauer SM: Pseudohermaphroditism, glomerulopathy, and Wilms tumor (Drash syndrome): Frequency in end-stage renal failure. J Pediatr 106:584, 1985.

168. Bialer MG, Penchaszadeh VB, Kahn E, et al: Female external genitalia and mullerian duct derivatives in a 46,XY infant with the Smith-Lemli-Opitz syndrome. Am J Med Genet 28:723, 1987.

169. Hamerton JL, Canning N, Ray M, et al: A cytogenetic survey of 14,069 newborn infants. I. Incidence of chromosome abnormalities. Clin Genet 8:223, 1975.

170. Smith HC, Seale JP, Posen S: Premature ovarian failure in a triple X female. J Obstet Gynecol Br Commonw 81:405, 1974.

171. Neri G: A possible explanation for the low incidence of gonosomal aneuploidy among the offspring of Triplo-X individuals. Am J Med Genet 18:357, 1984.

172. Collen RJ, Falk RE, Lippe BM, Kaplan SA: A 48,XXXX female with absence of ovaries. Am J Med Genet 6:275, 1980.

173. Gardner RJM, Veale AMO, Sands VE, et al: XXXX syndrome: Case report, and a note on genetic counselling and fertility. Human Genetik 17:323, 1973.

174. Monheit A, Francke U, Saunders B, et al: The penta-X syndrome. J Med Genet 17:392, 1980.

175. Russell P, Altshuler G: The ovarian dysgenesis of trisomy 18. Pathology 7:149, 1975.

176. Hansen J, Boyar RM, Shapiro LR: Gonadal function in trisomy 21. Horm Res 12:345, 1980.

177. Kennedy JF, Freeman MG, Benirschke K: Ovarian dysgenesis and chromosomal abnormalities. Obstet Gynecol 50:13, 1977.

178. Edmonds M, Killinger DW, Volpe R: Autoimmune thyroiditis, adrenalitis and oophoritis. Am J Med 54:782, 1973.

179. Vasquez AM, Kenny FM: Ovarian failure and antiovarian antibodies in association with hypoparathyroidism, moniliasis, Addison's and Hashimoto's diseases. Obstet Gynecol 41:414, 1973.

180. Coulam CB, Ryan RJ: Prevalence of circulating antibodies directed toward ovaries among women with premature ovarian failure. Am J Reprod Immunol Microbiol 9:23, 1985.

181. Irvine WJ, Cahn MMW: Immunological aspects of premature ovarian failure associated with Addison's disease. Lancet 2:883, 1968.

182. Kuki S, Morgan RL, Tucci JR: Myasthenia gravis and premature ovarian failure. Arch Intern Med 141:1230, 1981.

183. Collen RJ, Lippe BM, Kaplan SA: Primary ovarian failure, juvenile rheumatoid arthritis, and vitiligo. Am J Dis Child 133:598, 1979.

184. Sanders JE, Pritchard S, Mahoney P, et al: Growth and development following marrow transplantation for leukemia. Blood 68:1129, 1986.

185. Livesey EA, Brook CGD: Gonadal dysfunction after treatment of intracranial tumors. Arch Dis Child 63:495, 1988.

186. Chapman RM, Sutcliffe SB, Malpas JS: Cytotoxic-induced ovarian failure in women with Hodgkin's disease: I. Hormonal function. JAMA 242:1877, 1979.

187. Siris ES, Leventhal BG, Vaitukaitis JL: Effects of childhood leukemia and chemotherapy on puberty and reproductive function in girls. N Engl J Med 294:1143, 1976.

188. Parra A, Santos D, Cervantes C, et al: Plasma gonadotropins and gonadal steroids in children treated with cyclophosphamide. J Pediatr 92:117, 1978.

189. Kaufman FE, Kogut MD, Donnell GN, et al: Hypergonadotropic hypogonadism in female patients with galactosemia. N Engl J Med 304:994, 1981.

190. Skre H, Bassoe HH, Berg K, et al: Cerebellar ataxia and hypergonadotrophic hypogonadism in two kindreds. Chance concurrence, pleiotropism or linkage. Clin Genet 9:234, 1976.

191. Jones GS, DeMoraes-Ruehsen M: A new syndrome of amenorrhea in association with hypergonadotropism and apparently normal ovarian follicular apparatus. Am J Obstet Gynecol 104:597, 1969.

192. Evers JLH, Rolland R: The gonadotrophin resistant ovary syndrome: A curable disease? Clin Endocrinol 14:99, 1981.

193. Maxson WS, Wentz AC: The gonadotropin resistant ovary syndrome. Semin Reprod Endocrinol 1:147, 1983.

194. Farfel Z, Brickman AS, Kaslow HR, et al: Defect of receptor-cyclase coupling protein in pseudohypoparathyroidism. N Engl J Med 303:237, 1980.

195. Wolfsdorf JI, Rosenfield RL, Fang VS, et al: Partial gonadotrophin-resistance in pseudohypoparathyroidism. Acta Endocrinol 88:321, 1978.

10

THE TESTES: Disorders of Sexual Differentiation and Puberty

Dennis M. Styne

Since nonhuman primates and other mammals have hermaphroditic conditions we can be assured that early *Homo sapiens* suffered from the same disorders that are described below. The term *hermaphrodite* was first used in the third century BC and derives from the greek legend of Hermaphroditos, the son of Hermes and Aphrodite, admired by the nymph Salamacis, who so embraced him that, as Ovid wrote, they became permanently joined in a "single form, possessed of a dual nature, which could not be called male or female, but seemed to be at once both and neither."[1]

While the term *hermaphrodite* had not yet been coined, the first recorded mention of ambiguous genitalia is found on a Babylonian tablet from the seventh century BC on which was written: "When a woman gives birth to an infant that has no well marked sex, calamity and affliction will seize upon the land; the master of the house shall have no happiness."

Perhaps that is why Livy found that in 207 BC at Frusina (Italy) a baby of indeterminate sex was said to be "a disgusting and disgraceful portent" so that it was cast alive into the sea in a chest. We can take only small comfort that Pliny the Elder (171 BC) stated that "We call them Hermaphroditos. Formerly they were called androgynos and they were regarded as portents, but now they are regarded correctly as amusements." Presumably, being only amusements, the children were not put to physical death, but must have suffered great psychological trauma. Certainly our views have changed little in the last 2000 years, judging from the type of carnival side show exhibits that travel the country.

We now know that *intersexuality*, the general term for the conditions mentioned above, can be caused by a wide range of disorders of sexual differentiation. The testes or the adrenal glands are in most cases of major importance in the pathophysiology of the state, and the testes will therefore be a major focus of this chapter. We also consider the physiology and disorders of male puberty so that the continuum of development from conception to the attainment of reproductive capacity may be viewed.

NORMAL SEXUAL DIFFERENTIATION

The pioneering work of Jost developed the framework of our understanding of sexual differentiation. He demonstrated that a castrated mammalian fetus develops as a normal infantile phenotypic female.[2] At the stage where both wolffian and müllerian ducts coexist, high-dose testosterone crystals placed at the location of the ablated testes served to stimulate ipsilateral wolffian (male) duct development but had no effect on the müllerian (female) ducts, which remained. Jost thus established that an as-yet undiscovered testicular factor, a factor other than testosterone, was fundamental in normal male sexual development. This, added to the recently revealed understanding of the importance of the Y chromosome in male development, established the overall pattern of normal sexual development, a pattern we are ever closer to explaining in detail. We presently accept that in normal circumstances, chromosomal sex determines gonadal sex, which establishes phenotypic sex, which, possibly in conjunction with the response of the outside world to the phenotypic sex, determines gender identity of the individual. Each of these factors can go awry in disorders of sexual differentiation and each is considered in turn.

Chromosomal Sex

The human genome is contained within 22 paired autosomes and two sex chromosomes, the X and the Y chromosomes.[3] Chromosomes are classically studied by arraying them in the diploid metaphase state and staining them for various characteristics. Quinacrine mustard stains for fluorescent Q bands and Giemsa reagent is used to stain the centromeric region as C bands or stain the rest of the chromosome by a technique, resulting in G bands (Fig. 10–1). The distal end of the long arm of the Y chromosome also fluoresces brightly with quinacrine staining.[4] New techniques such as prome-

taphase banding can reveal abnormalities not seen on metaphase analysis.[5]

The Y Chromosome

The relatively small Y chromosome contains only 0.5 to 1.0 per cent of the diploid human genome and more than 50 per cent of the DNA sequences are repeated. Nonetheless, the genetic material contained on the short arm is crucial to sexual differentiation. The Y chromosome physically resembles the short acrocentric autosome in the chromosomes of group 6–12. The size of the Y chromosome varies in an inherited pattern between normal men, with most of the variation due to modification of the distal end of the long arm; the Y chromosome does not show great conservation of sequences between species or within individuals of the human species.[6] Part of this area of the long arm of the Y chromosome is fluorescent and accounts for the Y chromatin body; although originally this fluorescence

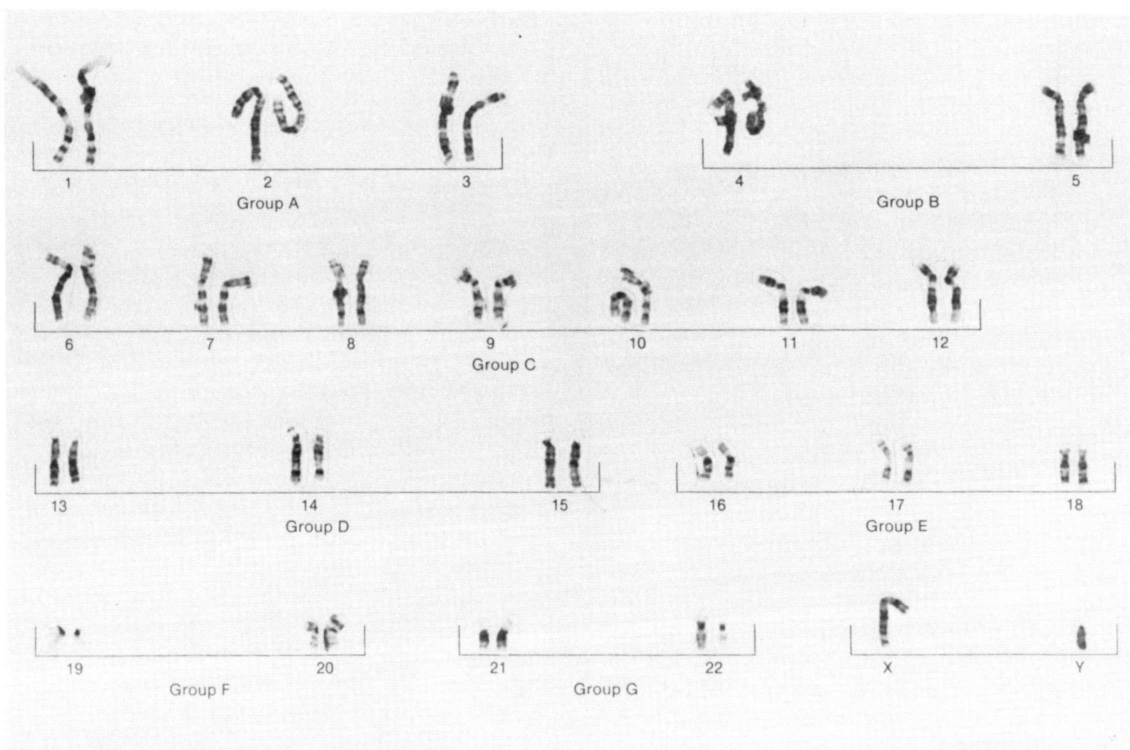

FIGURE 10–1. The normal chromosome constitution of a male analyzed on a Giemsa-stained prophase preparation. There are 22 paired autosomes and an X and a Y chromosome. The prophase method allows the delineation of more bands than the standard method, but the longer chromosomes tend to cross and tangle more. (Figure courtesy of cytogenetics laboratory, University of California Medical Center, Sacramento, CA.)

seemed a key to the detection of the Y chromosome in patients with ambiguous genitalia, the fluorescent Y body is absent in less than 1 per cent of normal men who have normal testes, indicating that it is not essential for testes formation.[7] One Y chromosome (45,Y) or two Y chromosomes without an X chromosome (46,YY) is incompatible with life; there must be at least one accompanying X chromosome in every individual. A succession of techniques has proved useful in studying the structure and activity of the Y chromosome over more than 50 years. Painter, in 1923, was the first to histologically note the presence of the Y and X chromosomes.[8] It was not until 1959 that it became evident that the presence of a Y chromosome caused male sexual development and the absence of a Y chromosome caused female development.[9] Exceptions to this rule became apparent when XX males and XY females were encountered. With the discovery that some deletions of the Y chromosome caused disorders of sexual differentiation and others did not, it was suggested that only a fragment of the Y chromosome was active in sexual determination. Methods of investigation of these fragments, such as simple karyotyping, banding, or fluorescent staining, all proved inadequate for the task, and new methods of studying the Y chromosome were developed.

The H-Y Antigen. An observation by Eichenwald and Silmser in 1955 laid the groundwork for the recognition of the H-Y antigen; they noted that skin transplants from males of a highly inbred mice strain were rejected by females of the same strains, although male-to-male or female-to-male transplants took.[10] In 1971, Goldberg et al. suggested that the H-Y antigen, which was also present in sperm, was responsible for such rejections.[11] Subsequently a wealth of evidence was produced to suggest that the H-Y antigen was the sex-determining antigen of the heterogametic gonad and was associated with the major histocompatibility antigens [in humans, the human leukocyte antigen (HLA) system].[12] Female inbred mice to which male skin is transplanted develop antibody to the H-Y antigen, and this phenomenon has been utilized for various types of serologic assays utilizing cytotoxicity, hemadsorption, hemagglutination, radiobinding, and other phenomena.[13] Because of the proliferation of techniques, results from different laboratories are not always comparable and indeed different "H-Y" antigens may be measured in different assays. H-Y antigen exhibits phylogenetic conservation and is found in XY female mice with testicular feminization, in XX male mice carrying the Sxr gene (sex-reversed gene), and in over 71 mammalian species and some lower phyla. The H-Y antigen, rather than the Y chromosome itself, was suggested to be the basis of testicular differentiation.[14]

Numerous intersex conditions express the H-Y antigen and further strengthened its presumed role in sexual differentiation. Thus, H-Y antigen is found by serologic testing in: the syndrome of androgen insensitivity, 17α-hydroxylase deficiency, 17β-hydroxysteroid dehydrogenase deficiency, 5α-reductase deficiency, and the syndrome of persistent müllerian structures. In some cases a reduced level of H-Y antigen is detected—for example, in 46,XX males, in some cases of 46,XX true hermaphroditism, in some cases of 46,XY gonadal dysgenesis and indeed in some cases of 45,X gonadal dysgenesis.[15] The genes for the H-Y antigen have been tentatively located in the short arm of the Y and of the X chromosomes.[16] H-Y antigen appears to be a protein of 17,000 daltons that binds to receptors on the gonads.

In vitro experiments have demonstrated that the bipotential gonad, when exposed to the H-Y antigen, will develop tubular structures similar to seminiferous tubules, but will develop into solid structures similar to follicles without the H-Y antigen.[17] H-Y antigen is present in epididymal fluid, apparently secreted from Sertoli cells of the testes. Receptors for the H-Y antigen are found on the gonad, with the majority of uptake noted in the homogametic gonad (ovary: XX in the human) presumably because there is full occupancy of the receptors in the heterogametic gonad (testis: XY in the human). Fetal bovine or murine gonads could be transformed into testicle-like cords after exposure to H-Y antigen. This is suggested as an explanation for the case of the freemartin, an originally female twin bovine fetus that becomes virilized and sterile and has testicularized ovaries as a result of its exposure to testosterone and H-Y antigen produced by the twin male fetus; these reach the freemartin by the common circulation of the twin fetuses.[18]

There are, however, studies that cast doubt upon the theory that the H-Y antigen is the primary factor in testes development.[19,20] Discrepancies are reported between the results of serologic H-Y typing and skin graft or cytotoxic T cell typing techniques, calling into question the common identity of the serologic H-Y antigen and the transplantation antigen detected by cytotoxic assays. Further, more cases of animals with testes but without expression of the H-Y antigen and non-testes-containing animals with H-Y antigen present are reported. It has been suggested that the H-Y antigen is important in spermatogenesis.[21] The actual role of the H-Y antigen in testes determination remains to be clarified.

The Testes-Determining Factor. Although the major portion of the Y chromosome does not undergo meiotic recombination, the distal end of the short arm of the Y chromosome (p), known as the pseudoautosomal region because of its recombinant behavior, does so with the distal short arm of the X chromosome.[22] Because of the lack of recombination over most of the length of the Y chromosome, it is not been possible to construct a classic genetic linkage map of the Y chromosome as has been done for the autosomes. Using an alternative technique of hybridization of restriction digested genomic DNA fragments to Y-DNA probes (Southern transfers), numerous patients with Y chromosome deletions were studied and a deletion map of the Y chromosome was constructed.[23] Eight deletion intervals of the Y chromosome were found, with interval 1 located close to the pseudoautosomal region; it appeared sufficient to cause testes differentiation because it was present in all patients with testes and was not present in those without testes. Further analysis mapped this fragment to the 1A2 region and a nucleotide probe (found in plasmid pDP1007) detected a highly conserved locus on both the mammalian Y and X chromosomes. The fragment on the X chromosome was also located on the short arm (p21–p22.3). This is the first time that similar DNA sequences were noted on both Xp and Yp, with the exception of the pseudoautosomal regions of X and Y. The highly conserved nature of the sequence suggests that it does not represent a pseudogene.

The action of the testes-determining factor (TDF) sequence on the X chromosome is unknown, but one scheme suggests that one active copy of the TDF is required to allow testicular formation: an XX female will inactivate one TDF copy according to the Lyon hypothesis, while an XY, an XXY, or other multiple X individual will retain one copy of the TDF to allow testes development. The presence of a 1.2-kilobase pair (kb) open reading frame indicates that this region of the Y chromosome codes for a protein and the predicted sequence contains a cysteine and histidine–rich protein that assumes a tetrahedral structure that binds a zinc cation, allowing the intervening residues to form a DNA-binding loop.[24] This predicted structure suggests that the TDF exerts its effects within the cell of origin, rather than being secreted to interact with a cell surface receptor of another cell.

The TDF gene maps to a different region of the Y chromosome than the gene expressing the H-Y antigen. In addition, the two gene products apparently act at different sites in the cell.

The TDF has not been found in XX true hermaphrodites nor in a few XX males. This suggests that testes may differentiate in the absence of the sex-determining portion of the Y chromosome and may develop as a result of autosomal or X-linked gene mutations downstream of the cascade of activity that starts with TDF.[25] It remains possible that the H-Y antigen is one of those factors that acts downstream of TDF. At present available evidence suggests that the sequence at 1A2 is the TDF.

The X Chromosome

The X chromosome is much longer than the Y and resembles the autosome of chromosome group 6–12: the X chromosome contains 5 per cent of the total DNA of the genome and shows a high degree of sequence conservation through evolution. Two X chromosomes are required for ovarian differentiation because 45,XO individuals have the streak gonads characteristic of Turner syndrome; further, an X chromosome is necessary in any karyotype having a Y chromosome because a 45,Y karyotype is a fatal anomaly. Regulatory or structural genes for the H-Y antigen and a gene for the cytosolic androgen receptor are present on the X chromosome. The long and sort arms of the X chromosome contain genes necessary for ovarian function, but the short arm appears to have genes necessary to prevent the short stature and the physical stigmata of 45,X Turner syndrome.[26]

Numerous other genes are contained on the X chromosome that are sex linked but not directly associated with sexual development. Thus, on the long arm of the X chromosome there are genes for hypoxanthine phoshoribosyltransferase, glucose-6-phosphate dehydrogenase, phosphoglycerate kinase, α-galactosidase, color blindness, hemophilia A, adrenoleukodystrophy, the site of the fragile X syndrome, and others.[27] In the pseudoautosomal region of the X chromosome there are genes for steroid sulfatase, XGa red cell antigen, and a H-Y–regulating gene.[28]

Except for the pseudoautosomal region, one of the two X chromosomes undergoes degeneration to assure that only one dose of X chromosome material is active in all cells: ova are exempt from this rule because both X chromosomes are necessary to allow normal ovarian development. This dosage compensation is dictated by the Lyon hypothesis, and the inactivated X chromosome forms the heteropycnotic region that stains darkly on the nuclear envelope, the Barr body.[29,30] Structurally abnormal X chromosomes are inactivated, as are all X chromosomes, after the first 12 to 18 days after fertilization; patients with an XX karyotype will have one Barr body, as will those with an XXY karyotype; those with an XY karyotype will have no Barr body; and those with an XXXY karyotype will have two Barr bodies. The inactivated chromosome will replicate later than the other X chromosome, and a structurally abnormal X chromosome will always be the last to replicate.[31] Trisomy of an autosome, such as chromosome 21 or 18, leads to striking physical abnormalities, whereas inactivation of extra X chromosomes leads to relatively few physical stigmata in an individual with an XXX or XXXX karyotype.

Gonadal Development

The bipotential fetal gonad begins as a thickening along the ventral cranial region of the mesonephros or primitive kidney at the 5-mm stage.[32] This gonadal ridge is located at the lower thoracic region. Mesenchymal cells invade this area early in gestation and give rise to the gonads, although celomic epithelium may also contribute to gonadal development. Primordial germ cells are found in the 4.5-day blastocyst[33] and in the yolk sac of the 17-day embryo. They migrate, assisted by ameboid motion, through the mesentery to the gonads.[34] Although there is some cell division during the

migration, once in the gonads the germ cells undergo mitosis and rapidly multiply; most of those that do not reach the gonad disappear but a minority are postulated to serve as precursors for extragonadal germ cell tumors postnatally.[35]

Testicular Development

Testicular development will occur in the presence of TDF prior to 9 weeks of gestation. In the absence of TDF, or if TDF is present only after the critical window of 9 weeks of gestation passes, an ovary will develop.[36]

The first stage of testicular differentiation is the formation of testicular cords consisting of Sertoli cell precursors packed tightly around germ cells, which are the future prespermatogonia or spermatogonia; this occurs between 6 and 7 weeks of development in the human fetus, fully 1½ months before the histologic differentiation of the ovary.[37] The cords remain in contact with the mesonephros until the remnant of the mesonephros itself turns into cords, the rete testis. The testicular cords soon retract from the celomic epithelium, which then forms an epithelium with an intact basal lamina, a structure that develops into the tunica albuginea. The presence of germ cells does not appear to be necessary for the formation of the testicular cords.

The diploid germ cells, the prespermatogonia, may undergo meiosis in the fetal testes, but they soon become quiescent and remain in meiotic arrest until puberty.[38] It is interesting to note that the ova in the fetal ovary undergo meiosis at a developmental stage when the fetal prespermatogonia enter the quiescent phase; it has been suggested that the mesonephros produces a meiosis-stimulating substance while the Sertoli cells produce a meiosis-inhibiting substance.[39] Numerous germ cells degenerate even if they reach the relative safety of the testicular cords.

Sertoli cells provide a location for support and proliferation of spermatogonia as well as a source of protein products for secretion; follicle-stimulating hormone (FSH) stimulates Sertoli cell metabolic activity. Sertoli cells are derived from the mesonephros and proliferate only during fetal life and in the neonatal period. When spermatogenesis begins, mitoses are no longer evident. The fetal and neonatal Sertoli cells are, as noted, the source of (antimüllerian factor) (AMF) while the adult Sertoli cell synthesizes sex hormone–binding globulin and inhibin. There are numerous physiologic similarities between Sertoli cells and granulosa cells: they are derived from the same embryonic tissue, they each have receptors for FSH and androgens, they each produce identical proteins such as inhibin and tissue plasminogen activator, they both synthesize estrogen from testosterone by FSH stimulation of aromatase activity, and both types of cells influence the development of the adjacent germinal cells.[40]

Leydig cells are the source of sex steroid production in the testes. They are derived from extracordal mesenchymal tissue soon after the testicular cords are formed, at about day 60, and make up more than 50 per cent of the volume of the testes by 14 to 16 weeks, the time of peak human chorionic gonadotropin (hCG) production.[41] As steroid producing cells, they develop smooth endoplasmic reticulum and increased numbers of mitochondria. Mitotic figures are rare in later development, so that the increase, and later decrease, in the number of Leydig cells with advancing gestation appears to be due to differentiation of Leydig cell precursors or regression of formed Leydig cells rather than cell division. The increase in the number of Leydig cells with development may be triggered by hCG or, later, fetal gonadotropins; the paucity of Leydig cells in anencephalic fetuses at term supports this contention.[42] Leydig cell numbers are reduced strikingly after birth and Leydig cells are difficult to visualize histologically until puberty.

The formation of a round shape of the testes is an important step in minimizing the feminizing effects of the mesenchymal tissue; forcing a mouse testis to remain in close contact with mesonephros causes diminished formation of testicular cords, premature meiosis of germ cells, and a toxic effect upon the testes.

Descent of the Testes. Testicular descent mainly occupies the last two thirds of gestation and can be divided into three stages.[43] In the first stage of testicular descent the peritoneal fold that attaches the testis to the abdominal wall degenerates and the gubernaculum (the ligament attaching the inferior part of the testes to the lower segment of the scrotum) shortens.[44] As the abdominopelvic region is growing rapidly, the testis is brought down to the anterior inguinal region. The increasing intra-abdom-

inal pressure then causes a herniation of the abdominal wall next to the inferior portion of the gubernaculum and thereby forms the processus vaginalis which then folds around the gubernaculum and forms the inguinal canal. Finally, the gubernaculum increases to the diameter of the testis, the proximal gubernaculum degenerates, drawing the testis into the scrotum through the processus vaginalis, and the proximal processus vaginalis degenerates, leaving the remaining processus vaginalis membranes to form the tunica albuginea.

Normal testes descend by the seventh month of gestation, so that 97.3 per cent of full-term infants and 79 per cent of premature infants have normally descended testes at birth.[45] During the first year there is a further incidence of descent of the testes, so that by 9 months of age 99.2 per cent of male infants have descended testes: the incidence of descended testes in young adult males rises to 99.8 per cent, suggesting little likelihood of a continuing incidence of spontaneous testicular descent after 9 months.[46] The right testis is more often undescended than the left.[47] Whichever testis is undescended in unilateral cryptorchidism, the contralateral testis usually undergoes compensatory hypertrophy to a larger than normal size for age.[48] Remarkably, some testes that are descended or retractile may ascend and become undescended testes 1 to 10 or more years after birth; a patent processus vaginalis may allow this phenomenon to occur in retractile testes and the processus may develop adhesions, trapping the testes in the undescended position.[49]

Histologic changes within undescended testes appear to occur only after 12 months of age.[50] The majority of undescended testes are inguinal; only one fourth are intra-abdominal.

The prevalence of retractile testes, which rise and fall within the inguinal canal, is unknown, but probably substantial: the inclusion of these patients in which the testes reside within the scrotum an appreciable portion of time into series of cryptorchid males may affect the conclusions drawn from such studies. It has been considered that retractile testes do not undergo the pathologic changes of undescended testes, but it has recently been shown that retractile testes that cannot descend below the upper part of the scrotum have decreased testicular volume, seminiferous tubule diameter, and numbers of spermatogonia compared to the contralateral descended testes. This observation suggests that there is a place for surgical treatment of retractile testes. Infertility is reported in adults with retractile testes.[51,52]

Lack of descent of the testes, or cryptorchidism, is associated with a 10-fold increase in the incidence of neoplasia in the affected testis[53]; it is generally assumed that this occurs as a result of damage to the testes caused by the increased temperature in the abdomen or high in the canal. Several lines of evidence suggest, however, that there is an intrinsic tendency for a cryptorchid testis to undergo malignant degeneration: (1) one third of carcinomas occurring in cryptorchid testes occurred after the orchiopexy was performed[54]; (2) in 20 per cent of patients with both a testicular carcinoma and cryptorchidism, the contralateral, descended testis was neoplastic[55]; and (3) the incidence of carcinoma in cryptorchid testes increases dramatically if the testes remain undescended during the growth phase of the testes prior to 10 years of age.[56]

Ovarian Development

While there is no histologic ovarian formation for more than a month after testicular differentiation, there is multiplication of the primordial germs cells, the precursors of the oogonia. At 12 weeks of gestation the fetal ovary begins to secrete estrogens.[57] The mesonephric tubules transform into the rete ovarii and infiltrate the gonadal area. The rete secretes a meiosis-inducing substance and, beginning at 11 to 12 weeks, peaking at 20 to 25 weeks, but continuing occasionally until 28 to 39 weeks, the oogonia enter meiotic prophase and become oocytes.[58] There are 6 to 7 million oocytes at peak development, but subsequent degeneration leads to only 2 million oocytes left at term in normal girls.[59] Follicles develop as granulosa cells form spheres around the oocytes under the stimulation of fetal gonadotropins; anencephalic fetuses have poorly or undeveloped follicles.

Phenotypic Sexual Development

Secretory Products of the Testes in Sex Determination

Antimüllerian Factor. Antimüllerian factor is produced by the fetal testes at a cru-cial time to cause the regression of the müllerian ducts that would ordinarily form the fallopian tubes, the uterus, and the upper part of the vagina.[60] It is a glycoprotein hormone dimer of 123,000 daltons that can be separated into monomers of 72,000 daltons with an isoelectric point of 6.0.[61] It is produced by the Sertoli cells of the seminiferous tubules. There is controversy as to whether AMF production is maximal only during the time of müllerian duct sensitivity or whether AMF secretion continues for some time thereafter; it appears that AMF secretion decreases by several months after birth to extremely low levels, detectable by only the most sensitive techniques.[62] The ovarian granulosa cells secrete AMF into follicular fluid in a manner similar to the analogous male Sertoli cells; the biologic role of AMF in the female is unknown, but clearly different than that of the male.[63] There is a narrow window of early responsiveness of müllerian ducts to AMF: limited data in the human fetus suggest lack of responsiveness by the 30-mm crown-rump length stage, with responsiveness noted at the 25-mm stage.[64] Antimüllerian factor appears to dissolve the basal membrane and cause mesenchymal condensation around the müllerian duct. There follows an important interaction as the epithelial cells diminish in number and the mesenchyme predominates in the area. Extracellular matrix constituents located near the basement membrane disappear just before the membrane itself disappears.[65] The superior part of the müllerian duct in the male becomes the appendix testis. Animal experiments show that diethylstibestrol antagonizes the effects of AMF upon müllerian ducts.[66]

Gonadal Steroids. Testosterone is the primary sex steroid produced by fetal and postnatal mammalian testes, with dihydrotestosterone (DHT) and estradiol the next most important steroid products, although precursors to these steroids are also secreted.[67] The adult testes secrete about 6 mg of testosterone per 24 hours, which indicates that the 25 µg of testosterone stored in a testes must turn over more than 200 times each day. Testosterone production commences with the histologic differentiation of the Leydig cells, just after the formation of the testicular cords.[68] Evidence from the rabbit suggests that early testosterone secretion is independent of gonadotropin stimulation, but such evidence is unavailable in the human fetus.[69] It is known that luteinizing hormone (LH) and hCG can stimulate human fetal testicular tissue at the 12th week of gestation, but this is after the major portion of sexual differentiation has occurred. It is clear that testosterone production thereafter, in the phase of penile growth, is gonadotropin dependent.[70]

The initial steps of gonadal sex steroid production are identical to those for glucocorticoid production; the final stages are where distinct testicular enzymes come into play.[71] Thus cholesterol is taken up as low-density lipoproteins (LDL) by receptor-mediated endocytosis and either stored or converted to free cholesterol to allow steroid synthesis. A series of enzymatic reactions follows, mainly utilizing the cytochrome P450 oxidases that reduce atmospheric oxygen with electrons donated from NADPH. The first step is rate limiting and involves the three activities of 20-hydroxylation, 22-hydroxylation, and cleavage of the side chain of cholesterol between carbon atoms 20 and 22; these tasks are accomplished by the P450scc (side-chain cleavage) enzyme, a mitochondrial enzyme responsive to hCG and previously called 20, 22-desmolase. The electron transfer to P450scc follows the path from NADPH to a flavoprotein named adrenodoxin reductase to the iron-sulfur protein adrenodoxin to the P450scc. Messenger RNA (mRNA) for insulin-like growth factor (IGF) II rises in parallel with mRNA for P450scc with stimulation of fetal testes, suggesting a paracrine role for IGF II in the steroidogenic process.

The pregnenolone resulting from the first step may be 17-hydroxylated by the P45017 enzyme in the endoplasmic reticulum to yield 17-hydroxypregnenolone and the 17-hydroxypregnenolone can then undergo 3β-hydroxysteroid dehydrogenation and isomerization to form 17-hydroxyprogesterone. Alternatively, pregnenolone can undergo 3β-hydroxysteroid dehydrogenation and isomerization of the double bond from the B ring to the A ring, thereby changing a Δ^5 compound (pregnenolone) to a Δ^4 compound (progesterone); the enzyme catalyzing this has not be characterized to date. The progesterone molecule can then be 17-hydroxylated in the same manner as pregnenolone to yield 17-hydroxyprogesterone. The P45017 enzyme that can 17-hydroxylate pregnenolone and progesterone has a second effect, that of lysing the 17-20 bond in 17-hydroxypregnenolone or in 17-hydroxyprogesterone, yielding dehydroepiandros-

terone (DHEA) or androstenedione, respectively. If DHEA, a Δ^5 compound, is produced, it can undergo transformation via 3β-hydroxysteroid dehydrogenase to a Δ^4 compound, androstenedione.

The steps listed above occur both in the adrenal gland and the gonad, whereas the steps that follow occur only in the testis (or ovary). Androstenedione may be converted to testosterone by the non-P450 enzyme variously called 17-ketosteroid reductase, 17-oxidoreductase, and 17β-hydroxysteroid dehydrogenase, which can also convert estrone to estradiol, and DHEA to androstenediol. Aromatase or P450aro, a P450 enzyme located in the endoplasmic reticulum, converts C_{19} androgenic steroids to C_{18} estrogenic steroids by two hydroxylations at the C_{19} methyl group and a third at the C_2 location with a loss of the C_{19} and aromatization of the A ring. Finally, testosterone may be converted to DHT, the active form that affects the sexual skin and other specific areas, by 5α-reductase, which is not a P450 enzyme. The human fetal testis has the greatest abundance of P450scc and P450c17 at 14 to 15 weeks of gestation and low values by 26 weeks of gestation, suggesting regulation by hCG, which follows a similar temporal pattern.[72] These enzymatic mRNAs are found in only minimal amounts in the fetal ovary, and this finding confirms the minimal role of this organ in fetal steroidogenesis.[73]

Testosterone exerts some direct effects upon the internal wolffian ducts and many other areas of the body, but the virilization of the external genitalia and the development of the penile urethra and prostate are caused by 5α-reduced testosterone or dihydrotestosterone (DHT).[74] This reduction occurs in cells containing the enzyme 5α-reductase after testosterone diffuses into the cell. After either DHT or testosterone binds to high-affinity receptor proteins, the complex undergoes transformation into a form that can interact with nuclear chromatin, which in turn causes increased transcription of structural genes and the appearance of mRNAs leading to translation and the appearance of new proteins, an anabolic effect. Several lines of evidence have demonstrated that the embryonic mesenchyme (stroma) contains androgen receptors and that this site of androgen action is the first that occurs during the formation of the male urogenital tract.[75]

More than 44 per cent of circulating testosterone is bound to sex hormone–binding globulin, while another 54 per cent is bound to albumin and other proteins; only 2 per cent or less is in the free form.[76] While it is the free form that is active, the time of transport through an organ and the half-life of dissociation from the binding proteins both play roles in the availability of testosterone to an organ, and probably more than 2 per cent of testosterone reaching an organ actually exerts bioactivity.

More than 90 per cent of testosterone and its metabolites are excreted in the urine. The products are 17-ketosteroids (40 per cent of total testosterone produced is excreted in this manner) and polar metabolites (50 per cent of total excreted). Testosterone may be irreversibly metabolized to DHT (6 to 8 per cent of total testosterone secretion is so converted), or be acted upon by aromatase to produce estradiol (0.3 per cent of total testosterone is so converted).[77] In the adult male, of an average total of 45 μg/day of estradiol produced, 17 μg are derived from aromatization of circulating testosterone, 22 μg from conversion of the far weaker estrogen estrone, and 6 μg from direct secretion of estradiol from the testes.[78] Approximately 300 μg of DHT per day is produced from 5α-reduction of plasma testosterone.

Development of the Internal Ducts

The wolffian ducts (named for Caspar Freidrich Wolff, who in 1759 noted the kidney progenitors in a chick embryo), or mesonephric ducts, first appear at 24 days as solid rods.[79] At 26 days, the rods become hollow and are attached to the cloaca, the terminal portion of the hindgut.[80] By 28 days, or soon thereafter, the wolffian ducts open in the ventral cloaca. The ventral cloaca gives rise to the urogenital sinus and the rectum and, as pressure increases within the wolffian ducts, the urogenital sinus ruptures to make an anterior opening. The wolffian ducts begin as the excretory ducts of the mesonephros but acquire androgen dependency after this time. The müllerian ducts (named for Johannes Müller, who first wrote about the structures) are also known as the paramesonephric ducts, because of their course parallel to the wolffian ducts.[81] They form at the sixth week from the caudal end of the mesonephros and elongate, possibly guiding the accompanying mesonephric ducts in their course to the urogenital

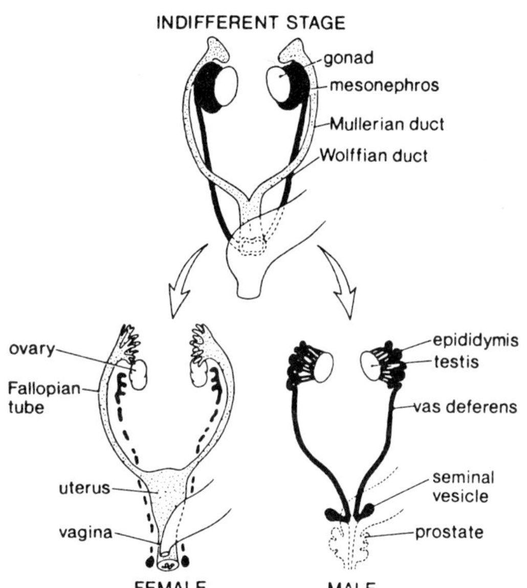

FIGURE 10–2. The differentiation of the internal genital ducts in the male and female. (Reproduced with permission of Dr. J. Wilson.)

sinus.[82] They are located in the tissue destined to become the broad ligament in the female. The paramesonephric ducts reach the urogenital sinus and fuse, outside first and inside thereafter, by the eighth week. Thus, prior to 8 weeks of gestation, the internal sexual ducts are bipotential, with both müllerian (or paramesonephric) and wolffian (or mesonephric) ducts present. This concludes the embryonic period, which lasts until the eigth week of gestation in the human; the fetal period follows.

Soon after the formation of testicular cords, AMF is produced and causes the regression of the müllerian ducts, except for the rostral end, which becomes the appendix testes. Shortly thereafter, the fetal Leydig cells begin the production of testosterone, which reaches locally high concentrations by diffusion, and stimulates growth and differentiation of the wolffian ducts into the epididymis and rete testes at the cranial end, and the vas deferens and seminal vesicles at the other[83] (Fig. 10–2). A portion of the remaining mesonephric duct between the seminal vesicle and the urethra develops into the ejaculatory duct. The prostate originates as a series of endodermal buds that are located off the urethra.[84]

In the absence of testosterone and AMF, the septum dividing the müllerian ducts at the ventral ends, which have already fused, canalizes. The vaginal plate forms to initially block the canal between the uterine lumen and the urogenital sinus, but later desquamates so that the canal becomes continuous.[85] The cervix is considered to be derived from the paramesonephric ducts while the urogenital sinus contributes to the lower portion of the vagina.[86] The upper portion of the paramesonephric ducts become the fallopian tubes. In the female, the wolffian ducts atrophy and the only remaining trace is Gartner's ducts. Because the internal male ducts are responsive to testosterone, normal internal male development does not require the conversion of testosterone to DHT, as does the development of the external genitalia. Abnormalities of the embryologic development of the ducts and their subsequent maturation lead to numerous types of congenital defects discussed late in the chapter.

These clear developmental patterns can be altered by accidents of nature or by the ingestion of exogenous agents. Thus a true hermaphrodite with a testis on one side and an ovary on the other will exhibit wolffian development and müllerian regression on the side with the testis and relatively normal female development on the other. A patient with a digenetic testes and inadequate AMF secretion may have müllerian structures of variable degrees present in addition to well-developed wolffian structures. Alternatively, a male with androgen resistance will produce AMF and have no müllerian structures, while the androgen resistance will preclude normal development of the wolffian ducts. A female with congenital adrenal hyperplasia will have endogenous androgen secretion but insufficiently high local testosterone concentrations to allow stimulation of wolffian structures; because she will have no AMF to cause regression of the müllerian structures she will have normal female internal ducts.

Development of the External Genitalia

Soon after the virilization of the internal sexual ducts of the male, development of the external genitalia commences at about 9 weeks; it is completed by 13 weeks of gestation.[87] In the presence of high concentrations of DHT, the anorectal distance increases and the genital tubercle, the bipotential predecessor to either a clitoris or a penis, elongates to become the corpora cavernosa and the glans penis[88] (Fig. 10–3) The scrotum forms by the midline fusion of

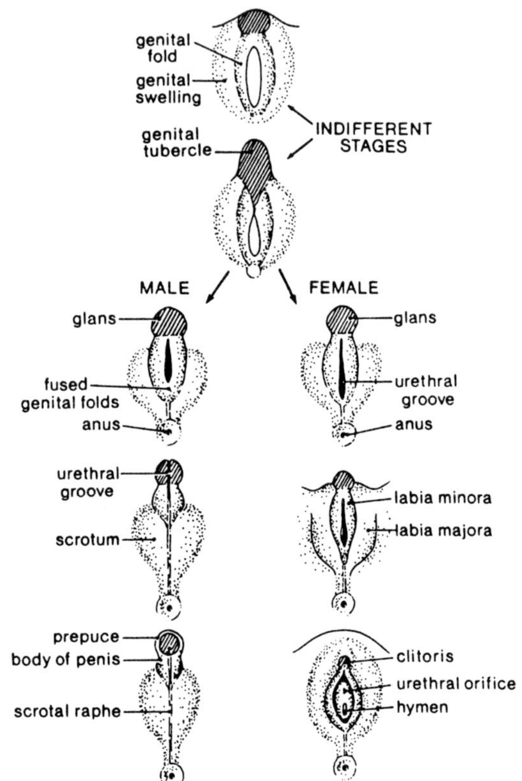

FIGURE 10–3. The differentiation of the external genitalia of the male and female. (Reproduced, with permission of Dr. J. Wilson.)

the two urogenital swellings. The bilateral urethral folds fuse over the urethral groove posteriorly to anteriorly at the penile raphe to form an enclosed penile urethra. The dorsal mesenchyme of the penis organizes into the paired corpora cavernosa and the ventral mesenchyme surrounds the urethra to form the corpus spongiosum. The formation of the penis and scrotum is complete by approximately 13 weeks and even extremely high concentrations of testosterone after this time cannot cause midline fusion of the urethral grove or scrotum, although the clitoris will enlarge. The urogenital sinus becomes the prostate and the bulbourethral glands under the influence of DHT. The vagina disappears in the male when the müllerian ducts are resorbed, although a prostatic utricle, the remains of the vagina, can be demonstrated by cystoscopy or contrast radiography.

In the absence of, or resistance to, DHT, the genital tubercle remains a clitoris, the urethral folds form the labia minora, the genital swellings form the labia majora and the urogenital sinus becomes the urethra and the lower one third of the vagina. In the female, the vesicovaginal septum enlarges and forms an opening of the vagina separate from the urethra.[89]

At the 13th week, the penis is about the same size as the clitoris.[90] Because of testosterone production from the fetal testes, the male penis grows much larger than the female clitoris. The testes are initially stimulated by hCG, which, although a maternal hormone, crosses the placenta in adequate amounts to exert a biologic effect upon the testes. As hCG concentration falls during the progression of gestation, fetal gonadotropins take over the role of testicular stimulation in the male. Because the gonadotropins do not cross the placenta, a fetus affected with hypothalamic gonadotropin deficiency will experience little testicular stimulation in the last two trimesters and the penis, although well formed, will be quite small.

Psychological Aspects of Sexual Differentiation: Gender Identity, Gender Role, Sexual Orientation, and Parenting

The role of nature versus nurture in the determination of personality, intelligence, and gender identity has been long debated. There is continuing controversy over the role of prenatal virilization in the determination of sexual dimorphism in behavior, sexual preference, and ideology in human beings.

Aromatization of testosterone to estradiol is the mode of androgen action in the hypothalamus and other areas of the brain.[91] Substantial evidence has been presented that prenatal virilization of the brain in rats changes lifelong patterns of gonadotropin secretion and sexual behavior.[92] While many binding studies have been done in rodents, few studies have been done on the human brain, and these have shown that there are no or few such receptors between 14 and 21 weeks of gestation.[93] Thus a mechanism for an effect of sex steroids upon the developing fetal human being is not established.

The factors constituting gender development are: *gender identity*, said to be firmly established by 18 to 24 months of age, the experience of one's self as male, female, or ambivalent; *gender role*, the behavior or activities indicating to others or self the degree to which an individual is male, female, or ambivalent: *adult sexual orientation*, the choice of gender of sexual objects; and *parenting*, the desire and capacity for child caretaking (an important trait for the survival of a species).[94] The study of intersexuality becomes confusing unless we clearly understand that an individual's gender identity is not based upon chromosomes, gonads, or internal ducts. Thus a 46,XY phenotypic female with androgen resistance having sexual relations with a 46,XY phenotypic male cannot be considered a homosexual individual, as would a 46,XY phenotypic male having sexual relations with another 46,XY phenotypic male.

Studies of girls with congenital adrenal hyperplasia (CAH) and prenatal androgenization, and other situations in which girls experience the prenatal administration of androgen, suggest that exposure to prenatal androgens causes a change in gender role expressed in increased physical activity levels, preference for boy playmates, tomboyism (expressed by themselves and others around them), a feeling that it may be more fun to be a boy, a preference for choosing a career as being more important or equal in importance to marriage, less of an interest in appearance and less preference in wearing a dress than pants, less interest in doll play, less interest in being pregnant, less interest in infant care, and less interest in wedding play than a control group of normal girls.[95] In most cases the girls retained a female gender identity, but recent data on a small group of patients shows a higher than expected incidence of bisexuality and homosexuality in prenatally virilized girls with CAH.[96] The boys with CAH had no observable differences from the control group of boys and had a heterosexual preference.[97] While these studies and others indicate that prenatal androgen exposure masculinizes gender role and possibly (but not definitely) sexual choice, the activities observed are within normal limits in the viewpoint of the 1980s as compared to the 1960s to 1970s, when the earlier investigations were performed. Studies of genotypic males with androgen resistance and female phenotype demonstrated unequivocal female gender role and identity, suggesting that lack of prenatal androgen effect allows a perfectly normal female gender development.[98] Girls with Turner syndrome who have lower levels of testosterone than normal girls (due to the lack of ovarian androgen secretion in Turner syndrome) seemed less interested in active play than matched female controls:

gender role and identity were unequivocally female and activity levels appeared more polarized away from male than seen in normal females.[99]

Other studies of children exposed to progesterone in utero demonstrated a tendency for males to be less active, suggesting that the progesterone antagonized the effects of the normal androgen secretion of the fetus.[100] A recent study comparing a small group of boys with significant idiopathic adolescent gynecomastia to a control group of males with CAH demonstrated an increased incidence of effeminate behavior (and increased teasing from peers) in early life and homosexuality and bisexuality later in the gynecomastia group compared to the CAH boys or normal boys; this has been interpreted to show that boys with gynecomastia, who the authors suggest are more sensitive to or produce more active estrogens, exhibit a lower degree of masculinization of their brain and therefore have a sexual preference less directed to the opposite sex.[101] Reports have been published in which differences in hormone levels or responses to stimulation were found in homosexual individuals compared to heterosexual individuals,[102] but widespread acceptance of the data or of its significance is lacking.

Studies of children with 5α-reductase deficiency, who are raised as girls but physically virilize at puberty, and can purportedly switch from a normal female to a normal male gender role and gender identity at the time of puberty, have been interpreted to show that prenatal androgen exposure directs the ultimate determination of gender identity and that gender identity can be changed even as late as the teenage years. Other studies on other groups of 5α-reductase–deficient individuals suggest that societal pressures exert far more influence than prenatal hormones in these patients.[103]

There is no apparent relationship between prenatal hormones and sexual orientation and parenting behavior.

The controversy on effects of prenatal virilization during a sensitive time period upon postnatal behavior in human beings and the subsequent interaction of social factors with this influence still must be resolved. It has been suggested that we not look at "whether or not hormones influence the development of the human brain but rather how experience interacts with the neural substrate to overcome or reinforce the organizational effects of gonadal steroids."[104]

The ovarian secretion of estrogen is discussed in Chapter 8. There appears to be little effect of the presence or absence of ovarian estrogen secretion in female sexual development.

ABNORMALITIES OF SEXUAL DIFFERENTIATION

Ambiguous Genitalia

The embryology described above demonstrates the continuum between development of male and female external genitalia. It is possible for a patient to have an appearance of a slightly virilized female or a slightly underdeveloped male, but it will become obvious in the following discussion that such appearances are not diagnostic of a specific condition; in fact it will become clear that even normal female (or occasionally normal male with "undescended testes") external genitalia are not diagnostic of a normal female (or occasionally a normal male) gonad or karyotype. However, there is a point at which it is no longer possible to categorize the individuals as normal males or females; these patients have ambiguous genitalia (Fig. 10–4). Rather than having a penis with a penile urethra or a clitoris they have the appearance of a phallic structure (often with ventral cordee binding downward) with a urethral opening on the ventral surface, generally at the base of the phallic structure. Rather than having a scrotum or labia majora they have rough, pigmented rugated scrotalized labia and instead of having a median raphe or an open vagina they have posterior fusion of the "vaginal" opening so that only a slitlike vaginal opening remains. Internally, rather than having complete absence or presence of the vesicovaginal septum, they will have a urogenital sinus of some size. Again it must be emphasized that all patients described above with normal male or female genitalia, with almost normal female or male genitalia, or with perfectly ambiguous genitalia can have a wide range of disorders; a difference in the completeness of an enzymatic block or the degree of function of the androgen receptor will account for the variability in appearance of different affected individuals.

Classification of these disorders is complex and several methods have been rec-

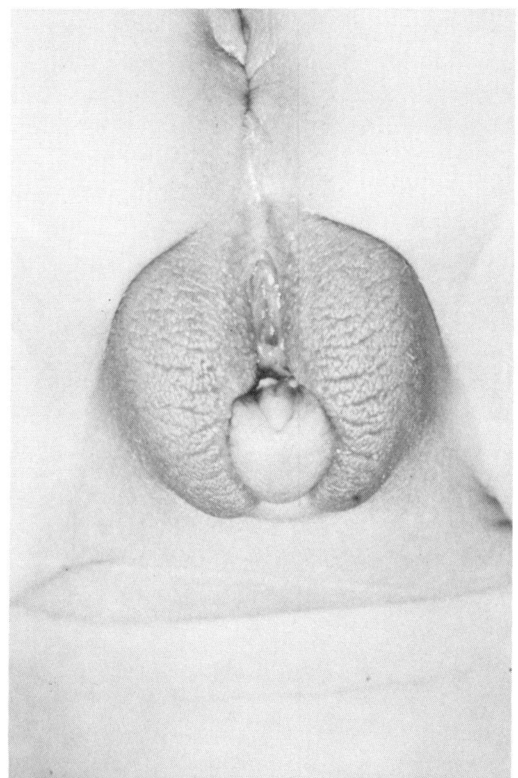

FIGURE 10–4. An example of ambiguous genitalia in a newborn. The phallic structure (actually an enlarged clitoris) is over 2 cm in length, and the perineal opening (actually a virilized vagina) is slitlike, with posterior fusion and a urogenital sinus. The labia majora are pigmented and rugated and appear to be an empty bifid scrotum. This 46,XX patient has congenital adrenal hyperplasia as a result of 21-hydroxylase deficiency but the appearance is ambiguous. An appearance similar to this may be found in most of the intersex conditions detailed in this chapter.

ommended. This discussion follows a classification of disorders of sexual differentiation based upon karyotype and gonad.[105]

Gonadal Disorders

True Hermaphroditism

The presence of both testicular and ovarian tissue in the same individual is necessary for the diagnosis of true hermaphroditism.[106] This condition is rare in the United States and Europe, but is the most common intersex condition in blacks of southern Africa.[107,108] Familial forms of true hermaphroditism are reported in Africa and elsewhere.[109]

The ovarian tissue must contain oocytes for the diagnosis to be true hermaphroditism. Presence only of ovarian stroma is an inadequate criterion. There may be a testis on one side and an ovary on the other (lateral; 30 per cent of patients), a testis or ovary on one side and an ovotestis on the other (unilateral; 50 per cent of patients), or bilateral ovotestes or even bilateral ovary and testes combinations (20 per cent of patients).[110] There is more often a testis on the right side than on the left side. The internal sexual ducts will be determined by the amount of functional testicular tissue. Secretion of AMF on one side will cause some degree of müllerian regression and the local secretion of high concentrations of testosterone will cause development of the wolffian ducts on the same side as the testis. If only an ovary is present on one side, there is a likelihood of a fallopian tube being present on that side with at least a hemiuterus. Approximately one half of patients develop a uterus, and the most common abnormality in uterine development is the absence of a cervix.[111]

The external genitalia are almost always ambiguous, although relatively normal male or female appearance is possible (Fig. 10–5). Testosterone secretion during the fetal period causes posterior fusion of the vagina, if a vagina has not been obliterated. Hypospadias, cryptorchidism, and often an inguinal hernia that contains either a gonad or a müllerian remnant may occur.

At puberty, breast development and menses often occur. Ovulation, pregnancy, and childbirth are reported in 46,XX true hermaphrodites, but no true hermaphrodites have exhibited male fertility.[112]

The majority of true hermaphrodites (75 per cent) have been raised in a male gender role because of the external appearance of the genitalia. However, over 50 per cent of patients have a 46,XX karyotype, with others demonstrating 46,XY, 46,XX/46,XY chimerism and still others having various types of mosaicism.[113] About 50 per cent of 46,XX true hermaphrodites demonstrate strong expression of the H-Y antigen and another 40 per cent decreased expression, while at least one subject had no such expression. No reported cases had detectable testes determining factor as defined above. It is suggested that patients with testes must have an autosomal or X-linked mutation whose products act with or downstream of TDF. The lack of the TDF sequence in XX true

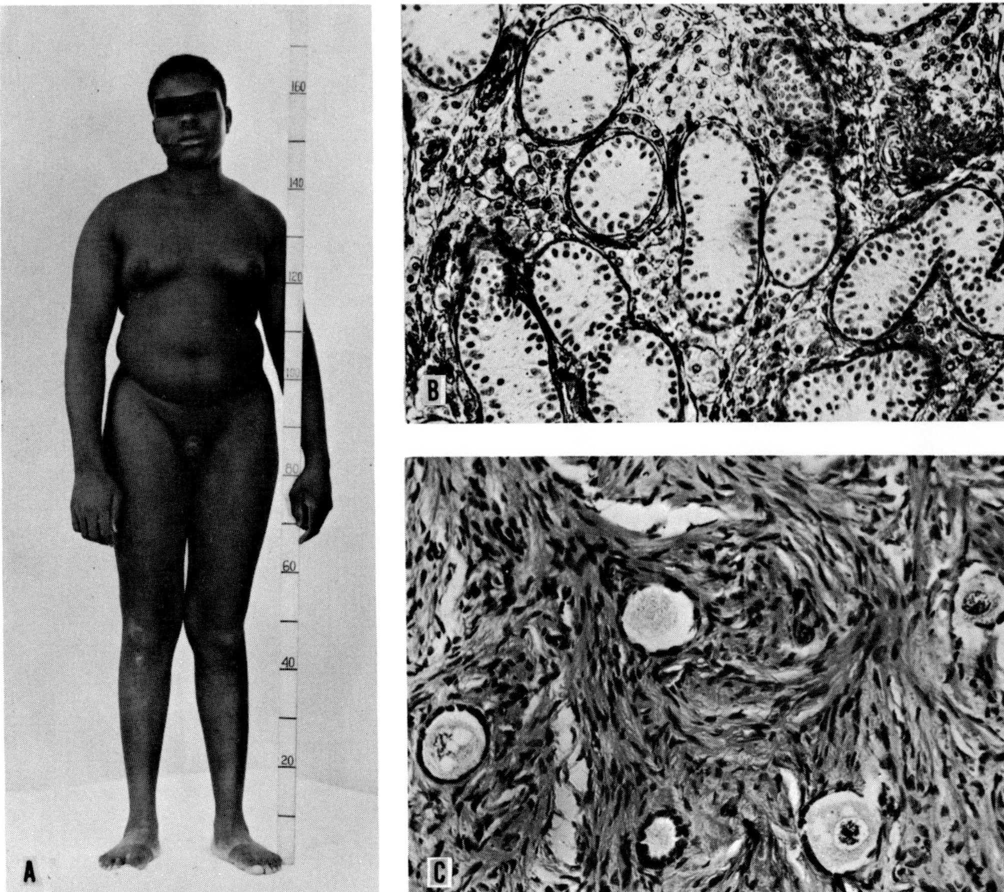

FIGURE 10–5. *A,* A 17-year-old true hermaphrodite with bilateral scrotal ovotestes, perineal hypospadias (partially repaired in the photograph), moderate bilateral gynecomastia and pubic hair (recently shaved in picture), sparse axillary hair, and no facial hair. The voice was high pitched. At operation there was a male type of urethra, bilateral scrotal fallopian tubes and ovotestes, and rudimentary bicornate uterus and vagina attached to the posterior urethra.

Photomicrographs show histopathology of demarcated ovarian and testicular portion of one ovotestis: *B,* immature seminiferous tubules lined with Sertoli cells and spermatogonia and Leydig cells; *C,* ova and follicles. (From Grumbach MM, Barr ML: Cytologic tests of chromosomal sex in relation to sexual anomalies in man. Recent Prog Horm Res 14:255, 1958, with permission.)

hermaphrodites contrasts with its presence in XX males and demonstrates the differing origins of the two conditions.

The diagnosis of true hermaphroditism will be made by the histologic examination of the gonads in a patient with ambiguous genitalia or evidence of heterosexual pubertal development. The newborn with the diagnosis of true hermaphrodism will have a gender identity assigned based upon the appearance of the external genitalia (adequacy of phallic length or difficulty of constructing a vagina) and the (unlikely) possibility of functional internal gonads. A patient over 18 months of age will generally have sexual structures and gonads removed or modified to conform with the gender identity already assigned. Thus, a patient to be raised as a female should have all testicular tissue removed and external genitalia altered to more closely appear female. A patient assigned a male gender identity should have ovaries and müllerian derivatives removed. All dysgenetic testicular tissue should be removed because of the high risk of tumor formation, especially in the ovotestes. However, if an intact and apparently normal testis is present, it may be retained if watched regularly for malignant degeneration. At the time of puberty, exogenous sex steroid therapy is indicated if the patient has not retained a function isosexual gonad.

Klinefelter Syndrome

Klinefelter syndrome, or the syndrome of seminiferous tubular dysgenesis, is the most common cause of testicular failure, with an incidence of 1:1000 males.[114] As a result of variable Leydig cell function, testosterone levels in affected patients vary from low to close to normal, so the onset of puberty often occurs at a normal age, but secondary sexual changes do not progress to the normal adult stage.[115] In all cases, seminiferous tubular function is impaired and absent spermatogenesis results. Before the onset of puberty, arm span is increased just as upper-to-lower segment ratio is decreased for age. Many prepubertal patients come to diagnosis as a result of personality disorders and mental retardation.[116] Prepubertal patients have small testes but the histology is generally normal at that age, except for a progressive tendency toward decreased numbers of spermatogonia. With the onset of puberty,

gonadotropin concentrations in the serum increase. The seminiferous tubules hyalinize and exhibit fibrosis, and there are adenomatous changes of the Leydig cells and impaired spermatogenesis.[117] Fertility has not been reported in the absence of a mosaic karyotype in Klinefelter syndrome. In puberty or in the adult, the testes are hard and small with length less than 3.5 cm, and histologic changes of hyalinization and fibrosis of the seminiferous tubules are found. Obvious gynecomastia is common in pubertal or adult subjects, probably as a result of an increased estradiol-to-testosterone ratio, and there is an increased incidence of breast carcinoma in Klinefelter syndrome.[118] The increased limb growth leads to a significantly decreased upper-to-lower segment ratio (less than 0.9 in Caucasians) and a tendency to tall stature[119] (Fig. 10–6). The relative lack of testosterone causes elevated serum LH and the lack of inhibin causes FSH to be especially elevated to castrate levels.

There is an increased incidence of advanced maternal age in the mothers of pa-

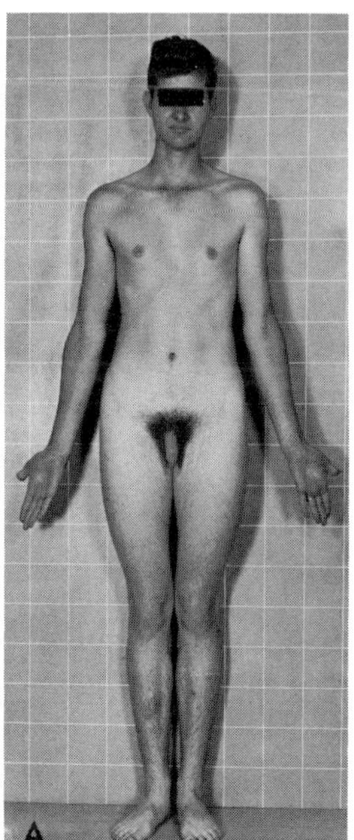
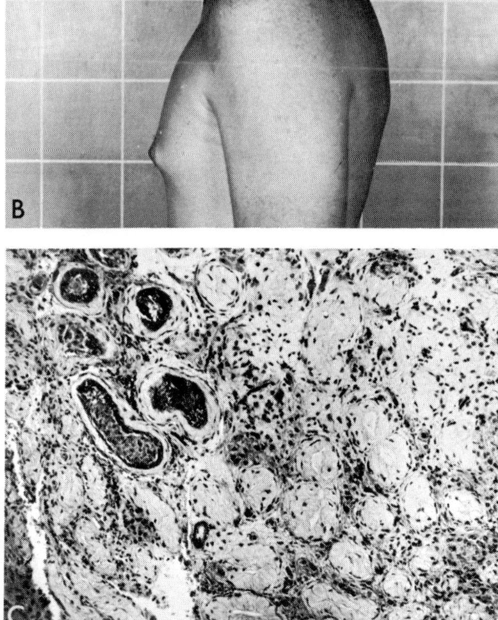
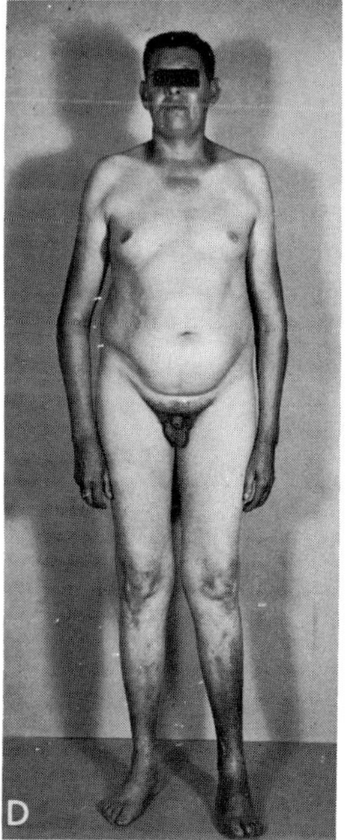

FIGURE 10–6. *A,* A 19-year-old with the syndrome of seminiferous tubule dysgenesis (Klinefelter syndrome). Karyotype was 47,XXY, gonadotropins were elevated, and testosterone levels were low-normal. Note normal virilization with long legs and (*B*) gynecomastia. Testes were small and firm and measured 1.8 × 0.9 cm. Testicular biopsy (*C*) revealed a severe degree of hyalinization of seminiferous tubules and Leydig cell "hyperplasia." *D,* A 48-year-old male with Klinefelter syndrome who came to medical attention because of severe leg varicosities. (From Grumbach MM, Conte FA: Disorders of sexual differentiation. *In* Wilson JD, Foster DW, (eds): Williams Textbook of Endocrinology. Philadelphia, WB Saunders Company, 1985, with permission.)

tients with Klinefelter syndrome.[120] It may be that the long diplotene stage of the maternal ovum predisposes to nondisjunction during the first or second meiotic prophase. There is evidence that both X chromosomes originate from the mother in more than 60 per cent of cases. In others, there may be mitotic nondysjunction in the fertilized ovum or meiotic nondysjunction during spermatogenesis.

Klinefelter syndrome is treated with androgen replacement as necessary (see "Treatment of Delayed Puberty" later in this chapter).

Numerous variants of Klinefelter syndrome are reported, with mosaicisms such as XY/XXY karyotypes or XXYY, XXXY, and XXXXY karyotypes.[121] XY/XXY mosaics have less obvious manifestations of Klinefelter syndrome and fertility has been reported in some of these patients. The other variants tend to have more severe mental retardation than found in XXY patients. Some, such as XXXXY patients have associated anomalies such as radioulnar synostoses, small genitalia and testes, unusual facies with prognathism, hypertelorism, strabismus, and other features, and severe mental retardation.

XX Males

More than 135 46,XX patients with a male phenotype are reported, but estimates of this karyotype appearing in 1:20,000 to 1:30,000 male infants are proposed.[122] It appears that there is transfer of part of the Y chromosome including the TDF sequence to the tip of the X chromosome during paternal spermatogenesis in some of these patients[123] and they have one maternal X and one paternal X chromosome; XX males are analogous to the sxr mouse model. Other explanations such as the loss of a Y chromosome in early development are also possible in some cases. XX males have H-Y antigen expression at lower levels than XY males.

Patients may have undescended testes (15 per cent) and hypospadias (10 per cent) and usually have small testes that may be soft early in life but become harder with age. Testicular histology reveals no spermatogonia, decrease in the diameter of the seminiferous tubules, and Leydig cell hyperplasia, similar to that in Klinefelter syndrome. However, these patients are shorter than those with Klinefelter syn-

drome, and in fact have heights and weights less than 46,XY phenotypic males in their families. They have less mental impairment than is found in Klinefelter syndrome. Testosterone production in the basal state and after hCG is low whereas gonadotropin secretion in the basal and gonadotropin-releasing hormone (GnRH)-stimulated states are high.

Turner Syndrome

Turner syndrome is described elsewhere (chapter 9). Patients lack a normal X chromosome (45,X karyotype) and their ovaries degenerate into streak structures. In the classic case, the phenotype is infantile female and does not strictly qualify as an abnormality of sexual differentiation. However, in patients with a Y cell line (45,X/46,XY, etc.) the genitalia may range from ambiguous to male and they have a strong predisposition to the development of a gonadal tumor as a result of testicular dysgenesis.

Fifteen cases have been reported of 45,X males who did not have mosaicism with a Y chromosome line. They do not have the physical characteristics of Turner syndrome but have normal male genitalia except for small and hard testes. At least two such patients had the TDF sequence transferred to autosome 15: thus the presence of TDF in a 45,X individual allowed the development of at least partially functioning testes.

Noonan (Pseudo-Turner) Syndrome

In pseudo-Turner syndrome (Noonan syndrome) an XY karyotype is found in male subjects (and an XX karyotype in females). The incidence is about 1:8000 live births.[124] This is a dominantly inherited condition with some features similar to Turner syndrome, such as webbed neck, ptosis, short stature, wide carrying angle of the arms, and lymphedema. There are also features different from Turner syndrome, such as triangular-shaped facies, pectus excavatum, right-sided heart disease such as pulmonic stenosis (Turner patients have left-sided heart disease such as coarctation of the aorta), and commonly, mental retardation (45,X patients usually have normal mentation). Affected males may have undescended testes that are often functionally impaired in testosterone and sperm production and may therefore have delayed puberty.

XX and XY Gonadal Dysgenesis

XX and XY gonadal dysgenesis, sometimes called pure gonadal dysgenesis, may be sporadic or familial.[125] Stature is normal and none of the dysmorphic features of Turner syndrome are present, although the gonads appear as streaks in both types of conditions. Eunuchoid proportions are common.

The phenotype is that of a sexually infantile female and the internal ducts are female in XX gonadal dysgenesis.[126] Rarely, there is some virilization as a result of androgen secretion from hilar cells of the ovary. Familial forms of XX gonadal dysgenesis follow an autosomal recessive pattern with variable effects on ovarian development; they may range from streaklike to hypoplastic ovaries. The autosomal pattern points out the importance of autosomes in the formation of the ovaries. Sensorineural deafness is found in some kindreds.[127] Other reported associations are microcephaly, arachnodactyly, renal failure, adrenal hyperplasia, primary hypogonadism as well as hypogonadotropic hypogonadism, mental retardation, myopathy, and cerebral ataxia. Gonadotropins are elevated and sex steroids low. Of course, amenorrhea is a feature.

XY gonadal dysgenesis leads to taller stature than found in XX gonadal dysgenesis.[128] If the gonadal dysgenesis is complete an infantile female appearance results, but if some Leydig cells remain functional there will be some pre- or postnatal virilization. Internal ducts are female in complete cases. There is variation in the degree of expression of the syndrome so that external and internal sexual features will vary. There is a high incidence of testicular tumor formation in XY gonadal dysgenesis. If familial, heredity follows the pattern of an X-linked recessive or male-limited autosomal-dominant trait with genetic heterogeneity.[129] Gonadotropins are elevated and testosterone low for a male, but often higher than usual in a normal female because of the retention of some testosterone secretory ability. Amenorrhea is noted in those patients raised as females. The presence of an XY karyotype indicates the necessity to undergo gonadectomy because of potential neoplastic degeneration of the dysgenetic testes.

At least four 46,XY female patients are reported with normal or short stature and features of Turner syndrome such as infantile lymphedema, webbed neck, wide-spaced nipples, and streak gonads, as well as gonadoblastoma in two patients. They had deletions of the short arm of the Y chromosome and absence of Y-specific DNA sequences.[130] Similar studies of other cases of XY gonadal dysgenesis may reveal smaller or different Y deletions.

The Drash syndrome arises as an abnormality of the genital ridge.[131] Thus there are problems with both sexual differentiation and kidney development. 46,XY patients have dysgenetic gonads (testes) or only fibrous streaks and therefore varying inhibition of müllerian and wolffian development internally and externally, microphallus, cryptorchidism, labioscrotal fusion, or even a normal female phenotype. All but one child have had a Y chromosome either in a 46,XY karyotype or a 46,XY mosaicism. The patients have nephropathy consisting of proteinuria, hypertension, nephrotic syndrome, and ultimately renal insufficiency; they have a predisposition to the development of Wilms tumor.[132] Thus male psuedohermaphrodites must be observed for the development of such tumors. Another syndrome that may share some common determinants consists of deletion of the short arm of the 11th chromosome, aniridia, mental retardation, and a high risk of nephroblastoma or gonadoblastoma in 46,X and 46,XY patients.[133]

The Dysgenetic Gonad and Neoplastic Formation.[134] There are two general classifications of patients subject to neoplastic degeneration of the gonads: those having a normal or abnormal Y chromosome associated with a dysgenetic gonad and those with undescended testes. Other rarer conditions can predispose a patient to testicular neoplasia as well.

The most common type of gonadal tumor considered here is the gonadoblastoma.[135] Except for three patients with a 46,XX karyotype, one with 45,X, two with 45,X/46,XX, four with structural abnormalities of the X chromosome, one with an autosomal deletion (#11), and two true hermaphrodites, reported patients with gonadoblastomas have a Y chromosome. It is possible that some of the patients listed as exceptions to this rule have undetected mosaicism with a Y chromosome or the TDF to account for development of the tumor.[136] Gonadoblastomas are found in syndromes of dysgenetic testes such as 46,XY gonadal dysgenesis and other syndromes of abnormal numbers of or structure of Y chromosomes. Gonadoblastomas are generally less than 8 mm in diameter, may develop calcification that will allow visualization by plain x-rays, and may secrete androgens or estrogens. Thus a patient with the syndrome of gonadal dysgenesis who was not expected to feminize but does may harbor a gonadoblastoma rather than a functional ovary. A gonadoblastoma itself poses little threat to the patient, but 50 per cent of them have associated dysgerminomas and another 10 per cent are associated with other malignant tumors. Dysgerminomas metastasize and are malignant partners of benign gonadoblastoma.[137] The incidence of gonadoblastomas in 46,XY gonadal dysgenesis is 33 per cent and this fact clearly argues for prophylactic gonadectomy in these patients.

Female Pseudohermaphroditism

Congenital Adrenal Hyperplasias[138,139]

The specifics of these conditions are discussed elsewhere (Chapter 6), but for the sake of completeness a short review is presented here.

3β-hydroxysteroid dehydrogenase deficiency causes the overproduction of the weak androgen DHEA and its sulfate (DHAS) and leads to virilization of the female fetus associated with salt loss and potassium retention.[140]

11-Hydroxylase deficiency causes virilization of the female fetus and resulting overproduction of deoxycorticosterone (DOC) causes hypertension, salt retention, and potassium loss; adrenal crisis is therefore rare because salt loss is not a feature.[141] However, glucocorticoid deficiency can cause hypoglycemia and shock under stress.

21-Hydroxylase deficiency is the most common type of CAH. Virilization of the female fetus to any degree is possible, and salt loss occurs in approximately 50 per cent of cases.[142] The late-onset form may cause virilization later in childhood or adolescence rather than at birth and is therefore a cause of precocious pubertal development rather than sexual ambiguity.[143]

Exposure of Mothers of Female Infants to Androgens and Progesterone. The window of vulnerability to virilization of the external genitalia was determined by the study of girls whose mothers had been treated with androgenic substances at various stages of gestation. Usually the medication consisted of progestational agents given to attempt to prolong a pregnancy threatened

with abortion. It was noted that such medications could cause posterior fusion of the vagina, scrotalization of the labia, and even some degree of fusion of the urethral folds if administered prior to 13 weeks of gestation; if administered after 13 weeks the androgen would only cause clitoral enlargement.[144]

The class of orally active progesterones that were administered to pregnant women and caused virilization of the female fetus included the 19-nortestosterones such as norethindrone, ethisterone, and norethynodrel. Testosterone and Danazol may have similar effects.[145] There are also several reported cases of stilbestrol causing virilization for unknown reasons (of course the possible development of clear cell adenocarcinoma of the vagina and cervix should preclude the use of stilbestrol in pregnancy).[146] The actual incidence of such virilization is low (probably less than 3 per cent of girls are affected) and the effects in virilized girls are dependent upon the medication used, the dose administered and the length of time it is given.

Female offspring of mothers with congenital adrenal hyperplasia, virilizing adrenal or ovarian tumors, luteoma, or luteal cyst of pregnancy may undergo virilization.[147] It has been suggested that some cases of virilization in newborn girls may be due to maternal luteal cysts that regressed after delivery. Since a fetus may be more responsive to androgens than the mother, the fetus may virilize but the mother may escape these effects.[148]

Teratologic Conditions Associated with Ambiguous Genitalia. The common embryonic derivation of the internal sexual ducts and the excretory system predisposes to concurrence of abnormal sexual development with anomalies of the kidneys and intestines. There is a large range of disorders of morphogenesis that include female pseudohermaphroditism.[149]

Male Pseudohermaphroditism

Leydig Cell Unresponsiveness to hCG

Leydig cell hypogenesis is reported in at least five cases and more recently has been termed *testicular unresponsiveness to hCG and LH*.[150,151] The patients have male pseudohermaphroditism with hypoplastic epididymis and vas deferens, absence or hypoplasia of wolffian ducts, minimal posterior vaginal fusion, a normal clitoris, absence of müllerian ducts, and intra-abdominal testes; some patients had normal female phenotype. Serum LH (and FSH) is remarkably elevated, while testosterone is low in the basal state and after hCG stimulation. Testicular histology reveals normal Sertoli cells and absence of Leydig cells.[152] There is an animal model of this condition known as the vestigial testes syndrome in the rat.[153]

Testicular Biosynthetic Defects

Defects Common to the Adrenal Gland and the Testes

20,22-Desmolase Deficiency (Side-Chain Cleavage Enzyme Deficiency).[154] In the pure form of deficiency of P450scc (side-chain cleavage enzyme) steroids cannot be formed from cholesterol. No glucocorticoids, mineralocorticoids, androgens, or estrogens are secreted, and signs of adrenal insufficiency occur in phenotypic infantile

female infants regardless of karyotype.[155] Partial defects are possible and such an affected child has ambiguous genitalia. Internal ducts will be female in a 46,XX individual, whereas a 46,XY individual will have no müllerian ducts because of the normal production of AMF but will have poorly developed wolffian derivatives because of lack of testosterone secretion (Fig. 10–7). The gonads will be in the abdomen, inguinal canal, or labia. There will be a blind vaginal pouch. The adrenal glands and gonads have large vacuolated cells, and because of this the condition was originally called lipoid adrenal hyperplasia. Inheritance is autosomal recessive. Diagnosis must be made quickly and will be indicated by the lack (or very low levels) of all steroid hormones in the basal or adrenocorticotropic hormone (ACTH)-stimulated state and elevated ACTH and plasma renin activity. Glucocorticoid and mineralocorticoid therapy must be administered or the child will die of adrenal failure.[156] Testes are subject to neoplastic formation and should be removed in

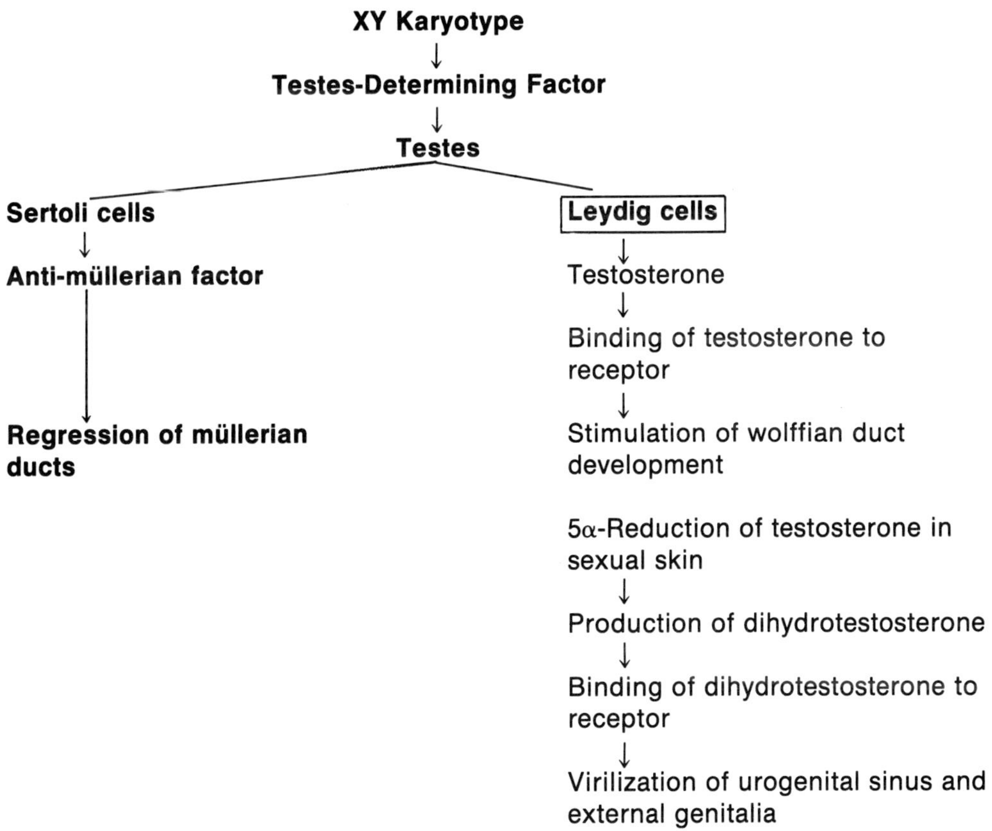

FIGURE 10–7. The results of a biosynthetic defect in testosterone production by the Leydig cells. The site of the defect is enclosed in a box. The substances and functions not in bold print are absent or subnormal.

patients raised as girls. Although the child will be infertile, there will be responsiveness to testosterone. The completely female genitalia will usually suggest that the child be raised as a female rather than undergo surgical reconstruction as male.

3β-Hydroxysteroid Dehydrogenase Deficiency.[157] The absence of 3β-hydroxysteroid dehydrogenase, the second in the cascade of enzyme reactions for steroid hormone production, leads to a lack of mineralocorticoid and glucocorticoid production with an excess of DHEA. Because 3β-hydroxysteroid dehydrogenase is necessary for testosterone production, males exhibit ambiguous genitalia as a result of lack of complete virilization while females exhibit ambiguous genitalia as a result of partial virilization. The enzymatic block may be incomplete, and various degrees of ambiguity of the genitalia are noted. The degree of loss of aldosterone production also varies between individuals.[158] 46,XY individuals produce AMF to cause regression of the müllerian ducts, and are reported to have normal wolffian ducts. In addition, 46,XY patients develop gynecomastia at puberty, possibly as a result of peripheral conversion of androgens to estrogens; they have elevated gonadotropin concentrations and diminished androgen production, leading to poor pubertal virilization and spermatogenic arrest.[159] Thus adrenal crisis in a child with ambiguous genitalia is compatible with 3β-hydroxysteroid dehydrogenase deficiency.

Classic diagnostic criteria, however, include decreased serum cortisol, elevated DHEA and DHAS in the basal or ACTH-stimulated state, increased urinary 17-ketosteroids (this test is rarely used with the advent of radioimmunoassays for serum metabolites), and elevated ACTH and plasma renin activity with hyponatremia and hypernatremia. It is important to note that salt loss may not be manifest until several days after birth. Treatment consists of replacement of glucocorticoids and mineralocorticoids.

17α-Hydroxylase Deficiency.[160] The inability to make 17-hydroxyprogesterone and 17-hydroxypregnenolone because of a deficiency of P450c17 impairs the production of glucocorticoids and sex steroids. Variable degrees of enzymatic block occur. Increased ACTH secretion drives the steroidogenic pathway toward mineralocorticoid production, but the excessive production of DOC,

corticosterone, 18-hydroxycorticosterone, and 18-hydroxy-DOC, all potent mineralocorticoids, causes salt retention and volume expansion that suppress renin production. This leads to decreased angiotensin and aldosterone secretion. Serum gonadotropins are elevated and sex steroids are low. Male pseudohermaphrodites with this disorder usually have female external genitalia but may resemble underdeveloped males in rare cases. Partial defects lead to formation of ambiguous genitalia in affected boys. At puberty, the lack of sex steroids usually causes a lack of secondary sexual development, but one case was reported with gynecomastia and some virilization.[161] Thus both 46,XX and 46,XY patients have infantile female genitalia and hypertension resulting from salt retention and hypokalemia.[162] The diagnosis is confirmed by increases in serum pregnenolone, progesterone, corticosterone, and DOC in the basal and ACTH-stimulated state and increased serum ACTH with decreased aldosterone and plasma renin activity. Gonadotropin concentrations are elevated. Treatment is accomplished by the replacement of glucocorticoids and sex steroids as necessary.

Defects Found Only in the Testes

17-Lyase Deficiency. The absence of the enzyme needed to convert C_{21} steroids to the C_{19} gonadal steroids leads to ambiguous genitalia or the appearance of underdeveloped genitalia in males and infantile female genitalia in females. Remarkably, the enzyme that catalyzes the 17-hydroxylation of progesterone and pregnenolone in adrenal and gonad, C450c17, also is responsible for 17,20-lyase activity of the gonad, although two separate clinical conditions result from the lack of either of the activities; no explanation for this observation is available to date. Wolffian ducts in 46,XY patients vary in appearance depending upon the amount of testosterone produced, which itself is dependent upon the degree of the enzymatic block; thus an infantile female genital appearance is possible, as is a male phenotype with undescended testes, micropenis, perineal hypospadias, and a bifid scrotum.[163] Müllerian ducts are absent in a 46,XY patient. A 46,XX patient with this defect will not progress through puberty, judging from the evidence of one reported case[164]; she had enlarged ovaries with primordial follicles and clusters of luteinized cells. This rare syndrome appears to have an autosomal-recessive inheritance. Laboratory analysis reveals low levels of serum testosterone, androstenedione, DHEA, and estradiol with elevated 17-hydroxyprogesterone, pregnenolone, and 17-hydroxypregnenolone levels in the basal or hCG-stimulated state; urinary excretion of pregnanetriolone, the urinary metabolite of serum 17-hydroxypregnenolone, is increased in those patients with this condition who have ambiguous genitalia. Cortisol and aldosterone production is normal. Gonadotropin concentrations are high.

17-Ketosteroid Reductase Deficiency. In 46,XY subjects with inability to convert androstenedione to testosterone and estrone to estradiol because of the lack of 17-ketosteroid reductase (or 17β-hydroxysteroid dehydrogenase) the external genitalia are female or slightly ambiguous with some clitoromegaly and posterior labioscrotal fusion. The testes are undescended or "labial."[165] At puberty there is a progressive virilization with clitoral enlargement, muscle development, and deepening of the voice. Gynecomastia occurs in some cases, presumably depending upon the degree of enzymatic block. Serum LH and FSH levels are high as a result of the absence of negative feedback inhibition. Androstenedione and estrone levels are high and testosterone and estradiol levels are low in the basal or hCG-stimulated condition. Histologic study demonstrates hyperplastic Leydig cells but decreased or absent sperm precursors in the seminiferous tubules. There are reported cases of 46,XY individuals who were raised as girls and converted to a male gender role at the time of virilization.[166] Inheritance appears autosomal recessive in the males diagnosed, although no females are reported. Patients have generally been assigned a female gender role and have been raised as females. Appropriate sex steroids are administered at puberty and gonadectomy is performed.

Syndromes of Androgen Resistance

The syndromes of androgen resistance range from phenotypic females with complete androgen resistance to phenotypic males manifesting only infertility.[167] While many of these defects have been completely characterized, others remain to be completely explained.

Complete Androgen Resistance. Cases of the complete syndrome of testicular feminization were reported early in the 19th century, but it was Lawson Wilkins who recognized the etiology in 1950 when a patient with amenorrhea and no pubic or axillary hair was demonstrated to be unresponsive to testosterone therapy.[168] Morris and Mahesh introduced the term *testicular feminization syndrome* in 1963.[169] Evidence from the tfm/y mouse indicated that such a syndrome could be caused by deficiency of androgen receptors[170] (Fig. 10–8), and a lack of DHT binding to fibroblasts from affected patients was soon shown to be the basic defect in human beings as well.[171]

The genetic code for the androgen receptor is located on the X chromosome near the centromere between Xq13 and Xp11.[172] The receptor binds testosterone, and even more avidly DHT.[173] A presumed mutation of a gene on the X chromosome is responsible for the syndrome of androgen resistance. The prevalence is estimated to be between 1:20,000 and 1:64,000 men, and it is the third most common cause of primary amenorrhea, after Turner syndrome and absence of the vagina. Some patients demonstrate decreased or absent androgen binding but others have normal amounts of androgen receptors; some of the latter group have abnormal temperature sensitivity of the receptor or lack of stability of the receptor.[174] There remain some patients that appear to have a completely normal amount of normally functioning androgen-binding receptors and these patients are suspected of having postreceptor defects in androgen action. As methods of study of androgen receptors are improved, presumably other abnormalities will be noted.[175] Family studies of complete androgen insensitivity follow the X-linked pattern, and fibroblasts of the mothers of patients with androgen insensitivity contain androgen receptors, consistent with the hypothesis that the abnormality of one X chromosome is the defect in the syndrome. It should be noted that an animal model of androgen resistance, the tfm mouse, has a mutation located on the X chromosome.

Patients with the complete syndrome of androgen resistance have a normal female phenotype at birth (Fig. 10–9) and may have unilateral or bilateral inguinal hernias (the sacs often contain testes) or labial masses. The clitoris resembles that of a normal female. During childhood and until puberty the child maintains a normal female appearance. However, at the time of puberty

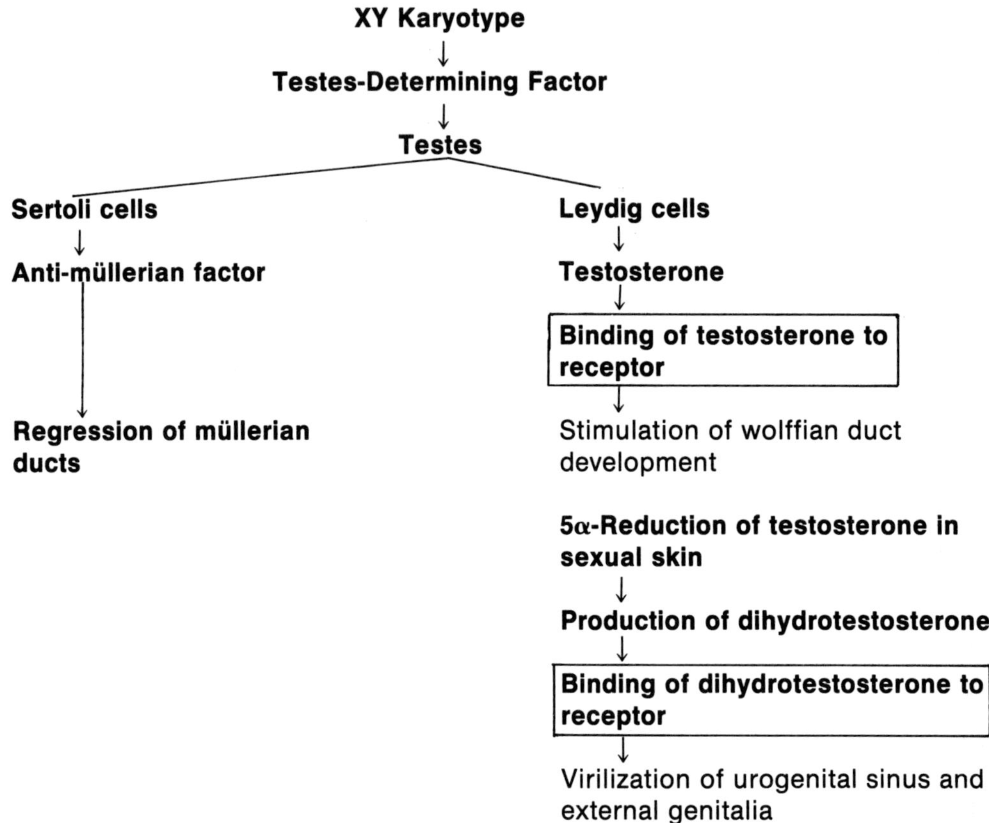

FIGURE 10–8. The syndrome of androgen resistance. The results of impaired binding of androgens to their receptors (testicular feminization syndrome). Refer also to legend for Figure 10–7.

feminization proceeds, but no menses or pubic or axillary hair development occurs.

Because of the normal production of AMF by the testes, müllerian remnants are atrophic and there are no oviducts or uterus; thus only the lower portion of the vagina remains. However, the wolffian structures are dependent upon testosterone and are themselves underdeveloped. No seminal vesicles and prostate are found and the vas deferens is only rudimentary. The testes contain hypoplastic seminiferous tubules but hyperplastic Leydig cells. Sperm formation is arrested in early phases.[176]

Gonadotropin concentrations in androgen resistance syndromes reflect the production and response to inhibin but lack of response to androgens. Thus LH is elevated and FSH is normal in the basal or GnRH-stimulated case. One patient was reported to have normal male negative feedback inhibition of LH secretion following androgen administration, but after orchiectomy demonstrated female-pattern positive feedback of estrogen upon LH secretion.[177] Others had a positive LH response to estradiol after gonadectomy and priming with chronic estradiol treatment.[178]

Circulating testosterone is elevated in androgen resistance as a result of the higher set-point in feedback sensitivity of LH secretion to testosterone and the resulting higher LH that stimulates the testes. Estradiol concentrations are likewise elevated for a normal male (but less than for a normal female) as a result of increased testicular secretion and peripheral conversion from testosterone. Dehydroepiandrosterone sulfate is normal because of its adrenal origin. Sex hormone–binding globulin (SHBG) is increased because of the increased estrogen production and not suppressed in spite of elevated testosterone concentrations due to the androgen insensitivity. The lack of response to androgens is responsible for the feminization in the presence of high circulating androgen concentrations.

Gender role and identity are unambigu-

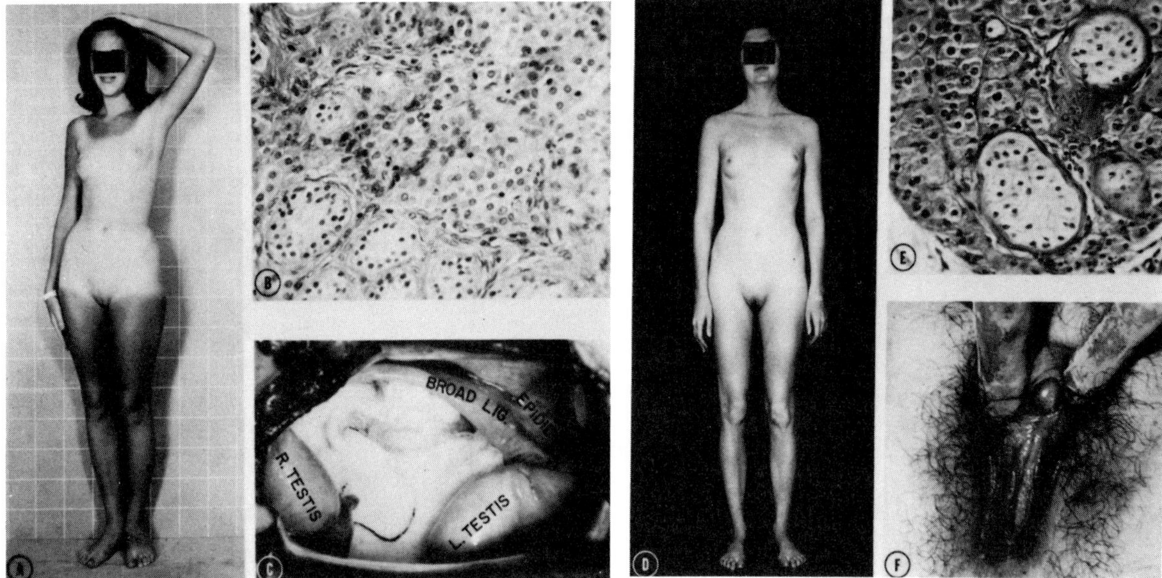

FIGURE 10–9. *A,* A 17-year-old patient with the complete syndrome of androgen resistance (testicular feminization). This phenotypic female has a 46,XY karyotype and complete absence of sexual hair with female secondary sexual characteristics. There is a small blind vagina. *B,* Testes exhibited Leydig cell hyperplasia, and seminiferous tubules lacked germinal elements. *C,* At laparotomy, abdominal testes, rudimentary wolffian structures, and no müllerian structures were found. *D,* Variant form of syndrome of androgen resistance in a 25-year-old female. Sexual hair is present although sparse. *E,* Testes exhibit Leydig cell hyperplasia. *F,* Clitoris is hypertrophied but there is no labial fusion. A shallow vagina ended blindly. At laparotomy, hypoplastic wolffian structures and absent müllerian structures were noted. (From Grumbach MM, Conte FA: Disorders of sexual differentiation. *In* Wilson JD, Foster DW (eds): Williams Textbook of Endocrinology. Philadephia, WB Saunders Company, 1985, with permission.)

ously female. Psychological tests confirm that gender role, reflected in activity levels, adult sexual orientation reflected in sex object choice, and parenting outlook are normally female in all patients assigned a female gender identity. Because these patients cannot respond to androgens, there is no reason to attempt to raise them as males. Because of the risk of the intra-abdominal testes becoming malignant, gonadectomy is ultimately indicated, but the question is at which stage should it be performed. The risk of malignancy is quite low until after the onset of puberty, and some argue that the testes should not be removed until after spontaneous puberty is reached.[179] Carcinoma in situ has been found in prepubertal patients, however.[180] The problem of deciding upon a pubertal, rather than a neonatal, time for gonadectomy involves the need for explaining to the patient the reason for the gonadectomy. If the testes are removed early, estrogen treatment should be started when puberty is expected to begin. The dose of estrogen should be low as in the treatment of hypogonadotropic hypogonadism (see pages 304, 305). Plastic surgical repair of the vagina may be necessary if it is inadequate for sexual intercourse.

Partial Androgen Resistance. Partial androgen resistance has been found to be the cause of a number of conditions and probably 10 per cent of patients with the syndrome of androgen resistance have this form.[181] The Reifenstien syndrome[182] of hereditary male pseudohermaphroditism (small phallus, ambiguous genitalia with perineoscrotal hypospadias, small testes, gynecomastia at puberty, and azoospermia) has been demonstrated to be comprised of a heterogeneous group of disorders, including patients with 5α-reductase deficiency and partial androgen insensitivity; phenotypic expression is likewise variable. The former is discussed below and the latter is included in this section. Other intersex conditions, such as the Lubs, Rosewater, and Gilbert-Dreyfus syndromes, probably fit into this category.

The endocrine manifestations of partial

androgen resistance are as may be expected; the serum androgen concentrations are raised above normal (but not usually as high as in complete androgen insensitivity), estrogen and LH concentrations are also high. Patients may have decreased or normal androgen binding ability as noted in the complete syndrome above. Some responsiveness to androgens allows some degree of virilization in these patients.

These patients, in contrast to those with complete androgen insensitivity, show some, but not complete, virilization at the time of puberty. They should therefore undergo gonadectomy at the time of diagnosis and be raised as females. Those older patients already raised as males may have to continue in that gender role, but must undergo considerable cosmetic reconstructive surgery.

Phenotypic Men with Azoospermia and Elevated Testosterone and LH. The last type of androgen resistance to be discussed is manifest in phenotypic men with azoospermia, elevated testosterone, and generally elevated LH concentrations.[183] Androgen receptors are decreased in the genital fibroblasts of these men but the phenotype and, in most cases, the serum LH, FSH, and testosterone concentrations are normal.

5α-Reductase Deficiency. Although this condition is often classified as an androgen resistance disorder, the androgen receptors are normal and an enzyme deficiency is the basis of the problem. The condition was originally descriptively termed *pseudovaginal perineoscrotal hypospadias* until the biochemical defect was uncovered.[184] A large kindred in which information has been traced back more than four generations was studied in the Dominican Republic.[185] In this area there is a high incidence of consanguinity and the condition can be traced to a mutation in one female ancestor of the present patients. 5α-Reductase deficiency is transmitted as an autosomal-recessive gene that manifests only in genetic males. As newborns, the children have a blind vaginal pouch and a small phallic structure bound ventrally in chordee with a hooded prepuce and tertiary hypospadias. Internally, wolffian ducts are found and müllerian duct regression is normal. Originally the children were raised as girls but, with the recognition of the syndrome, became known as *guevedoces* ("testicles at twelve") because of the virilization and descent of the testes from their intra-abdominal position to a labial lo-

cation at the time of puberty; in addition, they show deepening of the voice, muscular development, and increase in phallic size (Fig. 10–10). Spermatogenesis is reported, but the sperm ducts end blindly and fertility is not possible without surgical correction. Even with the virilization, the patients do not develop temporal balding, significant beard growth, or acne, suggesting that these features are dependent upon DHT. Gynecomastia does not develop at puberty, in contrast to some of the other syndromes in this section.

The ratio of serum testosterone to DHT is high in these patients (usually greater than 35 in contrast to 8 to 16 in normal adult males), and the discrepancy can be magnified by the use of hCG.[186–188] Stimulation of the testes with hCG leads to a very high serum testosterone-to-DHT ratio (greater than 74 in affected male children compared to 3 to 26 in controls), and urinary collections reveal a high 5β– to 5α-reduced steroid metabolite ratio. Further, there is low or absent 5α-reductase activity in fibroblasts from the genital region or in other tissue specimens. Activity of the 5α-reductase enzyme necessary for the conversion of testosterone to DHT in the sexual skin is either low or absent (Fig. 10–11). It may also have decreased affinity for testosterone, or may be unstable with a reduced affinity for NADPH. The serum testosterone concentration is normal or increased but 5α-DHT is low.[189,190] The phenotype does not appear to vary with the type of enzyme defect found. Affected females have normal female phenotypic development but similar biochemical abnormalities whereas heterozygotes have intermediate urinary steroid results. The cause for the virilization at puberty is unknown but it may be a result of the increasing testosterone secretion, which, by supplying large amounts of substrate, allows adequate DHT production by the small amount of 5α-reductase activity that persists.

The change in gender in these patients has awakened a large amount of controversy. Generally the concept that gender identity is determined irrevocably by 18 to 24 months of age holds true, but this condition is proposed as an exception to that rule. It has been stated that prenatal virilization allows these patients to begin life with a female gender role as dictated by the parents and others and then, with the rise of androgens and virilization at puberty, convert to

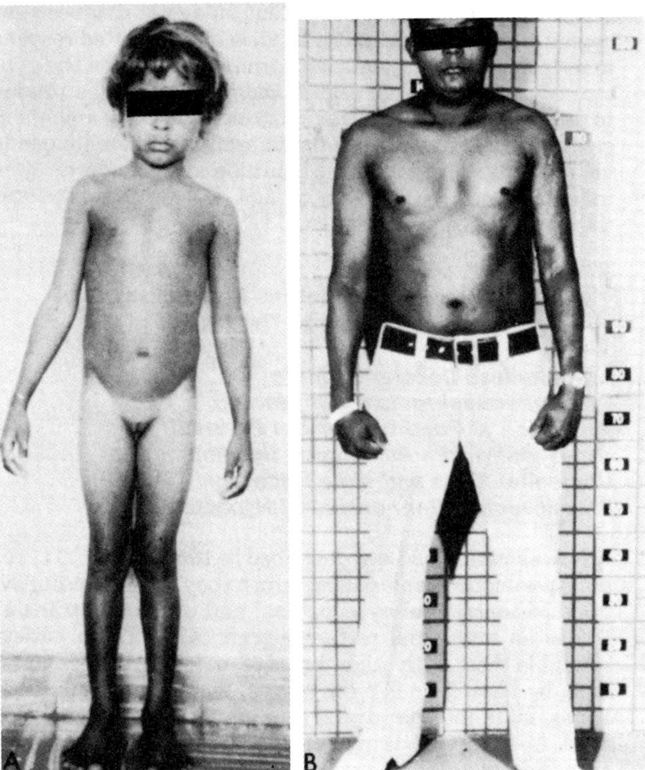

FIGURE 10–10. *A*, Prepubertal 46,XY child with 5α-reductase deficiency raised as a female. *B*, Postpubertal male with 5α-reductase deficiency who has virilized and changed gender identity. (From Peterson RE, Imperato-McGinley J, Gautier T, et al: Male pseudohermaphroditism due to 5α-steroid deficiency. Am J Med 62:170, 1977, with permission.)

a male gender role.[191] However, societal pressures in the community may intervene and it should be pointed out that in this village, as well as much of the undeveloped world, there are definite benefits to being a male as opposed to a female in terms of what a community expects of an individual. Further, after the first generation was observed, the village itself came to expect the gender change to occur and related to the child differently than to normal girls. A recent study of 14 individuals with 5α-reductase deficiency among the Sambia in New Guinea has yielded conclusions quite different from those proposed from the Dominican Republic studies. In New Guinea affected children are known at birth to be different and raised as males, although they are thought of as a third sexual category rather than male or female. At puberty they are fully accepted as males, in a gender role considered to be superior to that of a female in the area. Those children misdiagnosed at birth and raised as females are socially pressured into a male role at puberty as they virilize and suffer considerable psychosocial trauma in the process. These studies suggest that society rather than the prenatal hormonal environment directs the gender development.

Other kindreds have been studied and further psychological evaluation will be necessary to resolve the question of the determinants of gender role and identity.

Defects in Synthesis of Antimüllerian Factor

Cases of persistent müllerian ducts in phenotypic male 46,XY patients are reported; uterus and fallopian tubes are found in an inguinal hernia or discovered during laparotomy. The testes are usually undescended, may be hypoplastic, and have an increased incidence of malignant degeneration.[192] There are familial cases suggesting sex-limited autosomal-recessive of X-linked recessive patterns.

Maternal Ingestion of Progesterone and Estrogen. Animal evidence suggests that progesterone ingestion by a mother can feminize a male fetus, but proof of this tendency in the human being is incomplete. However, some studies have suggested a link between hypospadias and maternal progesterone intake.[193] Diethylstilbestrol (DES) may have effects upon a male fetus such as meatal stenosis, epididymal cysts, and hypoplasia of the testes. One case of male

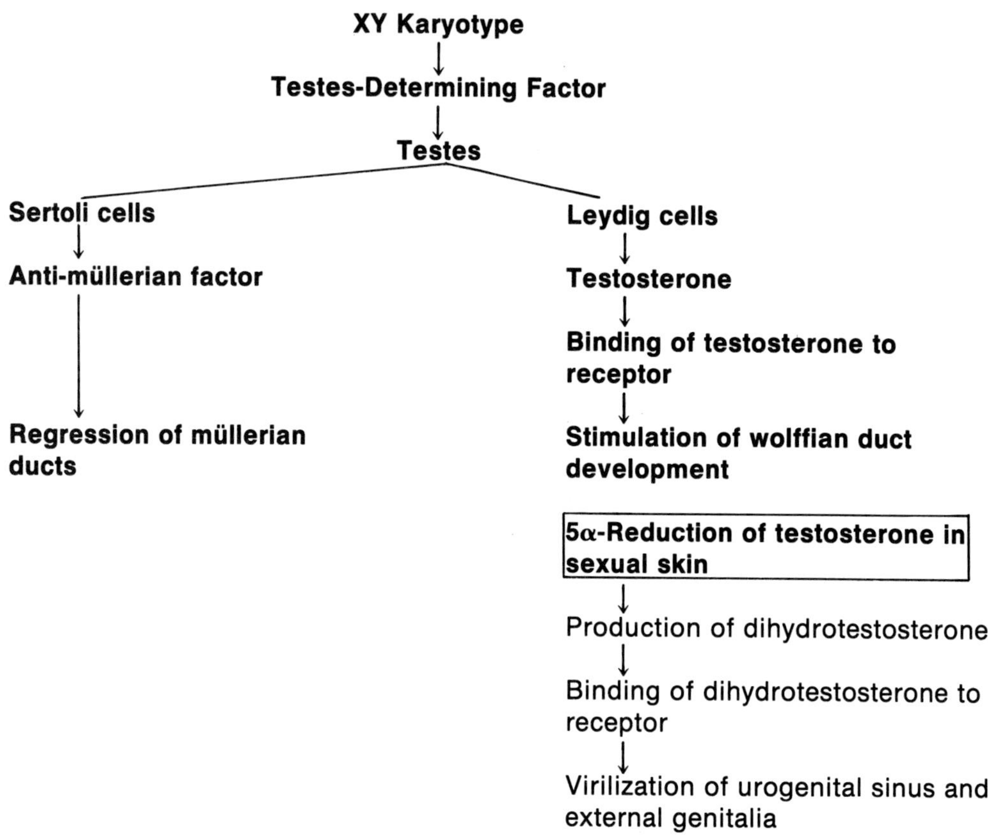

FIGURE 10–11. Abnormalities resulting from 5α-reductase deficiency. Refer also to legend for Figure 10–7.

pseudohermaphroditism has been reported, but there is little evidence to link DES with feminization.[194,195]

Unclassified Forms of Abnormal Sexual Development in Males

Hypospadias

Tertiary or perineoscrotal hypospadias is a feature of many of the syndromes discussed in this chapter, and such a finding should cause concern that there is an abnormality of sexual differentiation. However, first-degree or coronal or glandular hypospadias in an individual with an otherwise normal male phenotype in most cases appears to have no endocrine basis; the incidence of this anomaly is between 1:1000 and 8:1000 births.[196] There are reports of cases of minimal hypospadias associated with an abnormality of the androgen receptor, but the prevalence and importance of such a finding in a wider range of patients is unknown. 5α-Reductase activity is normal.[197]

Cryptorchidism

Some degree of cryptorchidism is common in many of the syndromes noted in this chapter. There is more than 25 per cent chance of presence of an intersex problem in patients with undescended testes and hypospadias, and the frequency increases if the disorder is bilateral and the hypospadias is severe.[198] Also, there is an increased incidence of cryptorchidism in hypogonadotropic hypogonadism. However, cryptorchidism can occur as an isolated finding, and the pathophysiology of undescended testes is discussed on page 372.

Anorchia

Congenital anorchia, or the vanishing testes syndrome, is defined as the absence of testes in an otherwise normal phenotypic male.[199] Because the penis is normally formed there must have been normal androgen production in the first 13 weeks of gestation, and if the penis is of normal newborn size the testes must have been functional for several weeks thereafter or the penis would not have grown. The testes are assumed to have atrophied, perhaps as a result of vascular compromise, before birth. Familial cases are reported, even twin cases.

Cases are also reported in which testes are absent in 46,XY patients in whom female internal and external differentiation or ambiguous development is found. These patients may have lost their testes before 13 weeks of gestation.[200] Recently two more cases have been reported with a 46,XY karyotype, a female phenotype similar to Turner syndrome, and deletions of crucial areas of the Y chromosome.[201]

Male Pseudohermaphroditism with Multiple Congenital Anomalies

The wolffian ducts may atrophy at the mesonephros stage so that the epididymis, ductus deferens, seminal vesicle, ureter, and kidney are lacking. After it has reached the cloaca, resorption of the wolffian duct can lead to absence of the epididymis, ductus epididymis, and proximal ductus deferens. Failure of development of the wolffian duct structures and rete testes is reported in as many as 1 per cent of patients with cryptorchid testes but is probably much rarer in patients with descended testes.[202]

Müllerian ducts may persist in otherwise normal males. A uterus and fallopian tubes may be located in a hernia sac; the patient may be infertile.[203]

In the syndrome of *lethal acrodysgenital dwarfism* failure to thrive, facial dysmorphism (anteverted nostrils and micrognathia), syndactyly, postaxial polydactyly, Hirschsprung disease, cardiac and renal anomalies, and ambiguous genitalia may be found. Many of the findings are similar to those of the Smith-Lemli-Opitz syndrome, but it has been been proposed that they are separate entities.[204]

Camptomelic dwarfism is a disorder of the epiphyseal cartilage leading to bending of the limbs, hypoplasia of the skeleton, cleft palate, micrognathia, failure to thrive, and other abnormalities. Three patients with ambiguous genitalia in spite of a 46,XY karyotype have been reported. The etiology of the developmental abnormality is unknown.[205]

In the *Najjar syndrome* ambiguous genitalia are found in association with cardiomyopathy and mental retardation. There are numerous other syndromes combining dys-

morphology and abnormalities of sexual differentiation.[206]

Unclassified Forms of Abnormal Sexual Development in Females

Absence of Vagina, Vaginal Atresia, and Atresia of Uterine Cervix

Congenital *absence of the vagina*, with a rudimentary uterus, is referred to as the Rokitasky-Kuster-Hauser syndrome.[207] In spite of this, there may be well-developed fallopian tubes. Absence of the uterus is always associated with absence of the vagina, but a small uterus may be found in cases where the vagina is absent. Diagnosis is usually made when primary amenorrhea occurs at puberty. As many as one third to one fourth of women with primary amenorrhea have this syndrome. Because the ovaries are normal, the patient will have normal secondary sexual development. Associated anomalies include unilateral renal agenesis or ectopic kidneys in 40 per cent, vertebral anomalies in 10 per cent, and some increase in the incidence of other skeletal or cardiac anomalies. It has been suggested that many of the cases of the Rokitasky-Kuster-Hauser syndrome with vertebral anomalies are actually manifestations of the VATER syndrome, which includes, Vertebral anomalies, Anal atresia, Tracheo-*E*sophageal fistula, and *R*adial limb dysplasia, as well as renal anomalies, cardiac anomalies, single umbilical artery, and abnormal genitalia such as bicornuate uterus and or vaginal atresia in the female (and hypospadias and bifid scrotum in the male).[208] The condition is probably sporadic, although familial cases are reported. Differential diagnosis of absence of the vagina includes vaginal atresia and the syndrome of androgen resistance.

Vaginal atresia differs from congenital absence of the vagina in that there is a failure of formation of the urogenital sinus and failure to canalize the solid vaginal plug.[209] Because there are no abnormalities of the müllerian structures, the uterus and ovaries are normal and normal secondary sexual development occurs. The diagnosis is usually made at puberty when there is obstruction to the flow of menstrual discharge to the vaginal opening and the increased pressure causes abdominal pain.

Atresia of the uterine cervix is exceptionally rare. It occurs in normally feminizing pubertal females with normal vaginal openings, but cramping and absence of vaginal bleeding occurring during menses.[210] Other anomalies of the vagina include transverse vaginal septum, which is one of the more common vaginal abnormalities, and longitudinal vaginal septum, which is quite rare in the absence of incomplete fusion of the müllerian derivatives.[211]

Incomplete müllerian fusion is rather common, with an prevalence of between 0.1 and 3 per cent of females.[212] The lack of fusion may lead to uterus unicornis (absence of one uterine horn with a normal vagina but often the absence of the contralateral kidney); uterus arcuatus (arcuate uterus with a flat fundus and a midline notch); uterus septus, with a longitudinal septum running the length of the uterus leading to two functional cavities; uterus subseptus, with the septum only in the caudal portion; uterus bicornis bicollis, with two cervices and usually one vagina; uterus didelphys with two completely separate cavities and fundi but one cervix, usually with a septate vagina; and finally separate hemiuteri, often with separate vaginas and possibly duplicated colon and anus. There are rare reported cases of true duplicated müllerian ducts with two separate uteri each of which has two fallopian tubes, in contrast to separate hemiuteri where each hemiuterus has only one fallopian tube. Rare syndromes combining abnormalities of müllerian fusion and other dysmorphic conditions have been reported, such as the hand-foot-uterus syndrome, camptobrachydactyly–longitudinal vaginal septum syndrome, Winter syndrome, Rudiger syndrome, cryptophthalamos syndrome, and müllerian aplasia–Klippel-Feil deformity with deafness.[213]

Diagnosis of Ambiguous Genitalia

The diagnosis of ambiguous genitalia is not for the amateur! The complex biochemistry and embryology of the formation of the genitalia are complicated, as are the potential difficulties encountered in the explanation of the diagnostic procedures and the ultimate diagnosis to the parents. It is, of course, in the delivery room when the first comments are made to the parents of a child with ambiguous genitalia, and in the excitement of the birth process it is easy to jump to conclusions for the assignment of sex, which will lead to repercussions later.

There is no place for guesswork in the diagnosis of ambiguous genitalia in a new-born; the appearance of external genitalia by itself will rarely enable one to make a diagnosis. Laboratory evaluation, often extensive in nature, is often necessary before an opinion regarding sex assignment can be given to the parents. Algorithms may be helpful, and two are supplied for the reader's use (Fig. 10–12), but a branched-chain approach to diagnosis, characteristic of algorithms, is not always possible.

The medical history will be important if it reveals maternal ingestion of androgenic substances or virilization of the mother for other reasons, the death of siblings in circumstances suggestive of congenital adrenal hyperplasia, the presence of infertility or lack of puberty, especially in an "aunt," or, in fact, the finding of ambiguous genitalia in another member of the family. Consanguineous marriages are more likely to produce a child with one of the disorders mentioned.

The physical examination may yield some important information even if the genitalia appear totally ambiguous at initial view. Stretched length and width of the phallic structure and the presence or absence of chordee should be noted. The degree of hypospadias and whether there is a common urogenital opening or whether the urethra is separate from the vaginal opening should be determined. The length of the vaginal opening and whether posterior fusion exists is noted, as well as the shape and texture of the skin of the labia majora or bifid scrotum. Spherical objects in the labia or bifid scrotum will suggest the presence of testes or ovotestes, but, as mentioned above, ovaries and uteri and tubes can herniate into the area. A careful rectal examination with the small finger may reveal the presence of a uterine cervix, although developing the ability to interpret findings on such an examination is not easy.

While it is clear that chromosomal sex does not determine correct gender assignment, a karyotype is invaluable. Such a study will take at least several days in the best of circumstances and should be started at the beginning of the diagnostic process so that the result will be available, if necessary, sooner. It is no longer recommended to do a buccal smear for sex chromatin determination because of inherent errors in technique and interpretation.

Ultrasound of the abdomen to determine the presence of uterus and ovaries should soon be done. The results will be most help-

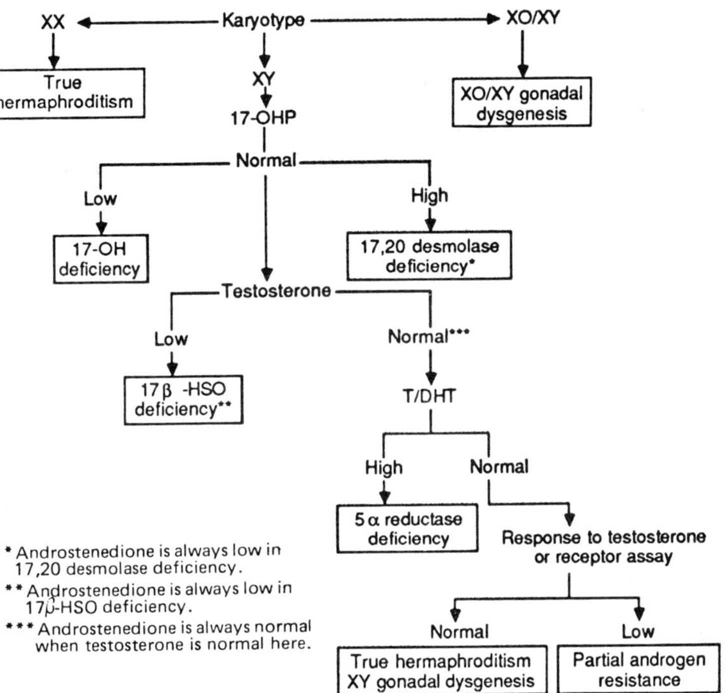

FIGURE 10–12. Diagnostic algorithms for patients with ambiguous genitalia in whom gonads are palpable (*top*) or are not palpable (*bottom*) on physical examination. It is essential to realize that variations of the classical appearance of these defects occur and that details found in the text or other sources should be consulted in addition to this simplified plan. (From Styne DM: Sexual differentiation. *In* Fitzgerald PA (ed): Handbook of Clinical Endocrinology. Greenbrae, CA, Jones Medical Publication, 1986, with permission.)

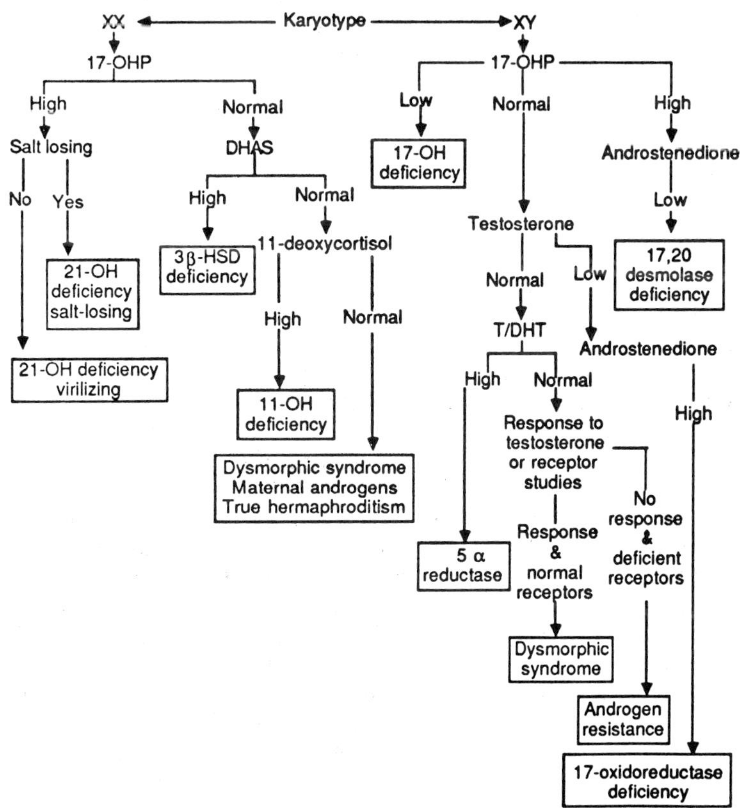

ful in determining whether AMF activity was present. Ultrasound evaluation of testicular size, shape, and contents may occasionally also be useful, particularly if a tumor is suspected.[214] While computed tomography (CT) or magnetic resonance imaging (MRI) could reveal the same information, such examinations are not warranted.

Steroid determinations will often be essential for diagnosis. These are now available for serum samples; it is no longer necessary or recommended to collect 24 hours of urine for steroid determinations in the majority of situations. Too often incomplete sample collection has led to incorrect diagnoses. A warning should be sounded regarding the choice of laboratories to perform the analysis. A few national endocrine laboratories can perform analyses correctly and quickly on small amounts of blood. These laboratories should be used rather than those with little experience in this area. Incorrect results or "QNS" results can tragically alter or delay the diagnosis. Some laboratories may, for example, have insensitive methods for androgen determinations because they usually deal with the diagnosis of infertility in males, requiring the differentiation of a testosterone value of 100 ng/dl from a value of 1000 ng/dl, rather than the necessity for the more sensitive differentiation between 20 and 100 ng/dl.

An initial blood sample should be sent for all steroid metabolites likely to be needed. Adrenal metabolites of interest include 17-hydroxyprogesterone, 11-deoxycortisol, DHEA and DHAS, and in some cases progesterone and pregnenolone. Salt losing will not be demonstrable until 3 to 7 days of age or later, but, if suspected, sodium and potassium level determinations may be supplemented by plasma renin activity determinations. Aldosterone, corticosterone, and in some cases 18-hydroxylated corticosterone levels can be measured if appropriate. If the diagnosis is most likely a form of congenital adrenal hyperplasia, the steroid concentrations will be high enough, as a result of endogenous ACTH stimulation, to allow diagnosis upon a basal value. Diagnosis of late-onset adrenal hyperplasia or the heterozygote state will require ACTH administration. A disorder of testosterone biosynthesis may be diagnosed from the basal state, but stimulation with 3000 U/m² of hCG intramuscularly and sampling 48 hours

later will often be useful in determining which steroids can be produced and which cannot. If the child is well past the newborn period, three doses of hCG per week for 2 weeks may be used to stimulate testicular secretion.

The diagnosis of androgen unresponsiveness is more time consuming. One method is to administer testosterone, 25 mg intramuscularly each month, for 3 months and observe the change in the stretched length and width of the penis. Androgen receptors may be determined in a sample of the patients fibroblasts from a skin biopsy, but this is only done in laboratories where research is being done in the area (see references 170–172 for locations). These procedures may take weeks or months to complete, but the information they yield is important because androgen insensitivity cannot be treated with androgens and the child cannot, therefore, be raised as a male.

Treatment of Ambiguous Genitalia

The first and unquestionably most important step in the treatment of a newborn with ambiguous genitalia is to avoid mentioning the sex of the child to the parents until a decision is made regarding the sex of rearing. A mistake at this point will often necessitate long-term counseling and reeducation of the parents in their relationship to the child. It is generally counterproductive to give the parents an encyclopedic explanation of the development of the genitalia because this may lead to misconceptions that will later have to be corrected. The question of karyotype should only be mentioned to minimize its importance in the outcome of the child. It is far better to describe "the baby" as being unfinished externally, rather than referring to a penis or clitoris. The internal organs are "baby" or "undeveloped gonads" rather than "testes" or "ovaries." No child is to be described as half-boy or half-girl: The child is either a boy or a girl. These cautions are made because each one of the mistakes cited is not uncommon.

The next step is to assign the sex of rearing, which is of course based upon the diagnosis, the ability to achieve functional sexual activity or fertility, and, in some cases, the firm preferences of the parents. Thus, a child with congenital adrenal hyperplasia will usually be raised as the chromosomal sex suggests, with glucocorticoid and mineralocorticoid therapy administered to stop the virilization (if present) or testosterone to promote virilization (if undervirilization is the problem); surgical therapy will then be required to repair the external appearance. If androgen resistance is the problem, a female sex will be assigned and, if some ambiguity of the external genitalia is present as a result of incompleteness of the androgen resistance, appropriate surgery must be performed. True hermaphrodites can be raised either as males or females, and the decision may be influenced by the presence of some normal functioning testicular or ovarian tissue. If the decision can go either way based upon the external appearance, and if surgical reconstruction of either normal male or female genitalia is possible, the parents may help in making the decision. A child who would be expected to be unable to function as a male because of a small probably untreatable, androgen unresponsive penis, whose parents insist upon raising a boy, may be assigned a male gender, but there is a great likelihood of development psychological problems in the future. The assignment of a name has lifelong influence and also requires care; there is no reason for the use of an ambiguous name in a child who has a definitive diag nosis and a known prognosis as to the best sex assignment.

The determination of how much to tell the parents about the diagnosis is also important. While it is appropriate to give full disclosure, the careless reference to the male karyotype in a patient with androgen resistance, rather than a careful discussion of the lack of importance of the chromosomes in the child's condition, is inappropriate. The reference to a blind vaginal pouch in a 46,XY patient with 5α-reductase deficiency may cause the parents to question the sex assignment and wonder whether they really have a son. In this increasingly sophisticated world it is necessary to offer the maximal information possible, but it is even more important to relate it in a compassionate and appropriate manner.

Psychological therapy will be indicated in many cases and should be offered. The experienced pediatric endocrinologist will often have the resources to counsel the family, but continued sessions may be indicated in some families. Sex reassignment after 18 months of age will lead to difficulties in most cases.

MALE PUBERTAL DEVELOPMENT

Endocrine Changes of Puberty

Because the hypothalamic-pituitary-gonadal axis is active in the fetal period and in childhood, the endocrine activity characteristic of puberty should be considered part of the continuum of development, rather than a de novo occurrence. The reawakening of gonadal function at puberty is known as *gonadarche*, and the increased adrenal androgen secretion is *adrenarche*. Much interest has focused upon the control of the onset of puberty, but a unifying theory has still eluded investigators.

The age of onset of puberty is not immutable. Historic records reveal the age of menarche over the last several centuries; menarche is removed from the onset of puberty by 2 to 3 years but can still serve as a guide to pubertal development. Aristotle was the first to reflect upon the age of onset of puberty; he noted that "when twice seven years old in most of the cases the male begins to engender seed and at the same time in the female the breasts swell and the so-called catamenia commences to flow."[215] This would suggest an age of menarche and ejaculation or erection only slightly delayed compared to modern times.[216,217] Genetic factors keep the age of onset of puberty rather constant within a family or a population.

Gonadarche

The pituitary gonadotropins, LH and FSH, are secreted into the systemic circulation in response to hypothalamic GnRH [or luteinizing hormone–releasing hormone (LHRH)], which reaches the pituitary gland via the hypothalamic-pituitary portal system (reviewed in ref. 218). Gonadotropin-releasing hormone is released episodically into the pituitary portal system in varying amplitudes and frequencies during different stages of development (and different stages of the menstrual cycle in females). This pulsatile activity originates in the arcuate nucleus, where a postulated hypothalamic pulse generator resides.[219] Animal and clinical experiments have shown that if the pulsatile nature of GnRH secretion is altered to a constant flow the pituitary gonadotrope decreases its affinity for GnRH and the number of GnRH receptors decreases, leading to a decrease of gonadotropin secretion (down-regulation).[220] Luteinizing hormone (or hCG, which is a virtually identical molecule with identical effects) stimulates testicular Leydig cell secretion of testosterone in boys and testosterone in turn exerts negative feedback inhibition of LH secretion. Follicle-stimulating hormone has little effect in boys until spermarche (the onset of maturation of spermatozoa), when it stimulates the Sertoli cells to support the development of spermatozoa.

In addition to their steroid products, both types of gonads produce a protein, inhibin, that exerts negative feedback inhibition on FSH secretion in both sexes. Inhibin is produced by the Sertoli cells of the seminiferous tubules of the testes and the granulosa cells of the follicles of the ovary.[221,222] Another protein product, AMF, which is described above, is also produced by the seminiferous tubules and follicles in males and females, respectively.

Hypothalamic GnRH and pituitary LH and FSH are present in the fetal hypothalamus in the first trimester of gestation.[223] By midgestation the pituitary portal system is completed, the GnRH-containing axon fibers reach the capillaries of the portal system, and hypothalamic peptides can reach the pituitary.[224] At 20 weeks of gestation GnRH secretion is maximal and stimulates active secretion of LH and FSH, which reach high serum concentrations similar to those found in castrate individuals. In the male fetus, testosterone increases and is responsible for the enlargement of the penis before birth, while LH is suppressed.

After birth there is a period of instability partially due to the withdrawal of maternal estrogens and partially due to the still-immature condition of the central nervous system (CNS) control mechanism. Thus LH and FSH concentrations reach pubertal levels in boys until 6 months of age.[225] Pulsatile LH secretion stimulates testosterone secretion in boys to concentrations over 150 ng/dl in the months after birth.[226]

After this period of instability in infancy, serum concentration of gonadotropins and sex steroids reach low values until the peripubertal period (just before secondary sexual development begins). In the newborn period, until about 2 to 4 years of age, chil-

dren without gonads or sex steroids, such as patients with Turner syndrome, have high serum gonadotropin concentrations compared to normal control children.[227]

At the peripubertal period the reverse phenomenon occurs; an increase in gonadotropin secretion takes place in the presence or absence of functional gonads.[228] The ability of a small dose of sex steroids to suppress gonadotropin secretion decreases at puberty. Administration of a few micrograms of estradiol may virtually eliminate gonadotropin secretion in a prepubertal child but exerts no effect on a pubertal subject.[229] Similarly, a small dose of opioids will completely suppress gonadotropin secretion in a prepubertal individual but have no effect in a pubertal individual.[230] At puberty gonadotropin concentrations first increase during sleep, when increased amplitude of pulsatile secretion of GnRH occurs every 60 to 90 min.[231] As puberty progresses the peaks of gonadotropin concentration occur more regularly throughout the day until no diurnal variation remains, and this pattern is maintained in the adult. Studies of large numbers of blood samples reveal that serum gonadotropin values are higher in the adult than in the prepubertal child but the pulsatile nature of gonadotropin secretion and the diurnal variation in early puberty makes the interpretation of single values difficult.[232,233] If a nadir in gonadotropin secretion occurs during sampling, a different interpretation will be reached than if a peak is captured; thus, unless the object is to determine if gonadotropins are in the castrate range in an agonadal individual, single samples will not be useful in the determination of which stage of puberty a child has reached (Fig. 10–13).

The concept of bioactivity measured in a bioassay as compared to immunoactivity measured in a standard radioimmunoassay is of interest at puberty. A slight change in the structure of LH or FSH, which may not be detected by the antibody used in a radioimmunoassay, may have a effect upon the binding of the hormone to the membrane-bound receptor of the cell in the bioassay and therefore change the biologic effect of the hormone. There is evidence of an increase in the bioactivity-to-immunoactivity ratio at the time of puberty.[234–236]

Gonadal steroid concentrations are low but detectable in the prepubertal period. Testosterone concentrations are less than 10 ng/dl in normal boys (Fig. 10–14). Nighttime

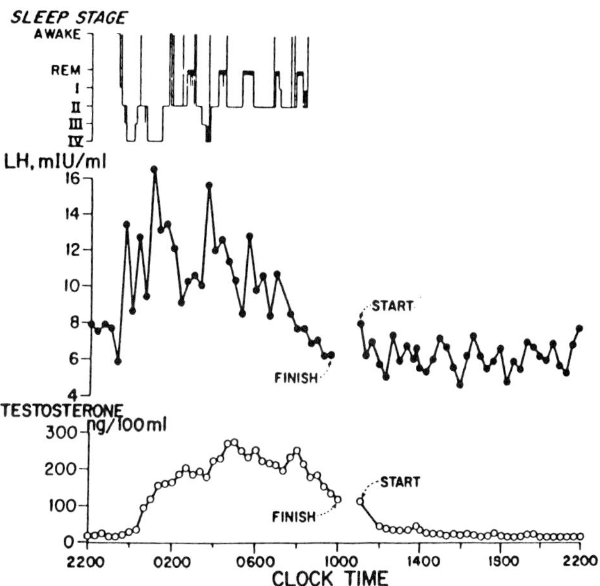

FIGURE 10–13. Plasma LH and testosterone measured in blood samples withdrawn every 20 min in a 14-year-old boy in pubertal stage 2. The histogram displaying sleep stage sequence is depicted above the period of nocturnal sleep. Sleep stages are 2 REM(−) with stages I–IV shown by depth of line graph. (From Boyar RM, et al: Simultaneous augmented secretion of luteininzing hormone and testosterone during sleep. J Clin Invest 54:609, 1974, with permission.)

elevations of testosterone are found following nighttime gonadotropin secretion in the earliest stages of puberty, and, as puberty progresses, the secretion becomes more regular until testosterone secretion occurs throughout the day and night by the time of late puberty.[237] Because of the presence of SHBG sex steroid concentrations are more constant throughout the day than are gonadotropin concentrations, but there is definite variation in estradiol levels so that concentrations may vary from 10 to 40 or 50 pg/ml within one 24-hour period; testosterone values may vary but not so strikingly. There is

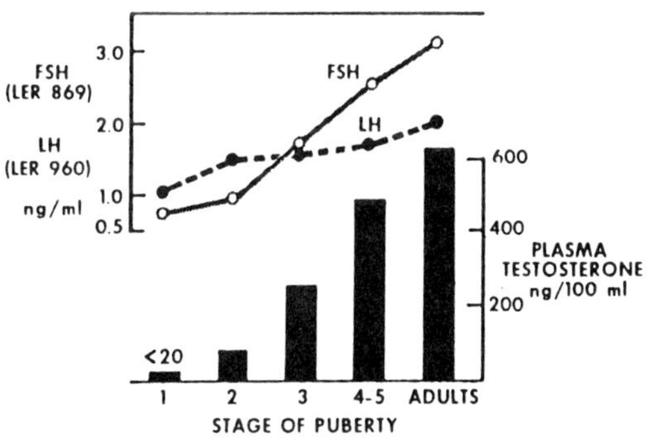

FIGURE 10–14. Mean plasma testosterone and gonadotropins in normal boys by stage of maturation and mean bone age for each stage. Most laboratories report LH and FSH values in terms of other standards, and the conversion is: for FSH (LER 869) 1 ng = 3 mIU; for LH (LER 960) 1 ng = 7.8 mIU. (From Grumbach, MM: Onset of puberty. *In* Berenberg SR (ed): Puberty, Biologic and Social Components. Leiden, H. E. Stenfert Kroese B. V., Publishers, 1975, p 1, with permission.)

a stepwise increase in serum sex steroid concentration with advancing stage of pubertal progression. Free sex steroids are the active moiety, but more than 97 per cent of sex steroids are noncovalently bound to SHBG; this process functionally inactivates the bound steroid.[238] SHBG concentration increases in girls during puberty as a result of estrogen stimulation, but serum values of SHBG decrease in boys because androgens decrease SHBG.[239] Higher percentages of androgens are bound in women, whereas androgens in men are less completely bound to SHBG and therefore are more active. This difference in SHBG and the 20-fold higher serum testosterone concentrations in men account for the 40-fold greater androgenic activity present in the serum of men than women.[240]

With increased GnRH stimulation, the pituitary storage of readily releasable gonadotropin increases. This is demonstrated by the gonadotropin secretory response to a bolus of exogenous GnRH. A 100-μg bolus of GnRH will cause a rise of LH greater than 16 MIU/ml in pubertal or adult subjects, whereas a far smaller rise is found in prepubertal subjects: the rise in LH after exogenous GnRH may be used as a reflection of pubertal status and of endogenous GnRH secretion.[241] Because females of all ages release more FSH than males, the FSH response to GnRH is not an adequate reflection of pubertal state. Subtle variations in gonadotropin secretion may not be diagnosed on GnRH testing, but in severely affected hypogonadotropic males this test will usually be useful.[242] Children with central precocious puberty can generally be diagnosed by the GnRH test as well.

The somatomedins are not strictly pubertal hormones but are of importance in the study of the pubertal growth spurt. Insulin-like growth factor I increases to concentrations higher than those of the adult at the time of puberty, although the actual concentrations of IGF I do not parallel the growth velocity during the pubertal growth spurt.[243,244] The increase in IGF I at puberty appears to be due to the increase in GH secretion during this stage; the GH secretion in turn is probably due to increased sex steroid secretion.[245]

Adrenarche

Serum concentrations of adrenal androgens begin to increase at 7 to 8 years of age, several years before the peripubertal rise in gonadotropin secretion can be demonstrated. The concentrations of the weak androgen DHEA and its sulfate DHAS begin to increase at 6 to 7 years in girls and 7 to 8 years in boys,[246] and continue to increase until midpuberty (Table 10–1). The control of adrenarche is separate from the mechanisms of gonadotropin stimulation, and LH and FSH have no effect upon DHEA or DHAS secretion.[247] Further, while ACTH must be present for adrenarche to occur, another unknown factor must also be operative to precipitate adrenarche. The timing of adrenarche is usually correlated with gonadarche, but they may occur on different time schedules or adrenarche may not occur at all (as in Addison disease) while gonadarche occurs normally.[248]

Male Physical Pubertal Development

In a normal male, the first sign of puberty is enlargement of the testes to greater than 2.5 cm. Testicular enlargement is mainly due to seminiferous tubule growth, but Leydig cell enlargement contributes as well. Androgens from the testes are the driving force behind secondary sexual development, although adrenal androgens play a role in normal puberty. Thus the development of genitalia and of pubic hair are best described separately. The Tanner method of describing the stages of pubertal development is widely accepted[249] (Fig. 10–15).

Several methods are used to determine the size of testes depending upon the preference of the clinic. The measurement of the length and width of the testes (carefully excluding the epididymis) either by comparison with a ruler or by calipers allows longitudinal records of growth with the expectation that a length greater than 2.5 cm is compatible with the onset of normal pubertal development. The testicular volume index is calculated by: [(length × width of the right testis) + (length × width of the left testis)] ÷ 2.[232]

Orchiometers are devices that allow direct comparison of the patient's testes with an oval of measured volume. The most popular is the Prader orchiometer, consisting of a set of solid or hollow ovals encompassing the range from infancy to adulthood (1 to 25 ml); the volumes of the testes are then recorded in the patient record, with a volume of 3 ml closely correlated with the onset of pubertal development.[250]

The range of onset of normal male puberty extends from 9 to 14 years if 2.5 standard deviations is used to define the limits. Boys complete pubertal development within 2 to

TABLE 10–1.   MEAN SERUM CONCENTRATIONS OF DHAS DURING CHILDHOOD*

Chronologic Age	1–6	6–8	8–10	10–12	12–14	14–16	16–20
Boys (μg/dl)	15.4 ± 6.8	18.8 ± 4.1	58.6 ± 10.1	126.4 ± 28.0	133.4 ± 22.2	264.3 ± 19.4	264.1 ± 61.8
Girls (μg/dl)	24.7 ± 11.1	30.4 ± 7.6	117.3 ± 41.7	112.7 ± 16.4	168.9 ± 19.3	253.5 ± 41.3	232.5 ± 49.8
Bone Age	**1–6**	**6–8**	**8–10**	**10–12**	**12–14**	**14–16**	**16–20**
Boys (μg/dl)	16.6 ± 6.1	36.3 ± 6.7	57.4 ± 8.5	125.0 ± 22.7	214.9 ± 30.1	403.4 ± 99.4	—
Girls (μg/dl)	2.5 ± 2.5	27.2 ± 9.6	—	112.9 ± 27.6	159.7 ± 26.3	261.0 ± 45.0	145.3 ± 32.2

* From Reiter EO, Fuldauer VG, Root AW: Secretion of the adrenal androgen, dehydroepiandrosterone sulfate, during normal infancy, childhood, and adolescence, in sick infants, and in children with endocrinologic abnormalities. J Pediatr 90:766, 1977.

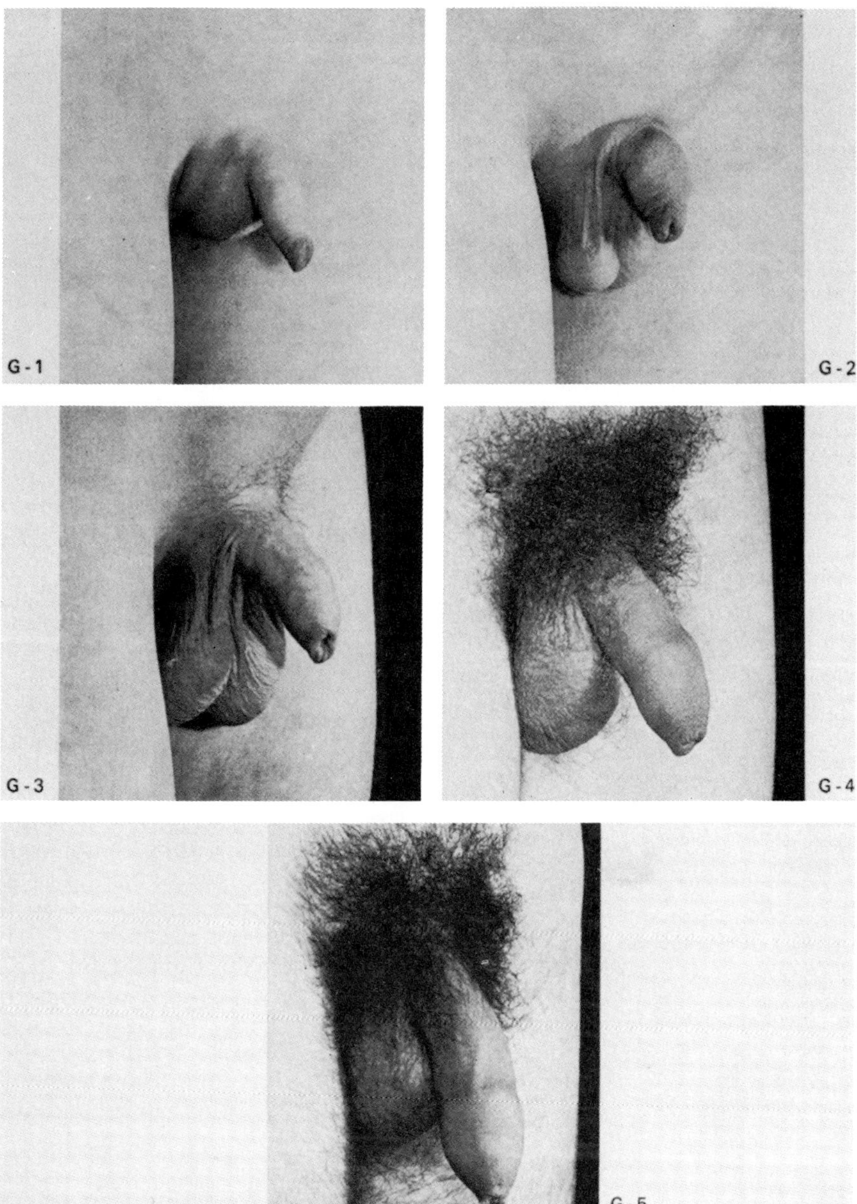

FIGURE 10–15. Stages of male genital development and pubic hair development, according to Marshall and Tanner and Reynolds and Wines. (Photographs reproduced with permission from van Wieringen JC, et al: Growth Diagrams. Groningen, Netherlands, Woplter-Noorhoff Publishing, 1971.)

Genital Development Stages

Stage 1: Preadolescent. Testes, scrotum, and penis are about the same size and proportion as in early childhood.

Stage 2: The scrotum and testes have enlarged; there is a change in the texture and also some reddening of the scrotal skin.

Stage 3: Growth of the penis has occurred, at first mainly in length but with some increase in breadth; there is further growth of testes and scrotum.

Stage 4: The penis is further enlarged in length and breadth with development of the glans. The testes and scrotum are further enlarged. The scrotal skin has further darkened.

Stage 5: Genitalia are adult in size and shape. No further enlargement takes place after Stage 5 is reached.

Pubic Hair Development Stages

Stage 1: Preadolescent. The vellus over the pubes is no further developed than that over the abdominal wall, (i.e., no pubic hair).

Stage 2: Sparse growth of long, slightly pigmented, downy hair, straight or only slightly curled, appearing chiefly at the base of the penis.

Stage 3: Hair is considerably darker, coarser, and curlier and spreads sparsely over the junction of the pubes.

Stage 4: Hair is now adult in type, but the area it covers is still considerable smaller than most adults. There is no spread to the medial surface of the thighs.

Stage 5: Hair is adult in quantity and type, distributed as an inverse triangle. The spread is to the medial surface of the thighs but not up the linea alba or elsewhere above the base of the inverse triangle. Most men will have further spread of public hair.

4.5 years with a mean of 3.25 years[251] (Fig. 10–16). The first appearance of spermatozoa in early morning urinary specimens is referred to as *spermarche*. This occurs at a mean age of 13.4 years, corresponding to gonadal stages 3 to 4 and pubic hair stages 2 to 4. In early or delayed puberty spermarche changes to an earlier or later age, accordingly.[252] The impressive increase in growth rate known as the pubertal growth spurt occurs late in puberty in boys, at gonadal stages 3 to 4. The acceleration of growth appears to be partially a result of increased growth hormone secretion at puberty and and partially a result of testosterone production.[253] Boys attain about 28 cm of growth during the pubertal growth spurt, and the 10-cm mean difference in adult stature between boys and girls is due to a greater pubertal growth spurt in boys and a greater height at the onset of peak height velocity in boys as compared to girls.[254] In prepuberty, boys and girls have the same lean body mass, skeletal mass, and body fat; adult males have 150 per cent of the average female lean and skeletal body mass and adult females have 200 per cent of the body fat of males. Males have twice the number of muscle cells as females as well as having 1.5 times the muscle mass.[255]

Delayed Puberty

Delay of puberty may indicate a temporary condition that spontaneously abates or is followed by a permanent lack of ability to progress through puberty. There is inadequate information on the lower limit of age of normal onset of puberty in the United States, but the upper limits of normal and the range of ages of menarche are known.[251,256] Assuming that 2.5 standard deviations above and below the mean define the normal age of onset of puberty, the term *delayed puberty* may be used to refer to the condition in a boy who has not initiated secondary sexual development by 14 years of age. It is still possible for the patient to be one of the 0.6 per cent of the normal population who will spontaneously enter puberty at a later age. By waiting until these ages to initiate a workup, the examining physician will decrease the likelihood of performing an evaluation unnecessarily. However, age of onset of puberty is not the only important criterion for normal puberty, and patients who do not progress in secondary sexual development after pubertal onset at the normal time must also be considered for evaluation.

Temporary Delayed Puberty

Constitutional Delay in Growth and Adolescence.[257]   This condition has been discussed in detail in Chapter 1. Only the pubertal aspects will be considered here.

Without a classic historical and physical presentation of constitutional delay in puberty, it is often difficult to differentiate temporary constitutional delay in puberty from permanent hypogonadotropic hypogonadism. Various tests have been proposed. A lack of increase in serum prolactin concentration after thyrotropin-releasing hormone (TRF) or chlorpromazine administration,

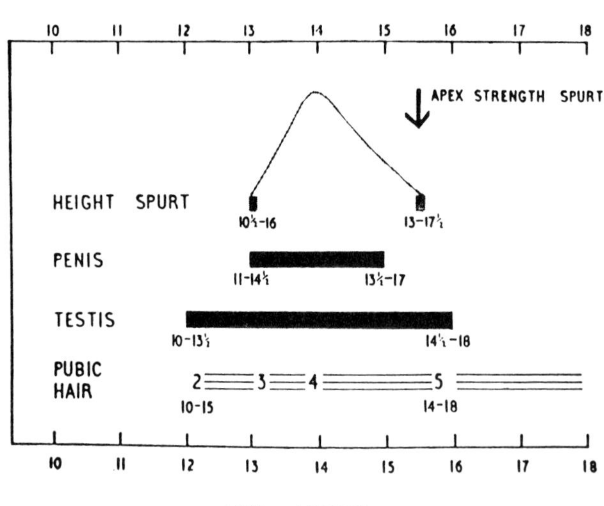

FIGURE 10–16.   Diagram of the sequence of events at puberty in males. An average is represented in relation to the scale of ages. The range of ages within which some of the changes occur is indicated by the figures below. These data are for British children but boys in the United States would normally enter puberty as early as 9 years or as late as 14 years. (From Marshall WA, Tanner JM: Arch Dis Child 45:13, 1970, with permission.)

and a smaller increase in LH concentration after repeated stimulation with GnRH than after the first dose of GnRH, are said to be characteristic of hypogonadotropic hypogonadism. An increase in serum DHAS concentration at the appropriate age of adrenarche combined with absence of an increase in concentrations of serum gonadotropins and testosterone at the expected time of gonadarche is said to occur in hypogonadotropic hypogonadism, whereas a delay in both adrenarche and gonadarche occurs in constitutional delay in puberty.[259,260] All these methods for differentiation of constitutional delay of puberty from hypogonadotropic hypogonadism have considerable overlap and have not proved to be useful, however, and are not recommended for this purpose.

The GnRH test, in which 100 μg of GnRH is administered and serum LH assayed at intervals for 120 min thereafter, does not help distinguish constitutional delay of puberty from the normal prepubertal state. However, approximately 6 months before secondary sexual development begins, the GnRH test will yield results similar to those obtained in normal pubertal patients[261] (Fig. 10–17). The difficulty in the use of the GnRH test is that it may fail to distinguish patients with constitutional delay, who are destined to undergo spontaneous pubertal development more than 6 months in the future, from those patients with hypogonadotropic hypogonadism, who will not undergo such development. In both cases the results of a GnRH challenge may be the same low response of LH. Clinical observation, sometimes for years, is required to uncover the ultimate outcome and differentiate between the two conditions.

Studies have shown that growth hormone secretion may temporarily decrease in patients with constitutional delay of growth at a time when growth rate decreases compared to age-matched controls, only to increase again to normal in 1 or 2 years when the pubertal growth spurt commences.[262] Some patients have received growth hormone therapy after the decreased growth hormone secretion was noted and they have shown at least a temporary increase in growth rate. It is difficult to prove that the increased growth was due to the growth hormone treatment and not a spontaneous occurrence. At present it is not possible to conclude if this therapy can increase the height of patients with constitutional delay in pu-

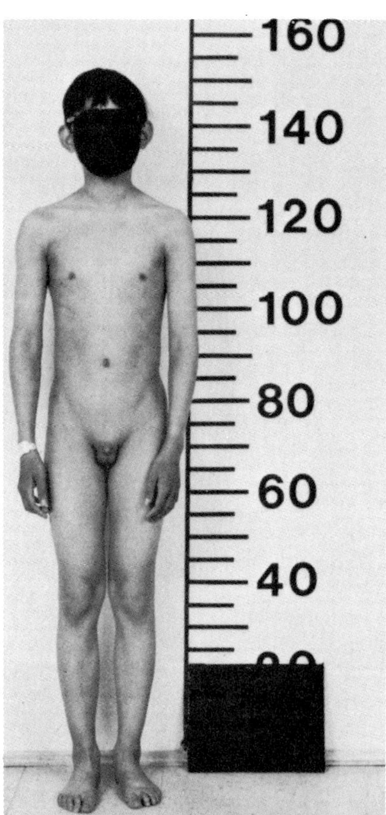

FIGURE 10–17. A male age 16 years and 2 months with constitutional delay in growth and puberty. His height was 149.5 cm (4 SD below the mean value for age); his upper-lower segment ratio of 1.1 (retarded for age). The phallus measured 6.0 × 1.6 cm and the testes 2.5 × 1.4 cm; the scrotum showed early thinning (at the beginning of genital stage 2); and there was no pubic hair (pubic hair stage 1). At a chronologic age of 15 years and 4 months, the bone age was 11 years and the sella turcica was normal. The plasma concentration of LH was 5.5 mIU/ml; that of FSH, 1.5 mIU/ml. On GnRH testing the plasma concentration of LH increased to 17 mIU/ml, and the testosterone rose from 52 to 77 ng/dl. The testes subsequently spontaneously enlarged, and the patient progressed through puberty. (From Styne DM, Grumbach MM: Puberty in the male and female. In Yen SSC, Jaffe RB (eds.): Reproductive Endocrinology. Philadelphia, WB Saunders Company, 1986, with permission.)

berty or if it advances the age of attainment of adult stature.

Permanent Conditions of Sexual Infantilism

Hypogonadotropic Hypogonadism. Permanent lack of onset of pubertal development within the time limits stated previously associated with low serum gonadotropins is defined as hypogonadotropic hypogonadism. This condition can be caused by abnormalities of the hypothalamus or pituitary gland. The patient will be of normal height if only gonadotropins are deficient, but the continued growth in the absence of epiphyseal fusion leads to eunuchoid proportions of long legs and arms and an upper-to-lower segment ratio well below 0.9. If the patient has growth hormone deficiency, growth rate will also be decreased.

Isolated Gonadotropin Deficiency.[263–265] Patients with isolated gonadotropin deficiency are of normal height until the adolescent age range, in contrast to those patients with constitutional delay in puberty and those with growth hormone deficiency. However, because of the lack of a pubertal growth spurt, hypogonadotropic patients have a growth rate less than that of a normal pubertal individual in the teenage years. Because their epiphyses are not closed at the normal age, they may continue to grow beyond the normal age of epiphyseal fusion and reach a normal adult height. They have characteristic eunuchoid proportions as noted above; they have an arm span more than 5 cm greater than height and a lower than normal upper-to-lower segment ratio (0.9 or more is normal for adult Caucasians[266]).

Patients with congenital midline defects may have hypothalamic-pituitary disorders, including gonadotropin deficiency.

In Kallmann syndrome hyposmia or anosmia (due to aplasia or hypoplasia of the olfactory lobes) is associated with gonadotropin deficiency[267] (Fig. 10–18). There is considerable heterogeneity so that within one family there can be patients with disorders of smell with normal gonadal function and others with abnormal gonadal function and normal sense of smell. Original reports suggested X-linked inheritance, but more recent studies show that there is autosomal-recessive or dominant inheritance with variable penetrance.[268] Associated abnormalities of Kallmann syndrome involve abnormalities of facial fusion, kidney formation, and metacarpal formation.

Sporadic or autosomal recessive isolated gonadotropin deficiency with normal sense of smell is reported more rarely than is Kallman syndrome. Some patients lack only normal LH secretion and although testosterone secretion is subnormal, they exhibit spermatogenesis (the fertile eunuch syndrome), whereas others do not secret FSH.[269]

X-linked congenital adrenal hypoplasia is associated with hypogonadotropic hypogon-

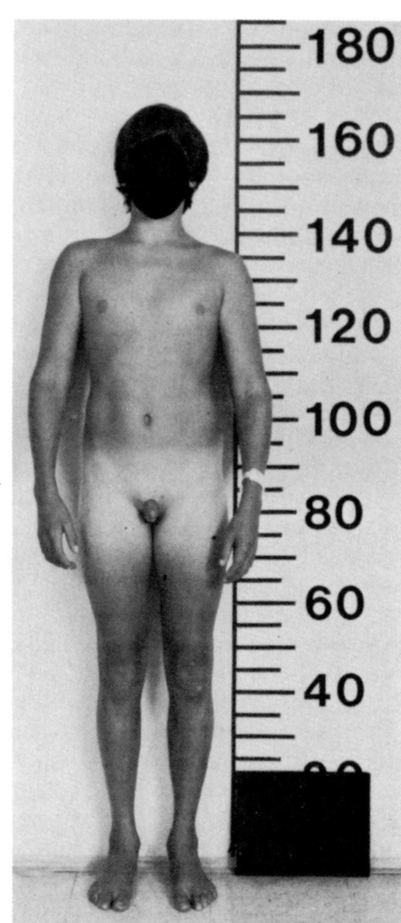

FIGURE 10–18. A boy of 15 years, 10 months, with isolated gonadotropin deficiency and anosmia (Kallmann syndrome). He had undescended testes, but after administration of a total of 10,000 units of hCG the testes descended and were palpable in the scrotum. Height has 163.9 cm (−1.5 SD); the upper-lower segment ratio was .86, which is eunuchoid. The phallus measured 6.3 × 1.8 cm, and the testes were 1.2 × 0.8 cm. The concentration of plasma LH was less than 2.3 mIU/ml; that of FSH, 3.6 mIU/ml; and that of testosterone, 16 mIU/dl. After 100 μg of GnRH the plasma LH was 4.5 mIU/ml and plasma FSH 7.2 mIU/ml. (From Styne DM, Grumbach MM: Puberty in the male and female. *In* Yen SSC, Jaffe RB (eds.): Reproductive Endocrinology. Philadelphia, WB Saunders Company, 1986, with permission.)

adism; other associations include glycerol kinase deficiency and muscular dystrophy.

Congenital Hypopituitarism. (See also Chapter 1) Untreated isolated growth hormone deficiency can delay the onset of puberty, and it may be difficult to tell which patient has gonadotropin deficiency accompanying growth hormone deficiency until the teenage years.[270] The presence of a microphallus (stretched penile length less than 2.5 cm compared to a normal mean length of 4 cm) in a newborn male may alert the examiner to growth hormone deficiency or gonadotropin deficiency, because either condition interferes with penile growth. The condition can be treated with low doses of testosterone (25. mg of testosterone enanthate intramuscularly every month for three doses) to enlarge the penis (both in length and width) without undue advancement of the bone age.[271] Although there are statements in the literature suggesting sex reversal and castration as a therapy for boys with congenital hypopituitarism with microphallus, the successful medical therapy of the microphallus in this condition strongly argues against such a course.

Abnormalities of the Central Nervous System. Hypothalamic-pituitary tumors may affect the secretion of gonadotropins as well as all other pituitary hormones. Thus delayed puberty in association with growth failure, hypothyroidism, adrenal insufficiency, or diabetes insipidus are found. Two characteristics strongly suggest the onset of a CNS tumor: late onset of pituitary deficiency and the combination of anterior and posterior pituitary defects.

Craniopharyngiomas are rare, but are the most common CNS tumor to affect endocrine function in the 6 to 14-year-old age group.[272] They are tumors of Rathke's pouch that originate in the pituitary stalk but spread to the suprasellar region as well as into the sella turcica. Patients characteristically complain of headache, visual loss, polyuria, and polydipsia. They may be found to have short stature, hypothyroidism, sexual immaturity even if of pubertal age, papilledema, and optic atrophy. Flecks of calcium will be found within the tumor in more than 80 per cent of cases by x-ray or CT scan. Craniopharyngiomas are usually cystic and contain cholesterol-laden "machinery oil" dark fluid. The sella is often eroded. Treatment by transsphenoidal microsurgery can be successful if the tumor is intrasellar. The transcranial approach is used for larger tumors, but they cannot usually be completely removed without causing neurologic sequelae. Because craniopharyngiomas are radiosensitive, a combination of surgery and radiation therapy is often employed.

Other extrasellar tumors of the CNS include germinomas (this tumor may also cause precocious puberty in boys through secretion of hCG). Germinomas often cause diabetes insipidus and visual defects. They are located in the pineal area, suprasellar hypothalamic area or elsewhere in the CNS. These tumors are highly radiosensitive.[273] Astrocytomas and gliomas (which may be isolated or associated with neurofibromatosis) may also cause hypopituitarism. Intrasellar adenomas are rare in childhood or adolescence but they may impair pituitary function. Hyperprolactinemia with or without a microadenoma or galactorrhea can delay the onset or progression of puberty, but successful therapy allows puberty to progress.[274,275]

Gonadotropin deficiency can occur in the histiocytosis X syndrome (Hand-Schuller-Christian disease),[276] granulomas caused by tuberculosis or sarcoid, postinfectious inflammation, and vascular lesions of the CNS.[277] Trauma due to accidents, child abuse, or surgery can affect hypothalamic-pituitary function, as can hydrocephalus.

Congenital defects of the CNS, including midline lesions, frequently cause hypothalamic pituitary disfunction. Optic dysplasia is diagnosed by the finding of small, pale optic disks usually surrounded by a dark margin (congenital optic dysplasia should not be confused with acquired optic atrophy, which is an ominous sign of a tumor) and is associated with impaired vision and subsequent pendular nystagmus.[278] Approximately 50 per cent of patients have absence of the septum pellucidum and the term *septo-optic dysplasia* has been coined to define this condition. Patients may be normal in terms of endocrine function, but others may have any combination of anterior and posterior pituitary deficiencies. Other midline defects may be found associated with endocrine deficiencies; cleft palate is one notable common type.

Radiation treatment for leukemia or head tumors that includes the fields the hypothalamic-pituitary area causes delayed onset of hypothalamic-pituitary defects.[279] Younger patients and those with higher radiation doses appear most susceptible. Endocrine defects are manifest 9 to 18 months after the radiation therapy. Growth hormone deficiency is the most common defect, but gonadotropin deficiency is possible.

Functional Disorders and Syndromes. The Prader-Willi syndrome is characterized by fetal and infantile hypotonia (the mother may note lack of fetal movements), short stature, massive obesity and lack of satiety, almond-shaped eyes and characteristic facies, small hands and feet (acromicria), deletion or translocation of chromosome 15 in 50 per cent of cases, mental retardation, and microphallus and undescended testes in males. This is a sporadically occurring condition.[280,281]

The Laurence-Moon-Biedl syndrome consists of polydactyly, obesity, short stature, mental retardation, and retinal pigmentation; this syndrome can be associated with either hypo- or hypergonadotropic hypogonadism.[282]

Weight loss due to chronic disease, malnutrition, and even dieting to less than 80 per cent of ideal weight can cause hypogonadotropic hypogonadism. Repair of the nutritional status will allow resumption of the pubertal process.[283]

Anorexia nervosa is a psychiatric disorder of disturbed body image associated with avoidance of food, regurgitation of food ingested, and performance of rituals around food.[284] Endocrine abnormalities include prepubertal gonadotropin secretion, prepubertal GnRH response pattern, increased serum growth hormone, low somatomedin, low triiodothyronine (T_3), low 1,25-OH-vitamin D, and increased 24,25-vitamin D.[285] Recently children have been reported with fear of obesity leading to compulsive dieting; this condition is said to be different from anorexia nervosa.[286]

Increased physical activity (primarily running) in adult males can cause decreased testosterone secretion; because male pubertal athletes do not seem to lack secondary sexual development it is doubtful that this situation causes delayed puberty.

Hypothyroidism can delay the onset of puberty and, if hypothyroidism occurs after the onset of puberty, stop the progression of puberty. Paradoxically, severe hypothyroidism can cause precocious pubertal development (Chapter 3).

Hypergonadotropic Hypogonadism. Primary testicular failure causes an increase in LH and FSH and is called hypergonadotropin hypogonadism. Patients may have congenital or acquired defects.

Klinefelter syndrome, or seminiferous tubular dysgenesis, is discussed on page 381. Patients usually enter puberty at a normal age, but inadequate testosterone secretion impairs the progression through puberty.

Mumps orchitis is a disease of patients of pubertal or older age.[287] Testicular atrophy is of greatest concern in this disorder, but appropriate immunization should further reduce the incidence of this rare complication.

Another viral infection noted to affect the testes is Coxsackie B virus.[288]

In the Sertoli cell only syndrome (germ cell aplasia, Del Castillo syndrome) normal virilization occurs but the patients have azoospermia and small testes as a result of the absence of the seminiferous tubules, which normally make up the bulk of the testes.[289] Histologic study reveals the seminiferous tubules to be lined with partially degenerated Sertoli cells with inclusion bodies and clear vacuoles.[290]

Low-dose radiotherapy may lead to decreased sperm counts, and the effects may be reversible with time. Doses less than 140 rads may cause oligospermia, and 140 to 300 rads are said to cause azoospermia, which may be reversible.[291] Doses of 1500 to 2000 rads cause considerable permanent damage to the germ cells, and although LH and FSH concentrations are elevated, testosterone concentrations may remain adequate to cause virilization.[292] When possible, the testes must be shielded from radiation (e.g., during radiographic study).

Chemotherapy with alkylating agents may cause testicular damage, with the degree of damage depending on the dose and age of the patient. Other forms of chemotherapy appear to be less damaging. Prepubertal patients are more resistant than older boys to the effects of chemotherapeutic agents. Generally Leydig cells have been thought to escape chemotherapy-induced damage, but reports have now demonstrated that they, too, may be involved.[293]

Only two pediatric patients have been reported as having testicular lymphangiectasis; one child had Noonan syndrome and the other, except for bilateral cryptorchidism, was normal.[294]

At least six prepubertal cases of epidermoid cysts of the testes are reported. If small enough, excisional biopsy appears appropriate because the cysts seem to follow a benign course, but larger ones may destroy enough testicular tissue to require orchiectomy. Dermoid cysts appear to be even rarer in childhood than epidermoid cysts.[295]

Macro-orchidism, starting as early as infancy, is associated with X-linked mental retardation and a fragile site on the long arm of the X chromosome (Xq,27fra).[296] Other associated anomalies include increased birth weight, high forehead, large ears, prognathism, pale irises, and an increased head circumference. Testicular biopsy has demonstrated normal Leydig and Sertoli cells, normal to slightly decreased spermatogenic cells, and an increase in testicular interstitial fluid.

Benign testicular enlargement without any of the other characteristics noted above is extremely rare. The testes of one such patient were completely normal on histologic examination.[297]

Testicular tenderness and swelling is a reported complication of Henoch-Schonlein purpura in 2 to 28 per cent of cases. Testicular symptoms may precede the cutaneous manifestations; because the symptoms may mimic testicular torsion, this association is of great importance.[298]

Diagnosis of Delayed Puberty

A diagnostic evaluation should be undertaken after the age of 14 years if puberty has not begun or after the cessation of progression of puberty in a boy who has already started secondary sexual development. When taking the medical history attention should be paid to chronic illness, nutritional disorders, birth or later trauma to the head, a history of infertility in members of the family, a history of consanguinity, and, of great importance, the age of menarche of the mother (or siblings) and the age of onset of puberty in the father (or siblings) and the heights of the parents and siblings.

The growth rate of the child is calculated from prior height measurements and the present stature and weight of the child is plotted in a growth chart. The arm span and upper-to-lower segment ratio (the distance from the symphysis pubis to the floor subtracted from the height) are determined. Physical exam should include a search for the presence of chronic disease or malnutrition. Signs of puberty, including acne, comedones, mustache, axillary hair, the stage of pubic hair, stretched penile length, length and width of the testes, and stage of genital development and tone of the voice should be noted. Neurologic examination should include visualization of optic disks and measurement of visual fields. The sense of smell must be tested to rule out the possibility of Kallmann syndrome.

Laboratory studies are first directed to determining whether concentrations of gonadotropins and testosterone are low or high to differentiate the broad areas of hypo- and hypergonadotropic hypogonadism. Screening chemistry panel, electrolytes, thyroxine (with protein binding correction), and prolactin measurements are performed.

A bone age determination may be useful in a short patient with suspected constitutional delay, but can only be used as a guide toward diagnosis. A lateral skull x-ray may reveal a craniopharyngioma if the sella is enlarged or if there is calcification, but if the diagnosis of craniopharyngioma or germinoma is suspected, a MRI or CT scan is necessary.

The differentiation of constitutional delay in puberty from hypogonadotropic hypogonadism is, as already mentioned, quite difficult (Table 10–2). In both conditions low serum gonadotropin and testosterone concentrations are found. Prepubertal patterns of GnRH testing and decreased episodic gonadotropin pulses until about 6 months before spontaneous pubertal development are found in the constitutional delay patients. Longitudinal observation is often required, sometimes until 18 years of age. As noted, at least one patient entered puberty spontaneously at 25 years of age. Constitutional delay patients tend to have low serum DHAS concentrations with low testosterone concentrations. In hypogonadotropic hypogonadal patients adrenarche and increasing DHAS concentrations occur at an appropriate age but gonadarche and increasing testosterone do not occur. At present no reliable method is available to distinguish constitutional delay from permanent hypogonadotropic hypogonadism.

Treatment of Delayed Puberty

The treatment of the conditions described above depends upon the diagnosis and whether there will be a temporary or permanent delay in pubertal development. Constitutional delay in puberty requires initial reassurance; often the boy and his parents will be relieved that no serious problem exists and no treatment is necessary. Many boys, however, are distressed about their shortness and immature appearance. If they are over 14 years of age, they can be offered low-dose testosterone therapy, which can cause them to look more mature without compromising their adult height.[299] High-dose testosterone was administered too often in the past and caused advancement of skeletal development leading to premature epiphyseal fusion and decreased final height. Low-dose therapy consists of 100 to 150 mg of testosterone enanthate given

TABLE 10–2.   DIFFERENTIAL DIAGNOSTIC FEATURES OF DELAYED PUBERTY AND SEXUAL INFANTILISM*

	Stature	Plasma Gonadotropins	GnRH Test: LH Response	Plasma Gonadal Steroids	Plasma DHAS	Karyotype	Olfaction
Constitutional delay in growth and adolescence	Short for chronological age, usually appropriate for bone age and for family growth patterns	Prepubertal, later pubertal	Prepubertal, later pubertal	Low, later normal	Low for chronologic age, appropriate for bone age	Normal	Normal
Hypogonadotropic Hypogonadism							
Isolated gonadotropin deficiency	Normal, absent pubertal growth spurt and eunuchoid proportions	Low	Prepubertal or no response	Low	Appropriate for chronologic age	Normal	Normal
Kallmann's syndrome	Normal, absent pubertal growth spurt and eunuchoid proportions	Low	Prepubertal or no response	Low	Appropriate for chronologic age	Normal	Anosmia or hyposmia
Idiopathic multiple pituitary hormone deficiencies	Short stature and poor growth since early childhood and eunuchoid proportions	Low	Prepubertal or no response	Low	Usually low	Normal	Normal
Hypothalamic-pituitary tumors	Decrease in growth velocity of recent onset	Low	Prepubertal or no response	Low	Normal or low for chronologic age	Normal	Normal
Primary Gonadal Failure							
Klinefelter's syndrome and variants	Normal to tall	High	Hyper-response at puberty	Low or normal	Normal for chronologic age	XXY or variant	Normal

* Modified from Styne DM, Grumbach MM: Puberty in the male and female. *In* Yen SSC, Jaffe RB (eds): Reproductive Endocrinology. Philadelphia, WB Saunders Company, 1986.

every 4 weeks for three doses. One month or sooner after the end of this regimen the boy should have signs of penile enlargement and pubic hair growth, and most will have a better self-image because of this development. After a 3-month wait to see if any spontaneous pubertal development occurs, another 3-month course may be started. With the passage of a year, as outlined above, many of the patients will undergo spontaneous development as they reach a bone age of 12 to 13 years. It is necessary to monitor skeletal age during treatment and to discontinue treatment if there is undue skeletal advancement.

Permanent hypogonadism requires continuing therapy and the treatment is the same as in primary hypogonadism or in hypogonadotropic hypogonadism. Testosterone enanthate should be given intramuscularly every 4 weeks in doses starting at 100 mg at an age when puberty normally begins, and the dose increased by 50 mg every 6 months to a dose of 200 to 300 mg (giving too much initially will cause priapism). If the boy has growth hormone deficiency, the testosterone is given in lower doses later in a regimen coordinated with the growth hormone therapy to assure maximal growth before epiphyseal fusion. Some boys are concerned that they do not have normal pubic hair development with testosterone; in these, the addition of hCG has been shown to promote thicker pubic hair growth.[300]

Methyl testosterone should not be given as it may be toxic to the liver. Other anabolic steroids have been recommended, but do not offer clear advantages over testosterone injections.

Hypogonadotropic hypogonadism can also be treated with a programmable pump, infusing GnRH episodically, recreating the pattern of the hypothalamic pulse generator.[301] This therapy is best reserved for the older patient who is being treated for infertility, because it is complicated and testosterone works well enough in promoting the appearance of puberty. Human chorionic gonadotropin and FSH can also be given to cause fertility in a male with functional testes who may lack a pituitary gland as a result of trauma or surgical removal.

Sexual Precocity in the Male

A boy exhibiting secondary sexual development before the age of 9 years is considered to have sexual precocity.[302] The diagnosis is true or central precocious puberty if the etiology is premature maturation of the hypothalamic-pituitary axis; if the etiology is autonomous secretion of sex steroids or autonomous secretion of hCG, the condition is incomplete precocious puberty. Regardless of the cause, patients will experience rapid growth and skeletal maturation and without treatment may demonstrate paradoxical tall stature as a child but cease growing at an early age and become a short adult.

True or Complete Precocious Puberty

The early onset of pubertal development when the sequence of endocrine events follows the normal course of hypothalamic-pituitary-gonadal activity of normal puberty is considered to be true or complete precocious puberty.

Constitutional Precocious Puberty. Some boys will normally begin puberty before the lower age limit of 9 years, without evidence of a disorder; these children simply lie at the younger age of the normal distribution of onset of puberty. There may be a family tendency toward such early development. These patients are not usually as young as patients afflicted with the following conditions.

Idiopathic Precocious Puberty. Idiopathic precocious puberty is a diagnosis of exclusion when no tumor or other definitive diagnosis is found. Affected children manifest all of the endocrine findings of normal puberty. Clinical progression may be rapid and continuous or slow and waxing and waning. Boys with this condition will first demonstrate testicular enlargement, as do normal boys at puberty. It is an interesting fact of our society that girls are brought for evaluation of idiopathic precocious puberty sooner in the course of the disorder than boys.

Central Nervous System Disorders. Boys more often have a diagnosable neurologic disorder as the etiology of their precocious puberty than they have idiopathic precocious puberty; this ratio is reversed in girls with precocious puberty. Hamartomas of the tuber cinereum are the most frequent type of CNS tumor to cause precocious puberty, and they are being more frequently found in patients because of the new noninvasive and sensitive CT and MRI scanning procedures available. Prior to availability of these techniques some these patients would have had the diagnosis of "idiopathic precocious puberty." Hamartomas are not progressive tumors and because of their sensitive location are not amenable to surgical removal. Medical therapy with GnRH agonists is the treatment of choice (Fig. 10–19). Hamartomas of the tuber cinereum may be diagnosed by their characteristic, often pediculated, appearance and location. They contain GnRH and presumably release it in a pulsatile pattern to cause precocious puberty.

Astrocytomas, ependymomas, and gliomas of the optic nerve or hypothalamus carry a less favorable prognosis than hamartomas of the tuber cinereum. Germinomas may activate the hypothalamic-pituitary axis and cause true precocious puberty similar to other tumors, or may secrete hCG and cause incomplete precocious puberty in boys. Germinomas are radiation sensitive. Precocious puberty may be the first sign of the tumor but headaches and visual disturbances may be among the early symptoms. Most space-occupying lesions or causes of increased intracranial pressure can cause true precocious puberty, probably by interfering with the inhibitory process controlling gonadotropin secretion. These conditions include granulomas, suprasellar cysts, hydrocephalus, and head trauma.

Because these tumors or CNS conditions can cause growth hormone deficiency in addition to precocious puberty itself, the possible combination of precocious puberty and growth hormone deficiency must be considered; patients affected with this combination may have a normal growth rate for chronologic age (because the testosterone stimulates growth and counters the growth hormone deficiency) but a growth rate inadequate for the stage of pubertal development (because the patients lack the combined effects of testosterone and growth hormone).

The McCune-Albright syndrome consists of the triad of irregularly shaped café-au-lait spots, fibrous dysplasia of the long bones (cysts are found on x-ray examination), and either true or incomplete precocious pu-

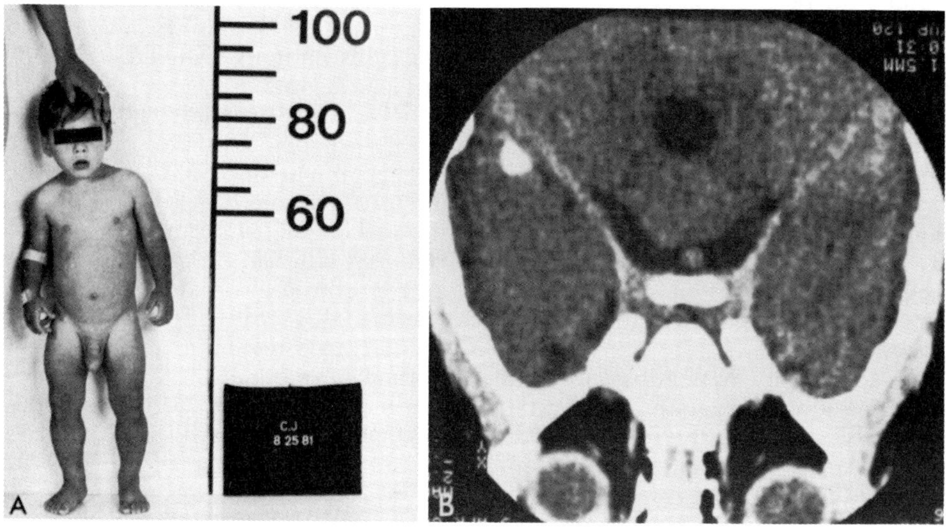

FIGURE 10–19. *A,* A 17-month-old male infant with a hamartoma of the tuber cinereum and true precocious puberty. At 8 months of age, secondary sexual development was noted, and the patient was misdiagnosed as having congenital virilizing adrenal hyperplasia. He was treated with glucocorticoids, which slowed his growth but did not affect his sexual development and bone age advancement. When he was first seen at 17 months, his height was 84.2 cm (−1 SD); his weight was 14.8 kg (−2.2 SD); the pubic hair stage was II; the penis was 10.4 × 2.2 cm; the testes were 1.5 × 2.8 cm; and the scrotum was thinned and rugose. The bone age was 4⁹⁄₁₂ years. After GnRH administration, the LH level rose from 3.9 to 24 mIU/dl, the FSH level from 1.5 to 3.6 mIU/ml, and the testosterone level from 409 to 450 ng/dl. The DHAS was 17 µg/dl (preadrenarchal value). The patient was treated with a potent long-acting GnRH agonist (D-Trp⁶Pro⁹NEt-GnRH), which resulted in arrest of his pubertal advancement and a striking decrease in the plasma concentration of testosterone, LH pulses, and the response to exogenous GnRH.

B, Computed tomography scan of the patient, demonstrating a 1.5-cm mass posterior and rostral to the dorsum sellae, which depresses the floor of the third ventricle. (From Styne DM, Grumbach MM: Puberty in the male and female. *In* Yen SSC, Jaffe RB (eds.): Reproductive Endocrinology. Philadelphia, WB Saunders Company, 1986, with permission.)

berty.[303,304] It is possible that autonomous gonadal function and sex steroid secretion occurs first and this sex steroid production leads to maturation of the hypothalamic-pituitary axis and true precocious puberty. Patients may also have other evidence of autonomous endocrine function such as gigantism, autonomous ovarian activity, nodular adrenal hyperplasia, Cushing syndrome, and thyrotoxicosis.[305,306] When central precocious puberty is found in the McCune-Albright syndrome, treatment with GnRH agonists is effective, but if incomplete precocious puberty is present it is not. However, testolactone, an aromatase inhibitor, has been shown to be useful in a recent study in girls.[307]

Neurofibromatosis, or von Recklinghausen syndrome, is inherited in an autosomal pattern and is also characterized by café-au-lait spots; these are smoother than those found in McCune-Albright syndrome.[308]

(Fig. 10–20). A basic feature is the overgrowth of nerve sheaths and fibrous tissue elements. Freckling of the axilla and subcutaneous sessile or deeper plexiform lesions of the skin are found. The neurofibromas that develop with time can mold the bones and cause such problems as cysts, pseudoarthroses, hemihypertrophy and bowing, scoliosis, and facial and skull defects.[309] The neurofibromas or associated gliomas of the CNS may cause precocious or delayed puberty.

Profound hypothyroidism can cause either delayed puberty or, paradoxically, precocious puberty.[310] Testicular enlargement is seen and, rarely, galactorrhea. Treatment with thyroid hormone will reverse the condition (see Chapter 3).

Any virilizing condition can cause maturation of the hypothalamic-pituitary axis. While the androgen may suppress gonadotropin secretion, removal of the source of an-

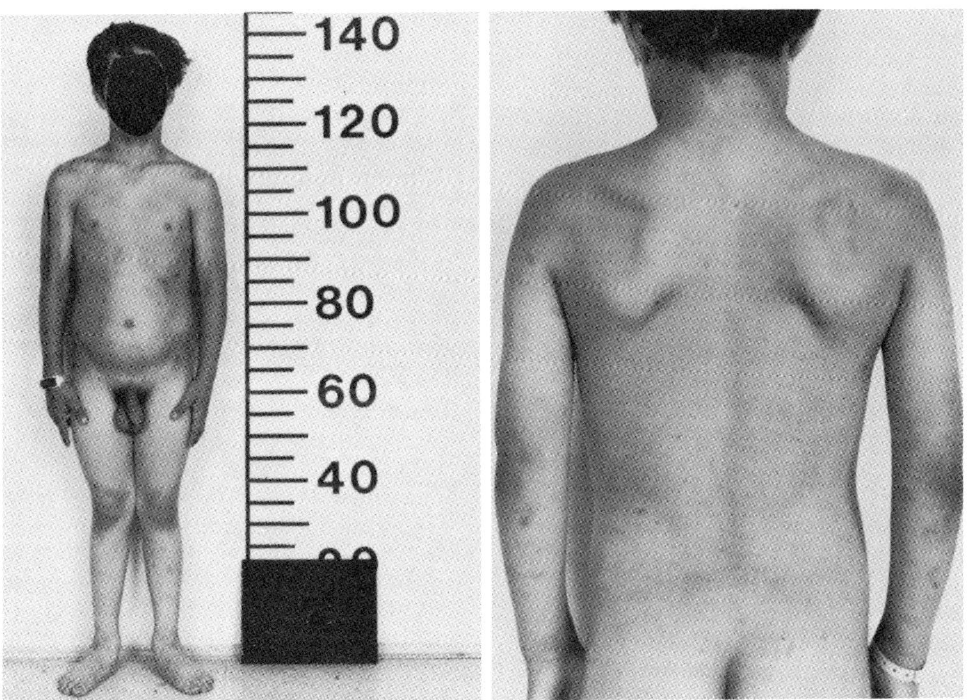

FIGURE 10–20. A boy of 8 years and 8 months of age with neurofibromatosis and precocious puberty, associated with a hypothalamic glioma. He had tonic-clonic seizures at 2½ years and rapid growth starting at 4 years; an enlarged penis and testes and the presence of pubic hair were first noted at 7½ years. At this time, his height was 139.9 cm (+1.4 SD); the phallus was 9 × 3 cm; the right testis measured 5.5 × 3.2 cm and the left 5.4 × 2.9 cm. He had stage 3 pubic hair and 24 large café-au-lait spots. Computed tomography and pneumoencephalography revealed a 1.5 × 2.5-cm hypothalamic mass, which was treated with irradiation. The plasma concentration of LH was 3.9 mIU/ml; that of FSH, 1.2 mIU/ml; and that of testosterone, 221 ng/dl. After 100 μg of intravenous GnRH, the peak concentration of LH was 38 mIU/ml; that of FSH, 4.2 mIU/ml; and that of testosterone, 1.4 ng/dl. (From Styne DM, Grumbach MM: Puberty in the male and female. *In* Yen SSC, Jaffe RB (eds.): Reproductive Endocrinology. Philadelphia, WB Saunders Company, 1986, with permission.)

drogen will allow true precocious puberty to occur. This situation may develop after the institution of treatment for congenital adrenal hyperplasia, after the removal of adrenal androgen-secreting tumors, and after the cessation of androgen therapy for various disorders such as anemia.

Incomplete Precocious Puberty

Pubertal development can occur without maturation of the hypothalamic-pituitary axis. Thus, males can virilize with precocious puberty either by autonomous secretion of sex steroids or by production of hCG, which will cause Leydig cell testosterone secretion. An important physical finding in many types of incomplete precocious puberty is the lack of testicular enlargement compared to that found in true precocious puberty; an important endocrine characteristic is the lack of a pubertal gonadotropin response to GnRH.

Autonomous Androgen Production. Androgen secretion can occur because of adrenal enzyme defects involving 21-hydroxylase or 11-hydroxylase, as noted earlier in this chapter, or by adrenal carcinomas as described elsewhere in this volume (Chapter 6). If adrenal hyperplasia is inadequately treated, adrenal rests that may be present in the testes are susceptible to ACTH stimulation, and will enlarge, giving the testes an irregular appearance, and secrete androgens.

Interstitial cell tumors of the testes are rare, but will secrete testosterone and lead to unilateral enlargement of a testes.

Another recently described cause of incomplete precocious puberty in boys is familial gonadotropin-independent sexual precocity with premature Leydig cell maturation, also named testotoxicosis because of parallelism to TSH-independent thyroid activity in thyrotoxicosis.[311,312] This is a sex-limited autosomal recessive disorder that affects only boys. Serum testosterone concentration is quite high and serum LH and FSH are suppressed. There is no LH response to GnRH. Histologic examination of the testes reveals Leydig cell maturation and sometimes hyperplasia; spermatogenesis is also found in some cases. Treatment with GnRH is initially ineffectual. Ketoconazole is a fungicidal agent with a side effect of inhibition of steroidogenesis; when used in this disorder it can decrease androgen production.[313] Later, as a result of the androgen ex-

erting maturational effects upon the hypothalamic-pituitary axis, true precocious puberty may follow, and GnRH may be used successfully at that stage of therapy.[314] The testes in the initial stages will be slightly enlarged over 2.5 cm but will not be as large as found in true precocious puberty.

Human chorionic gonadotropin-secreting tumors cause Leydig cell stimulation in boys and some testicular enlargement. Such conditions include hepatomas or hepatoblastomas as well as teratomas or chorioepitheliomas of the gonads, mediastinum, retroperitoneum, or pineal gland.[315] As noted, germinomas of the pineal gland may secrete hCG and can cause precocious puberty in boys, although this will not occur in girls.

Iatrogenic precocious puberty occurs in boys exposed to androgens through medication prescribed or through the addition of androgens to other substances, like geriatric vitamins. The administration of hCG to a boy for undescended testes will also cause androgen secretion and, if prolonged, will produce signs of precocious puberty.

Diagnosis Of Precocious Puberty

The medical history of the patient with precocious puberty will be helpful in the differential diagnosis of precocious puberty (Table 10–3). Evidence should be sought regarding CNS injuries at birth or later, exposure to sex steroids, the age of puberty in and the height of the mother, father, and siblings, and the occurrence of precocious puberty other family members.

Physical examination should determine the height and weight of the child, height corrected for parents' heights, and height velocity compared to the normal for age. The stage of gonadal and pubic hair development and the presence of acne, comedones, mustache, axillary hair development, and odor should be noted. Particular attention is paid to the size and shape of the testes. In true precocious puberty the testes will first enlarge symmetrically, whereas in Leydig cell tumors or adrenal rests there is asymmetrical and nodular enlargement. The skin should be searched for café-au-lait spots of neurofibromatosis or McCune-Albright syndrome, and for neurofibromas. A neurologic examination should include the optic disks, visual fields, and signs of increased intracranial pressure.

Skeletal age should be determined. Lateral skull x-rays will usually not dem-

TABLE 10–3.   DIFFERENTIAL DIAGNOSIS OF SEXUAL PRECOCITY*

	Serum Gonadotropin Concentration	GnRH Test: LH Response	Serum Sex Steroid Concentrations	Gonadal Size	Miscellaneous
True Precocious Puberty (Premature reactivation of hypothalamic GnRH pulse generator)	Prominent LH pulses, initially during sleep	Pubertal LH response	Pubertal values of testosterone or estradiol	Normal pubertal testicular enlargement or ovarian and uterine enlargement (by sonography)	CT scan of brain to rule out a CNS tumor or other abnormality; skin examination and skeletal survey for McCune-Albright syndrome
Incomplete Sexual Precoscity (Pituitary gonadotropin-independent), Males Chorionic gonadotropin–secreting tumor in males	High hCG	Elevated LH but prepubertal LH response	Pubertal value of testosterone	Slight to moderate uniform enlargement of testes	Hepatomegaly suggests hepatoblastoma; CT scan of brain if chorionic gonadotropin–secreting CNS tumor suspected
Leydig cell tumor in males	Low-prepubertal	Prepubertal LH response	Very high testosterone	Irregular asymmetric enlargement of testes	
Familial testoxicosis	Low-prepubertal	Prepubertal LH response	Pubertal values of testosterone	Testes symmetric and larger than 2.5 cm but smaller than expected for pubertal development; spermatogenesis occurs	Familial; probably sex-limited, autosomal dominant trait
Premature adrenarache	Prepubertal	Prepubertal LH response	Prepubertal testosterone; DHAS or urinary 17-ketosteroid values appropriate for pubic hair stage	Testes prepubertal	Onset usually after 6 years of age; more frequent in brain-injured children

* Modified from Styne DM, Grumbach MM: Puberty in the male and female. *In* Yen SSC, Jaffe RB (eds): Reproductive Endocrinology, Saunders 1986.

onstrate the types of tumors that cause precocious puberty except for rare craniopharyngiomas that precipitate precocious puberty that may be revealed by calcification or distortion of the sella turcica. A MRI or CT scan of the head with particular attention to the hypothalamic-pituitary region is generally indicated in a patient with true precocious puberty.

Endocrine analysis in precocious puberty includes determinations of serum concentrations of gonadotropins, testosterone, and possibly DHAS. A GnRH test is indicated in the diagnosis of a patient who appears to have central precocious puberty. Nocturnal sampling for peaks of LH and FSH is useful, but usually difficult in most clinical situations. Determination of thyroxine and TSH is diagnostic in cases of apparent severe hypothyroidism causing precocious puberty.

Patients without enlargement of the testes and virilization may have congenital adrenal hyperplasia, and appropriate adrenal androgen determinations are indicated (see Chapter 6). Cushing disease may also be accompanied by virilization, and glucocorticoid excretion should be measured.

Treatment of Precocious Puberty

True precocious puberty can be controlled with the new GnRH agonists that initially stimulate pituitary gonadotropins and then "down-regulate" gonadotropin secretion.[316–318] These agents are administered daily by subcutaneous or intranasal routes but the newer depot preparations may be given less frequently. Within a few days gonadotropin secretion in the basal or GnRH-stimulated state decreases, and testosterone secretion decreases within 1 to 2 weeks. Rapid growth decreases, as does skeletal development rate, and predicted adult height increases. The GnRH agonists are not presently licensed for use in central precocious puberty, but at the time of this writing companies are applying for orphan drug status. Many pediatric endocrinologists are using Lupron, which is approved in the United States for use in prostatic carcinoma, after obtaining Investigational New Drug status (IND) and informed consent from the parents of the patients. This agent is used in doses of 20 to 50 μg/kg daily, a dose higher than necessary for some of the agents used initially, such as D-trp^{6}pro^9-NET-GnRH. Gonadotropin-releasing hormone agonists are ineffectual in many cases of McCune-Albright syndrome in the stage of incomplete precocious puberty; other patients with true precocious puberty are responsive to the agent. Patients with testotoxicosis are unresponsive to GnRH agonists and should be treated first with ketoconazole. Medroxyprogesterone acetate, a progestational agent, has been used for decades in the treatment of true precocious puberty, but with the advent of the GnRH agonists it appears no longer indicated.

Gonadotropin-independent sexual precocity can best be treated with ketoconazole, an antifungal agent that also inhibits steroidogenesis. These patients may then experience true precocious puberty because of the effects upon the hypothalamus of the prior, chronic exposure to androgens. At this later stage, GnRH agonists become useful in therapy. Ketoconazole used as above has not been demonstrated to cause clinical adrenal insufficiency. Ketoconazole has not been approved for treatment of sexual precocity. If it is to be used, proper procedures must be followed to obtain informed consent.

Psychological management is important in these boys, who may have increased activity levels and aggressiveness. Boys with precocious puberty usually do not try to engage in heterosexual activity, but may masturbate in public. The situation is aggravated by the large size of the child, who appears older and from whom more mature behavior and intelligence are expected. Although intelligence does not advance concurrently with body size, if it seems appropriate for the given situation the child may be advanced in school so that he may be with children closer to his size.

Aside from inhibiting the release of testosterone the therapy of incomplete precocious puberty should be directed at the cause, such as ablation of tumors.

Variations of Early Pubertal Development

Premature Adrenarche

Premature adrenarche (previously called premature pubarche) is a benign, self-limited condition. It is heralded by the appearance of a small amount of pubic hair, comedones, axillary hair, or odor usually after the age of 6 years. Increased secretion of the adrenal androgens DHEA and DHAS occurs earlier in this condition than in normal puberty.[319] Thus a boy of 7 or 8 years who has Tanner stages II to III pubic hair will characteristically have a DHAS value ordinarily found in a 13-year-old boy. The signs of virilization are always mild and the rest of pubertal development will occur at a normal age. There may be small increase in growth rate along with a slight advancement of bone age. This condition appears more frequently in girls than boys, and must be differentiated from sexual precocity.

Pubertal Gynecomastia

Transient increase in glandular breast tissue is said to occur in as many as 40 per cent of normal boys during the pubertal period. Usually starting in early puberty, before adult concentrations of testosterone are reached, the process typically resolves within 2 years, but in some cases it may last longer and cause significant concern in parents and in the patient. Obese subjects characteristically appear more affected; they may have a reduction in the adipose tissue component of the gynecomastia by reducing their weight. The etiology of pubertal gynecomastia has been the subject of study for decades and conflicting results abound. Implicated in the process in some studies but contradicted in others have been a higher estrogen-to-androgen ratio,[320] elevated prolactin concentrations, episodic elevations of estrogens, and increased sensitivity of receptors to circulating estrogens; a unifying theory has not yet been generally accepted.

Gynecomastia may also occur in pathologic conditions detailed elsewhere in this chapter. Thus Klinefelter syndrome,[321] anorchia or acquired testicular failure, biosynthetic defects in testosterone production, androgen receptor defects,[322] and a rare condition of increased activity of peripheral aromatase are associated with gynecomastia.[323] Gynecomastia is an adverse reaction to several drugs, including cimetidine, spironolactone, digitalis, and phenothiazines, and may occur with marihuana ingestion. Gynecomastia also occurs with the ingestion of estrogens from meat treated with estrogen or from pills contaminated with estrogen (in one case from a prior production of estrogen on the same machinery in the factory).[324] Further, treatment with hCG, testosterone, or estrogens may cause the development of breast tissue. Hyperprolactinemia may cause nipple discharge, but not gynecomastia per se.

The treatment of gynecomastia depends upon the cause and duration. Routine pubertal gynecomastia should be treated with reassurance and psychosocial support because resolution should occur relatively quickly. It is useful to have the boy avoid changing or showering in public to eliminate the ridicule of peers. In prolonged cases, with no sign of remission in 2 years, therapy may be considered. In permanent conditions of gynecomastia listed above, therapy may be offered earlier.

Surgical glandular and adipose tissue removal has been the mainstay of therapy in those patients requiring treatment; the approach has recently been circumareolar and the surgery leaves little noticeable scarring. Reports have begun to appear suggesting liposuction as an alternative, but the safety and efficacy of this approach is unproven in adolescents. Medical therapy with clomiphene citrate, Tamoxiphen, Danazol, and testosterone or dihydrotestosterone heptanoate[325] have been reported to be successful, but in most cases controlled studies or confirmatory reports have been lacking.

TESTICULAR TUMORS

In addition to their occurrence in dysgenetic and cryptorchid testes (previously discussed in this chapter), tumors may arise in testes that are originally normal. Symmetric, regular testicular enlargement is characteristic of the early stages of pubertal development, but testicular tumors may also cause testicular enlargement. Tumors are usually painless and generally can be easily differentiated from pubertal enlargement because of their irregularity and hardness to palpation. Testicular torsion or infections are usually characterized by pain and hydroceles by the ability to transilluminate the swollen area; associated infection or hydrocele may conceal the presence of a tumor and a tumor should be at least considered even if one of these more benign diagnoses is made. Diagnosis is usually dependent upon histologic examination, although imaging modalities such as ultrasound have a good degree of diagnostic value prior to surgery.[326] Less than 5 per cent of testicular tumors present in childhood and they represent 1.5 per cent of all childhood cancers.[327,328]

Testicular tumors of germinal cell origin are the most common in childhood. Embryonal carcinomas of the testes are the single most common testicular tumor in childhood, and are malignant and rapidly growing. There are the adult forms, the infantile yolk sac tumors and, if differentiated elements are present, teratocarcinomas. α-Fetoprotein concentration in the serum is high and may serve as a marker as to the presence of the tumor and the efficacy of therapy. Surgery is commonly employed, although chemotherapy similar to that used in teratomas may be appropriate in some cases. Seminomas are rarely seen prior to the young adult period, but seminomas or dysgerminomas may be found in a dysgenetic gonad with a gonadoblastoma. Well-differentiated teratomas of the testes in childhood are generally benign and generally occur prior to 3 years of age. They may contain cysts and solid tissue with elements of bone, cartilage, fibrous and adipose tissue, or squamous epithelium. Surgical removal is the recommended treatment. Teratocarcinomas or malignant anaplastic teratomas occur in older boys, generally during puberty, and will require chemotherapy and radiotherapy; β-hCG may serve as a tumor marker in this condition.

Rhabdomyosarcomas are muscular tumors arising in the cord structures, and may present as masses separate from the testicular tissue itself. Other tumors of the vasculature (hemangiomas), the fibrous tissue (fibromas), and the smooth muscle of arteries (leiomyomas) are rarely reported in the testes of children.

Sertoli cell tumors may occur in childhood and are generally benign. They are said to be responsible for development of incomplete precocious puberty but the relationship is hard to explain.

Leydig cell tumors are quite rare, and may cause incomplete precocious puberty as a result of testosterone production. Crystals of Reinke are found on histologic examination in some cases but are not invariably present.

Embryonic adrenal rest tissue may enlarge under stimulation from ACTH in untreated adrenal hyperplasia and simulate a neoplasm of the testes. Glucocorticoid replacement will decrease ACTH concentrations and cause the rest to shrink.

Leukemia may involve the testes by infiltration with tumor cells. Histologic evidence for involvement may be found long before swelling is detected. Lymphoma is considerably rarer but is reported in the testes.

REFERENCES

1. Gordon H: Ancient ideas about sex differentiation. *In* Vallet HL (ed): Genetic Mechanism of Sexual Development. New York Academic Press, 1979, p 1.
2. Jost A: Problems of fetal endocrinology: The gonadal and hypophyseal hormones. Recent Prog Horm Res 8:379, 1953.
3. Stern C: The genetics of sex determination in man. Int Congr Genet 2:1121, 1961.
4. Golomb HM, Bahr GF: Analysis of an isolated metaphase plate by quantitative electron microscopy. Exp Cell Res 68:65, 1971.
5. Ikeuchi T: Cytogentics. Cell Genet 38:56, 1984.
6. Cooke H: Repeated sequence specific to human males. Nature 262:182, 1976.
7. Pearson P: The use on new staining techniques for human chromosome identification. J Med Genet 9:264, 1972.
8. Painter T: Studies in mammalian spermatogenesis. II. The spermatogenesis of man. J Exp Zool 37:291, 1923.
9. Ford CE, Miller OJ, Polani PE, de Almeida JC, Briggs JH: A sex-chromosome anomaly in a case of gonadal dysgenesis (Turner's syndrome). Lancet 1:711, 1959.
10. Eichwald EJ, Silmser CR: Untitled communication. Transplant Bull 2:148, 1955.
11. Goldberg EH, Boyse EA, Bennett D, Scheid M, Carswell EA: Serological demonstration of H-Y (male) antigen on mouse sperm. Nature 232:478, 1971.
12. Wachtel SS: Human sexual development. J Endocrinol Invest 7:663, 1984.
13. Koo GC: Serology of H-Y antigen. Hum Genet 58:18, 1981.
14. Wachtel SS, Ohno S, Koo GC, Boyse EA: Possible role for H-Y antigen in the primary determination of sex. Nature 257:235, 1975.
15. Hall JL, Wachtel SS: Primary sex determination: Genetics and biochemistry. Mol Cell Biochem 33:49, 1980.
16. Wachtel SS: The dysgenetic gonad: Aberrant testicular differentiation. Biol Reprod 22:1, 1980.
17. Ford CE: Cytogenetics and sex determination in man and mammals J Biosoc Sci Suppl 2:7, 1970.
18. Ohno S, Christian LC, Wachtel SS, et al: Hormone-like role of H-Y antigen in bovine freemartin gonads. Nature 261:597, 1976.
19. Simpson E, Chandler P, Goulmy E, Disteche CM, Ferguson-Smith MA, Page DC: Separation of the genetic loci for the H-Y antigen and for testis determination on human Y chromosome. Nature 317:692, 1987.
20. McLaren A, Simpson E, Tomonari K, Chandler P, Hogg H: Male sexual differentiation in mice lacking H-Y antigen. Nature 312:552, 1984.
21. Burgoyne P, Levy ER, McLaren A: Spermatogenic failure in mice lacking H-Y antigen. Nature 320:170, 1986.
22. Chandley AC, Goetz P, Hargreave TB, Joseph AM, Speed RM: On the nature and extent of XY pairing at meiotic prophase in man. Cytogenet Cell Genet 38:241, 1984.
23. Page DC: Sex reversal: Deletion mapping of the male-determining function of the human Y chromosome. Cold Spring Harbor Sym Quant Biol 51:229, 1986.
24. Page DC, Mosher R, Simpson EM, Fisher EMC,

Mardon G, Pollack J, McGillivray B, de la Chapelle A, Brown LG: The sex-determining region of the human Y chromosome encodes a finger protein. Cell 51:1091, 1987.

25. Vergnaud G, Page DC, Simmler M-C, Brown L, Rouyer F, Noel B, Botstein D, de la Chapelle A, Weissenbach J: A deletion may pf the human Y chromosome based on DNA hybridization, Am J Hum Genet 38:330, 1986.

26. Ferguson-Smith MA: Karyotype-phenotype correlations in gonadal dysgenesis and their bearing on the pathogenesis of malformations. J Med Genet 2:142, 1965.

27. McKusick VA: Mendelian Inheritance in Man: Catalogs of Autosomal Dominant, Autosomal Recessive, and X-linked Phenotypes. 6th ed. Baltimore, Johns Hopkins University Press, 1983.

28. Polani PE: Pairing of the X and Y chromosomes. Non-inactivation of X-linked genes, and the maleness factor. Hum Genet 60:207, 1982.

29. Lyon MF: X-chromosome inactivation and developmental patterns in mammals. Biol Rev 47:1, 1972.

30. Barr ML, Bertram EG: A morphological distinction between neurones of the male and female, and the behavior of the nucleolar satellite during acceleration of nucleoprotein synthesis. Nature 163:676, 1949.

31. Grumbach MM, Morishima A, Taylor JH: Human sex chromosome abnormalities in relation to DNA replication and heterochromatinization. Proc Natl Acad Sci (USA) 49:581, 1963.

32. Haseltine FP, Ohno S: Mechanisms of gonadal differentiation. Science 211:1212, 1981.

33. McKay DG, Hertig AT, Adams EC, et al: Histochemical observations on the germ cells of the human embryo. Anat Rec 117:201, 1953.

34. Witschi E: Contrib Embryol Carnegie Inst. 32:67, 1948.

35. Friedman NB, Van de Velde RL: Germ cell tumors in man, pleiotropic mice, and continuity of germplasm and somatoplasm. Hum Pathol 12:772, 1981.

36. Baker TG, O WS: Development of the ovary and oogenesis. Clin Obstet Gynaecol 3:3, 1976.

37. Guraya SS: Recent progress in the morphology, histochemistry, biochemistry, and physiology of developing and maturing mammalian testis. Int Rev Cytol 62:187, 1980.

38. Guraya SS: Recent progress in the morphology, histochemistry, biochemistry, and physiology of developing and maturing mammalian ovary. Int Rev Cytol 51:49, 1977.

39. Jost A, Magre S, Cressent M: *In* Mancini RE, Martini L (eds): Male Fertility and Sterility. New York, Academic Press, p 1, 1974.

40. Fritz IB: Comparison of granulosa and sertoli cells at various stages of maturation: Similarities and differences. *In* Channing CP, Segal SJ (eds): Intraovarian Control Mechanisms. New York, Plenum Press, vol 147, p 357, 1982.

41. Jirasek JE: Development of the Genital System and Male Pseudohermaphroditism. Baltimore, Johns Hopkins University Press, 1971.

42. Kaplan SL, Grumbach MM: Pituitary and placental gonadotropins and sex steroids in the human and sub-human primate fetus. J Clin Endocrinol Metab 47:487, 1978.

43. Griffin JE, Wilson JD: Disorders of the testes and male reproductive tract. *In* Wilson JD, Foster DW (eds): Williams Textbook of Endocrinology. 7th ed. Philadelphia, WB Saunders Company, p 259, 1985.

44. Backhouse KM: The gubernaculum testis Hunteri: Testicular descent and maldescent. Ann R Coll Surg Engl 35:15, 1964.

45. Scorer GC: The descent of the testes. Arch Dis Child 39:605, 1976.

46. Czeizel A, Erodi E, Toth J: Genetics of undescended testes. J Urol 126:528, 1981.

47. Sudmann E: The undescended testis: A clinical and histological study. Acta Chir Scand 137:815, 1971.

48. Laron Z, Zilka E: Compensatory hypertrophy of testicle in unilateral cryptorchidism. J Clin Endocrinol 29:1409, 1969.

49. Robertson JFR, Azmy AF, Cochran W: Assent to ascent of the testis. Br J Urol 61:146, 1988.

50. Gaudia E, Paggiarino D, Carpino F: Structural and ultrastructural modifications of cryptorchid testes. J Urol 131:292, 1984.

51. Ito H, Kataumi Z, Yanagi S, Kawamura K, Sumiya H, Fuse H, Shimazaki J: Changes in the volume and histology of retractile testes in prepubertal boys. Int J Androl 9:161, 1986.

52. Nistal M, Paniagua R: Infertility in adult males with retractile testes. Fertil Steril 41:395, 1984.

53. Rutgers JL, Scully RE: Pathology of the testis in intersex syndromes. Semin Diagn Pathol 4:275, 1987.

54. Chilvers C, Dudley NE, Gough MH, et al: Undescended testes: The effect of treatment subsequent risk of subfertility and malignancy. J Pediatr Surg 21:691, 1986.

55. Johnson DE, Woodhead DM, Pohl DP, Robison JR: Cryptorchism and testicular tumorigenesis. Surgery 63:919, 1968.

56. Martin DC. Malignancy in the cryptorchid testis. Urol Clin North Am 9:371, 1982.

57. George FW, Wilson JD: Conversion of androgen to estrogen by the human fetal ovary. J Clin Endocrinol Metab 47:550, 1978.

58. Peters H: Migration of gonocytes into the mammalian gonad and their differentiation. Philos Trans R Soc [Biol] 259:91, 1970.

59. Baker TG: A quantitative and cytological study of germ cells in human ovaries. Proc R Soc 158:417, 1963.

60. Josso N, Picard JY, Tran D: The anti-mullerian hormone. Recent Prog Horm Res 33:117, 1977.

61. Picard JY, Josso N: Purification of testicular anti-Mullerian hormone allowing direct visualization of the pure glycoprotein and determination of yield and purification factor. Mol Cell Endocrinol 34:23, 1984.

62. Josso N, Tran D, Picard JY, Vigier B: Physiology of anti-Mullerian hormone: In search of a new role for an old hormone. *In* Tsafriri A, Eshkol A (eds): Development and Function of Reproductive Organs. New York, Raven Press, p 73, 1986.

63. Vigier B, Picard JY, Tran D, Legal L, Josso N: Production of anti-Mullerian hormone: Another homology between Sertoli and granulosa cells. Endocrinology 114:1315, 1984.

64. Josso N, Picard JY: Anti-mullerian hormone. Physiol Rev 66:1038, 1986.

65. Ikawa H, Trelstad RL, Hutson JM, Manganaro TF, Donahoe PK: Changing patterns of fibronectin, laminin, type IV collagen and a basement

membrane proteoglycan during rat Mullerian duct regression. Dev Biol 102:260, 1984.

66. Donahoe PK, Budzik GP, Trelstad R, Mudgett-Hunter M, Fuller A JR, Hutson JM, Ikawa H, Hayashi A, MacLaughlin D: Mullerian-inhibiting substance: An update. Recent Prog Horm Res 38:279, 1982.

67. Hammond GL, Ruokonen A, Kontturi M, et al: The simultaneous radioimmunoassay of seven steroids in human spermatic and peripheral venous blood. J Clin Endocrinol Metab 45:16, 1977.

68. Siiteri PK, Wilson JD: Testosterone formation and metabolism during male sexual differentiation in the human embryo. J Clin Endocrinol Metab 38:113, 1974.

69. George FW, Simpson ER, Milewich L, Wilson JD: Studies on the regulation of steroid hormone biosynthesis in fetal rabbit gonads. Endocrinology 105:1100, 1979.

70. Kaplan SL, Grumbach MM, Aubert ML: The ontogenesis of pituitary hormones and hypothalamic factors in the human fetus: Maturation of central nervous system regulation of anterior pituitary function. Recent Prog Horm Res 32:161, 1976.

71. Miller WL: Molecular biology of steroid hormone synthesis. Endocr Rev 9:295, 1988.

72. Voutilainen R, Miller WL: Human Mullerian inhibitory factor messenger ribonucleic acid is hormonally regulated in the fetal testis and in adult granulosa cells. Mol Endocrinol 1:604, 1987.

73. Voutilainen R, Miller WL: Developmental expression of genes for the steroidogenic enzymes P450scc (20,22 desmolase), P450c17 (17 alpha-hydroxylase/17,20 lyase) and P450c21 (21-hydroxylase) in the human fetus. J Clin Endocrinol Metab 63:1145, 1986.

74. Wilson JD, Lasnitzki I: Dihydrotestosterone formation in fetal tissues of the rabbit and rat. Endocrinology 89:659, 1971.

75. George FW, Noble JF, Wilson JD: Female feathering in Sebright cocks is due to conversion of testosterone to estradiol in skin. Science 213:557, 1981.

76. Dunn JF, Nisula BC, Rodbard D: Transport of steroid hormones: Binding of 21 endogenous steroids to both testosterone-binding globulin and corticosteroid-binding globulin in human plasma. J Clin Endocrinol Metab 53:58, 1981.

77. MacDonald PC, Madden JD, Brenner PF, et al: Origin of estrogen in normal men and in women with testicular feminization. J Clin Endocrinol Metab 49:905, 1979.

78. Ito T, Horton R: The source of plasma dihydrotestosterone in man. J Clin Invest 50:1621, 1971.

79. Wolff CF: "Theoria Generationis (1759)." Zweiter Theil (Entwicklung der Thiere, Allgemeines). Translated from German by P. Samassa. W. Engelmann, 1896.

80. Torrey TW: The early development of the human nephros. Contrib Embryol Carnegie Inst 35:175, 1954.

81. Muller J: "Bildungsgeschichte de genitalien aus anatomischen untersuchungen an embryonen des menschen und der thiere." Dusseldorf, Arnz, 1830.

82. Faulconer RJ: Observations on the origin of the Mullerian groove in human embryos. Contrib Embryol Carnegie Inst 34:159, 1951.

83. Lipsett MB, Tullner WW: Testosterone synthesis by the fetal rabbit gonad. Endocrinology 77:273, 1965.

84. Kellokumpo-Lehtinen P, Santti R, Pelliniema LJ: Correlation of early cytodifferentiation of the human fetal prostate and Leydig cells. Anat Rec 196:263, 1980.

85. Forsberg J-G: Derivation and differentiation of the vaginal epithelium. Lund, Institute of Anatomy, 1963.

86. O'Rahilly RO: The development of the vagina in the human. Birth Defects 13(2):123, 1977.

87. Grumbach MM, Ducharme JR: The effects of androgens on fetal sexual development. Androgen-induced female pseudohermaphrodism. Fertil Steril 11:157, 1960.

88. Wilson JD, Griffin JE, George FW, et al: The role of gonadal steroids in sexual differentiation. Recent Prog Horm Res 37:1, 1981.

89. Gondos B: Development of the reproductive organs. Ann Clin Lab Sci 15:363, 1985.

90. Feldman KW, Smith DW: Fetal phallic growth and penile standards for newborn male infants. J Pediatr 86:395, 1975.

91. Gorski RA: Gonadal hormones and the perinatal development of neuroendocrine function. In Martini L, Ganong WF (eds): Frontiers in Neuroendocrinology. New York, Oxford University Press, p 237, 1971.

92. Gorski RA: Sexual dimorphisms of the brain. J Anim Sci 61(3):38, 1985.

93. Abramovich DR, Davidson IA, Longstaff A, Pearson CK: Sexual differentiation of the human mid-trimester brain. Eur J Obstet Gynecol Repro Biol 25:7, 1987.

94. Baker SW: Psychosexual differentiation in the human. Biol Reprod 22:61, 1980.

95. Money J, Ehrhardt AA: Man and Woman, Boy and Girl: The Differentiation and Dimorphism of Gender Identity from Conception to Maturity. Baltimore, John Hopkins University Press, 1972.

96. Money J, Schwartz M, Lewis VG: Adult erotosexual status and fetal hormonal masculinization and demasculinization: 46,XX congenital virilizing adrenal hyperplasia and 46,XY androgen-insensitivity syndrome compared. Psychoneuroendocrinology 9:405, 1984.

97. Ehrhardt AA, Baker SW: Fetal androgens, human central nervous system differentiation, and behavioral sex differences. In Friedman RC, Richart RM, Vande Wiele RL (eds): Sex Differences in Behavior. New York, John Wiley & Sons, p 53, 1974.

98. Masica D, Money J, Ehrhardt AA: Fetal feminization and female gender identity in the testicular feminizing syndrome of androgen insensitivity. Arch Sex Behav 1:131, 1971.

99. Ehrhardt A, Greenberg N, Money J: Female gender identity and absence of fetal gonadal hormones: Turner's syndrome. Johns Hopkins Med J 126:327, 1970.

100. Reinisch JM, Karow WG: Prenatal exposure to synthetic progestins and estrogens: Effects on human development. Arch Sex Behav 6:257, 1977.

101. Money J, Lewis VG: Homosexual/heterosexual status in boys at puberty: Idiopathic adolescent gynecomastia and congenital virilizing adrenocorticism compared. Psychoneuroendocrinology 7:339, 1982.

102. Dorner G: Neuroendocrine response to estrogen and brain differentiation in heterosexuals, homosexuals and transsexuals Arch Sex Behav 17:57, 1988.

103. Herdt GH, Davidson J: The Sambia "Turnim-Man": Sociocultural and clinical aspects of gender formation in male pseudohermaphrodites with 5 alpha reductase deficiency in Papua, New Guinea. Arch Sex Behav 17:33, 1988.

104. Gorski RA: Sexual differentiation of the brain: Possible mechanisms and implications. Canad J Physiol Pharmacol 63:577, 1985.

105. Grumbach MM, Conte FA: Disorders of sexual differentiation. *In* Wilson JD, Foster DW (eds): Williams Textbook of Endocrinology. 7th ed. Philadelphia, WB Saunders Company, p 312, 1985.

106. van Niekerk WA: True hermaphroditism. An analytic review with a report of a 3 new cases. Am J Obstet Gynecol 126:890, 1976.

107. Van Niekerk SA: True Hermaphroditism: Clinical, Morphologic, and Cytogenetic Aspect. New York, Harper & Row, 1974.

108. Ramsay M, Bernstein R, Zwane E, Page DC, Jenkins T: XX true hermaphroditism in souther african blacks: An enigma of primary sexual differentiation. Am J Hum Genet 43:4, 1988.

109. Gallegos AJ, Guizar E, Armendaves S, Cortes-Gallegos V, Cervantes C, et al: Familial true hermaphroditism in three siblings: Plasma hormonal profile and in vitro steroid biosynthesis in gonadal structure. J Clin Endocrinol Metab 42:653, 1976.

110. van Niekerk WA: True hermaphrodism. *In* Josso N (ed): The Intersex Child. Pediatric and Adolescent Endocrinology, Vol 8. Basel, Karger, p 80, 1981.

111. Jones HW Jr, Park IJ: Intersex. Clin Obstet Gynecol 20:545, 1977.

112. Kim MH, Gumpel JA, Graff P: Pregnancy in a true hermaphrodite. Obstet Gynecol (Suppl) 53:405, 1979.

113. van Niekier WA, Retief AE: The gonads of human true hermaphrodites. Hum Genet 58:117, 1981.

114. Jacobs PA: The incidence and etiology of sex chromosome abnormalities in man. Birth Defects 15:3, 1979.

115. Ahmad KN, Dykes JRW, Ferguson-Smith MA, et al: Leydig cell volume in chromatin-positive Klinefelter's syndrome. J Clin Endocrinol Metab 33:517, 1971.

116. Robinson A, Lubs HA, Bergsma D: Summary of clinical findings: Profiles of children with 47,XXY, 47,XXX and 47XYY karyotypes. Birth Defects 15:261, 1979.

117. Ferguson-Smith MA: The prepubertal testicular lesions in chromatin positive Klinefelter's syndrome (primarily microorchidism) as seen in mentally handicapped children. Lancet 1:219, 1959.

118. Harnden DG, Maclean N, Langlands AO: Carcinoma of the breast and Klinefelter's syndrome. J Med Genet 8:460, 1971.

119. Stewart DA, Netley CT, Park E: Summary of clinical findings of children with 47,XXY, 47,XXY and 47,XXX karyotypes. Birth Defects 18:1, 1982.

120. Ferguson-Smith MA, Mack WS, Ellis PM, et al: Parental age and the source of the X chromosomes in XXY Klinefelter's syndrome. Lancet 1:46, 1964.

121. Leonard JM, Paulsen CA, Ospina LF, et al: The classification of Klinefelter's syndrome. *In* Vallet HL, Porter IH (eds): Genetic Mechanisms of Sexual Development. New York, Academic Press, p 407, 1978.

122. de la Chapelle A: Analytic review: Nature and origin of males with XX sex chromosomes. Am J Hum Genet 24:71, 1972.

123. Andersson M, Page DC, la Chapelle AD: Chromosome Y-specific DNA is transferred to the short arm of X chromosome in human XX males. Science 233:786, 1986.

124. Noonan J: Hypertelorism with Turner phenotype. A new syndrome with associated congenital heart disease. Am J Dis Child 116:373, 1968.

125. Harnden DG, Stewart JSS: The chromosomes in a case of pure gonadal dysgenesis. Br Med J 2:1285, 1959.

126. McDonough PG, Byrd JR, Tho PT, et al: Phenotypic and cytogenetic findings in eighty-two patients with ovarian failure—changing trends. Fertil Steril 28:638, 1977.

127. Simpson JL: Disorders of Sexual Differentiation: Etiology and Clinical Delineation. New York, Academic Press, 1976.

128. Sawyer GIM: Male pseudohermaphrodism: A hitherto undescribed from. Br Med J 2:709, 1955.

129. Simpson JL, Blagowidow N, Martin AO: XY gonadal dysgenesis: Genetic heterogeneity based upon observation, H-Y antigen status and segregation analysis. Hum Genet 58:91, 1981.

130. Diteche CM, Casanova M, Saal H, Freidman C, Sybert V, Graham J, Thuline H, Page DC, Fellous M: Small deletions of the short arm of the Y chromosome in 46XY females. Proc Natl Acad Sci (USA) 83:7841, 1986.

131. Drash A, Sherman F, Hartmann WH, et al: A syndrome of pseudohermaphroditism, Wilm's tumor, hypertension, and degenerative renal disease. J Pediatr 76:585, 1970.

132. Manivel JC, Sibley RK, Dehner LP: Complete and incomplete Drash syndrome: A clinicopathologic study of five cases of a dysontogenetic-neoplastic complex. Hum Pathol 18:80, 1987.

133. Turleau C, de Grouchy J, Dufier JL, et al: Aniridia, male pseudohermaphroditism, gonadoblastoma, mental retardation and del 11p13. Hum Genet 57:300, 1981.

134. Verp MS, Simpson JL: Abnormal sexual differentiation and neoplasia. Cancer Genet Cytogenet 25:191, 1987.

135. Scully RE: Gonadoblastoma. Cancer 25:1340, 1970.

136. Talerman A, Jarabak J, Amarose AP: Gonadoblastoma and dysgerminoma in a true hermaphrodite with 46,XX karyotype. Am J Obstet Gynecol 140:475, 1981.

137. Talerman A: Germ cell tumors of the ovary. *In* Blaustein, A (ed): Pathology of the Female Genital Tract. 2nd ed. New York, Springer-Verlag, p 602, 1982.

138. Miller WL, Levine LS: Molecular and clinical advances in congenital adrenal hyperplasia. J Pediatr 111:1, 1987.

139. White PC, New MI, Dupont B: Congenital adrenal hyperplasia. N Engl J Med 278:695, 1968.

140. Bongiovanni AM: The adrenogenital syndrome with deficiency of 3 beta-hydroxysteroid dehy-

drogenase. J Clin Endocrinol Metab 50:586, 1980.

141. Zachmann M, Tassinari D, Prader A: Clinical and biochemical variability of congenital adrenal hyperplasia due to 11 beta hydroxylase deficiency. A study of 25 patients. J Clin Endocrinol Metab 56:222, 1983.

142. New MI, Dupont B, Pang S, et al: An update of congenital adrenal hyperplasia. Recent Prog Horm Res 37:105, 1981.

143. New MI: The HLA system in congenital adrenal hyperplasia. *In* Styne DM, Brook CGD (eds): Current Concepts in Pediatric Endocrinology. New York, Elsevier, p 28, 1987.

144. Grumbach MM, Ducharme JR, Moloshok RE: On the fetal masculinizing action of certain oral progestins. J Clin Endocrinol Metab 19:1369, 1959.

145. Ishizuka N, Kawashima Y, Nakanishi T, et al: Statistical observations on genital anomalies of newborns following the administration of progestins to their mothers. Obstet Gynecol Surv 19:496, 1964.

146. Bongiovanni AM, Di George AM, Grumbach MM: Masculinization of the female infant associated with estrogenic therapy alone during gestation: Four cases. J Clin Endocrinol Metab 19:1004, 1959.

147. Murset G, Zachmann M, Prader A, et al: Male external genitalia of a girl caused by a virilizing adrenal tumor in the mother. Acta Endocrinol 65:627, 1970.

148. Hensleigh PA, Woodruff JD: Differential maternal-fetal response to adrogenizing luteoma or hyperreactio luteinalis. Obstet Gynecol Surv 33:262, 1978.

149. Park IJ, Johanson A, Jones HW, et al: Special female hermaphroditism associated with multiple disorders. Obstet Gynecol 39:100, 1972.

150. Berthezene F, Forest MG, Grimaud JA, Claustrat B, Mornex R: Leydig-cell agenesis: A cause of male pseudohermaphroditism. N Engl J Med 295:969, 1976.

151. Perez-Palacios G, Scaglia H, Kofman-Alfaro S, et al: Inherited male pseudohermaphrodism due to gonadotropin unresponsiveness. Acta Endocrinol 98:148, 1981.

152. David R, Yoon D, Landin L, et al: A syndrome of gonadotropin resistance possibly due to an LH receptor defect (abstr). Endocr Soc 468:197, 1983.

153. Bardin CW, Bullock LP, Sherins RJ, et al: Androgen metabolism and mechanism of action in male pseudohermaphrodism: A study of testicular feminization (Part II). Recent Prog Horm Res 29:65, 1973.

154. Camacho AM, Kowarski A, Migeon CJ, et al: Congenital adrenal hyperplasia due to a deficiency of one of the enzymes involved in the biosynthesis of pregnenolone. J Clin Endocrinol Metab 28:153, 1968.

155. Koizumi S, Kyoya S, Mujawaki T, Kidani H, Funabashi T, et al: Cholesterol side chain cleavage enzyme activity and cytochrome P450 content in adrenal mitochondria of a patient with congenital lipoid hyperplasia (Prader disease). Clin Chim Acta 77:301, 1977.

156. Hauffa BP, Miller WL, Grumbach MM, et al: Deficiency of 20,22-desmolase complex (cholesterol side-chain cleavage activity): Growth, development, and steroidal findings in a patient successfully treated for 18 years. Clin Endocrinol 23:481, 1985.

157. Zachmann M, Vollmin JA, Murset G, et al: Unusual type of congenital adrenal hyperplasia probably due to deficiency of 3 beta-hydroxysteroid dehydrogenase. Case report of a surviving girl and steroid studies. J Clin Endocrinol Metab 30:716, 1970.

158. Pang S, Levine LS, Stoner E, Opitz JM, Pollack MS, et al: Nonsalt-losing congenital adrenal hyperplasia due to 3 beta-hydroxysteroid dehydrogenase deficiency with normal glomerulose function. J Clin Endocrinol Metab 56:808, 1983.

159. Janne O, Perheenutpa J, Viinikka L, et al: Plasma and urinary steroids in an eight-year-old boy with 3 beta-hydroxysteroid dehydrogenase deficiency. J Clin Endocrinol Metab 31:162, 1970.

160. Jones HW Jr, Lee PA, Rock JA, et al: A genetic male patient with 17 alpha-hydroxylase deficiency. Obstet Gynecol 59:254, 1982.

161. New MI: Male pseudohermaphrodism due to 17 alpha-hydroxylase deficiency. J Clin Invest 49:1930, 1970.

162. Jones HW Jr, Lee PA, Rock JA, et al: A genetic male patient with 17 alpha hydroxylase deficiency. Obstet Gynecol 59:254, 1982.

163. Zachmann M, Werder EA, Prader A: Two types of male pseudohermaphroditism due to 17,20 desmolase deficiency. J Clin Endocrinol Metab 55:487, 1982.

164. Larrea F, Lisker R, Banuelos R, et al: Hypergonadotropic hypogonadism in an XX female subject due to 17,20 desmolase deficiency. Acta Endocrinol 103:400, 1983.

165. Sawz JM, de Peretti E, Morera AM, et al: Familial male pseudohermaphroditism with gynecomastia due to a testicular 17-ketosteroid reductase defect. I. In vitro studies. J Clin Endocrinol Metab 32:604, 1971.

166. Imperato-McGinley J, Peterson RE, Stoller R, et al: Male pseudohermaphroditism secondary to 17-hydroxysteroid dehydrogenase deficiency: Gender role change with puberty. J Clin Endocrinol Metab 49:391, 1979.

167. Griffin JE, Wilson JD: Syndromes of androgen resistance. Hosp Pract August 15, p 159, 1987.

168. French FS, Van Wyk JJ, Baggett B, et al: Further evidence of a target organ defect in the syndrome of testicular feminization. J Clin Endocrinol Metab 26:493, 1966.

169. Morris JM, Mahesh VB: Further observations on the syndrome, "testicular feminization." Am J Obstet Gynecol 87:731, 1963.

170. Goldstein JL, Wilson JD: Studies on the pathogenesis of the pseudohermaphroditism in the mouse with testicular feminization. J Clin Invest 51:1647, 1972.

171. Keenan BX, Meyer WJ III, Hadijian AJ, et al: Syndrome of androgen insensitivity in man: Absence of 5 alpha-dihydrotestosterone binding protein in skin fibroblasts. J Clin Endocrinol Metab 38:1143, 1974.

172. Migeon BR, Brown TR, Axelman J, Migeon CJ: Studies of the locus for androgen receptor: Localization on the human X chromosome and evidence for homology with the Tfm locus in the mouse. Proc Natl Acad Sci (USA) 78:6339, 1981.

173. Maes S, Sultan C, Zerhouni N, Rothwell SW, Migeon CJ: Role of testosterone binding to the

androgen receptor in male sexual differentiation of patients with 5 alpha-reductase deficiency. J Steroid Biochem 11:1385, 1979.

174. Wilson JD, Griffin JE, Leshin M, MacDonald PC: The androgen resistance syndromes: 5 Alpha-reductase deficiency, testicular feminization, and related disorders. *In* Stanbury JB, Wyngaarden JB, Frederickson DS, Goldstein JL, Brown MS (eds): The Metabolic Basis of Inherited Disease, New York, McGraw Hill, p 1001, 1983.

175. Griffin JE, Kovacs WJ, Wilson JD: Characteristics of androgen resistance. *In* Bruchovsky N, Chapdelaine, Neumann F (eds): Regulation of Androgen Action. The Proceedings of an International Symposium. Berlin, Congressdruck R. Bruckner, p 127, 1985.

176. Muller J: Morphometry and histology of gonads from twelve children and adolescents with the androgen insensitivity (testicular feminization) syndrome. J Clin Endocrinol Metab 49:785, 1984.

177. Gooren LJG: Reversal of the LH response to oestrogen administration after orchiectomy in a male subject with the androgen insensitivity syndrome. Horm Metab Res 19:138, 1987.

178. Goretzlehner G, Wodrig W, Sas M, Morvay J, Scholtz B, Wever A, Schmidt W: The modulating effect of estrogens on luteinizing hormone release in complete androgen insensitivity syndrome before and after gonadectomy and cyclic steroid application. Exp Clin Endocrinol 90:99, 1987.

179. Manuel M, Katayama K, Jones HW Jr: The age of occurrence of gonadal tumors in intersex patients with a Y chromosome. Am J Obstet Gynecol 124:293, 1976.

180. Muller J, Skakkebaek NE: Testicular carcinoma in situ testis in children with the androgen insensitivity (testicular feminization) syndrome. Br Med J 1:1419, 1984.

181. Griffin JE, Wilson JD: The syndrome of androgen resistance. N Engl J Med 302:198, 1980.

182. Reifenstein EC Jr: Hereditary familial hypogonadism. Clin Res 3:86, 1947.

183. Aiman J, Griffin JE, Gazak JM, et al: Androgen insensitivity as a cause of infertility in otherwise normal men. N Engl J Med 300:223, 1979.

184. Optiz JM, Simpson JL, Sarto EG, et al: Pseudovaginal perineoscrotal hypospadias. Clin Genet 3:1, 1972.

185. Imperato-McGinley JL, Peterson RE: Male pseudohermaphroditism: The complexities of male phenotypic development. Science 186:1213, 1974.

186. Savage MO, Preece MA, Jeffcoate SL, Ransley PG, Rumsby G, Mansfield MD, Williams DI: Familial male pseudohermaphroditism due to deficiency of 5 alpha-reductase. Clin Endocrinol 12:397, 1980.

187. Peterson RE, Imperato-McGinley J, Gautier T, et al: Male pseudohermaphroditism due to steroid 5 alpha-reductase deficiency. Am J Med 62:170, 1977.

188. Pang S, Levine LS, Chow D, et al: Dihydrotestosterone and its relationship to testosterone in infancy and childhood. J Clin Endocrinol Metab 48:821, 1979.

189. Moore RJ, Griffin JE, Wilson JD: Diminished 5 alpha reductase activity in extracts of fibroblasts cultured from patients with familial incomplete male pseudohermaphroditism, type 2. J Biol Chem 250:7168, 1975.

190. Leshin M, Griffin JE, Wilson JD: Hereditary male pseudohermaphroditism associated with an unstable form of 5 alpha-reductase. J Clin Invest 62:685, 1978.

191. Imperato-McGinley J, Peterson RE, Gautier T, Sturla E: Androgens and the evolution of male gender identity among male pseudohermaphrodites with 5α-reductase deficiency. N Engl J Med 300:1233, 1979.

192. Brook CGD, Wagner H, Zachmann M, et al: Familial occurrence of persistent mullerian structures in otherwise normal males. Br Med J 1:771, 1973.

193. Aarskog D: Maternal progestins as a possible cause of hypospadias. N Engl J Med 300:75, 1979.

194. Driscoll SG, Taylor SH: Effects of prenatal maternal estrogen on the male urogenital system. Obstet Gynecol 56:537, 1980.

195. Kaplan NM: Male pseudohermaphrodism: Report of a case, with observations on pathogenesis. N Engl J Med 261:641, 1959.

196. Sweet RA, Schrott HG, Kurland R, et al: Study of the incidence of hypospadias in Rochester, Minnesota, 1940–1970, and a case control comparison of possible etiologic factors. Mayo Clin Proc 49:52, 1974.

197. Svensson J, Snochowski M: Androgen receptor levels in preputial skin from boys with hypospadias. J Clin Endocrinol Metab 49:340, 1979.

198. Rohatgi M, Menon PSN, Verma IC, et al: The presence of intersexuality in patients with advanced hypospadias and undescended gonads. J Urol 137:263, 1987.

199. Connors MS, Styne DM: Familial functional anorchia. A review of etiology and management. J Urol 133:1049, 1985.

200. Cleary RE, Caras J, Rosenfield R, et al: Endocrine and metabolic studies in a patient with male pseudohermaphrodism and true agonadism. Am J Obstet Gynecol 128:862, 1977.

201. Disteche CM, Casanova M, Saal H, Freidman C, Sybert V, Graham J, et al: Deletions of the short arm of the Y chromosome in 6 XY females. Proc Natl Acad Sci (USA) 83:7841, 1986.

202. Nelson RE: Congenital absence of the vas deferens: A review of the literature and report of three cases. J Urol 63:176, 1950.

203. Emery CB, Goldstein AMB, Morrow JW: Congenital absence of vas deferens with ipsilateral urinary anomalies. Urology 4:201, 1974.

204. Le Merrer M, Briard ML, Girard S, Mulliez N, Moraine C, Imbert MC: Lethal acrodysgenital dwarfism: A severe lethal condition resembling Smith-Lemli-Opitz syndrome. J Med Genet 25:88, 1988.

205. Hovmoller L, Osuna A, Eklof O, Fredga K, Hjerpe A, et al: Camptomelic dwarfism. A genetically determined mesenchymal disorder combined with sex reversal. Hereditas 86:51, 1977.

206. Jones KL: Smith's Recognizable Patterns of Human Malformations. 4th ed. Philadelphia, WB Saunders Company, 1988.

207. Bryan AL, Nigro JA, Counseller VS: One hundred cases of congenital absence of vagina. Surg Gynecol Obstet 88:79, 1949.

208. Smith DW: Male genital defects in patterns of malformation. Birth Defects 14(6C):57, 1978.

209. Sarto GE, Simpson JL: Abnormalities of the Mullerian and Wolffian duct systems. Birth Defects 14(6C):37, 1978.

210. Scott JR, Galask R, Yannone ME: Congenital atresia of the uterine cervix. Int J Gynaecol Obstet 9:249, 1971.

211. Bowman JA Jr, Scott RB: Transverse vaginal septum. Report of four cases. Obstet Gynecol 3:441, 1954.

212. Semmens JP: Congenital anomalies of female genital tract. Functional classification based on review of 56 personal cases and 500 reported cases. Obstet Gynecol 19:328, 1962.

213. Polishuk WZ, Ron MA: Familial bicornuate and double uterus. Am J Obstet Gynecol 119:982, 1974.

211. Finkelstein MS, Rosenberg HK, Snyder HM, Duckett JW: Ultrasound evaluation of scrotum in pediatrics. Urology 27:1, 1986.

215. Aristotle: De generatione animalium. *In* Tanner JM (ed): A History of the Study of Human Growth. Cambridge, England, Cambridge University Press, p 7, 1981.

216. Tanner JM: A History of the Study of Human Growth. Cambridge, England, Cambridge University Press, p 286, 1981.

217. Wyshak G, Frisch RE: Evidence for a secular trend in age of menarche. N Engl J Med 306:1033, 1982.

218. Styne DM, Grumbach MM: Puberty in the male and female: Its physiology and disorders. *In* Yen SSC, Jaffe RB (eds): Reproductive Endocrinology. 2nd ed. Philadelphia, WB Saunders Company, p 313, 1986.

219. Knobil E, Plant TM: The neuroendocrine control of gonadotropin secretion in the female rhesus monkey. *In* Ganong WF, Martini L (eds): Frontiers in Neuroendocrinology, vol 4. New York, Raven Press, 1978.

220. Clayton RN, Catt KJ: Gonadotropin-releasing hormone receptors: Characterization, physiological regulation and relationship to reproductive function. Endocr Rev 2:186, 1981.

221. Steinberger A, Steinberger E: Secretion of an FSH-inhibiting factor by cultured Sertoli cells. Endocrinology 98:918, 1976.

222. Channing CP, Anderson LD, Hoover DJ, Kolena J, Osteen KG, Pomerantz SH, Tanabe K: The role of nonsteroidal regulators in control of oocyte and follicular maturation. Recent Prog Horm Res 38:331, 1982.

223. Kaplan SL, Grumbach MM, Aubert ML: The ontogenesis of pituitary hormones and hypothalamic factors in the human fetus: Maturation of central nervous system regulation of anterior pituitary function. Recent Prog Horm Res 32:161, 1976.

224. Gluckman PD, Grumbach MM, Kaplan SL: The neuroendocrine regulation and function of growth hormone and prolactin in the mammalian fetus. Endoc Rev 2:363, 1981.

225. Faiman C, Winter JSD: Gonadotropins and sex hormone patterns in puberty: Clinical data. *In* Grumbach MM, Grave GD, Mayer FE (eds): Control of the Onset of Puberty. New York, John Wiley & Sons, p 32, 1974.

226. Forest MG, de Peretti E, Bertrand J: Hypothalamic-pituitary-gonadal relationships in man from birth to puberty. Clin Endocrinol 5:551, 1976.

227. Conte FA, Grumbach MM, Kaplan SL: A diphasic pattern of gonadotropin secretion in patients with the syndrome of gonadal dysgenesis. J Clin Endocrinol Metab 40:670, 1975.

228. Conte FA, Grumbach MM, Kaplan SL, Retier EO: Correlation of LRF-induced LH and FSH release from infancy to 19 years with the changing patterns of gonadotropin secretion in agonadal patients: Relation to the restraint of puberty. J Clin Endocrinol Metab 50:1163, 1981.

229. Kelch RP, Kaplan SL, Grumbach MM: Suppression of urinary and plasma follicle-stimulating hormone by exogenous estrogens in prepubertal and pubertal children. J Clin Invest 52:1122, 1973.

230. Mauras N, Veldhuis JD, Rogol AD: Role of endogenous opiates in pubertal maturation: Opposing actions of naltrexone in prepubertal and late pubertal boys. J Clin Endocrinol Metab 62:1256, 1986.

231. Boyar R, Finkelstein J, Roffwarg H, Kapen S, Weitzman, Hellman L: Synchronization of augmented luteinizing hormone secretion with sleep during puberty. N Engl J Med 287:582, 1972.

232. August GP, Grumbach MM, Kaplan SL: Hormonal changes in puberty. III. Correlation of plasma testosterone, LH, FSH, testicular size and bone age with male pubertal development. J Clin Endocrinol Metab 34:319, 1972.

233. Jenner MR, Kelch RP, Kaplan SL, Grumbach MM: Hormonal changes in the puberty. IV. Plasma estradiol, LH, and FSH in prepubertal children, pubertal females, and in precocious puberty, premature thelarche, hypogonadism, and in a child with a feminizing ovarian tumor. J Clin Endocrinol Metab 34:521, 1972.

234. Lucky AW, Rich BH, Rosenfield RL, Fang VS, Roche-Bender N: LH bioactivity increases more than immunoreactivity during puberty. J Pediatr 92:205, 1980.

235. Reiter EO, Beitens IZ, Optrea T, Gutai JP: Bioassayable luteinizing hormones during childhood and adolescence and in patients with delayed pubertal development. J Clin Endocrinol Metab 54:155, 1982.

236. Burstein S, Schaff-Glass E, Glass J, Rosenfield RL: The changing ratio of bioactive to immunoreactive luteinizing hormone (LH) through puberty principally reflects changing LH radioimmunoassay dose-response characteristics. J Clin Endocrinol Metab 61:508, 1985.

237. Boyar RM, Rosenfeld RS, Kapen S, Finkelstein JW, Roffwarg HP, Weitzman ED, Hellman L: Simultaneous augmented secretion of luteinizing hormone and testosterone during sleep. J Clin Invest 54:609, 1974.

238. Anderson DC: Sex hormone-binding globulin. Clin Endocrinol 3:39, 1974.

239. Bartsch W, Horst H-J, Derwahl K-M: Interrelationships between sex hormone-binding globulin and 17 beta-estradiol, testosterone, 5 alpha-dihydrotestosterone, thyroxine and triiodothyronine in prepubertal and pubertal girls. J Clin Endocrinol Metab 50:1053, 1980.

240. Horst H-J, Bartsch W, Dirksen-Thededs I: Plasma testosterone, sex hormone binding globulin capacity and per cent binding of testoste-

rone and 5 alpha-dihydrotestosterone in prepubertal, pubertal and adult males. J Clin Endocrinol Metab 45:522, 1977.

241. Roth JC, Kelch RP, Kaplan SL, Grumbach MM: FSH and LH response to luteinizing hormone-releasing factor in prepubertal and pubertal children, adult males and patients with hypogonadotropic and hypergonadotropic hypogonadism. J Clin Endocrinol Metab 35:926, 1972.

242. Santor N, Filicori M, Crowley WF Jr: Hypogonadotropic disorders in men and women: Diagnosis and therapy with pulsatile gonadotropin-releasing hormone. Endocr Rev 7:11, 1986.

243. Rosenfield RI, Furlanetto RW, Bock D: Relationship of somatomedin-C concentrations to pubertal changes. J Pediatr 103:723, 1983.

244. Luna AM, Wilson DM, Wibbelsman CJ, Brown RC, Nagashima RJ, Hintz RL, Rosenfeld RG: Somatomedins in adolescence: A cross-sectional study of the effect of puberty on plasma insulin-like growth factor I and II levels. J Clin Endocrinol Metab 57:268, 1983.

245. Harris DA, Van Vliet G, Egli CA, Grumbach MM, Kaplan SL, Styne DM, Vainsel M: Somatomedin-C in normal puberty and in true precocious puberty before and after treatment with a potent LRF-agonist: Evidence for an effect of estrogen and testosterone on somatomedin-C concentrations. J Clin Endocrinol Metab 61:152, 1985.

246. Reiter EO, Fuldauer VG, Root AW: Secretion of the adrenal androgen, dehydroepiandrosterone sulfate, during normal infancy, childhood, and adolescence, in sick infants, and in children with endocrinologic abnormalities. J Pediatr 90:766, 1977.

247. Grumbach MM, Richards HE, Conte FA, Kaplan SL: Clinical disorders of adrenal function and puberty: An assessment of the role of the adrenal cortex in normal and abnormal puberty in man and evidence for an ACTH-like pituitary adrenal androgen stimulating hormone. In Serio M (ed): The Endocrine Function of the Human Adrenal Cortex. Serono Symposium. New York, Academic Press, 1977.

248. Sklar CS, Kaplan SL, Grumbach MM: Evidence for dissociation between adrenarche and gonadarche: Studies in patients with idiopathic precocious puberty, gonadal dysgenesis, isolated gonadotropin deficiency, and constitutionally delayed growth and adolescence. J Clin Endocrinol Metab 51:548, 1980.

249. Marshall WA, Tanner JM: Variations in the pattern of pubertal changes in boys. Arch Dis Child 45:13, 1970.

250. Largo RH, Prader A: Pubertal development in Swiss boys. Helv Paediatr Acta 38:211, 1983.

251. Harlan WR, Grillo GP, Cornoni-Huntley J, Leaverton PE: Secondary sex characteristics of boys 12 to 17 years of age: The US Health Examination Survey. J Pediatr 95:293, 1979.

252. Nielsen CT, Skakkebaek NE, Richardson DW, Darling JA, et al. Onset of the release of spermatozoa (spermarche) in boys in relation to age, testicular growth, pubic hair, and height. J Clin Endocrinol Metab 62:532, 1986.

253. Aynsley-Green A, Zachmann M, Prader A: Interrelation of the therapeutic effects of growth hormone and testosterone on growth in hypopituitarism. J Pediatr 89:992, 1976.

254. Tanner JM, et al: The adolescent growth spurt of boys and girls of the Harpenden Growth Study. Ann Hum Biol 3:109, 1976.

255. Cheek DB: Body composition, hormones, nutrition and adolescent growth. In Grumbach MM, Grave GD, Mayer FE (eds): Control of the Onset of Puberty. New York, John Wiley & Sons, p 424, 1974.

256. Harlan WR, Harlan EA, Grillo GP: Secondary sex characteristics of girls 12 to 17 years of age: The US Health Examination Survey. J Pediatr 96:1074, 1980.

257. Horner JM, Thorsson AV, Hintz RL: Growth deceleration patterns in children with constitutional short stature: An aid to diagnosis. Pediatrics 62:529, 1978.

258. Bauman A: Markedly delayed puberty or Kallmann's syndrome variant. J Androl 7:224, 1986.

259. Spitz IM, Hirsch HJ, Trestian S: The prolactin response to thyrotropin-releasing hormone differentiates isolated gonadotropin deficiency from delayed puberty. N Engl J Med 308:575, 1986.

260. Partsch C-J, Hermanussen M, Sippell WG: Differentiation of male hypogonadotropic hypogonadism and constitutional delay of puberty by pulsatile administration of gonadotropin-releasing hormone. J Clin Endocrinol Metab 60:1196, 1985.

261. Job JC, Garnier PE, Chaussain JL, Milhaud G: Elevation of serum gonadotropins (LH and FSH) after releasing hormone (LH-RH) injection in normal children and in patients with disorders of puberty. J Clin Endocrinol Metab 35:473, 1972.

262. Penny R, Blizzard RM: The possible influence of puberty on the release of growth hormone in three males with apparent isolated growth hormone deficiency. J Clin Endocrinol Metab 34:82, 1972.

263. Santen RJ, Paulse CA: Hypogonadotropic eunuchoidism. I. Clinical study of the mode of inheritance. J Clin Endocrinol Metab 36:47, 1973.

264. Santen RJ, Paulsen CA: Hypogonadotropic eunuchoidism. II. Gonadal responsiveness to exogenous gonadotropins. J Clin Endocrinol Metab 36:55, 1973.

265. Van Dop C, Burstein S, Conte FA, Grumbach MM: Isolated gonadotropin deficiency in boys: Clinical characteristics and growth. J Pediatr 111:684, 1987.

266. McKusick V: Hereditable Disorders of Connective Tissue. 4th ed. St. Louis, CV Mosby, 1972.

267. Kallmann F, Schonfeld WA, Barrera WS: Genetic aspects of primary eunuchoidism. Am J Ment Defic 48:203, 1944.

268. Meriam GR, Beitins IZ, Bode HH: Father to son transmission of hypogonadism with anosmia. Am J Dis Child 131:1216, 1977.

269. McCullagh EP, Beck JC, Schaffenberg CA: A syndrome of eunuchoidism with spermatogenesis, normal urinary FSH and low or normal ICSH ("fertile eunuchs"). J Clin Endocrinol Metab 13:489, 1953.

270. Tanner JM, Whitehouse RH: A note on the bone age at which patients with true isolated growth hormone deficiency enter puberty. J Clin Endocrinol Metab 41:788, 1975.

271. Burstein S, Grumbach MM, Kaplan SL: Androgen responsiveness is important in the management of microphallus. Lancet 2:983, 1979.

272. Thomsett MJ, Conte FA, Kaplan SL, Grumbach MM: Endocrine and neurologic outcome in childhood craniopharyngioma: Review of effect of treatment in 42 patients. J Pediatr 97:728, 1980.

273. Dayan AD, Marshall AHE, Miller AA, Pick FH, Rankin NE: Atypical teratomas of the pineal and hypothalamus. J Pathol Bacteriol 92:1, 1966.

274. Koenig MP, Zuppinger K, Leichti B: Hyperprolactinemia as a cause of delayed puberty: Successful treatment with bromocriptine. J Clin Endocrinol Metab 45:825, 1977.

275. Sklar CA, Grumbach MM, Kaplan SL, Conte FA: Hormonal and metabolic abnormalities associated with central nervous system germinoma in children and adolescents and the effect of therapy: Report of 10 patients. J Clin Endocrinol Metab 51:548, 1980.

276. Vogel JM, Vogel P: Idiopathic histiocytosis: A discussion of eosinophilic granuloma, the Hand-Schuller-Christian syndrome, and the Letterer-Siwe syndrome. Semin Hematol 9:349, 1972.

277. Asherson RA, Jackson WPU, Lewis B: Abnormalities of development associated with hypothalamic calcification after tuberculous meningitis. Br Med J 2:839, 1965.

278. Kaplan SL, Grumbach MM, Hoyt WF: A syndrome of hypopituitary dwarfism, hypoplasia of optic nerves, and malformation of prosencephalon: Report of 6 patients. Pediatr Res 4:480 (A), 1970.

279. Richards GE, Wara WM, Grumbach MM, Kaplan SL, et al: Delayed onset of hypopituitarism: Sequelae of therapeutic irradiation of central nervous system, eye, and middle ear tumors. J Pediatr 89:553, 1976.

280. Ledbetter DH, Mascarello JT, Riccardi VM, Harper VD, Airhart SD, Strobel RJ: Chromosome 15 abnormalities and the Prader-Willi Syndrome: A follow-up report of 40 cases. Am J Hum Genet 34:278, 1982.

281. Tolis G, Lewis W, Verdy M, Friesen HG, Solomon S, Paglis G, Pavlatos F, Fessas PH, Rochefort JG: Anterior pituitary function in the Prader-Labhart-Willi (PLW) syndrome. J Clin Endocrinol Metab 39:1061, 1974.

282. Bauman ML, Hogan GR: Laurence-Moon-Biedl Syndrome. Am J Dis Child 126:119, 1973.

283. Vigersky R, Anderson AE, Thompson RH, Loriaux DL: Hypothalamic dysfunction in secondary amenorrhea associated with simple weight loss. N Engl J Med 297:1141, 1977.

284. Schwabe AD, Lippe BM, Chang RJ, Peps MA, Yager J: Anorexia nervosa. Ann Intern Med 94:371, 1981.

285. Beaumont PJV, George GCW, Pimstone BL, Vinik AI: Body weight and the pituitary response to hypothalamic releasing hormones in patients with anorexia nervosa. J Clin Endocrinol Metab 43:487, 1976.

286. Pugliese MT, et al: Fear of obesity: A cause of short stature and delayed puberty. N Engl J Med 309:513, 1983.

287. Beard CM, Benson RC Jr, Kelalis PP, Elveback LR, Kurland LT: The incidence and outcome of mumps orchitis in Rochester, Minnesota, 1935 to 1974. Mayo Clinic Proc 52:3, 1977.

288. Jamieson WM, Prinsley DM: Bornholm disease in the tropics. Br Med J 2:47, 1947.

289. Rothman CM, Sims CA, Stotts CL: Sertoli cell-only syndrome 1982. Fertil Steril 38:388, 1982.

290. Guay AT, Tuthill RJ, Woolf PD: Germinal cell aplasia: Response of luteinizing hormone (LH), follicle-stimulating hormone (FSH), and testosterone to LH/FSH-releasing hormone with histopathologic correlation. Fertile Steril 28:642, 1977.

291. Lushbaugh CC, Casakett GW: The effects of gonadal irradiation in clinical radiation therapy: A review. Cancer 37:1111, 1976.

292. Byrd R: Late effects of treatment of cancer in children. Pediatr Clin North Am 32:835, 1985.

293. Rivkees SA, Crawford JD: The relationship of gonadal activity and chemotherapy-induced gonadal damage. JAMA 259:2123, 1988.

294. Nistal M, Paniagua R, Bravo MP: Testicular lymphangiectasis in Noonan's syndrome. J Urol 131:759, 1984.

295. Cotter M, Lampert IA, Salm R: Epidermoid cysts of testis. Clin Oncol 10:149, 1984.

296. Sutherland GR, Ashforth PL: X-linked mental retardation with macro-orchidism and the fragile site at Xq 27 or 28. Hum Genet 48:117, 1979.

297. Breen DH, Braunstein GD, Neufeld N, Kudish H: Benign macro-orchidism in a pubescent boy. J Urol 125:589, 1981.

298. Sahn DJ, Schwartz AD: Schonlein-Henoch syndrome: Observations of some atypical clinical presentations. Pediatrics 49:114, 1972.

299. Rosenfeld RG, Northcraft GB, Hintz RL: A prospective randomized study of testosterone treatment of constitutional delay of growth and development in male adolescents. Pediatrics 69:681, 1982.

300. Clopper RR, Mazur T, MacGillivray MH, et al: Data on virilization and heterosexual behavior in male hypogonadotropic hypopituitarism during gonadotorpin and androgen treatment. J Androl 4:303, 1983.

301. Santoro N, Filicori M, Crowley WF Jr: Hypogonadotropic disorders in men and women: Diagnosis and therapy with pulsatile gonadotropin-releasing hormone. Endocr Rev 7 (1):11, 1986.

302. Styne DM, Grumbach MM: Puberty in the male and females: Its physiology and disorders. In Yen SSC, Jaffe RB (eds): Reproduction Endocrinology, Physiology, Pathophysiology and Clinical Management. Philadelphia, WB Saunders Company, p 189, 1978.

303. Albright F, Butler AM, Hampton AO, Smith P: Syndrome characterized by osteitis fibrosa disseminata, areas of pigmentation and endocrine dysfunction, with precocious puberty in females. N Engl J Med 216:727, 1937.

304. Danon M, Robboy SH, Kim S, Scully R, Crawford JD: Cushing syndrome, sexual precocity and polyostotic fibrous dysplasia (Albright syndrome) in infancy. J Pediatr 87:917, 1975.

305. Lightner ES, Penny R, Frasier SD: Growth hormone excess and sexual precocity in polyostotic fibrous dysplasia (McCune-Albright syndrome): Evidence for abnormal hypothalamic function. J Pediatr 87:922, 1975.

306. Lee PA, Van Dop C, Migeion CJ: McCune-Albright syndrome. Long-term follow-up. JAMA 256:2980, 1986.

307. Feuillan PP, Foster CM, Pescovitz OH, Hench KD, et al: Treatment of precocious puberty in the McCune-Albright syndrome with the aro-

matase inhibitor testolactone. N Engl J Med 315:1115, 1986.

308. Saxena KM: Endocrine manifestations of neurofibromatosis in children. Am J Dis Child 120:265, 1970.

309. Fienman NL, Yakovac WC: Neurofibromatosis in childhood. J Pediatr 76:339, 1970.

310. Van Wyk JJ, Grumbach MM: Syndrome of precocious menstruation and galactorrhea in juvenile hypothyroidism: An example of hormonal overlap in pituitary feedback. J Pediatr 57:416, 1960.

311. Rosenthal SM, Grumbach MM, Kaplan SL: Gonadotropin independent familial sexual precocity with premature Leydig and germinal cell maturation ("familial testotoxicosis"): Effects of a potent luteinizing hormone-releasing factor agonist and medroxyprogesterone acetate therapy in four cases. J Clin Endocrinol Metab 57:571, 1983.

312. Wierman ME, et al: Puberty without gonadotropins. N Engl J Med 312:65, 1985.

313. Holland FJ, et al: Ketoconazole in the management of precocious puberty not responsive to LHRH-analogue therapy. N Engl J Med 312:1023, 1985.

314. Holland FJ, Kirsch SE, Selby R: Gonadotropin-independent precocious puberty ("testotoxicocosis"): Influence of maturational status on response to ketoconazole. J Clin Endocrinol Metab 64:328, 1987.

315. Braunstein GD, Bridson WE, Glass A, Hull EW, McIntire KR: In vivo and in vitro production of human chorionic gonadotropin and alpha-fetoprotein by a virilizing hepatoblastoma. J Clin Endocrinol Metab 35:857, 1972.

316. Styne DW, et al: Treatment of true precocious puberty with a potent luteinizing hormone-releasing factor agonist: Effect on growth, sexual maturation, pelvic sonography, and the hypothalamic-pituitary-gonadal axis. J Clin Endocrinol Metab 61:142, 1985.

317. Pescovitz OH, Comite F, Hench K, Barnes K, et al: The NIH experience with precocious puberty: Diagnostic subgroups and response to short-term luteinizing hormone releasing hormone analogue therapy. J Pediatr 108:47, 1986.

318. Boepple PA, Mansfield MJ, Wierman ME, Rudlin CR, et al: Use of potent, long acting agonist of gonadotropin-releasing hormone in the treatment of precocious puberty. Endocr Rev 7:24, 1986.

319. Grumbach MM, Richards HE, Conte FA, Kaplan SL: Clinical disorders of adrenal function and puberty: An assessment of the role of the adrenal cortex in normal and abnormal puberty in man and evidence for an ACTH-like pituitary adrenal androgen stimulating hormone. *In* Serio M (ed): The Endocrine Function of the Human Adrenal Cortex. Serono Symposium, New York, Academic Press, 1977.

320. Moore DC, Schlaepfer LV, Paunier L, Sizonenko PC: Hormonal changes during puberty: V. Transient pubertal gynecomastia: Abnormal androgen-estrogen ratios. J Clin Endocrinol Metab 58:492, 1984.

321. Salbenblatt JA, Bender BG, Puck MH, Robinson A, et al: Pituitary-gonadal function in Klinefelter syndrome before and during puberty. Pediatr Res 19:82, 1985.

322. Grino PB, Griffin JE, Cushard WG Jr, Wilson JD: A mutation of the androgen receptor associated with partial androgen resistance, familial gynecomastia, and fertility. J Clin Endocrinol Metab 66:754, 1988.

323. Hemsell DL, Edman CD, Marks JF, Siiteri PK, MacDonald PC: Massive extraglandular aromatization of plasma androstenedione resulting in feminization of a prepubertal boy. J Clin Invest 60:455, 1977.

324. Cook CD, McArthur JW, Berenberg W: Pseudoprecocious puberty in girls as a result of estrogen ingestion. N Engl J Med 248:671, 1953.

325. Eberle AJ, Sparrow JT, Keenan BS: Treatment of persistent pubertal gynecomastia with dihydrotestosterone heptanoate. J Pediatr 109:144, 1986.

326. Finkelstein MS, Rosenberg HK, Snyder HM 3d, Duckett JW: Ultrasound evaluation of scrotum in pediatrics. Urology 27:1, 1986.

327. Myers RP: Tumors and related disorders of the male genital tract. *In* Kelalis PP, King LR, Belman AB (eds): Clinical Pediatric Urology. Philadelphia, WB Saunders Company, p 937, 1976.

328. Williams DI: Gonadal tumors. *In* Williams DI, Johnston JH (eds): Paediatric Urology. London, Butterworth Scientific, p 549. 1982.

11

PARATHYROID AND VITAMIN D–RELATED DISORDERS

Francis Mimouni and Reginald C. Tsang

THE PARATHYROIDS

Parathyroid Physiology

Preproparathyroid hormone (prepro-PTH) is first synthesized in the parathyroid gland as an 115–amino acid polypeptide with a molecular weight of 14,000. The "pre" peptide of 25 amino acids is attached to the NH_2 terminus of pro-PTH. When the "pre" peptide is removed, pro-PTH remains as a 90–amino acid polypeptide with a molecular weight of 10,200. The "pro" peptide fragment contains six amino acids attached to the NH_2-terminus of PTH, and when this fragment is removed, PTH remains as the 84–amino acid (molecular weight 9500) polypeptide, located in secretory granules prior to discharge into the circulation. The NH_2-terminus of PTH (amino acid-1) is the biologically active end of the hormone. The COOH-terminus (amino acid-84) is biologically inactive.

When PTH is released into the circulation via the parathyroid venous effluent, it is rapidly cleaved to smaller fragments of molecular weights 4000 and 7000. The 7000–molecular weight fragments are biologically inactive because they lack the NH_2-terminus, but the 4000–molecular weight fragments include the NH_2-terminus and are potent. Catabolism of PTH occurs primarily in the liver and kidney. Synthetic PTH fragments with the amino acid sequence 1–34 have the full biologic potency of native PTH, both in vitro and in vivo.

Hypocalcemia stimulates and hypercalcemia suppresses PTH synthesis and secretion. Acute decreases in blood magnesium also stimulate and acute increases suppress PTH secretion, although the effects are less than that of calcium on a molar basis. The major target organs of PTH are bone and kidney (Fig. 11–1). At target cells, adenylate cyclase activity is stimulated with production of cyclic AMP; at the same time intracellular calcium concentration is increased. In bone, PTH activity requires vitamin D; osteoclastic activity is increased and osteoblastic activity decreased, initially. Calcium and phosphorus are mobilized from bone to the extracellular space. With long-term PTH administration, there is a secondary rise in osteoblastic activity, which, in concert with increased osteoclastic activity, results in increased bone remodeling and turnover. In the kidneys, PTH causes increased reabsorption of calcium, and phosphaturia by decreased renal tubular phosphate reabsorption. Increased renal excretion of sodium, bicarbonate, glucose, and amino acids also occurs. The PTH effect on increasing intestinal calcium and phosphorus absorption is probably secondary to its facilitation of conversion of 25-hydroxyvitamin D (25-OHD) to 1,25-dihydroxyvitamin D $[1,25(OH)_2D]$. The combined effects of PTH on bone, kidney, and, indirectly, the intestine, are to raise serum calcium concentrations. Serum phosphorus is decreased, since the phosphaturic effect exceeds the serum phosphorus–raising effect of PTH on bone, and (indirectly) the intestine.

Radioimmunoassay is the most sensitive method for measuring circulating PTH concentrations. However, assays vary in their recognition of various sites in the PTH molecule. Assays recognizing the NH_2-terminus or the entire molecule appear to be useful in detecting acute changes in PTH secretion. Assays recognizing the biologically inactive COOH-terminus are more useful in measuring PTH in chronic hyperparathyroidism, since large amounts of COOH-terminus fragments are present in blood.

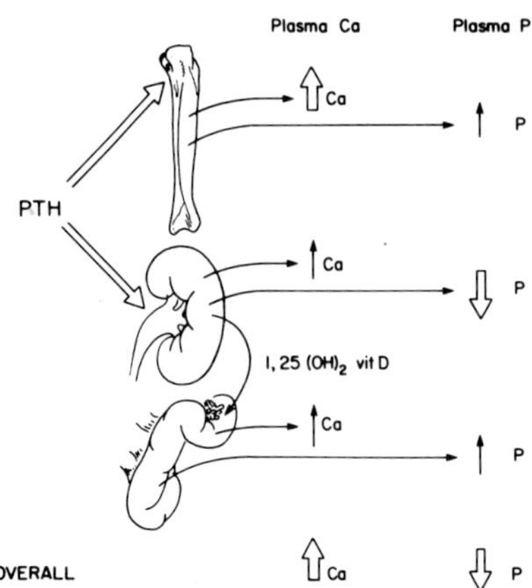

FIGURE 11–1. Action of parathyroid hormone on target tissues (bone, kidney and intestine). Net effect is increase in plasma calcium and decrease in plasma phosphorus. (From Tsang RC, Noguchi A, Steichen JJ: Pediatric parathyroid disorders. Pediatr Clin North Am 26:223, 1979.)

Circadian rhythms in serum PTH concentrations occur, the highest concentrations being found between 2 and 4 A.M. This factor should be taken into account when comparisons of PTH concentrations are made on different days.

Parathyroid Function in the Perinatal Period[2]

Calcium is transferred across the placenta by an active mechanism, requiring energy, and against a concentration gradient.[3] Fetal calcium requirements reach up to 150 mg/kg weight in the last trimester.[4] At that time, a significant increase in serum $1,25(OH)_2D$ concentration occurs in the maternal circulation, presumably to maintain maternal calcium economy.[5] An increase in maternal serum immunoreactive PTH has also been reported ("physiologic" hyperparathyroidism of pregnancy), but is still controversial.[3,6]

There seems to be maternal-fetal autonomy for parathyroid function; PTH does not cross the placenta in either direction. Calcium is actively transported from mother to fetus and presumably is the cause of fetal hypercalcemia. Fetal serum PTH concentrations have been reported to be low or normal; some degree of suppression of fetal parathyroid function would be expected from the high fetal serum calcium concentrations. The fetal parathyroids appear to be partially responsive to hypocalcemic stimulation. Also, fetal bone resorption and renal phos-

phaturia appear to occur in response to fetal PTH.

After birth, serum PTH concentrations increase, presumably in response to the abrupt withdrawal of transplacental calcium and decrease in extracellular calcium concentration. The postnatal increase in serum PTH concentrations is less marked in premature infants, and premature infants appear to have a smaller parathyroid response to a hypocalcemic stimulus when compared with more mature infants. Postnatal age is another important variable affecting neonatal parathyroid function. The degree of parathyroid response to a hypocalcemic stimulus increases significantly with postnatal age, and overcomes the effect of decreased gestational age.[7]

The suppression of neonatal serum PTH concentrations by hypercalcemia has not been adequately studied. Regimens of treatment or prevention of neonatal hypocalcemia [using oral or intravenous calcium, or $1,25(OH)_2D$] that do not result in hypercalcemia are not associated with suppression of serum PTH concentrations. Elevations of neonatal serum magnesium concentrations as a consequence of maternal hypermagnesemia have been associated with suppression of serum PTH concentrations; however, neonatal serum calcium concentrations in this condition appear to be in creased, possibly because of a direct effect of magnesium on calcium homeostasis.

VITAMIN D

Physiology of Vitamin D[8–10]

Under ultraviolet irradiation, provitamin D_3 in the skin is converted to previtamin D_3. Previtamin D_3 thermally isomerises to vitamin D_3 in the skin (Fig. 11–2), a slow process (24 hours). A carrier globulin in the blood, vitamin D binding protein, transports vitamin D_3 from the skin to the liver. In the liver vitamin D_3 is hydroxylated to 25-hydroxyvitamin D_3; 25-hydroxyvitamin D_3 in turn is hydroxylated in the kidney to 1,25-dihydroxyvitamin D_3. The final hydroxylation is facilitated by decreased calcium, decreased phosphorus, or increased PTH; other possible facilitators include prolactin, growth hormone, estrogen, progesterone, and testosterone.

1,25-Dihydroxyvitamin D_3 increases in-

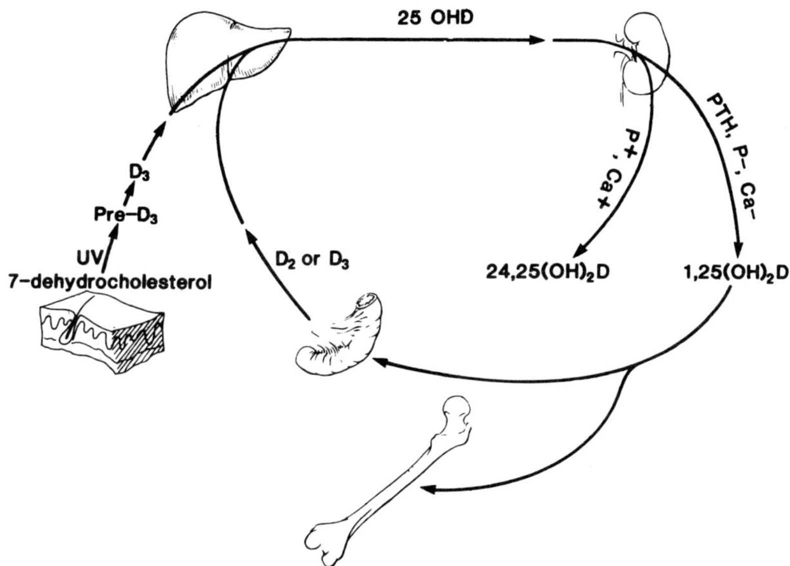

FIGURE 11–2. Vitamin D₃ is produced in the skin: pro-vitamin D (7-dehydrocholesterol) is converted to pre-vitamin D₃ under ultraviolet irradiation. Pre-vitamin D₃ isomerizes to D₃ gradually, and D₃ is released into the circulation. Hepatic 25-hydroxylation produces 25-hydroxyvitamin D₃. Renal 1α-hydroxylation produces 1,25-dihydroxyvitamin D₃, stimulated by calcium lack, phosphate lack, and parathyroid hormone (PTH). 1,25-Dihydroxyvitamin D₃ results in stimulation of intestinal calcium and phosphorus absorption and mobilization of calcium from bone. (From Tsang RC, Greer F, Steichen JJ: Perinatal vitamin D metabolism. Clin Perinatol, 8:287, 1981.)

testinal calcium and phosphorus absorption, mobilizes calcium and phosphorus from bone, and possibly retains calcium and phosphorus through its renal effect. The combined effects of 1,25(OH)₂D are to increase calcium and phosphorus retention and enhance the conditions for bone mineralization. 1,25-Dihydroxyvitamin D fulfills the criteria for classification as a hormone. It is synthesized in the body and transported to distant target organs, and control of its production is regulated by a feedback mechanism.

In the kidney, 24,25-dihydroxyvitamin D[24,25(OH)₂D] is also produced from 25-hydroxyvitamin D₃. This metabolite is produced in conditions of normal availability of calcium and phosphorus and its production is stimulated by 1,25-dihydroxyvitamin D₃. Possible functions of 24,25-dihydroxyvitamin D₃ are intestinal calcium transport, chondrocyte protein synthesis, and bone mineralization.

In this chapter the term "vitamin D" is used for vitamin D₃ (derived from animal sources) and vitamin D₂ (vegetable sources), since the metabolic transformations and activities are similar and since most assays do not distinguish between the two forms of vitamin D.

Vitamin D in the Perinatal Period

Maternal serum 1,25(OH)₂D concentrations become elevated during pregnancy.[4] The cause of the elevation is unclear but may be related to the transfer of calcium to the fetus, which would result in a fall in extracellular calcium concentration and stimulation of parathyroid activity. Decreased calcium and increased PTH[11] would result in increased production of 1,25(OH)₂D. The elevation of serum 1,25(OH)₂D coincides with the increased need for calcium (and phosphorus) during pregnancy and the increased calcium absorption and retention that occurs.[12] It is speculated that calcium transfer across the placenta triggers the production of PTH and 1,25(OH)₂D, which would act in concert at the bone site to mobilize calcium from bone to the extracellular space, thereby correcting any tendency toward hypocalcemia; in addition, 1,25(OH)₂D would enhance intestinal absorption of calcium and phosphorus and thus replenish any depletion of maternal mineral stores.

Vitamin D and 25-OHD appear to cross the placenta from mother to fetus.[13] 1,25-Dihydroxyvitamin D also appears to cross the placenta, although the quantities transported are not clearly defined.[14] The placenta itself also synthesizes 1,25(OH)$_2$D from 25-OHD,[15] but it is not clear whether this production contributes to the elevation of maternal serum 1,25(OH)$_2$D concentrations, or whether 1,25(OH)$_2$D may affect the placental transport of calcium. There is an ATP-dependent calcium uptake process that has been recently identified in purified human placental membranes; this process may be involved in the transport of calcium from mother to fetus.[16]

In the neonatal period, serum 25-OHD concentrations generally undergo little change. Premature infants may have decreased serum concentrations,[17] although the significance of the finding is unclear. Serum 1,25(OH)$_2$D concentrations, however, increase from birth to 24 hours of age in full-term infants (Fig. 11–3).[4] The factors leading to the increase in serum 1,25(OH)$_2$D are unclear but may be related to the decrease in serum calcium concentrations and increase in PTH concentrations that occur normally in this period. Because the increase in 1,25(OH)$_2$D coincides with the time when infants receive increasing amounts of milk, it is possible that production of the active metabolite of vitamin D is increased to meet the needs for more efficient intestinal absorption of calcium and phosphorus in the newborn period.[18]

Vitamin D and Breast Milk

Concentrations of vitamin D in human milk are low, ranging from 12 to 60 IU/L.[19-21] High concentrations of a water-soluble or sulfated compound of vitamin D have been reported,[22] but the bioactivity of this compound is weak[23] and its presence in human milk is questionable.[24] Most of the bioactivity in human milk is from vitamin D itself and 25-OHD, while very little is from 1,25 or 24,25(OH)$_2$D.[23-25]

Breast milk vitamin D concentrations correlate significantly with maternal dietary intake of vitamin D.[21] Similarly, maternal ul-

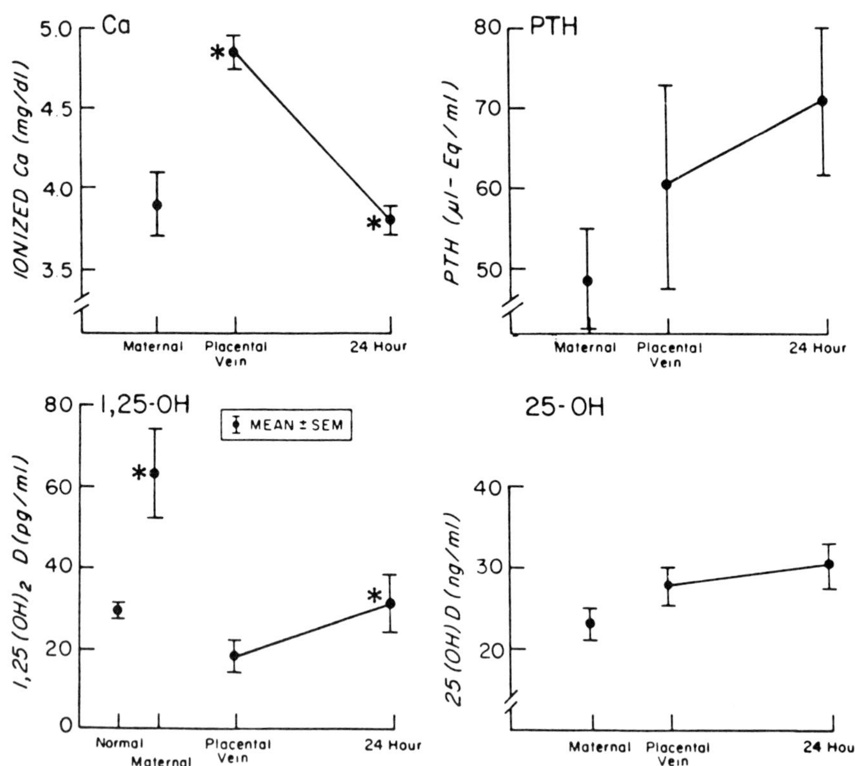

FIGURE 11–3. In term pregnancies, maternal serum 1,25(OH)$_2$D concentrations are increased. Umbilical vein 1,25(OH)$_2$D concentrations are low but reach normal adult concentrations by 24 hours of age. (From Steichen JJ, Tsang RC, Gratton TL, et al: Vitamin D homeostasis in the perinatal period. N Engl J Med 302:315, 1980.)

traviolet B exposure may affect breast milk vitamin D content.[26] Marked racial differences of breast milk vitamin D concentrations have been reported,[21] and it has been suggested that dark skin pigmentation as well as low ultraviolet B exposure may result in reduced breast milk vitamin D concentrations.[21]

In a prospective, double-blind study of term infants exclusively breast-fed and randomized to either daily 400 IU vitamin D supplements or placebo, it was noted that bone mineral content and serum 25-OHD concentrations were lower in the placebo group at 6 months of age.[27] Thus, it appears that breast milk contains very little vitamin D of significant biologic activity, and we suggest that vitamin D supplementation (400 IU/day) be considered in exclusively breast-fed infants, particularly those with dark skin complexion or with little sunshine exposure.

Calcitonin Physiology[28]

Calcitonin is produced mostly by the C cells of the thyroid gland, which are embryologically derived from the neural crest; it is a 32–amino acid molecule. At the bone site, calcitonin has an anti-PTH effect and decreases the amount of calcium and phosphate released from bone. Calcitonin also has calciuric and phosphaturic affects; thus its overall effects are to decrease serum calcium and phosphate concentrations. The main factor regulating the secretion of calcitonin is serum calcium concentration, which has an effect opposite to that on PTH secretion. An acute rise in serum calcium stimulates calcitonin release, and a fall in serum calcium concentration supresses its secretion. Other factors that increase the production of calcitonin include increases in circulating magnesium and increases in gastrointestinal hormones such as gastrin, glucagon, and pancreozymin. Since these hormones are released by the presence of food in the gastrointestinal tract, it has been suggested that the gastrointestinal hormones—calcitonin system helps prevent marked increases in serum calcium concentration during food intake. However, the relative importance of calcitonin in the regulation of mineral metabolism is unclear. There is no known disease related to calcitonin deficiency. Thyroidectomized patients have very little disturbance in their calcium metabolism and at most, when infused with calcium intravenously, demonstrate higher serum calcium concentrations than control patients. Syndromes involving excess circulating calcitonin do not produce hypocalcemia.

Concentrations of serum calcitonin in fetal animals and human newborns are very high. The serum calcitonin concentrations increase further after birth, but its role in neonatal hypocalcemia is unproven.

Syndromes of Decreased Parathyroid Hormone Secretion (Hypoparathyroidism) or Action (Pseudohypoparathyroidism)

Classification

In *hypoparathyroidism*, PTH production is decreased or absent.[29] Hypocalcemia and hyperphosphatemia are the major diagnostic clues, which presumably relate to deficient calcium release from bone, deficient calcium and increased phosphate reabsorption in the kidney, and indirectly [through decreased renal $1,25(OH)_2D$ production] decreased intestinal calcium absorption. The various situations in which hypoparathyroidism may be encountered are described in a later paragraph.

In *pseudohypoparathyroidism* (PHP) a combination of the biochemical features of hypoparathyroidism (i.e., hypocalcemia and hyperphosphatemia) and an end-organ resistance to PTH occurs.[29] In this syndrome, PTH secretion is increased, presumably as a result of chronic hypocalcemia. Specific dysmorphic features and mental retardation, initially described by Albright et al.[30] and comprehensively discussed by Bronsky et al.[31] are present in varying degrees of severity.

Different subtypes of PHP seem to be related to different pathophysiologic mechanisms.[29,32]

In PHP type I, PTH is unable to elicit cyclic AMP production in target cells; administration of exogenous PTH does not increase urinary cyclic AMP production. In 60 per cent of patients with PHP type I, there is a 40 to 50 per cent reduction in the N protein of erythrocytes, platelets, or cultured fibroblasts; the N protein couples a number of membrane receptors, including that for PTH to adenylate cyclase. These patients, classified as PHP type IA, usually present the dysmorphic features described by Albright (see later). The N protein appears to be present universally in cells,[33] and some patients with PHP type IA are affected by other endocrinopathies (presumably due to end-organ resistance), such as abnormal thyroid response to thyroid-stimulating hormone (TSH) and hypothyroidism, hypogonadism, and decreased cyclic AMP generation in response to glucagon.[34] In these patients, end-organ resistance appears to be progressive over the first 2 to 3 years of life, with dysmorphic features and possible migratory calcifications preceding hypocalcemia and elevation of serum PTH concentrations.[35] In one study, a circulating factor was identified that inhibits biologic activity of PTH at the level of the kidney.[36]

In PHP type IB patients, the N protein content of cells is normal, and no dysmorphic features are found. In these patients, the exact molecular basis for PTH resistance is as yet undetermined.

A wide spectrum of skeletal or renal end-organ resistance to PTH has been reported: in some patients with PHP type I, end-organ resistance is found in the kidney, but the bone is normally responsive. These patients, classified as PHP type I with osteitis fibrosa, or pseudohypo-hyperparathyroidism, have a combination of hypocalcemia and hyperphosphatemia with skeletal signs of hyperparathyroidism.[37] Patients with skeletal, but no renal resistance (pseudo-pseudohypoparathyroidism) present the constitutional features of PHP without hypocalcemia or hyperphosphatemia. In these patients, skeletal defects may be more severe in the female as a result of early epiphyseal closure.[29]

In PHP type II, cyclic AMP production in urine is normally elicited by PTH, but phosphaturic response is profoundly decreased.[29] The end-organ resistance is presumed to be due to defective tubular response to cyclic AMP.[29] Interestingly, in these patients, restoration of normocalcemia by treatment with vitamin D and calcium also restores the phosphaturic response to PTH.[38]

Etiology, Inheritance, and Associated Disorders

Hypoparathyroidism. Hypoparathyroidism may occasionally be familial; in such cases, it is usually inherited as an X-linked recessive trait and males are affected early (first month of life).[39] However, autosomal-dominant and autosomal-recessive patterns of inheritance also have been reported.[40] Rarely, congenital hypoparathyroidism is associated with ring chromosome 16 or 18p or 22p syndrome.[41]

Congenital aplasia or hypoplasia of the parathyroid glands may occur sporadically, in isolated fashion, or within the spectrum of the DiGeorge syndrome, where immunologic deficiency (from thymic hypoplasia or aplasia), cardiovascular defects, and craniofacial anomalies are variably combined.[42] DiGeorge syndrome arises from embryologic failure (of unknown etiology) of the third and fourth pharyngeal pouches.[41]

At any time during childhood to adulthood, parathyroid gland failure may present as an autoimmune disorder. It is frequently associated with the presence of antibodies to the parathyroid in the serum and with mucocutaneous candidiasis.[43] Other related disorders may occur in these patients, such as adrenal insufficiency, diabetes mellitus, lymphocytic thyroiditis, pernicious anemia, and gonadal atrophy.[44] (See also Chapters 3, 4, 6, 8, and 10.) Steatorrhea may cause magnesium deficiency, which complicates further both the diagnosis and the treatment.

Transient neonatal hypoparathyroidism may be seen in preterm infants[45] or in infants of diabetic mothers.[46] In the latter infants, it is believed to be largely due to magnesium deficiency (see later). Transient neonatal hypoparathyroidism also may be a consequence of chronic fetal parathyroid gland suppression resulting from maternal hypercalcemia, and in several instances has led to the discovery of the maternal disorder (e.g., parathyroid adenoma).[47] It may also occur sporadically, and disappear over a few weeks to a few months.[48] It is unclear, however, if disappearance of manifestations of the disorder is due to complete remission or to a compensated state.[48]

Magnesium deficiency leads to a state of both inadequate PTH production and end-organ resistance to PTH, presumably as a result of effects on the magnesium-dependent adenylate cyclase involved in both secretion and action of PTH.[49] An autosomal recessive disorder of intestinal magnesium absorption has been described that leads to severe hypocalcemia in the first few weeks of life.[50]

Finally, hypoparathyroidism may be iatrogenic (following subtotal or total thyroidectomy) or a consequence of progressive destruction of parathyroid tissue by iron deposition due to iron overload (in hemolytic anemias).[51]

Pseudohypoparathyroidism. Pseudohypoparathyroidism is probably inherited as an X-linked dominant trait with variable expression, although an autosomal dominant form has also been described.[52] Associated disorders, as discussed above, include hypothyroidism and gonadal failure. Patients also may have decreased hepatic cyclic AMP generation in response to glucagon infusion, although they do not suffer from episodes of hypoglycemia. Presumably, different cyclic AMP concentrations are needed for the mediation of responses to different hormones. Diabetes mellitus also has been reported to occur at unusually high rates in patients with PHP.[53]

Clinical Features

Signs Common to Hypoparathyroidism and Pseudohypoparathyroidism. Tetany, convulsions (grand mal, petit mal, or focal seizures), carpopedal spasm, muscle cramps and twitching, paresthesias, and laryngeal stridor are usually the presenting features of both types of hypoparathyroidism. Tetany may be precipitated by menstruation.[54] Chvostek's (provoked facial muscle twitching), and less commonly Trousseau's (provoked carpopedal spasm), signs may be present as manifestations of latent tetany. The skin may be dry and coarse; maculopapular skin eruptions, eczematous dermatitis, and exfoliative erythroderma may occur. The hair is often brittle with areas of alopecia. The nails are thin and brittle. Characteristic nail changes directly related to hypocalcemia are smooth transverse grooves, reversible with restoration of serum calcium to normal. Dental and enamel hypoplasia occur in both PHP and hypoparathyroidism, and occasionally are associated with thickened lamina dura.

Signs That May Help Distinguishing between the Two Disorders. The most comprehensive clinical description of hypoparathyroidism and PHP was given by Bronsky and colleagues (Fig. 11–4).[31] Children with PHP Ia are short and thick set, and have round faces and short, thick necks. The digits of the fingers and toes are short and stubby, and because of shortened metacar-

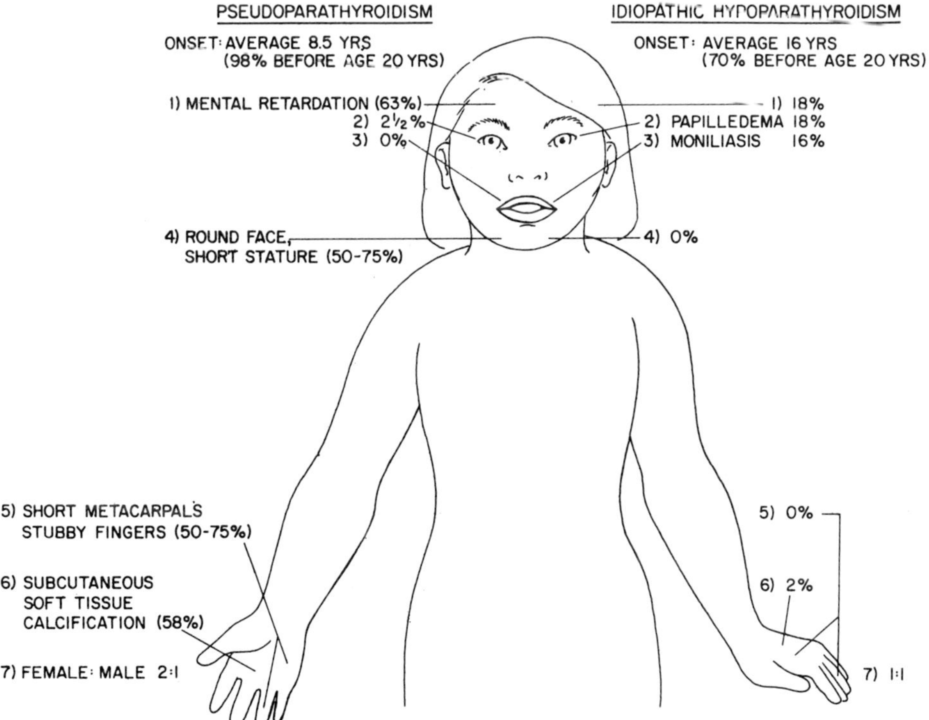

FIGURE 11–4. Pseudohypoparathyroidism contrasted with idiopathic hypoparathyroidism. (Based on Bronsky et al.[31])

pals, the skin over the knuckles is dimpled (Fig. 11–5). Classically, the index finger is longer than the middle finger because the second metacarpal is not affected by metacarpal shortening. None of these features is typical for patients with hypoparathyroidism. Subcutaneous soft tissue calcifications are a prominent feature of PHP but not of hypoparathyroidism. The calcified lesions may occur in any part of the body, although the extremities are the typical sites. Mental retardation is a much more prominent feature of PHP than of hypoparathyroidism. There appears to be less retardation when onset of disease is later and when there is less delay in the diagnosis and treatment. Swings of emotion, loss of memory, depression, and confusion may occur. Papilledema, presumably related to increased intracranial pressure, may occur in hypoparathyroidism but is rare in PHP. Bilateral lamellar cataracts may occur in both hypoparathyroidism and PHP. Moniliasis of the nails and mouth occurs in hypoparathyroidism but is rare in PHP. Moniliasis of the nails results in irregular pitting of nails and flakiness that are not corrected by restoration of normocalcemia.

Radiologic Features

The radiologic signs are much more prominent in PHP than in hypoparathyroidism. Subcutaneous bone formation may occur as punctate or granular lesions, especially in the extremities. Shortened metatarsal and metacarpal bones are characteristic of PHP,

with sparing of the second digit. The bones are wide, with widened medullary canals and coarse trabecular patterns. In PHP, thickening of the calvarium may occur. In the brain, symmetric punctate calcifications are seen in basal ganglia areas. In contrast, but rarely, in prolonged unrecognized hypoparathyroidism, there may be signs of osteomalacia, presumably related to deficiency of $1,25(OH)_2D$. In PHP type I with osteitis fibrosa, typical hyperparathyroid bone resorptive lesions are present.

Diagnosis[1]

The diagnosis of hypoparathyroidism is made from signs and symptoms in association with decreased serum calcium and increased serum phosphorus concentrations. Hypoparathyroidism appears to be a more severe biochemical disorder than PHP. Signs of associated disorders may be evident. Familial patterns especially may be present in PHP.

Plasma PTH levels will be low in hypoparathyroidism but high in PHP. Whereas the end-organ response to PTH in PHP is decreased, considerable variations in responsiveness occur. In the classical (type I) PHP, there is bone and renal unresponsiveness to PTH: urinary cyclic AMP and urinary phosphate excretion are not increased after PTH administration. Type II PHP is similar except that urinary cyclic AMP responsiveness is present without the phosphaturic response; presumably, cyclic AMP is generated but this does not lead to phos-

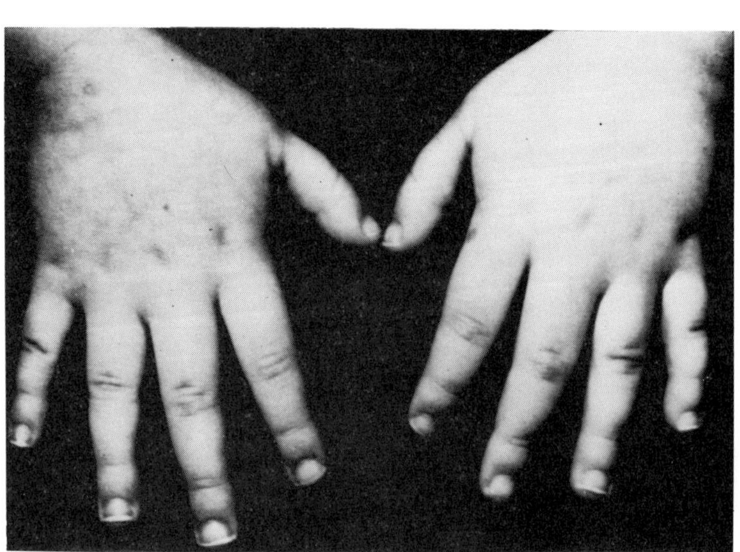

FIGURE 11–5. Hands of child with pseudohypoparathyroidism, with stubby short fingers, and dimpled skin due to shortened metacarpals. (From Tsang RC, Noguchi A, Steichen JJ: Pediatric parathyroid disorders. Pediatr Clin North Am 26:223, 1979.)

phaturia. In PHP with isolated skeletal resistance, skeletal unresponsiveness is associated with normal renal responsiveness; however, the skeletal responsiveness is improved with $1,25(OH)_2D$ therapy. In PHP with osteitis fibrosa, bone responsiveness is present, and elevated serum PTH levels produce the picture of hyperparathyroid bone disease; in spite of the bone responsiveness, however, serum calcium remains low. In "pseudoidiopathic hypoparathyroidism" (or "hypoparathyroidism with ineffective PTH,"), responsiveness to exogenous PTH is present but there is no responsiveness to endogenous PTH. Finally, in "pseudo-PHP" the phenotypic features of PHP are present but serum calcium and phosphorus are normal, and both bone and renal responsiveness to PTH are intact.[1]

To test for end-organ responsiveness in children, PTH, 200 units, is administered. The dose for infants is 5 to 15 units/kg. Timed urinary collections are made prior to (ideally two 60-min collections) and after PTH injection (two 30-min, followed by three 60-min collections). Urinary cyclic AMP is normally increased in the first 30 min after PTH injection and phosphaturia occurs soon thereafter. In hypoparathyroid patients and normal subjects, cyclic AMP excretion increases 10-fold when compared with control urines; in PHP there is no increase or less than a twofold increase. The increase in phosphaturia in hypoparathyroidism following PTH injection is fourfold to sixfold compared with less than twofold in PHP.[55] Tests for the calcemic responsiveness to PTH are less well standardized; previous studies using large repeated doses of PTH (e.g., PTH, 200 units every 8 hours for 4 to 7 days) are potentially dangerous, because serum calcium levels may reach 15 to 18 mg/dl in responsive subjects. Calcemic and phosphaturic responses to PTH may be augmented with vitamin D therapy.[56,57]

Treatment

At the time of clinical presentation, since the main problem is generally tetany or seizures associated with hypocalcemia, intravenous calcium salts are the treatment of choice. A dose of 2 ml/kg body weight of 10 per cent calcium gluconate (9.4 mg elemental calcium/ml) is generally sufficient for acute correction of hypocalcemia. Follow-up intravenous therapy with 10 per cent calcium gluconate 5 to 8 ml/kg/day gives 50 to 75 mg calcium/kg/day; the higher dose is suitable for infants less than two years, and the lower dose for older children. During the acute phase, serum calcium levels should be measured once or twice daily.

Vitamin D therapy is begun when the diagnosis of hypoparathyroidism is confirmed. A major biochemical problem in hypoparathyroidism is decreased production of 1,25-dihydroxyvitamin D_3 because of decreased renal hydroxylase activity resulting presumably from lack of PTH stimulation.[58] Vitamin D therapy is directed primarily toward restoration of serum 1,25-dihydroxyvitamin D_3 concentrations and optimal intestinal calcium absorption.[59] This can be accomplished by administration of 1,25-dihydroxyvitamin D_3 itself, which bypasses the renal hydroxylation block,[60] or by large doses of 25-hydroxyvitamin D_3[61] or vitamin D_3 (Fig. 11–2). The initial dose of 1,25-dihydroxyvitamin D_3 is approximately 0.03 to 0.08 μg/kg/day, up to a maximum 1 to 2 μg/day. These doses approximate the normal requirement for 1,25-dihydroxyvitamin D_3. The dose of 25-hydroxyvitamin D_3, however, is 3 to 6 μg/kg/day or 30 times the physiologic requirement of 0.15 μ/kg/day. Similarly, the dosage of vitamin D_3 required to control hypoparathyroidism ranges from 50,000 to 100,000 units (1000 to 2000 units/kg); or more than 100 times the "physiologic requirement" (1 μg of vitamin D_3 has 40 units of activity). These dosage requirements reflect the degree of block in renal hydroxylase activity in hypoparathyroidism. Rarely, massive doses of vitamin D metabolites, including 900 μg of 25-hydroxyvitamin D_3 or 6 μg of 1,25-dihydroxyvitamin D_3 may be required to correct hypocalcemia.

The theoretical advantage of 1,25-dihydroxyvitamin D_3 is its rapid onset of action and short half-life. However, it is possible that other metabolites of vitamin D may play important physiologic roles.[62] 25-Hydroxyvitamin D_3 is intermediate in its onset of action and half-life between 1,25-dihydroxyvitamin D_3 and vitamin D_3. Vitamin D_3, the mainstay of treatment for hypoparathyroidism,[63] has an onset of action of 7 to 14 days and a comparably long half-life. If hypercalcemia develops, it is more serious with vitamin D_3 therapy because it persists for a longer time.

Treatment with vitamin D metabolites should be begun with low doses, with stepwise increase and careful daily monitoring of serum calcium values until normal levels are achieved. When levels have stabilized, monthly blood sampling, then 3-monthly, and finally 6-monthly blood sampling can be performed. It is safer to keep serum calcium levels between 8.5 to 9 mg/dl rather than higher because of the significant morbidity from overdosage and hypercalcemia (particularly central nervous system damage and nephrocalcinosis). Six-monthly to yearly evaluation of renal function and blood pressure should be carried out to detect possible renal toxicity. Serum magnesium levels should be measured at 3- to 6-monthly intervals to detect hypomagnesemia, which if present may raise the requirements for vitamin D. Six-monthly measurements of plasma 25-OHD levels and, with increasing availability of the assay, plasma $1,25(OH)_2D$ levels, will allow better assessment of the dosage of vitamin D.

Oral calcium supplementation is also useful. Doses of 50 mg elemental calcium/kg (or 530 mg calcium gluconate/kg) up to a maximum of about 1 gm of calcium (10 gm calcium gluconate) can be used in three or four divided doses. Higher doses can result in diarrhea. Calcium supplementation is not essential, but its use may facilitate the attainment of optimal serum calcium levels. When hypercalcemia occurs or is imminent, discontinuing the calcium intake and decreasing or discontinuing vitamin D administration may help to avert damage from hypercalcemia. Vitamin D toxicity can occur even after prolonged stabilization of serum calcium,[64] possibly because of amelioration of bone disease.

If serum magnesium levels fall below 1.5 mg/dl, magnesium salt supplementation should be given. The usual dose is 7 to 15 mg of elemental magnesium/kg (or 70 to 150 mg of magnesium sulfate/kg). The requirement for vitamin D may be increased by anticonvulsant therapy, probably because of lowered plasma 25-OHD concentrations.

The prognosis for hypoparathyroidism is good, provided vitamin D overdosage is avoided. Mental retardation should be preventable with early diagnosis and optimal management.

Neonatal Hypocalcemia[65,66]

"Early" Neonatal Hypocalcemia

"Early" neonatal hypocalcemia occurs within the first 3 days of life and is an accentuation of the normal fall in serum calcium concentrations experienced by all infants after birth. One third of premature infants and infants with birth asphyxia and half of infants of diabetic mothers have serum calcium concentrations less than 7 mg/dl. The nadir of serum calcium concentration occurs from 24 to 48 hours of age.

In premature infants, the major pathogenetic factor appears to be decreased parathyroid responsiveness at a time when maternal-fetal calcium transport is abruptly discontinued[45,67] (Fig. 12–6). The role of vitamin D metabolites is unclear, but serum calcitonin elevation may aggravate the hypocalcemia.[68] Hypocalcemia in infants with birth asphyxia has been attributed to endogenous phosphorus release into the extracellular space.[69] Increased levels of calcitonin may also be contributory.[70] In infants of diabetic mothers hypomagnesemia occurs; the condition is directly related to the severity of maternal diabetes and is associated with hypocalcemia and decreased parathyroid function.[71] Since magnesium deficiency may occur in diabetes, neonatal magnesium deficiency is thought to be a cause of neonatal hypocalcemia.[72]

"Late" Neonatal Hypocalcemia

Classical "infantile tetany" is neonatal hypocalcemia occurring usually after a week of age in an infant ingesting cow's milk formula. The high phosphate content of cow's milk formulas results in hyperphosphatemia and secondarily, hypocalcemia and "tetany."[73] Ingestion of cereals, which have

---

FIGURE 11–6. Hypoparathyroidism in "early" neonatal hypocalcemia. Serum parathyroid hormone (PTH) levels in term infants, premature infants, and infants of diabetic mothers (Class A and insulin-dependent Classes B, C, and D). In term infants, a mild decrease in serum total and ionized calcium after birth is associated with an appropriate increase in serum PTH. In premature infants and in infants of insulin dependent mothers, there is no significant increase in serum PTH levels in spite of marked falls in serum calcium. In infants of Class A diabetic mothers the PTH response is equivocal in the face of a fall in serum calcium. (From Tsang RC, et al: Parathyroid function in infants of diabetic mothers. J Pediatr 86:399, 1975, and Tsang RC, et al: Neonatal parathyroid function. J Pediatr 83:728, 1973.)

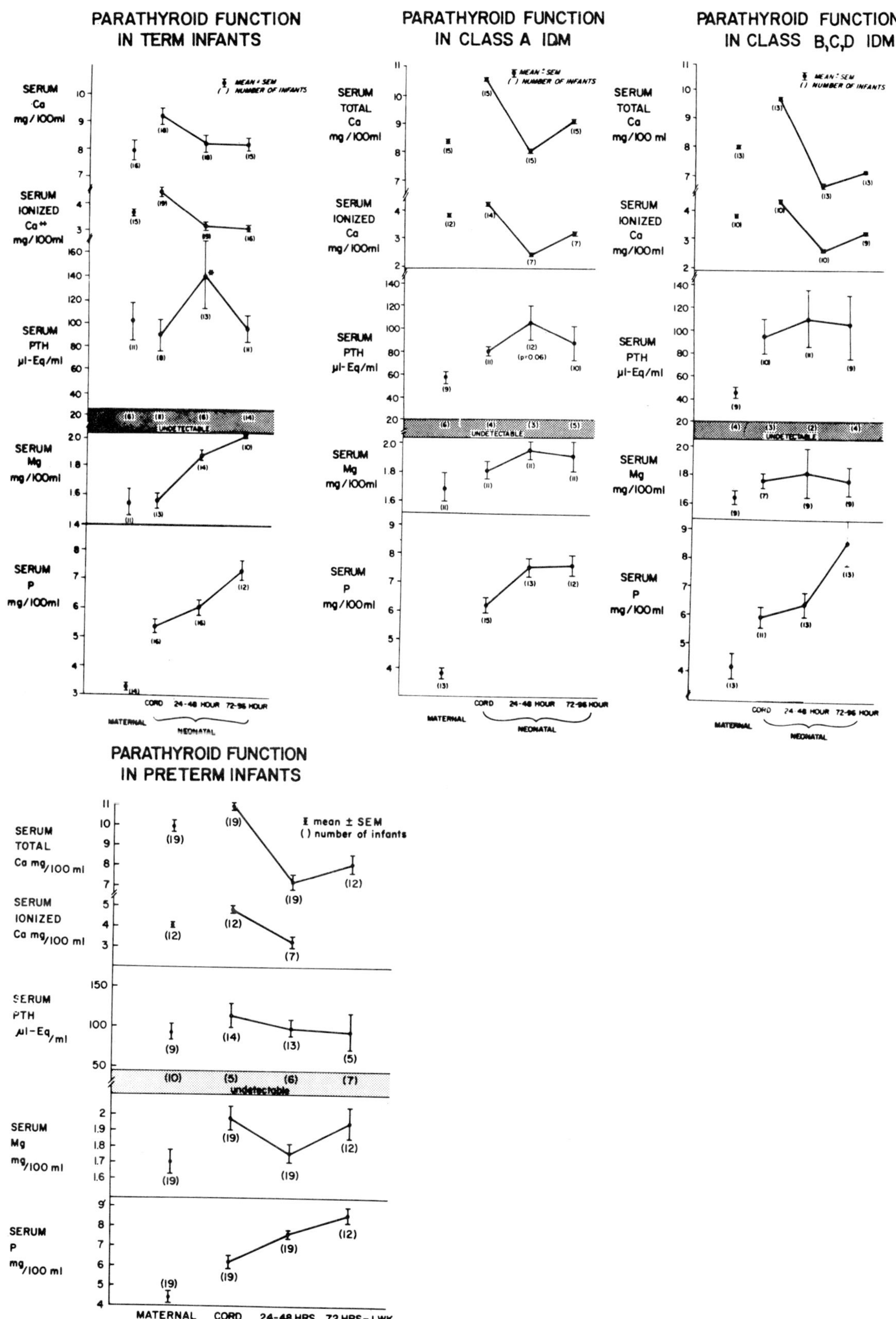
PARATHYROID FUNCTION
IN TERM INFANTS
MEAN ± SEM
( ) NUMBER OF INFANTS
SERUM
Ca
mg/100ml
SERUM
IONIZED
Ca++
mg/100ml
SERUM
PTH
µl-Eq/ml
UNDETECTABLE
SERUM
Mg
mg/100ml
SERUM
P
mg/100ml
MATERNAL
NEONATAL
CORD   24-48 HOUR   72-96 HOUR

PARATHYROID FUNCTION
IN CLASS A IDM
MEAN ± SEM
( ) NUMBER OF INFANTS
SERUM
TOTAL
Ca
mg/100ml
SERUM
IONIZED
Ca
mg/100ml
SERUM
PTH
µl-Eq/ml
(p=0.06)
UNDETECTABLE
SERUM
Mg
mg/100ml
SERUM
P
mg/100ml
MATERNAL
NEONATAL
CORD   24-48 HOUR   72-96 HOUR

PARATHYROID FUNCTION
IN CLASS B,C,D IDM
MEAN ± SEM
( ) NUMBER OF INFANTS
SERUM
TOTAL
Ca
mg/100 ml
SERUM
IONIZED
Ca
mg/100ml
SERUM
PTH
µl-Eq/ml
UNDETECTABLE
SERUM
Mg
mg/100ml
SERUM
P
mg/100ml
MATERNAL
NEONATAL
CORD   24-48 HOUR   72-96 HOUR

PARATHYROID FUNCTION
IN PRETERM INFANTS
mean ± SEM
( ) number of infants
SERUM
TOTAL
Ca mg/100 ml
SERUM
IONIZED
Ca mg/100 ml
SERUM
PTH
µl-Eq/ml
undetectable
SERUM
Mg
mg/100 ml
SERUM
P
mg/100 ml
MATERNAL   CORD   24-48 HRS   72 HRS-1 WK

relatively high phosphate content, also may lead to hypocalcemia.[74] Maternal vitamin D deficiency appears to aggravate the tendency to late neonatal hypocalcemia.

Neonatal hypomagnesemia may be due to specific intestinal malabsorption of magnesium. Magnesium deficiency leads to decreased parathyroid secretion, decreased response of bone to PTH, or decreased release of calcium from bone. Males appear to be more commonly affected, and the clinical presentation includes irritability, muscle twitching, eye rolling movements, and convulsions.[75]

Chronic diarrhea may lead to malabsorption of calcium. Theoretically, vitamin D malabsorption may occur, and 25-OHD and $1,25(OH)_2D$ malabsorption also may occur, since there are enterohepatic circulations of these metabolites. In infants with severe diarrhea, treatment of acidosis with bicarbonate has been associated with hypocalcemia. In acidosis, calcium is mobilized from bone to extracellular space and may be lost in the urine. When alkali treatment is given, calcium release from bone is decreased and hypocalcemia can occur.

Idiopathic hypoparathyroidism may present in the neonatal period, as may neonatal hypoparathyroidism secondary to maternal hyperparathyroidism (see earlier discussion). Hypovitaminosis D rickets may present with hypocalcemia, although the presentation is usually after the first few months of life (see earlier discussion).

Decreases in Ionized Calcium

Citrate complexes blood calcium and lowers the concentration of ionized calcium. When citrated blood is used for "exchange" blood transfusion, serum ionized calcium is decreased during the procedure. Free fatty acids may complex calcium in blood and decrease ionized calcium, if present in high concentrations. In alkalosis, ionized calcium is decreased because of decreased dissociation of calcium from serum protein.

Treatment[65,66]

Prevention of early neonatal hypocalcemia may be achieved with oral calcium supplementation (elemental calcium 75 mg/kg/day). In infants who cannot tolerate enteric feeding, $1,25(OH)_2D$ may be a possible alternative, although great care should be exercised in its administration.

Seizures can be treated with 10 per cent calcium gluconate (2 ml/kg) given cautiously intravenously over 10 min, with constant monitoring of the heart rate. In neonates, skin sloughing, tissue necrosis, and calcifications can occur from extravasation of calcium salts into the soft tissue. Maintenance amounts of calcium (oral or intravenous calcium gluconate) can be given at a dosage of 75 mg of elemental calcium/kg/day in neonates and 50 mg/kg/day in older infants.

Calcium chloride should be avoided because it may result in metabolic acidosis. Oral calcium gluconate is preferred over Neocalglucon, since the syrup base of the latter is hyperosmolar and leads to diarrhea. Care should be exercised in infants receiving digitalis because of the potentiating effects of calcium on digitalis toxicity. If intravenous catheters are used for calcium infusions, they should not be placed near the heart because of the danger of cardiac standstill from inadvertent rapid calcium infusions. The intravenous tubing also should be clearly labeled as containing calcium, so that any "flushing" of the tubing can be done judiciously without causing a bolus of calcium to be administered. Ideally, termination of therapy should be done gradually by halving the intravenous rate successively on 2 days before discontinuation. Presence of "rebound" hypercalcemia should be checked for at least a day later. Intra-arterial infusions of calcium are dangerous and have been associated with tissue necrosis.

In "late" neonatal hypocalcemia due to high-phosphate diet, a formula containing low amounts of phosphate (such as Similac PM 60/40) or breast milk should be used and rice cereals should be eliminated. In primary hypomagnesemia, hypocalcemia cannot be controlled by calcium alone. Initially, magnesium sulfate (50 per cent) can be given intramuscularly in a dosage of 0.2 ml kg every 8 to 12 hours. Serum magnesium levels should be measured every 12 hours until normal levels are found. Oral magnesium sulfate supplementation of 0.2 to 1.2 ml/kg day can be given as a maintenance dose for conditions with magnesium malabsorption.[75]

Hyperparathyroidism
Primary Hyperparathyroidism

Primary hyperparathyroidism is generally a disease of adult life rather than childhood.

The genesis of primary hyperparathyroidism is obscure.[76] Familial hyperparathyroidism has been described.[77] Familial hyperparathyroidism may be part of the syndrome of multiple endocrine adenomatosis: pancreatic islet cell adenomas, gastrin-secreting tumors, pituitary tumors, and adrenal cortical adenomas (see Chapter 6). Neonatal familial hyperparathyroidism has been assumed to be inherited in an autosomal-recessive manner.[78] However, father-to-daughter transmission has occurred occasionally and this is consistent with autosomal-dominant inheritance.[79]

The clinical manifestations of primary hyperparathyroidism[80] are (1) gastrointestinal, (2) central nervous system, (3) neuromuscular, (4) osseous, and (5) renal. Gastrointestinal manifestations, primarily related to the degree of hypercalcemia, are nausea, vomiting, abdominal discomfort, constipation, and signs of pancreatitis. Central nervous system symptoms, resulting from hypercalcemia, are delusions, confusion, hallucinations, impaired memory, lack of interest and initiative, depression and varying levels of consciousness.[81] Neuromuscular manifestations, presumably on a neuropathologic basis, include weakness, easy fatigability and muscle atrophy, especially of the proximal muscles of the lower limbs, twitching of the tongue resembling fasciculations, and paresthesias in the extremities. Osteolytic activity of PTH produces bone symptoms, including vague bone pains. Renal changes are polyuria and polydipsia related to the hypercalcemia and increased filtered calcium, renal colic from renal stones, and hypertension. Hypercalcemia may be diagnosed by careful ophthalmologic examination of the corneoscleral junction for corneal calcification.

Radiographs show generalized bone demineralization, subperiosteal resorption in the phalanges (Fig. 11–7) and clavicles, lytic skull lesions ("salt and pepper patterns"), loss of the lamina dura in dental films, cysts in the pelvic and long bones, and chondrocalcinosis. Signs of nephrocalcinosis or renal stones may occur.

Hypercalcemia (particularly elevations of ionized calcium) and hypophosphatemia are present, often associated with hyperchloremic acidosis. Increased serum alkaline phosphatase levels are found. Decreased fractional renal tubular reabsorption of phosphate, less than 80 per cent, is a classical finding in hyperparathyroidism, but

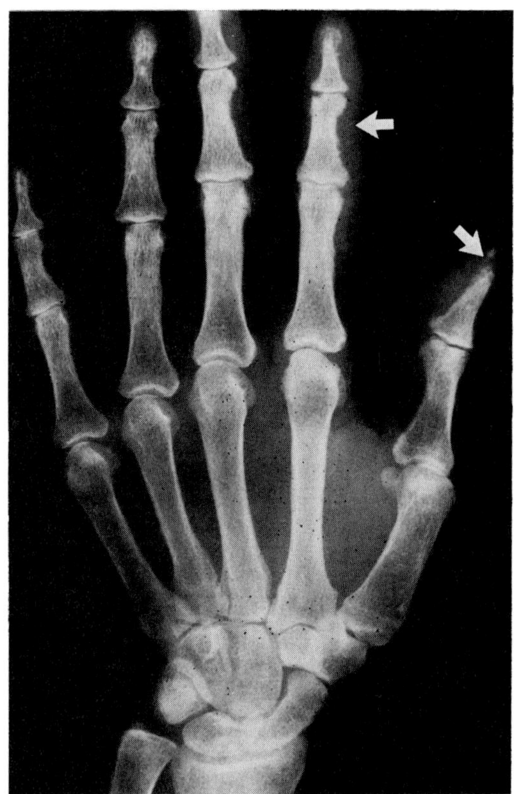

FIGURE 11–7. Hyperparathyroidism secondary to renal failure: subperiosteal resorption on radial edge of phalanges and resorption of phalangeal tufts (see arrows). (From Tsang RC, Brown DR: The parathyroids. *In* Kelley V (ed): Practice of Pediatrics. Vol 1. New York, Harper & Row, 1979, p 1.)

the overlap with normal subjects is great.[82] Hyperaminoaciduria can be present and urinary cyclic AMP excretion is increased. Defective urinary concentration or acidification and impaired renal function occur more often in children than adults.[83] Radioimmunoassays for PTH using COOH-terminal–recognizing antisera are valuable in the diagnosis of hyperparathyroidism.

Symptoms of neonatal primary hyperparathyroidism are poor feeding, weight loss, dehydration, hypotonia, respiratory distress from poorly developed rib cage, and anemia. Bone resorption, disturbed epiphyseal osteogenesis, widespread fibrosis of the marrow cavity, and fractures of the long bones occur. Hypercalcemia is more pronounced and renal lithiasis less common in infancy compared with later childhood. Aminoaciduria may be seen. In infancy the histologic pattern of parathyroid hyperplasia is more common, whereas in later childhood parathyroid adenoma is more common.

Parathyroid adenomas are removed surgically. Treatment of parathyroid hyperplasia is subtotal parathyroidectomy. After extensive and careful search for the parathyroids, three and a half or three and three quarters of the four parathyroid glands are removed. The major problem in parathyroidectomy is that, if insufficient parathyroid tissue is removed, reexploration at the second operation becomes extremely difficult. In adults, sonography, selective thyroid vein catheterization, and measurements of thyroid venous plasma PTH levels have helped to localize the hyperparathyroid tissue.

Secondary Hyperparathyroidism[1]

Hypocalcemia of maternal origin, or caused by intestinal, hepatic and renal disease may lead to hyperparathyroidism.

Maternal. Maternal hypoparathyroidism may result in neonatal hyperparathyroidism. When maternal hypoparathyroidism is untreated or poorly treated, maternal hypocalcemia is thought to lead to intrauterine fetal hypocalcemia. Chronic fetal hypocalcemia stimulates fetal parathyroid hyperfunction, and neonatal hyperparathyroidism continues after birth. In the few reported instances, signs of hyperparathyroidism (vomiting and failure to thrive) were minimal. Serum calcium was normal or increased up to 16.5 mg/dl, serum phosphorus was normal, (greater than 4.3 mg/dl), and bone demineralization and lytic bone lesions were found.[84,85] The disorder is transient, since the hypocalcemic stimulus for hyperparathyroidism is removed after birth. In instances with severe hypercalcemia, treatment with glucocorticoids, calcitonin, and furosemide diuretics may be needed.

Intestinal and Hepatic. In vitamin D–deficiency rickets or "hepatic" rickets, secondary hyperparathyroidism occurs in response to hypocalcemia. The secondary hyperparathyroidism compounds the rachitic bone picture (see later discussion). Also, in hypocalcemia due to high dietary phosphate, secondary hyperparathyroidism may occur and presumably helps to normalize serum calcium concentrations.

Renal. Osteodystrophy in uremia is related to disordered vitamin D metabolism and secondary hyperparathyroidism.[86]

Hypercalcemia

Hypercalcemia of Nonparathyroid Etiology[1]

In hypercalcemia of nonparathyroid etiology, parathyroid function is generally suppressed. The signs and symptoms are predominantly those of hypercalcemia (central nervous system and gastrointestinal), and bone changes are generally absent.

Tumors. Hepatoma, lung cancer, malignancy with bone metastases, adrenal pheochromocytoma, renal cancer, fibrosarcoma, and leukemia have been associated with hypercalcemia. Possible causes for tumor-related hypercalcemia include ectopic parathyroid tissue, tumoral secretion of a PTH-like hormone, a prostaglandin (PGE_2) with osteoclastic activity, and an "osteoclast-stimulating factor."[1]

Nonparathyroid Endocrine Causes. Hypercalcemia occurs in 10 per cent of thyrotoxic subjects, possibly through increased bone resorption.[87] Conditions with decreased glucocorticoid secretion, such as abrupt steroid withdrawal or Addison disease, may be associated with hypercalcemia, probably because of a lack of the hypocalcemic effect of corticosteroids.[88]

Familial Hypocalciuric Hypercalcemia

Also called "benign" familial hypercalcemia, this autosomal-dominant disorder does not usually lead to clinical signs of hypercalcemia.[89] There is a low frequency of complications, which are mainly chondrocalcinosis and pancreatitis. However, infants born to mothers with familial hypocalciuric hypercalcemia may (1) inherit the disorder; (2) develop true, severe neonatal hyperparathyroidism; and (3) develop neonatal tetany from chronic parathyroid gland suppression. The pathophysiology of this disorder is poorly understood, and it may be linked to both excessive renal conservation of calcium and a genetic defect in the regulation of PTH secretion.[90]

Exogenous Causes. Vitamin A or D faddism is an important cause of hypercalcemia[91] (see vitamin D disorders). Thiazide-induced hypercalcemia is thought to be related to increased calcemic response to parathyroid hormone. In adults, thiazide-related hypercalcemia is the commonest form of hypercalcemia that is detected by laboratory "screening" procedures.[92] The milk alkali syndrome is a rare cause of hypercalcemia. Affected patients typically receive large amounts of milk and alkali for treatment of peptic ulcers. Serum calcium may rise several weeks after therapy is begun,[93] and there is great variability in the severity of the syndrome.[94]

Hypercalcemia occurs in adolescents, particularly males, who are immobilized for fractures or burns. Urinary calcium excretion rises within 2 or 3 days, and an increase in serum calcium is found in 4 or 5 days.[95] Increased bone mineral loss and negative calcium balance occur. Serum PTH levels are normal or elevated.[96] Hypercalcemia may lead to nephrocalcinosis, hypertension, and possibly hypertensive encephalopathy.

Hypercalcemia can develop in infants with extensive subcutaneous fat necrosis, particularly resulting from traumatic delivery of large infants. Subcutaneous necrosis generally involves the areas subjected to greatest pressure: shoulders, back, upper arms, and outer thighs. With forceps deliveries, the cheeks typically are affected. The lesions become indurated, red or violaceous, and fluctuant. Hypercalcemia is thought to be related to mobilization of calcium from the necrotic areas into the extracellular space. The signs of hypercalcemia occur usually one or several weeks after birth, with vomiting, lethargy or irritability, and fever. As the fat necrosis resolves, serum calcium levels revert to normal.[97]

Idiopathic Infantile Hypercalcemia

Idiopathic infantile hypercalcemia (IHH) a peculiar syndrome of hypercalcemia may occur during the first year of life and resolve within a few months to a few years. This condition may, however, be severe and even fatal in a few patients. Idiopathic infantile hypercalcemia may be isolated or associated with the features of Williams syndrome[98,99] (elfin facies, mental retardation, and supravalvular aortic stenosis); however, not all patients with Williams syndrome have IIH. It is, however, possible that these patients may have had hypercalcemia during the fetal or early neonatal life before the diagnosis of Williams syndrome was recognized. Rarely, IIH may occur together with the "blue diaper" syndrome, an inborn error of tryptophan metabolism leading to indicanuria.[100]

The etiology of IIH is unknown. Patients have increased calcium retention,[101] result-

ing in hypercalcemia within the first 2 to 4 years of life. Idiopathic infantile hypercalcemia and vitamin D intoxication have some similarities, and some studies have suggested that vitamin D may play a role in the pathogenesis of IIH. Pregnant rabbits given high doses of vitamin D give birth to offspring with generalized vascular lesions, some of which resemble supravalvular aortic stenosis.[102] At a period during which vitamin D supplementation through fortified commercial milk, cereals, and vitamin D supplements may have been as high as 4000 IU/day in Great Britain, a high incidence of IIH was reported.[103] Also, Williams syndrome has been found in infants of mothers who had received 500,000 units of vitamin D during pregnancy in Germany.[104] However, mothers treated with very high doses of vitamin D or other D metabolites for hypoparathyroidism or for vitamin D–dependent rickets delivered infants with hypercalcemia that was very limited in time and intensity.[105] In most cases of Williams syndrome, the dietary history does not confirm excessive vitamin D intake by the mother during pregnancy or the infant in early extrauterine life. Measurements of serum vitamin D activity or vitamin D metabolites have been reported as showing normal, decreased, or increased concentrations.[106–108] Hypersensitivity to vitamin D was suggested in a study in which fibroblasts from infants with IIH were shown to be highly susceptible to metachromasia when exposed to vitamin D and calcium.[109] Recently, it has been suggested that calcitonin deficiency may be an etiologic factor in IIH.[110] From these conflicting reports it is evident that a need exists to investigate patients with IIH more thoroughly primarily in the active, hypercalcemic phase of the syndrome.

Congenital Hypokalemia with Hypercalciuria

Some prematurely delivered infants with a maternal history of polyhydramnios develop episodes of fever, failure to thrive, vomiting, diarrhea, and renal electrolyte and water wastage.[111] A renal tubular defect leads to hypokalemia, polyuria, isosthenuria, hypercalciuria, hypercalcemia, and metabolic alkalosis. Osteopenia and nephrocalcinosis are frequent complications. Hyperprostaglandinuria occurs, and treatment with indomethacin, an inhibitor of PGE_2 formation, leads to significant improvement of both biochemical and clinical features. It is unclear if this condition is distinct from the Bartter syndrome.[111]

Treatment of Hypercalcemia[1]

Since central nervous system and renal damage may result from untreated hypercalcemia, it is important that effective treatment be carried out immediately. Removal of the primary etiology for hypercalcemia should be attempted. Hydration (at least 200 to 250 ml/kg/day) and furosemide diuretics (1 mg/kg every 6 hours) will result in calciuresis and amelioration of hypercalcemia. Excessive urinary losses of sodium, potassium, phosphate, and magnesium may occur. Thiazide diuretics should not be used because of their potential hypercalcemic effects.

Corticosteroids (hydrocortisone 1 mg/kg every 6 hours) effectively decrease serum calcium concentrations, probably through reduction in intestinal absorption of calcium. However, the onset of action may be delayed for several days. Calcitonin (10 units/kg intravenously) may be helpful for acute treatment. It acts primarily by blocking PTH-induced bone resorptive activity and facilitating calciuria. The maximal effect is seen in an hour. Infusions of calcitonin need to be repeated every 4 hours because the effects are transient. Calcitonin administered intramuscularly with a gelatin vehicle has a longer lasting effect. Because calcitonin is extracted from the salmon, antibodies to the hormone may be detected following initiation of therapy. However, human (recombinant DNA) calcitonin is now available for therapeutic use. Mithramycin, which blocks bone resorptive activity, is useful also in the treatment of hypercalcemia. The onset of action occurs in a day or two and the effect persists for a day. The doses used (25 mg/kg intravenously for 4 hours) are much lower than those used for treatment of neoplasias. Potential side effects include thrombocytopenia, and hepatic and renal toxicity. Phosphates are not recommended in the treatment of hypercalcemia, because deposition of calcium phosphate salts in soft tissue may occur. In conditions in which PGE_2 production may be excessive, indomethacin or aspirin may be effective in reducing production of this metabolite.

Disorders Related to Vitamin D, Calcium, or Phosphorus Deficiency

Vitamin D–Deficiency (Hypovitaminosis D) Rickets[112]

Poor sunlight exposure in infants without vitamin D supplementation continues to be the major cause of rickets in infancy. Reports of rickets have come from different parts of the world. In Cape Town, South Africa, infants wrapped up for protection from the sun have developed rickets[113]; in Ethiopia, infants who developed rickets were kept indoors in the dark in houses with shutters closed or no windows. When these infants were carried outdoors on the backs of their mothers, a cloak was placed over them to protect them from "evil eyes."[114] In Melbourne, Australia, rickets was reported in infants born of Mediterranean immigrants who were reluctant to expose infants to the sun.[115] In Manitoba, Canada, Indian children with apparent lack of sunshine exposure have been reported to have rickets.[116] As expected in a disease related to sunshine exposure, the incidence of rickets is generally highest in winter months.[113]

From published reports, infants with rickets usually were receiving milk that was not fortified with vitamin D,[113,116–119] or were receiving prolonged breast feeding.[118,120] Rickets in Asian immigrant children in the United Kingdom has been thought to be related to ingestion of the Hindu ethnic foods ghee (a butter product) and phytate-rich chapaties[121] (a bread). When ghee is produced from butter, vitamin D may be destroyed; phytate also is associated with decreased intestinal calcium and phosphorus absorption and possibly has a direct adverse effect on bone mineralization.

Rickets is three times more common in males than in females.[117,120] Typical signs of rickets include craniotabes, frontal skull bossing, rachitic rib rosary (enlarged costochondral junctions), widened ribs, bowed legs, and muscle weakness. There appear to be three stages in the progression of the disease. In stage 1, serum calcium concentrations are low but serum phosphorus concentrations are normal. In stage 2, serum calcium concentrations are restored to normal ranges because of compensatory hyperparathyroidism. However, serum phosphorus concentrations are low with hyperphosphaturia and hyperaminoaciduria from hyperparathyroidism; typical rachitic bone features are present. In stage 3, both serum calcium and phosphorus concentrations are low and bone disease is florid because of the combined effect of mineral deficiency and hyperparathyroidism[122] (Table 11–1).

Serum 25-OHD concentrations are generally less than 15 ng/ml in severe rickets and less than 20 ng/ml in the earliest hypocalcemic phase of rickets.[123] Serum alkaline phosphatase is elevated and bone radiographs show cupping and fraying of the metaphyseal ends of long bones, widened distance between the metaphysis and epiphysis, bone demineralization, and thinning of the cortical bone. Demineralization of the skull can occur; cortical lines outlining the facial structures and the floor of the anterior fossa become indistinct, and the lamina dura of the teeth may not be evident.

Vitamin D, 400 IU, is the standard recommended daily allowance for infants for prevention of rickets. Treatment of vitamin D deficiency rickets is accomplished with vitamin D or its metabolites. Oral vitamin D 5000 to 10,000 IU/daily, 25-OHD 0.12 to 0.2 μg/kg/day and 1,25 $(OH)_2D$ 0.05 to 0.06 μg/kg/day[118] may be used. Serum calcium, phosphorus, and alkaline phosphatase concentrations should be measured at least once a week initially to assess the efficacy of treatment and to help in prevention of toxicity.

Rickets and Osteopenia of Prematurity

Radiologic signs of rickets may develop in more than 30 per cent of very low birth weight (less than 1500-gm) preterm infants.[124] Usually, these infants are very immature and sick. The cause of rickets (or osteopenia) of prematurity, is still debated, and probably multifactorial. Vitamin D deficiency does not seem to play a role in most cases, since serum 25-OHD concentrations (the best indicator of vitamin D status) generally are within the normal range.[125,126] Defective renal 1-hydroxylation of vitamin D does not seem to be the cause, since serum $1,25(OH)_2D$ concentrations are increased in this condition.[125] However, relative end-organ resistance to $1,25(OH)_2D$ may be contributory since, compared to adults, considerably higher doses of $1,25(OH)_2D$ are necessary to elicit a calcemic response in premature infants.[127,128] Nevertheless, the major etiologic factor seems to be related to mineral (calcium and phosphorus) deficiency.[129,130] Indeed, intakes of calcium and phosphorus in these infants are usually much lower than the fetal intrauterine accretion rates (normally up to 150 mg calcium/kg/day and 75 mg phosphorus/kg/day in the last trimester of pregnancy[131]), particularly if the infants are sick, with limited enteral intake, or receiving total parenteral nutrition for prolonged periods. Longitudinal measurements of bone mineral content (BMC) by photon absorptiometry have been particularly useful to demonstrate that the bones are undermineralized when preterm infants are fed a standard proprietary formula.[129,130] However, when adequate mineral intake (approximating intrauterine mineral accretion rates) is supplied,[129] reduced BMC is prevented (Fig. 11–8).

A particular situation occurs in preterm infants fed human milk.[132,133] Calcium and especially phosphorus concentrations present in human milk appear to be inadequate for these infants,[132] and rickets with severe hypophosphatemia and hypercalcemia may develop. Presumably, hypercalcemia and hypercalciuria are due in part to hypophosphatemia-induced increased $1,25(OH)_2D$ production, with subsequent increase in bone resorption. Fortification of human milk with "home-made," or commercially available, preparations rich in calcium and phosphorus has been proposed, in

TABLE 11–1.   STAGES OF HYPOVITAMINOSIS D RICKETS

		Vitamin D Deficiency			
	PTH	*Serum CA*	*Serum P*	**Bone**	**Urine**
I	Uncompensated	↓	N	Minimal changes	—
II	Increased	N	↓	Rickets	Aminoaciduria Phosphaturia
III	? Unresponsive bone	↓	↓	Florid	Aminoaciduria Phosphaturia

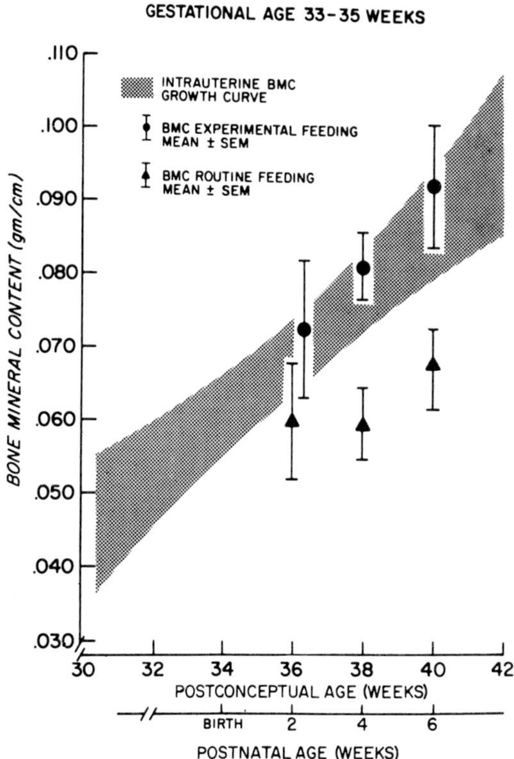

FIGURE 11–8. Bone mineral content of premature infants given routine feedings is markedly decreased from that expected in utero. High calcium and phosphorus formulas result in bone mineralization rate comparable to that expected in utero. (From Steichen JJ, Gratton TL, Tsang RC: Osteopenia of prematurity. J Pediatr 96:528, 1980.)

order to prevent this type of rickets, but results of clinical trials have been conflicting.[134–136]

Other etiologic factors for osteopenia of prematurity have been suggested. Among them are cholestasis induced by total parenteral nutrition,[137] hypersulfatemia also from total parenteral nutrition,[138] aluminum intoxication due to aluminum contamination of products administered parenterally,[139] and urinary calcium losses due to chronic furosemide therapy.[140]

Treatment of osteopenia of prematurity includes prevention by optimization of mineral and vitamin D intake and avoidance of calciuric diuretics. In general, osteopenia of prematurity will heal progressively once adequate mineral intake is achieved. In severe cases, whenever possible, a daily intake of 200 mg elemental calcium/kg body weight and of 100 mg elemental phosphorus/kg body weight is advisable in order to hasten healing.

Rickets Associated with Hepatic Disease

The liver has a prime role in vitamin D metabolism. Vitamin D absorption is bile salt-facilitated.[141] 25-Hydroxylation of vitamin D occurs mainly in the liver; an active enterohepatic circulation of 25-OHD exists. 25-Hydroxyvitamin D is reabsorbed from the intestine in a process facilitated by bile salts.[142] Thus, decreased plasma 25-OHD concentrations and rickets may occur in hepatic disease, presumably from vitamin D malabsorption, decreased production of 25-OHD, and decreased enterohepatic circulation of 25-OHD. As in most other forms of rickets, secondary hyperparathyroidism may occur,[143] presumably in response to hypocalcemia, which helps to restore serum calcium to normal. Cirrhosis of the liver, neonatal hepatitis, biliary atresia, and cholestasis associated with parenteral hyperalimentation may lead to "hepatic rickets." Phenobarbital and dilantin use can lead to decreased serum 25-OHD and rickets, thought to be caused by increased metabolism of 25-OHD.[2]

Treatment with 25-OHD or 1,25(OH)$_2$D would theoretically bypass the hepatic defect in 25-OHD metabolism. The doses of 25-OHD (approximately 4 to 5 μg/kg/day orally[144] and 1,25(OH)$_2$D (parenteral 0.2 μg/kg/day[145]) that have been used to effect healing are still relatively high, since "physiologic requirements" for these metabolites are approximately 0.15 μg/kg/day and 0.05 μg/kg/day, respectively. The reason for the higher requirements is unclear. Alternatively, vitamin D (2000 to 10,000 IU/day) can be given.[146]

Vitamin D–Dependent Rickets

Vitamin D dependency is characterized by the combination of clinical and biochemical features of vitamin D–deficient rickets (VDDR) in the absence of vitamin D deficiency. It is often hereditary, transmitted in an autosomal-recessive manner.[147] Two independent forms of VDDR exist.[147]

VDDR Type I.[147,148] This condition is characterized by extremely low serum 1,25(OH)$_2$D concentrations, as a result of deficient renal 1α-hydroxylation. When administered at "physiologic doses," 1,25(OH)$_2$D (or its analog 1α-hydroxyvitamin D) is very effective in resolving the clinical and biochemical features of rickets.

Treatment includes massive doses of vitamin D (1.25 to 2.5 mg/day or 50,000 to 100,000 IU/day) or 25-OHD (400 to 900 µg/day). The large requirements are probably necessary to overcome or bypass the metabolic block in renal 1α-hydroxylation of 25-OHD. "Physiologic" doses of 1,25(OH)$_2$D, however (1 µg/day), are successful in treating the rickets. The synthetic analog of 1,25(OH)$_2$D, 1α-hydroxyvitamin D, at doses of 0.5 to 2 µg/day, achieves similar results.[149]

Production of 1,25(OH)$_2$D also is impaired in renal failure.[150] The "osteodystrophy" in uremia is related to both a lack of 1,25(OH)$_2$D and secondary hyperparathyroidism (see earlier discussion).

VDDR Type II. In this condition, 1,25(OH)$_2$D production by the kidney is normal, or even supranormal. However, end-organ resistance to 1,25(OH)$_2$D is present. In some but not all kindreds, rickets is accompanied by total alopecia from birth.[105,151–165] There is a great heterogeneity in the clinical features.[165] Variable degrees of rickets, hypocalcemia, secondary hyperparathyroidism, and end-organ resistance to vitamin D metabolites coexist.[165] In some patients, favorable responses to pharmacologic doses of native vitamin D, 25-hydroxyvitamin D$_3$, 1α-hydroxyvitamin D$_3$, 1,25-dihydroxyvitamin D$_3$,[105,152,154,156,159,161–163] or 24,25-dihydroxyvitamin D$_3$[160] have been reported. Other patients are unresponsive to similar therapeutic trials,[152,153,157] or become completely refractory to vitamin D metabolites with time.[152] Some patients appear to undergo spontaneous improvement and remission after 7 to 9 years of age,[158] whereas in others, death within the first 3 years of age may occur as a consequence of pulmonary complications or hypocalcemic convulsions.[152,160]

Studies of cultured skin fibroblasts of these patients have demonstrated 1,25(OH)$_2$D receptor or postreceptor defects.

Treatment of VDDR type II is very difficult because of decreased or absent response to vitamin D metabolites. Recently, there has been a successful attempt to cure rickets and promote normal mineralization by the use of long-term parenteral calcium and phosphorus supplementation;[151] striking clinical and radiologic improvement has occurred during high-dose oral calcium therapy.[164] More data are required to determine if improvement using either of these methods was spontaneous or truly related to therapy.

X-Linked Dominant Hypophosphatemic Rickets

Although sporadic cases are occasionally reported, renal hypophosphatemic rickets is usually transmitted as an X-linked dominant trait.[165] The hemizygous male is usually more severely affected than the heterozygous female, whose normal allele modifies the expression of the abnormal gene.[166] Hypophosphatemia is the major metabolic feature of the disease, and is caused by an isolated defect in phosphate reabsorption in the proximal tubule. Intracellular phosphate may be relatively well conserved, and this may be the reason for the absence of elevation of serum 1,25(OH)$_2$D concentration and the lack of hypotonia in spite of significant hypophosphatemia. The exact mechanism responsible for defective 25-OHD 1α-hydroxylation in the kidney is unclear.[166]

Clinically, growth failure is the dominant feature, and the rachitic features (bone deformities) predominate in the lower limbs.[167] The disease seems to be latent over the first few months of life, and develops progressively thereafter. Characteristic dentine defects lead to microchannels that are a port of entry for infection (tooth abscesses)[168] (Fig. 11–9).

In untreated individuals hypocalcemia and secondary hyperparathyroidism are usually absent.[169] The considerable urinary phosphate losses are a major clue in the diagnosis. Tubular reabsorption of phosphate varies from 42 per cent to 72 per cent (normal in children over 85 per cent to 90 per cent), in spite of the hypophosphatemia.[170] Craniosynotoses may occur, possibly linked to vitamin D metabolite intoxication.[171]

The treatment of choice consists of a combination of phosphate salts and calcitriol.[169,172–174] Calcitriol decreases the phosphate supplement requirements (presumably by increasing intestinal phosphate absorption) and prevents hypocalcemia, and hence secondary hyperparathyroidism (a frequent occurrence when phosphate alone is used). Additionally, the combination of 1,25(OH)$_2$D and phosphate salts improves both growth plate and endosteal bone surface mineralization while the latter is unaffected by treatment with phosphate

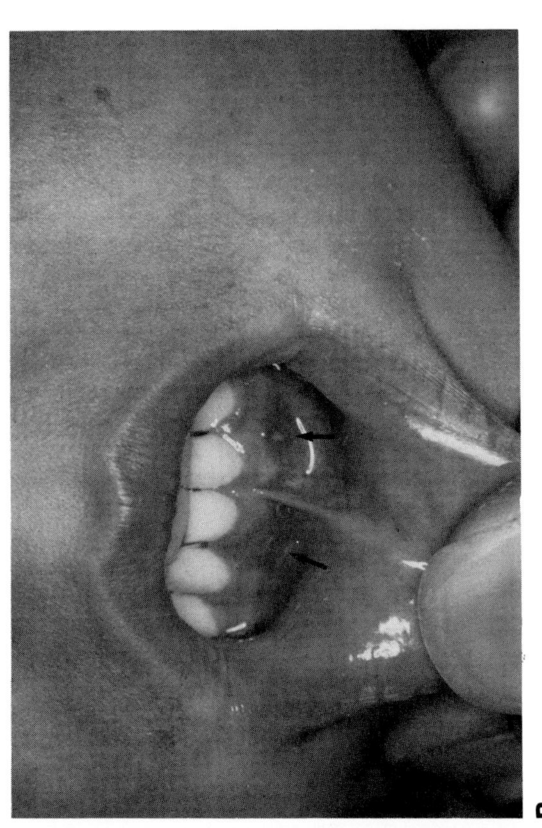

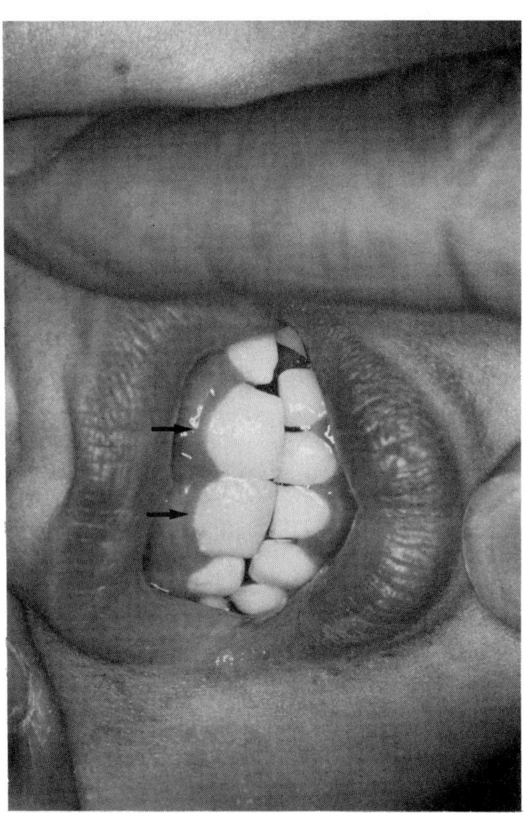

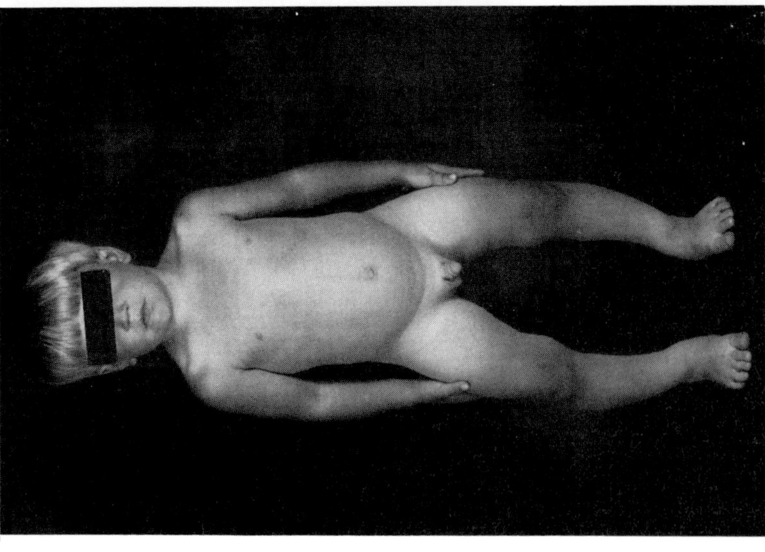

FIGURE 11–9. (*Legend on facing page.*)

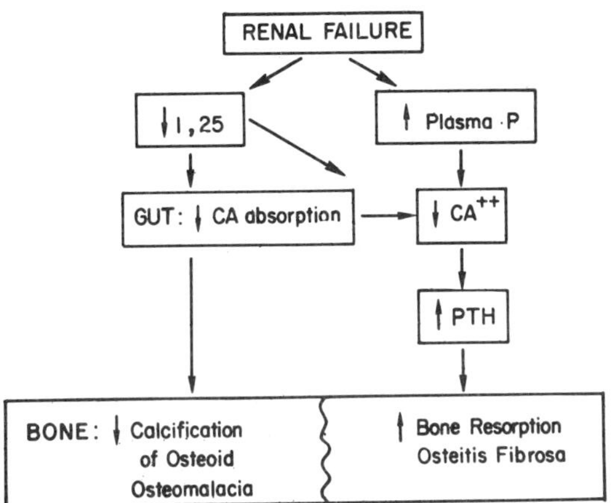

FIGURE 11–10. Pathogenesis of renal osteodystrophy. Decreased production of 1,25(OH)$_2$D and secondary hyperparathyroidism result in disordered bone metabolism. (From Tsang RC, Noguchi A, Steichen JJ: Pediatric parathyroid disorders. Pediatr Clin North Am 26:223, 1979.)

alone.[169] Various schedules of treatment have been proposed, but in general patients should be monitored frequently to prevent iatrogenic hypercalcemia and/or hypercalciuria.[166,172–174]

Other Forms of Phosphopenic Rickets

Hypophosphatemic rickets may occur in the Fanconi syndrome (aminoaciduria, glycosuria, and phosphaturia). Phosphaturia is the major component of the syndrome and results in hypophosphatemia and rickets. Cystinosis,[175] tyrosinosis, heavy metal poisoning (cadmium and lead), glycogenosis, and multiple myeloma are causes of the syndrome.[112] Vitamin D, 25,000 to 50,000 IU/ daily, normalizes serum phosphorus concentrations and results in healing of rickets. In renal tubular acidosis, the basic distal tubular defect occurs with secondary decrease in phosphate reabsorption.[176] Correction of the bicarbonate deficit, without vitamin D therapy, decreases phosphate loss and resolves the rickets.

Mesenchymal "nonendocrine" tumors in bone, soft tissue, or skin have resulted in hypophosphatemia and rickets. A tumor-derived humoral substance that results in decreased renal phosphate reabsorption[177,178]

and decreased 1,25(OH)$_2$D production[179] has been proposed as the cause of rickets.

Renal tubulopathy can occur as a result of acute neonatal asphyxia and neonatal renal vascular accidents. Decreased renal tubular phosphate reabsorption, hypophosphatemia, and rickets may occur in the first year of life.[180] Vitamin D, 20,000 to 25,000 units daily, is effective in treatment.

Calciopenic Rickets

Low calcium intake as a cause of rickets is probably extremely rare. Anecdotal cases have been reported in a rural population from South Africa[181] and in an infant receiving formula with lamb's milk base (calcium, 1 mg/dl phosphorus, 17 mg/dl).[182] However, in these two studies concomitant phosphorus lack or hypophosphatemia, respectively, as an additional factor in the causation of rickets was not ruled out.

Renal Osteodystrophy

In chronic renal failure, severe bone disease may occur, including osteopenia, fractures, and ectopic calcifications. With time, patients become resistant to vitamin D therapy, and require considerable increases in the doses of vitamin D. The causes of renal osteodystrophy probably are multiple (Fig. 11–10), involving decreased intestinal calcium absorption (secondary to decreased renal 1,25(OH)$_2$D production),[183,184] increased bone resorption (subsequent to secondary hyperparathyroidism),[183] increased mineral bone losses induced by acidosis, and aluminum intoxication due to contamination by this metal of dialysis systems.[185]

Persistence of hyperparathyroidism may occur in 20 per cent of uremic subjects after renal transplantation. Hyperparathyroidism may last for 2 to 3 years. Elevation of serum ionized calcium concentrations appears to be a sensitive method to detect persistent hyperparathyroidism.[186] Hypercalcemia is most severe in the first 2 weeks after renal transplantation.[187]

Treatment of secondary hyperparathyroidism and osteodystrophy includes the use of vitamin D or its metabolites, and

---

FIGURE 11–9. X-linked dominant hypophosphatemic rickets. Note bowing of legs (A); dental abscesses (arrows) at roots of lower incisors (B); and mottled appearance of enamel in upper two incisors (arrows) due to dentin defects (C). (From Mimouni F, Mughal Z, Tsang RC, et al: X-linked dominant hypophosphatemic rickets. Am J Dis Child 142:191, 1988. Copyright 1988, American Medical Association.)

"phosphate binders" administered orally. Vitamin D, 30,000 to 50,000 units daily,[188] or 1,25(OH)$_2$D in physiologic doses are used in order to restore normal circulating levels of the active vitamin D metabolite. Hypercalcemia may occur but is less persistent following administration of 1,25(OH)$_2$D than of vitamin D.[189,190] Phosphate binders (Amphogel) and a low-phosphate diet help to reduce the degree of hyperphosphatemia and consequent hyperparathyroidism. Dialysis with solutions of high calcium (above 6 to 7 mg/dl) will help suppress parathyroid overactivity; high magnesium concentrations also can be used but are of little additional value when dialysate calcium is above 7 mg/dl.[191] In severe instances and in persistent hyperparathyroidism after renal transplantation, parathyroidectomy may be needed.[190]

REFERENCES

1. Tsang RC, Noguehi A. Steichen JJ: Pediatric parathyroid disorders. Pediatr Clin North Am 26:223, 1979.
2. Tsang RC, Erenberg AP: Calcium homenatasis in the newborn—the calciotropic hormones: parathyroid hormone, calcitonin and vitamin D. *In* Moss AJ (ed): Pediatrics Update. Elsevier, New York, p 193, 1980.
3. Pitkin RM: Calcium metabolism in pregnancy and the preinatal period: A review. Am J Obstet Gynecol 151:99, 1985.
4. Steichen JJ, Tsang RC, Gratton TL, et al: Vitamin D homeostasis in the perinatal period—1,25-dihydroxy-vitamin D in maternal, cord and neonatal blood. N Engl J Med 302:315, 1980.
5. Kumar R, Cohen WR, Silva P, et al: Elevated 1,25 dihydroxyvitamin D plasma levels in normal human pregnancy and lactation. J Clin Invest 63:342, 1979.
6. Mimouni F, Tsang RC, Hertzberg V, et al: Parathyroid hormone (PTH) and 1,25-dihydroxyvitamin D (1,25(OH)$_2$D) changes in normal and insulin-dependent diabetic (IDD) pregnancies. J Am Coll Nutr 6:433, 1987.
7. Dincsoy MY, Tsang RC, Laskarzewski P, et al: The role of magnesium and postnatal age on parathyroid hormone responses during "exchange" blood transfusion in the newborn period. J Pediatr 00:000, 1982.
8. Bikle DD, Morrissey RL, Zolock DT: The mechanism of action of vitamin D in the intestine. Am J Clin Nutr 32:2322, 1979.
9. DeLuca HF: Metabolism of vitamin D: Current status. Am J Clin Nutr 29:1258, 1976.
10. Haussler MR, McCain TA: Basic clinical concepts related to vitamin D metabolism and action. N Engl J Med 297:974, 1041, 1977.
11. Cushard WG, Creditor MA, Canterbury JM, et al: Physiologic hyperparathyroidism in pregnancy. J Clin Endocrinol Metabol 34:767, 1972.
12. Heany RD, Skillman TG: Calcium metabolism in normal human pregnancy. J Clin Endocrinol Metabol 33:661, 1971.
13. Haddad JG Jr, Boisseau V, Avioli L: Placental transfer of vitamin D$_3$ and 25-hydroxycholecalciferol in the rat. J Lab Clin Med 77:908, 1971.
14. Schedewie H, Tsang RC, Slikker W, et al: Maternal-fetal crossover of 1,25-(OH)$_2$ vitamin D in subhuman primates. Proc. VII International Conference on Calcium Regulating Hormones, Keystone, Colorado, 1980 (abstract).
15. Whitsett JA, HO M, Tsang RC, et al: Synthesis of 1,25-dihydroxyvitamin D$_3$ by human placenta in vitro. J Clin Endocrinol Metab 53:484, 1981.
16. Whitsett JA, Tsang RC: Calcium uptake and binding by membrane fractions of human placenta: ATP-dependent calcium accumulation. Pediatr Res 14:769, 1980.
17. Hillman LS, Haddad JG: Perinatal vitamin D metabolism II: Serial 25-hydroxyvitamin D concentrations in sera of term and premature infants. J Pediatr 86:928, 1975.
18. Tsang RC, Greer F, Steichen JJ: Perinatal vitamin D metabolism: The transition from fetal to neonatal life. Clin Perinatol 8:287, 1981.
19. Leerbeck E, Sondegaard H: Total content of vitamin D in human milk and cow's milk. Br J Nutr 44:7, 1980.
20. Reeve LE, Chesney RW, DeLuca HF: Vitamin D of human milk: Identification of biologically active forms. Am J Clin Nutr 36:122, 1982.
21. Specker BL, Tsang RC, Hollis BW: Effect of race and diet on human milk vitamin D and 25-hydroxyvitamin D. Am J Dis Child 139:1134, 1985.
22. Lakdawala DR, Widdowson EM: Vitamin D in human milk. Lancet 1:167, 1977.
23. Reeve LE, DeLuca HF, Schnoes HK: Synthesis and biological activity of vitamin D$_3$ sulfate. J Biol Chem 256:823, 1981.
24. Hollis BW, Roos BA, Draper HH, et al: Vitamin D and its metabolites in human and bovine milk. J Nutr 111:1240, 1981.
25. Greer FR, Ho M, Dodson D, et al: Lack of 25-hydroxy-vitamin D and 1,25-dihydroxyvitamin D in human milk. J Pediatr 99:233, 1981.
26. Greer FR, Hollis BW, Crips DJ, et al: Effects of maternal ultraviolet B irradiation on the vitamin D content of human milk. J Pediatr 105:431, 1984.
27. Greer FR, Searcy JE, Levin RS, et al: Bone mineral content and serum 25-hydroxyvitamin D in a double-blind study of breast-fed infants with and without supplemental vitamin D. J Pediatr 98:696, 1981.
28. Clemens TL, Holick MF: Recent advances in the hormonal regulation of calcium and phosphorus in adult animals and humans. *In* Holick MF, Gray TK, Anast CS (eds): Perinatal Calcium and Phosphorus Metabolism. Amsterdam, Elsevier, p 1, 1983.
29. Alon U, Chan JC: Hypocalcemia from deficiency of and resistance to parathyroid hormone. Adv Pediatr 32:439, 1985.
30. Albright F, Burnett CH, Smith PHG: Pseudohypoparathyroidism: An example of "Sealbright-Bantam syndrome." Endocrinology 30:922, 1942.
31. Bronsky D, Kushner DS, Dubin A, et al: Idiopathic hypoparathyroidism and pseudohypoparathyroidism: Case reports and review of the literature. Medicine 37:317, 1958.

32. Radeke H, Auf'Mkolk B, Juppner H, et al: Multiple pre- and post receptor defects in pseudohypoparathyroidism (A multicenter study with twenty-four patients). J Clin Endocrinol Metab 162:393, 1986.
33. Spiegel AM, Levine MA, Aurbach GD, et al: Deficiency of hormone receptor-adenylate cyclase coupling protein: Basis for hormone resistance in pseudohypoparathyroidism. Am J Physiol 243:E37, 1982.
34. Brickman AS, Carlson HE, Levin SR: Responses to glucagon infusion in pseudohypoparathyroidism. J Clin Endocrinol Metab 63:1354, 1986.
35. Tsang RC, Venkataraman P, Ho M, et al: The development of pseudohypoparathyroidism: Involvement of progressively increasing serum parathyroid hormone concentrations, increased 1,25-dihydroxyvitamin D concentrations, and "migratory" subcutaneous calcifications. Am J Dis Child 138:654, 1984.
36. Loveridge N, Tschopp F, Born W, et al: Separation of inhibitory activity from biologically active parathyroid hormone in patients with pseudohypoparathyroidism type I. Biochim Biophys Acta 889:117, 1986.
37. Kidd GS, Schjaaf M, Adler RA: Skeletal responsiveness in pseudohypoparathyroidism: A spectrum of clinical disease. Am J Med 68:772, 1980.
38. Rodriguez HJ, Villarseal H, Klahr S, et al: Pseudohypoparathyroidism type II: Restoration of normal renal responsiveness to parathyroid hormone by calcium administration. J Clin Endocrinol Metab 39:693, 1974.
39. Peden V: True idiopathic hypoparathyroidism as a sex-linked recessive trait. Am J Hum Genet 12:323, 1960.
40. Bronsky D, Kiamoku RT, Waldstein SS: Familial idiopathic hypoparathyroidism. J Clin Endocrinol 18:61, 1968.
41. DiGeorge AM: Disorders of the parathyroid glands. In Behrman RE, Vaughan VC (eds): Nelson Textbook of Pediatrics. 12th ed. Philadelphia, WB Saunders Company, p 1432, 1983.
42. Conley ME, Beckwith JB, Mancer JFK, et al: The spectrum of DiGeorge syndrome. J Pediatr 94:883, 1979.
43. Blizzard RM, Chee, D, Davis W: The incidence of parathyroid and other antibodies in the sera of patients with idiopathic hypoparathyroidism. Clin Exp Immunol 1:119, 1966.
44. Eisenbarth G, Wilson P. Ward F, et al: HLA type and occurrence of disease in familial polyglandular failure. N Engl J Med 298:92, 1978.
45. Tsang RC, Chen IW, Freidman MA, et al: Neonatal parathyroid function role of gestational age and postnatal age. J Pediatr 83:728, 1973.
46. Noguchi A, Eren M, Tsang RC: Parathyroid hormone in hypocalcemic and normocalcemic infants of diabetic mothers. J Pediatr 97:112, 1980.
47. Hartenstein H, Gardner LI: Tetany of the newborn associated with maternal parathyroid adenoma. N Engl J Med 274:266, 1966.
48. Bainbridge R, Mughal Z, Mimouni F, et al: Transient congenital hypoparathyroidism: How transient is it? J Pediatr 111:866, 1987.
49. Levine BS, Coburn JW: Magnesium, the mimic/antagonist of calcium. N Engl J Med 310:1253, 1984.
50. Friedman M, Hatcher G, Watson L: Primary hypomagnesaemia with secondary hypocalcaemia in an infant. Lancet 1:703, 1967.
51. Flynn DM, Fairney A, Jackson D, et al: Hormonal changes in thalassemia major. Arch Dis Child 51:828, 1976.
52. VanDop C, Bourne HR, Neer RM: Father to son transmission of decreased N's activity in pseudohypoparathyroidism type IA. J Clin Endocrinol Metab 59:825, 1984.
53. Drezner MK, Neelon FA: Pseudohypoparathyroidism. In Stanbury JB, Wyngaarden JB, Frederickson DS, et al (eds): The Metabolic Basis for Inherited Disease. New York, McGraw-Hill, p 1508, 1983.
54. Woodhouse NJY: Hypocalcemia and hypoparathyroidism. Clin Endocrinol Metabol 3:323, 1974.
55. Tsang RC, Brown DR: The parathyroids. Practice of Pediatrics In Kelly V (ed): vol 1. New York, Harper and Row, 1979.
56. Metz SA, Baylink DJ, Hughes MR, et al: Selective deficiency of 1,25-dihydroxycholecalciferol. A cause of isolated skeletal resistance to parathyroid hormone. N Engl J Med 297:1084, 1977.
57. Stogman W, Fischer JA: Pseudohypoparathyroidism. Disappearance of the resistance to parathyroid extract during treatment with vitamin D. Am J Med 59:140, 1975.
58. Drezner MK, Neelon FA, Haussler M, et al: The probable cause of hypocalcemia and metabolic bone disease in pseudohypoparathyroidism. J Clin Endocrinol Metabol 42:621, 1976.
59. Rosen JF, Fleischman AR, Finberg L, et al: 1,25 dihydroxycholecalciferol: Its use in the long term management of idiopathic hypoparathyroidism in children. J Clin Endocrinol Metabol 45:457. 1977.
60. Werder EA, Kind HP, Egert F, et al: Effective long term treatment of pseudohypoparathyroidism with oral 1α-hydroxy- and 1,25 dihydroxycholecalciferol. J Pediatr 89:266, 1976.
61. Kooh SW, Fraser D, DeLuca HF, et al: Treatment of hypoparathyroidism and pseudohypoparathyroidism with metabolites of vitamin D. N Engl J Med 293:840, 1975.
62. Bordier P, Rychwaert A, Marie R, et al: Vitamin D metabolites and bone mineralization in man. In Norman AW, Schaefer K, Coburn JW, et al (eds): Vitamin D, Biochemical, Chemical and Clinical Aspects Related to Calcium Metabolism. Berlin, Walter de Gruyter, 1977.
63. Kind HP, Handysides A, Kooh SW, et al: Vitamin D therapy in hypoparathyroidism and pseudohypoparathyroidism: Weight-related dosages for initiation of therapy and maintenance therapy. J Pediatr 90:1006, 1977.
64. Bell NH, Stern PH: Hypercalcemia and increases in serum hormone value during prolonged administration of 1α, 25-dihydroxyvitamin D. N Engl J Med 298:1241, 1978.
65. Tsang RC, Steichen JJ, Brown DR: Perinatal calcium homeostasis: Neonatal hypocalcemia and bone demineralization. Clin Perinatol 4:385, 1977.
66. Tsang RC, Steichen JJ, Chan GM: Neonatal hypocalcemia, mechanism of occurrence and management. Crit Care Med 5:56, 1977.
67. David L, Anast C: Calcium metabolism in newborn infants. J Clin Invest 54:287, 1974.
68. David L, Salle B, Chopard P, et al: Studies on

circulating immunoreactive calcitonin in low birth weight infants during the first 48 hours of life. Helv Pediatr Acta 32:39, 1977.

69. Tsang RC, Chen I, Atkinson W, et al: Neonatal hypocalcemia in birth asphyxia. J Pediatr 84:428, 1974.

70. Schedewie HK, Odell WD, Fisher DA, et al: Parathormone and perinatal calcium homeostasis. Pediatr Res 13:1, 1979.

71. Tsang RC, Strub R, Steichen J, et al: Hypomagnesemia in infants of diabetic mothers: Perinatal studies. J Pediatr 89:115, 1976.

72. Tsang RC, Brown DR, Steichen JJ: Diabetes and calcium: *In* Merkatz IR, Adam PA (eds): Calcium disturbances in infants of diabetic mothers. New York, Grune & Stratton, 1979.

73. Oppe TE, Redstone D: Calcium and phosphorus levels in healthy newborn infants given various types of milk. Lancet 1:1045, 1968.

74. Tsang RC, Donovan EF, Steichen JJ: Calcium physiology and pathology in the neonate. Pediatr Clin North Am 23:611, 1976.

75. Tsang RC: Neonatal magnesium disturbances. A review Am J Dis Child 124:282, 1972.

76. Reiss E, Canterbury JM: Genesis of hyperparathyroidism. Am J Med 50:679, 1971.

77. Marx SJ, Powell D, Shimkin PM, et al: Familial hyperparathyroidism: mild hypercalcemia in at least nine members of a kindred. Ann Intern Med 78:371, 1973.

78. Hillman DA, Scriver CR, Pedvis S, et al: Neonatal familial primary hyperparathyroidism. N Engl J Med 270:483, 1964.

79. Spiegel AM, Harrison HE, Marx SJ, et al: Neonatal primary hyperparathyroidism with autosomal dominant inheritance. Pediatrics 90:269, 1977.

80. Mallette LE, Bilezikian JP, Heath DA, et al: Primary hyperparathyroidism: Clinical and biochemical features. Medicine 53:127, 1974.

81. Brown GM: Psychiatric and neurologic aspects of endocrine disease. Hosp Pract 1975:71, 1975.

82. Anderson P, Mosekilde: Tubular resorption of phosphate and calcium in primary hyperparathyroidism. Acta Med Scand 191:565, 1972.

83. Malek RS, Kelalis PP: Urologic manifestations of hyperparathyroidism in childhood. J Urol 115:717, 1976.

84. Bronsky D, Kiamko R, Moncada R, et al: Intrauterine hyperparathyroidism secondary to maternal hypoparathyroidism. Pediatrics 42:606, 1972.

85. Landing BH, Kōmashita S: Congenital hyperparathyroidism secondary to maternal hypoparathyroidism. J Pediatr 77:842, 1970.

86. Roof BS, Piel CF, Rames L, et al: Parathyroid function in uremic children with and without osteodystrophy. Pediatrics 53:404, 1974.

87. Rude RK, Oldham SB, Singer FR, et al: Treatment of thyrotoxic hypercalcemia with propanolol. N Engl J Med 294:431, 1976.

88. Farrell PM, Rikkers H, Moel D: Cortisol dihydrotachysterol antagonism in a patient with hypoparathyroidism and adrenal insufficiency: Apparent inhibition of bone resorption. J Clin Endocrinol Metabol 42:953, 1976.

89. Foley TP, Harrison HC, Arnaud CD, et al: Familial benign hypercalcemia. J Pediatr 81:1060, 1972.

90. Arnaud CD: Familial benign hypercalcemia: Na-

91. Fisher G, Skillern PG: Hypercalcemia due to hypervitaminosis A. JAMA 227:1413, 1974.

92. Heedman P-A, Stenstrom G: Clinical findings in patients with hypercalcemia. Acta Med Scand 193:167, 1973.

93. Wenger J, Kirsner JB, Palmer WL: Editorial. The milk-alkali syndrome. Am J Med 24:161, 1958.

94. David NJ, Verner JV, Engel FL: The diagnostic spectrum of hypercalcemia. Am J Med 33:88, 1962.

95. Heath H III, Earll JM, Schaaf M, et al: Serum ionized calcium during bed rest in fracture patients and normal men. Metabolism 21:633, 1972.

96. Lerman S, Canterbury JM, Reiss E: Parathyroid hormone and the hypercalcemia of immobilization. J Clin Endocrinol Metabol 45:425, 1977.

97. Barltrop D: Hypercalcemia associated with neonatal subcutaneous fat necrosis. Arch Dis Child 38:516, 1963.

98. Beuren AJ, et al: Syndrome of supravalvular aortic stenosis, peripheral pulmonary stenosis, mental retardation and similar facial appearance. Am J Cardiol 13:471, 1964.

99. Black JA, Bonham C, Carter RE: Association between aortic stenosis and facies of severe infantile hypercalcaemia. Lancet 2:745, 1963.

100. Drummond KN, et al: The blue diaper syndrome: Familial hypercalcemia with nephrocalcinosis and indicanuria. Am J Med 37:928, 1964.

101. Forbes GB, Bryson MF, Manning J, et al: Impaired calcium homeostasis in the infantile hypercalcemia syndrome. Acta Paediatr Scand 61:305, 1972.

102. Friedman WF, Roberts WC: Vitamin D and the supravalvular aortic stenosis syndrome: The transplacental effects of vitamin D on the aorta of the rabbit. Circulation 34:77, 1966.

103. Forfar JO, et al: Idiopathic hypercalcaemia of infancy: Clinical and metabolic studies with special reference to the aetiological role of vitamin D. Lancet 1:981, 1956.

104. Forbes GB: Vitamin D in pregnancy and the infantile hypercalcemic syndrome. Pediatr Res 13:1382, 1979.

105. Marx SJ, Swart EG Jr, Hamstra AJ, et al: Normal intrauterine development of the fetus of a woman receiving extraordinarily high doses of 1,25-dihydroxyvitamin D$_3$. J Clin Endocrinol Metab 51:1138, 1980.

106. Chesney RW, DeLuca HF, Gertner JM: Increased plasma 1,25-dihydroxyvitamin D in infants with hypercalcemia and elfin facies. N Engl J Med 3113:889, 1985.

107. Garabedian M, et al: Elevated plasma 1,25-dihydroxyvitamin D concentrations in infants with hypercalcemia and in elfin facies. N Engl J Med 312:948, 1985.

108. Taylor AB, Stern PGH, Bell NH: Abnormal regulation of circulating 25-hydroxyvitamin D in the Williams syndrome. N Engl J Med 306:972, 1982.

109. Becroft DMO, Chambers D: Supravalvular aortic stenosis—infantile hypercalcemia syndrome: In vitro hypersensitivity to vitamin D$_2$ and calcium. J Med Genet 13:223, 1976.

110. Culler FL, Jones KL, Deftos LJ: Impaired cal-

citonin secretion in patients with Williams syndrome. J Pediatr 107:720, 1985.

111. Seyberth HW, et al: Congenital hypokalemia with hypercalciuria in preterm infants: A hyperprostaglandinuric tubular syndrome different form Bartter syndrome. J Pediatr 107:694, 1985.

112. Harrison HE, Harrison HC: Rickets then and now. J Pediatr 87:1141, 1975.

113. Robertson I: Survey of clinical rickets in the infant population in Cape Town 1967–1968. S Afr Med J 43:1072, 1969.

114. Mumaziev N: Rachitis in children up to 2 years of age in Addis Ababa (Ethiopia) and some peculiarities in its clinical picture. Folia Med 10:198, 1968.

115. Mayne V, McCredie D: Rickets in Melbourne. Med J Aust 2:873, 1972.

116. Dilling LA, Ellestad-Sayed J, Coodin FJ, et al: Growth and nutrition of preschool Indian children in Manitoba: I Vitamin D deficiency. Can J Public Health 69:248, 1978.

117. Lapatsanis P, Deliyanni V, Doxiadis S: Vitamin D deficiency rickets in Greece. J Pediatr 73:195, 1968.

118. Miller CG, Chutkan W: Vitamin D deficiency rickets in Jamaican children. Arch Dis Child 51:214, 1976.

119. Nichols BL, Montandon C, Potts E: Nutritional rickets among indigent children in Houston. Texas Med 66:74, 1970.

120. Ladatan AAO, Adeniyi A: Rickets in Nigerian children—response to vitamin D. J Trop Med Hyg 78:206, 1975.

121. Goel KM, Sweet EM, Logan RW, et al: Florid and subclinical rickets among immigrant children in Glasgow. Lancet 1:1141, 1976.

122. Fraser D, Kooh SW, Scriver CR: Hyperparathyroidism as the cause of hyperamino-aciduria and phosphaturia in human vitamin D deficiency. Pediatr Res 1:425, 1967.

123. Arnaud SB, Stickler GB, Haworth JC: Serum 25-hydroxyvitamin D in infantile rickets. Pediatrics 57:221, 1976.

124. Callerbach JC, Sheehan MB, Abramson SJ, Hall RT: Etiologic factors in rickets of very low birth weight infants. J Pediatr 98:800, 1981.

125. Steichen JJ, Tsang RC, Greer FR, et al: Elevated serum 1,25-dihydroxyvitamin D concentrations in rickets of very low-birth-weight infants. J Pediatr 99:293, 1981.

126. Hoff N, Haddad J, Teitelbaum S, et al: Serum concentrations of 25-hydroxyvitamin D in rickets of extremely premature infants. J Pediatr 94:460, 1979.

127. Koo WWK, Tsang RC, Poser JW, et al: Elevated serum calcium and osteocalcin levels from calcitriol in preterm infants. Am J Dis Child 140:1152, 1986.

128. Venkataraman PS, Tsang RC, Steichen JJ, et al: Early neonatal hypocalcemia in extremely preterm infants: High incidence, early onset, and refractoriness to supraphysiologic doses of calcitriol. Am J Dis Child 140:1000, 1986.

129. Greer FR, Steichen JJ, Tsang RC: Effects of increased calcium, phosphorus and vitamin D intake on bone mineralization in very low birth weight infants fed formulas with Polycose and medium-chain triglycerides. J Pediatr 100:951, 1982.

130. Steichen JJ, Gratton TL, Tsang RC: Osteopenia

131. Greer FR, Tsang RC: Calcium, phosphorus, magnesium, and vitamin D requirements for the preterm infant. *In* Tsang RC (ed): Vitamin and Mineral Requirements in Preterm Infants. New York, Marcel Dekker, p 99, 1985.

132. Forbes GB: Nutritional adequacy of human breast milk for premature infants. *In* Lebenthal E (ed): Textbook of Gastroenterology and Nutrition in Infancy. New York, Raven Press, p 321, 1981.

133. Rowe J, Rowe D, Horak E, et al: Hypophosphatemia and hypercalciuria in small premature infants fed human milk: Evidence for inadequate dietary phosphorus. J Pediatr 104:112, 1984.

134. Carey DE, Rowe JC, Goetz CA, et al: Growth and phosphorus metabolism in premature infants fed human milk, fortified human milk, or special premature formula. Am J Dis Child 141:511, 1987.

135. Greer Fr, McCormick A: Improved growth and bone mineralization in premature infants fed fortified mother's own milk. J Pediatr 112:961, 1988.

136. Gross SJ: Bone mineralization in preterm infants fed human milk with and without mineral supplementation. J Pediatr 111:450, 1987.

137. Pereira FR, Sherman MS, DiGucoma J: Hyperalimentation cholestasis. Am J Dis Child 135:842, 1981.

138. Cole DEC, Zlotkin SH: Increased sulfate as an etiological factor in the hypercalciuria associated with total parenteral nutrition. Am J Clin Nutr 37:108, 1983.

139. Sedman AB, Klein GL, Merritt RJ, et al: Evidence of aluminum loading in infants receiving intravenous therapy. N Engl J Med 312:1337, 1985.

140. Venkataraman PS, Han BK, Tsang RC, et al: Secondary hyperparathyroidism and bone disease in infants receiving long term furosemide therapy. Am J Dis Child 137:1157, 1983.

141. Schachter D, Finkelstein JD, Kowarski S: Metabolism of vitamin D: I Preparation of radioactive vitamin D and its intestinal absorption in the rat. J Clin Invest 43:787, 1964.

142. Arnaud SB, Goldsmith RS, Lambert PW, et al: 25-hydroxyvitamin D_3: evidence of an enterohepatic circulation in man. Proc Soc Exp Biol Med 149:570, 1975.

143. Kobayashi A, Kawai S, Utsunomiya T, et al: Hyperparathyroidism in hepatobiliary disease in infancy. Eur J Pediatr 121:5, 1975.

144. Daum F, Rosen JF, Roginsky M, et al: 25-hydroxycholecalciferol in the management of rickets associated with extrahepatic biliary atresia. J Pediatr 88:1041, 1976.

145. Heubi JE, Tsang RC, Steichen JJ, et al: 1,25-dihydroxyvitamin D_3 in hepatic osteodystrophy. J Pediatr 94:977, 1979.

146. Scriver CR: Commentary: Vitamin D dependency. Pediatrics 45:361, 1970.

147. Silver J, Landau H, Bab I, et al: Vitamin D-dependent rickets types I and II: Diagnosis and response to therapy. Isr J Med Sci 21:53, 1985.

148. Fraser D, Kooh SW, Kind HP, et al: Pathogenesis of hereditary vitamin D-dependent rickets. An inborn error of vitamin D metabolism involving defective conversion of 25-hydroxyvitamin D to

1,25-dihydroxyvitamin D. N Engl J Med 289:817, 1973.

149. Balsan S. Garabedian M, Courtecuisse V. et al: Long term therapy with 1α-hydroxyvitamin D₃ in children with pseudo-deficiency rickets. Clin Endocrinol 7 Suppl:225s, 1977.

150. Mawer EB, Backhouse J, Taylor CM, et al: Failure of formation of 1,25-dihydroxycholecalciferol in chronic renal insufficiency. Lancet 1:626, 1973.

151. Balsan S, Garabedian M, Larchet M, et al: Long-term nocturnal calcium infusions can cure rickets and promote normal mineralization in hereditary resistance to 1,25-dihydroxyvitamin D. J Clin Invest 77:1661, 1986.

152. Balsan S, Garabedian M, Liberman UA, et al: Rickets and alopecia with resistance to 1,25-dihydroxyvitamin D: Two different cellular defects. J Clin Endocrinol Metab 57:803, 1983.

153. Beer S, Tieder M, Kohelet D, et al: Vitamin D resistant rickets with alopecia: A form of end organ resistance to 1,25-dihydroxyvitamin D. Clin Endocrinol 14:395, 1981.

154. Brooks MH, Bell NH, Love L, et al: Vitamin D-dependent rickets type II. Resistance of target organs to 1,25-dihydroxyvitamin D. N Engl J Med 298: 996, 1978.

155. Fraser D, Scriver CR: Familial forms of vitamin D–resistant rickets revisited; X-linked hypophosphatemia and autosomal recessive vitamin D dependency. Am J Clin Nutr 29:1315, 1976.

156. Brooks MH, Stern PH, Bell NH: Vitamin D-dependent rickets type II (letter). N Engl J Med 302:810, 1980.

157. Feldman D, Chen T, Cone C, et al: Vitamin D resistant rickets with alopecia: Cultured skin fibroblasts exhibit defective cytoplasmic receptors and unresponsiveness to 1,25(OH)₂D₃. J Clin Endocrinol Metab 55:1020, 1982.

158. Hochberg Z, Benderli A, Levy J: 1,25-dihydroxyvitamin D resistance, rickets, and alopecia. Am J Med 77:805, 1984.

159. Kudoh T, Kumagai T, Uetsuji N, et al: Vitamin D-dependent rickets: Decreased sensitivity to 1,25-dihydroxyvitamin D. Eur J Pediatr 137:307, 1981.

160. Liberman UA, Samuel R, Halabe A, et al: End-organ resistance to 1,25-dihydroxy-cholecalciferol. Lancet 1:504, 1980.

161. Marx SJ, Spiegel AM, Brown EM, et al: A familial syndrome of decrease in sensitivity to 1,25-dihydroxyvitamin D. J Clin Endocrinol Metabol 47:1303, 1978.

162. Tsuchiya Y, Matsua N, Cho M, et al: An unusual form of vitamin D-dependent rickets in a child: Alopecia and marked end-organ hyposensitivity to biologically active vitamin D. J Clin Endocrinol Metab 51:685, 1980.

163. Zerwekh JE, Glass EK, Jowsey J, et al: An unique form of osteomalacia associated with end organ refractoriness to 1,25-dihydroxyvitamin D and apparent defective synthesis of 25-hydroxyvitamin D. J Clin Endocrinol Metab 49:171, 1979.

164. Sakati N, Woodhouse NJY, Niles N, et al: Hereditary resistance to 1,25-dihydroxyvitamin D: Clinical and radiological improvement during high-dose oral calcium therapy. Horm Res 24:280, 1986.

165. Burnett CHG, Deut CE, Harper C, et al: Vitamin D resistant rickets: Analysis of 24 pedigrees with hereditary and sporadic cases. Am J Med 36:322, 1964.

166. Lyles KW, Drezner MK: Parathyroid hormone effects on serum 1,25-dihydroxyvitamin D levels in patients with X-linked dominant hypophosphatemic rickets: Evidence for abnormal 25-hydroxyvitamin D-1 hydroxylase activity. J Clin Endocrinol Metab 54:368, 1982.

167. Chan JC, Alon U, Hirschman GM: Renal hypophosphatemic rickets. J Pediatr 106:533, 1985.

168. Mimouni F, Mughal Z, Tsang RC, et al: X-linked dominant hypophosphatemic rickets. Am J Dis Child 142:191, 1988.

169. Glorieux FH, Marie PJ, Pettifor JM, et al: Bone response to phosphate salts, erogocalciferol, and calcitriol in hypophosphatemic vitamin D-resistant rickets. N Engl J Med 303:1023, 1980.

170. Alon U, Chan JC: Effects of PTH and 1,25(OH)₂D on tubular handling of phosphate in hypophosphatemic rickets. J Clin Endocrinol Metab 58:671, 1984.

171. Carlsen NLT, Krasilnikoff PA, Eiken M: Premature cranial synostosis in X-linked hypophosphatemic rickets: Possible precipitation by 1-alpha OH-Cholecalciferol intoxication. Acta Paediatr Scand 73:149, 1984.

172. Chesney RW, Mazess RB, Rose P, et al: Long-term influence of calcitriol (1,25-dihydroxyvitamin D) and supplemental phosphate in X-linked hypophosphatemic rickets. Pediatrics 71:559, 1983.

173. Santos F, Vernon-Smith MJ, Chan JCM: Hypercalciuria associated with long-term administration or calcitriol (1,25-dihydroxyvitamin D₃)—Action of chlorothiazide. Am J Dis Child 140:139, 1986.

174. Tsuru N, Chan JCM, Chinchilli V: Renal hypophosphatemic rickets: Growth and mineral metabolism after treatment with calcitriol (1,25-dihydroxyvitamin D₃) and phosphate supplementation. Am J Dis Child 141:108, 1987.

175. Etches P, Pickering D, Smith R: Cystinotic rickets treated with vitamin D metabolites. Arch Dis Child 52:661, 1977.

176. Harrison HE, Chisolm JJ Jr, Harrison HC: Congenital renal tubular acidosis. Am J Dis Child 96:588, 1958.

177. Aschinbert LC, Solomon LM, Zeis PM, et al.: Vitamin D–resistant rickets associated with epidermal nevus syndrome: Demonstration of a phosphaturic substance in the dermal lesions. J Pediatr 91:56, 1977.

178. Fukumoto Y, Tarui S, Tsukiyama K, et al: Tumor-induced vitamin D-resistant hypophosphatemic osteomalacia associated with proximal renal tubular dysfunction and 1,25-dihydroxyvitamin D deficiency. J Clin Endocrinol Metabol 49:873, 1979.

179. Bricker NS: On the pathogenesis of the uremic state. An exposition of the "trade off" hypothesis. N Engl J Med 286:1093, 1972.

180. Stark H, Geiger R: Renal tubular dysfunction following vascular accidents of the kidneys in the newborn period. J Pediatr 83:933, 1973.

181. Pettifor JM, Ross P, Wang J, et al: Rickets in children of rural origin in South Africa: Is low dietary calcium a factor? J Pediatr 92:320, 1978.

182. Kooh SW, Fraser D, Reilley BJ, et al: Rickets due

to calcium deficiency. N Engl J Med 297:1264, 1977.

183. Chan JC, Oldham SB, DeLuca HF: Effectiveness of 1 alpha hydroxyvitamin D_3 in children with renal osteodystrophy associated with hemodialysis. J Pediatr 90:820, 1977.

184. Postlethwaite RJ, Houston IB: Bone disease in children with chronic renal failure: Therapy with 1 alpha hydroxyvitamin D_3. Clin Endocrinol 7:1175, 1977.

185. Hood SA, Clark WF, Hodsman AB, et al: Successful treatment of dialysis osteomalacia and dementia, using Desferrioxamine infusions and oral 1-alpha hydroxycholecalciferol. Am J Nephrol 4:369, 1984.

186. Geis WP, Popovtzer MM, Corman JL, et al: The diagnosis and treatment of hyperparathyroidism after renal transplantation. Surg Gynecol Obstet 137:997, 1973.

187. David DS, Sakai S, Brennan BL, et al: Hypercalcemia after renal transplantation. Long term follow-up data. N Engl J Med 289:398, 1973.

188. Potter DE, Wilson CJ, Ozonoff MB: Hyperparathyroid bone disease in children undergoing long-term hemodialysis; treatment with vitamin D. J Pediatr 85:60, 1974.

189. Brickman AS, Sherrard DJ, Jowsey J, et al: 1,25-dyhydroxycholecalciferol. Effects on skeletal lesions and plasma parathyroid hormone levels in uremic osteodystrophy. Arch Intern Med 134:883, 1974.

190. Parfitt AM: The spectrum of hypoparathyroidism. J Clin Endocrinol Metabol 34:152, 1972.

191. Ritz E, Lenhard V, Bommer J, et al: The effect of dialysate magnesium concentration on serum PTH levels in patients on maintenance hemodialysis. Klin Wochenschr 52:51, 1974.

INDEX